Health IT and EHRs
Principles and Practice
Sixth Edition

Margret K. Amatayakul, MBA, RHIA, CHPS, CPHIT, CPEHR, CPHIE, FHIMSS

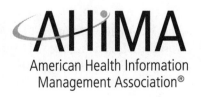

American Health Information
Management Association®

ISBN: 978-1-58426-529-0
AHIMA Product No.: AB102615

AHIMA Staff:
Chelsea Brotherton, MA, Assistant Editor
Katherine M. Greenock, MS, Production Development Editor
Pamela Woolf, Director of Publications

Cover image: ©Mmaxer/Shutterstock.com

American Health Information Management Association
233 North Michigan Avenue, 21st Floor
Chicago, Illinois 60601-5809
ahima.org

Brief Contents

Detailed Contents

About the Author

Margret K. Amatayakul, MBA, RHIA, CHPS, CPHIT, CPEHR, CPHIE, FHIMSS has more than 40 years of experience in national and international healthcare information management. She is a leading authority on electronic health record (EHR) strategies and has extensive experience in EHR selection, project management, and optimization for their use in a meaningful way. After having served as director of medical record services at the Illinois Eye and Ear Infirmary, associate professor at the University of Illinois at the Medical Center, associate executive director of the American Health Information Management Association, and executive director of the Computer-based Patient Record Institute, Ms. Amatayakul formed the consulting firm, Margret\A Consulting, LLC, in 1999 to assist providers, health plans, and vendors with EHR and associated regulatory practices, including HIPAA transactions and code sets, privacy, and security; meaningful use incentive programs, and health reform initiatives. She also served as adjunct professor at the College of St. Scholastica and is on the advisory council of the University of Illinois at Chicago College of Applied Health Sciences. She provides health information systems technology consulting services, freelance writing, and educational programming to the healthcare industry.

Preface

The amount of change from one edition of this book to the next continues to be monumental. Since the 2013 update to the fifth edition was published, EHRs have been adopted by the vast majority of hospitals, many physician practices, and an increasing number of other types or provider settings. In fact, the federal government's meaningful use (MU) incentive program that was the key topic of the fifth edition is being supplanted in the federal government by a focus on the broader scope of health information technology (health IT) in general. Though not without some measure of complaints and controversy, the industry:

- Has seen unprecedented amounts of federal funding put toward incentivizing adoption of EHR, providing associated workforce training, and supporting research in best health IT practices. These incentives are now transitioning into components of reimbursement under health reform initiatives; much as quality measures—such as avoidance of certain types of readmissions and reducing emergency department visits—have influenced Medicare payments.

- Is focusing EHR efforts on optimizing their use, replacing "starter" EHRs with more robust systems, and acquiring complementary health IT to ensure that every aspect of information use within a given setting is automated. While there remains considerable concern over the usability of EHR systems and their potential for unintended consequences, provider settings are focusing on workflow and process improvement to improve use and reduce risk. Vendors are also looking into ways to make it easier for users to use these systems.

- Is expanding the scope of health IT beyond EHR within a given entity to finding ways to better share health information across the continuum of care and with patients. Interoperability, or the ability for disparate systems to exchange data, continues to be a challenge. But new ways to share information are being found. A variety of health information exchange services support provider-to-provider sharing of health information. Patient consent structures and data/information governance processes have also enabled enhanced use of clinical information—for personalized medicine, quality improvement, and clinical research. Is integrating clinical information with administrative and financial information in an effort to achieve greater value for healthcare spending. Health reform initiatives focused on finding best practices that reduce cost and improve the quality of care and patient experience of care depend on accurate and standardized data. Value-based payment, as the mechanism for paying providers under health reform, is focused on paying for positive outcomes, not just what services are provided. This is a significant shift in how healthcare is reimbursed and will require significant focus on the quality of data in the EHR and data from improved revenue cycle management, It is also being recognized that health depends not only on the medical care which a person receives, but on a person's life style. Information about health and social determinants of health are being brought together as population health.

Objectives of this Practical Guide

This sixth edition is being renamed *Health IT and EHRs* as a result of the expanded scope of the technology needed for all health information collection and use. The sixth edition is also focused more on serving as a textbook in addition to serving as a reference work for readers who work in any health setting, whether a healthcare provider organization, vendor, health plan, or policy-maker. The book introduces the full scope of health IT in chronological fashion, covering the information systems development life cycle, strategic planning, goal setting workflow and process mapping, change management, vendor selection, project management, and implementation, training, and ongoing maintenance of EHR and other health IT systems. It also addresses the essential elements of data infrastructure, information technology, privacy and security, and interoperability for all forms of health IT. Finally, there is considerable expansion in chapters covering techniques to achieve value with health IT in various acute care, ambulatory care, and specialty care settings as well as for consumer health IT, enterprise content and record management as an EHR bridge technology, revenue cycle management, and population health. Those familiar with the fifth edition of *Electronic Health Records: A Practical Guide for Professionals and Organizations* will find that some of the chapters have been moved around, consolidated, or expanded in the sixth edition. Two chapters have been added, on revenue cycle management and population health, given expanded interest in integrating information on clinical, administrative or financial, and social determinants of health.

Chapter 1 defines health IT and the EHR, summarizes the key elements of the federal government's programs for incentivizing use of EHRs, and explains the origins of EHR and its future directions and envisioned benefits. It also provides a framework and conceptual model of the components comprising EHR in a provider setting and the components comprising health IT. These frameworks serve as references throughout the remaining chapters in the book. Chapter 2 provides grounding in general systems theory and the systems development life cycle to reinforce that an EHR is not a single application but, rather, a system of health IT components that must work together and with other health IT components. Chapter 3 addresses the purpose, scope, and governance of strategic planning for health IT, including how to construct and document a migration path that addresses not only hardware and software but the people, policy, and process issues needed to achieve success with health IT.

Chapter 4 introduces the concept of healthcare value and the US focus on the Triple Aim goals for EHR and health IT. It encourages the application of a process to set both SMART and STRETCH goals and to monitor achievement. Types of benefits of health IT are described and ways to measure benefits, including how to compile a total cost of ownership and return on investment analysis for EHR and other health IT. Chapter 5 identifies the importance and scope of workflow and process improvement, providing detailed information on how to use workflow and process mapping tools, ensure process improvement through managing team empowerment, group facilitation, and process improvement techniques. Chapter 6 focuses on change management for health IT. It discusses the nature of health IT change and the need for change management, planning for communications, and creating change leaders. Chapters 7 through 9 cover the various aspects of health IT vendor selection and contract negotiation; project management; and systems implementation, training, and ongoing maintenance. These tasks in various degrees are performed with every acquisition of health IT – whether a new system or a replacement. Chapter 7 provides information on conducting a vendor selection, including critical tasks of due diligence, contract negotiation, and contract management throughout the duration of systems implementation. Chapter 8 focuses on project management, another task that is conducted for every new, modified, or replaced information system. The scope and characteristics of an EHR or other health IT project are described, especially with respect to human resource requirements, organizational structures, team-building characteristics, and skills sets for being or hiring a successful project manager. Chapter 9 covers health IT implementation planning and management, including risk management. The importance of infrastructure preparedness, configuration management, testing, data and chart conversions, and ongoing strategies for successful adoption and optimization of health IT are described.

Chapters 10 through 13 cover more of the technical aspects of health IT and EHRs. Chapter 10 describes the data, information, and file structures necessary for an EHR and other health IT, It defines the role of data infrastructure in the creation of the data-information-knowledge-wisdom continuum; describes types of data, their formats, and process requirements; discusses vocabulary standards; distinguishes between types of data architectures; defines data management and data modeling; describes the importance of a data dictionary and metadata; and discusses the importance of governance, data quality, and data integrity. Chapter 11 provides a primer on computer concepts, communications technologies, internet services, data storage and retrieval, and emerging technologies. Chapter 12 is devoted completely to privacy and security, explaining federal privacy and security standardization efforts, discussing breach management and notification, reviewing Red Flags and Payment Card Industry Data Security as applicable to certain health-related organizations, and identifying emerging privacy and security threats and suggesting strategies for addressing them. Chapter 13 on interoperability describes the maturity of interoperability, describes technical standards, explains the role of semantic interoperability, introduces standard messaging protocols, and emphasizes the importance of process interoperability for healthcare. Chapter 13 also covers health information exchange, including organizational structures, architectures, and services; and explains how providers may share data over the nationwide health information exchange called eHealth Exchange.

Chapters 14 through 18 focus on specific types of EHR applications, with an emphasis on optimizing their use. Chapter 14 describes optimization strategies for the acute care EHR components of results management, point of care documentation, computerized provider order entry and barcode medication administration, clinical decision support, and reporting. Chapter 15 describes EHR in the ambulatory care environment, with an emphasis on comparing and contrasting acute and ambulatory EHRs, functions of an EHR in the ambulatory setting, and recommending tactics for optimizing use of EHR in an ambulatory setting. Chapter 16 covers EHR in specialty organizations, focusing on the nursing home, home health, and behavioral health facilities, but also addressing the full scope of special facility needs for EHRs. Chapter 17 focuses on PHRs, describing their attributes, functionality, and supporting standards. The current state of PHR utilization, benefits and barriers for adoption, policies and practices that may aid in overcoming barriers to use, describes mobile health devices, and discusses the impact of consumer empowerment on PHRs and their role in value-driven healthcare initiatives. Chapter 18 addresses enterprise content and record management as an EHR bridge technology, also describing how electronic content management technologies fit into the overall strategic health IT migration path.

Finally, chapters 19 and 20 provide content that is new to the sixth edition of this book. Chapter 19 on revenue cycle management is included to emphasize the importance of revenue cycle management in integrating administrative and financial data with clinical data in the current push to value-based payment. The chapter describes revenue cycle management challenges, enhancements to HIPAA transactions, and opportunities for health IT to better support revenue cycle management for health reform. Chapter 20 defines population health and its scope, including health IT needed for population health management, tools to support quality measurement for improved health outcomes, and discusses the importance and use of big data and healthcare analytics to measure quality of care, cost, and experience of care and provide intelligence for continuous improvement.

As suggested by the ever-accelerating pace of change in health IT and EHR, a textbook should be considered a means to understand basic concepts and promote best practices—including the need to keep current. There are many factors that influence the dynamics of health IT and EHR, including technology advances, continuous product improvement, user acclimation to health IT and EHR, and public policy—especially a new administration at the federal government which can shift emphasis seemingly without warning. Readers are encouraged to continue their pursuit of knowledge about health IT and EHR by continuously scanning the web for new information. That said, it is important to note that any websites listed in this book were current and valid as of the date of publication. However, web page addresses and the information on them may change or disappear at any time and for any number of reasons. The reader is encouraged to perform general web searches to locate information where site addresses listed here are no longer valid.

Note to academic educators: Instructor materials for this book include lesson plans, chapter slides, test banks, EHR simulation modules, and other useful resources. Visit http://www.ahima.org/publications/educators.aspx for further instruction. If you have any questions regarding the instructor materials, please contact AHIMA Customer Relations at (800) 335-5535 or submit a customer support request at https://secure.ahima.org/contact/contact.aspx.

Acknowledgments

The first edition of this book acknowledged the contribution of Rita Finnegan, past president and former executive director of AHIMA. It was Ms. Finnegan who brought me into the field of health information management (HIM) and achieved AHIMA support for the Institute of Medicine's first patient record study that led to my involvement in the formation of the Computer-based Patient Record Institute (CPRI) and extended my network of associates and influence well beyond traditional boundaries.

As noted in subsequent editions of this book, that network has only continued to grow and be enriched by many colleagues, clients, and students who teach me so much. These opportunities help me to achieve my professional goal of seeing EHRs become the basic supporting infrastructure for healthcare, now enhanced with many other forms of health IT. This sixth edition with its dual focus on EHR and health IT occurred largely as result of the unprecedented investment by the federal government in supporting EHR acquisition and implementation and then moving rapidly to health reform initiatives that depend heavily on data derived from EHRs and processed by other forms of health IT in many new ways. Challenges still remain, but significant progress is being seen.

Finally, a book is not a realization of one's passion without expressing appreciation to those who made a direct contribution to the work. The staff and reviewers from AHIMA kept me on my toes. With each edition, there are many unidentified persons who review the book and offer suggestions that are greatly appreciated. It is especially helpful to have input from students' perspective. As with previous editions of the book, two students who conducted their management practicum with me, Amanda Turek and Mika Ishikawa, offered recommendations for content and help with case studies for the instructor's manual. Finally, my husband, Paul, is the ever-present force that keeps me going and makes this work so special to me. My sincere thanks to all.

AHIMA Press would like to thank Linda C. Galocy, MS, RHIA, and Dr. Neisa R. Jenkins, EdD, RHIA for their technical reviews of this title.

Online Resources

For Academic Instructors

AHIMA provides supplementary materials for approved academic educators who use this book in their classes. Materials include curriculum map, test bank questions and answers, and Power-Point slides. Visit **http://www.ahimapress.org/Amatayakul5290** and click the link to download the files. Please do not enter the scratch-off code from the interior front cover, as this will invalidate your access to the instructor materials. If you have any questions regarding the instructor materials, contact AHIMA Customer Relations at (800) 335-5535 or submit a customer support request at https://secure.ahima.org/contact/contact.aspx.

Chapter 1
Introduction to Health IT

Key Terms

American Recovery and Reinvestment Act of 2009 (ARRA)

Bar code medication administration record (BC-MAR)

Basic EHR

Centers for Medicare and Medicaid Services (CMS)

Certified EHR technology (CEHRT)

Clinical data repository (CDR)

Clinical data warehouse (CDW)

Clinical decision support (CDS) system

Clinical documentation system

Clinical messaging system

Clinician

Computerized provider order entry (CPOE)

Connectivity system

Context sensitive

Core clinical systems

Data mining

Discrete data

Document imaging system (DIMS)

Electronic document/content management (ED/CM) system

Electronic document management system (EDMS)

Electronic health record (EHR)

Electronic medical record (EMR)

Electronic medication administration record (EMAR)

Enterprise-wide MPI (EMPI)

Executive decision support

E-visits

Five rights of medication administration

Health information exchange (HIE)

Health information network

Health information technology (health IT)

Health Information Technology for Economic and Clinical Health Act (HITECH)

HIE organization (HIO)

Home monitoring

Human-computer interfaces (HCI)

Inference engine

Integrated delivery network (IDN)

Interoperability

Intranet

Knowledge sources

Laboratory information system (LIS)

Meaningful use (MU)

Medication management system

National Quality Forum (NQF) Health Outcomes Policy Priorities

Natural language processing

Office of the National Coordinator for Health Information Technology (ONC)

Personal health record (PHR)

Pharmacy information system (PIS)

Picture archiving and communication systems (PACS)

Platform

Point-of-care (POC) charting

Portal

Predictive modeling

Print file

Radio frequency identification (RFID)

Radiology information system (RIS)

Registries

Reporting

Report writers

Results management system

Rules engine (also called inference engine)

Smart peripherals

Source system

Storage area network (SAN)

Storage system
Structured data
Supporting infrastructure
System
Telehealth
Unstructured data
Wireless on wheels
Workflow technology

Learning Objectives

- Define health IT and the EHR.

- Summarize the key elements of the federal government's programs for incentivizing use of EHRs.

- Explain the origins of the EHR and its future directions.

- Describe how the envisioned benefits of health IT have been achieved to date.

- Describe a framework and conceptual model of the components comprising the EHR in a provider setting.

- Describe a framework and conceptual model of the components comprising health IT.

Health information technology (health IT) is defined as "the application of information processing involving both computer hardware and software that deals with the storage, retrieval, sharing, and use of healthcare information, data, and knowledge for communication and decision making" (HRSA n.d.). Health IT is not new; however, because health IT can include highly sophisticated systems that require transformative change, adoption has been a slow process. In 2004, the federal government recognized the slow pace of adoption in general, and electronic health records (EHRs) in particular. A national goal for EHR adoption by 2014 was set, but the pace of change did not immediately increase. In 2006, Healthcare Information Management and Systems Society (HIMSS) Analytics found that only 3.6 percent of US hospitals had two of the core components of an EHR: computerized provider order entry (CPOE) and bar code medication administration record (BC-MAR) systems to support improved medication management. By 2008, the number of hospitals with such applications had increased to just 5.8 percent (HIMSS 2006–2015). Then, in 2009, the **American Recovery and Reinvestment Act (ARRA)** and the **Health Information Technology for Economic and Clinical Health Act (HITECH)** introduced financial incentives for hospitals and physicians to make meaningful use of federally **certified EHR technology (CEHRT)**. (In federal parlance, CEHRT moves beyond a **basic EHR**, which includes computerized documentation but offers minimal or no clinical decision support that alerts clinicians of potential issues with their patients.) This federal incentive program, which is often referred to simply as **meaningful use (MU)**, has resulted in significantly improved use of EHRs and other forms of health IT. By the end of 2015, HIMSS Analytics reported that 62 percent of hospitals had CPOE and BCMAR, with another 31 percent having additional health IT beyond what is required for MU. Furthermore, approximately 36 percent of physician offices had adopted EHRs by this point in time (HIMSS 2006–2015).

When considering these statistics, it should be noted that HIMSS uses an analytical structure that is generally, but not specifically, consistent with MU. Therefore, HIMSS data on rates of health IT adoption are different than those reported by the federal government. The **Office of the National Coordinator for Health Information Technology (ONC)** is the agency within the US Department of Health and Human Services (HHS) designated to serve as the primary resource for the United States on the adoption of health IT and promotion of a nationwide health information exchange. According to ONC's healthIT.gov dashboard, 75 percent of all nonfederal acute care hospitals had adopted a basic EHR as of December 31, 2015, and 97 percent of such hospitals had possession of CEHRT that meets ONC requirements for MU, including the increasingly sophisticated clinical decision support required as MU moves through its staged adoption requirements. HIIMSS statistics about EHR adoption also vary from the government's statistics about MU because the **Centers for Medicare and Medicaid Services (CMS)**, which administers Medicare, Medicaid, Children's Health Insurance Program, and the Health Insurance Exchange Marketplace, provides the measures of usage requirements to earn the MU monetary incentives (or incur reimbursement adjustment penalties), but the extent to which actual use includes workarounds or equates to the degree of desired value from EHR is variable. EHRs represent a huge change for hospitals and physician offices. They require a significant investment in time, money, process change, and human factor reengineering to be successful. EHRs in particular change how **clinicians** (a collective term used to describe physicians, nurses, and all other healthcare professionals who deliver care directly to patients) perform not only their documentation but how they practice medicine. Furthermore, the process of implementing health IT is ongoing, as constantly changing clinical knowledge and increasing expectations require continual maintenance and enhancements.

Scope of Health IT

As defined at the start of this chapter, health IT is an expansive concept, which includes EHRs as well as additional forms of information technology, such as data warehousing and analytics, apps on mobile phones, personal health records, health information exchange, and many others. The definition of health IT also continues to evolve in response to technological changes, regulatory requirements, and political priorities. There is considerable work to be done to enhance EHR products, especially in moving toward new generations of the technology and in optimizing their use to gain full value (Wallace 2014). Additionally, the federal government is pressing forward to encourage the use of health data from EHRs and other sources (such as financial systems, health plans, public health resources, personal health records and monitoring devices, disease registries, and genomic research) to improve the quality, cost, and experience of care in the United States. In 2014, the ONC laid out a vision in *Connecting Health and Care for the Nation: A 10-Year Vision to Achieve an Interoperable Health IT Infrastructure*. In 2015, it provided the *Federal Health IT Strategic Plan: 2015–2020* (ONC 2015a) and delivered the detailed *Connecting Health and Care for the Nation: A Shared Nationwide Interoperability Roadmap* (ONC 2015b). Recognizing that there needs to be ever greater attention on privacy and security in an interoperable environment, ONC works with HHS Office for Civil Rights (OCR) and the National Institute of Standards and Technology (NIST) to ensure that the healthcare community has appropriate privacy and security resources (see chapter 12).

EHR Definition

Defining the EHR has not been simple. Even as progress in implementing EHRs has been made, there continues to be a mix of different terminology, sometimes in an attempt to differentiate among types of products, other times resulting from force of habit and perhaps an unwillingness to change.

For example, in hospitals, the term *electronic medical record* (EMR) may be used to describe systems based on **electronic document management systems (EDMSs)**, which are storage solutions based on digital scanning technology in which source documents are scanned to create digital images of the documents that can be stored electronically. Hospitals may even state that they have both an EMR (that is, the EDMS) and an EHR, referring to systems that meet MU requirements. Alternatively, physicians' offices frequently use EMR to describe EHR systems in their offices, even when those systems are highly sophisticated. Physicians may use the term EMR out of habit, but they may also use it to keep the focus on medical care as opposed to the broader scope of healthcare, which encompasses disease prevention and wellness.

In 2008, the federal government asked the National Alliance for Health Information Technology (NAHIT) to develop definitive definitions to distinguish between EMR and EHR. These definitions are as follows (NAHIT 2008):

- **Electronic medical record:** An electronic record of health-related information on an individual that can be created, gathered, managed, and consulted by authorized clinicians and staff within one healthcare organization.

- **Electronic health record:** An electronic record of health-related information on an individual that conforms to nationally recognized interoperability standards and that can be created, managed, and consulted by authorized clinicians and staff across more than one healthcare organization.

Today, the federal government has adopted the term *EHR* exclusively. An EMR is more limited than an EHR, which is an information system framework rather than a single application. An EHR can be implemented in a variety of ways, providing many different functions, and achieving a multiplicity of purposes.

In sum, the federal government's present definition of EHR encompasses functions identified by the Institute of Medicine (IOM; now known as Health and Medicine Division [HMD] of the National Academies of Science, Engineering, and Medicine) in its early efforts to define the term, which suggested that the functions performed by an EHR serve to collect and integrate data from multiple sources, capture and enable use of data at the point of care, and support clinical decision making (IOM 1991). MU enhances those fundamental elements by adding support for quality measurement and reporting and for the enablement of health information exchange. When these five elements are embodied in components that work in harmony, the result may be considered the EHR as now required under MU and as illustrated in figure 1.1.

MU Incentive Program

The federal government's MU incentive program has driven the widespread adoption of EHR technology in the United States. While many are calling for significant changes in the program or for the program to be dropped (which a representative of CMS observed early in 2016 could happen by the end of 2016 [Miliard 2016]), the program created a foundation of functionality for all providers (Halamka 2015).

There were three primary components (and associated regulations) to the MU incentives program: a certification program for EHR technology, standards and criteria for CEHRT, and objectives and measures for earning incentives.

ONC HIT Certification Program

ONC oversees the ONC HIT Certification Program to ensure EHR technology is tested and certified as meeting standards and criteria (ONC 2015c). This program establishes the requirements

Figure 1.1.   Fundamental functions of EHR

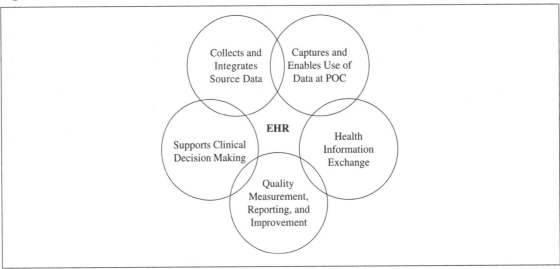

for accredited testing laboratories (ATLs) and authorized certification bodies (ACBs) and uses the American National Standards Institute (ANSI) National Voluntary Laboratory Accreditation Program (NVLAP) to accredit testing laboratories. NIST develops test procedures and conformance test tools based on the ONC's EHR certification criteria (Snelick and Taylor 2013). The process of testing and certification is illustrated in figure 1.2.

ONC Standards and Criteria for CEHRT

Regulations from ONC define the standards and criteria that CEHRT must meet (45 CFR 170(b)). Criteria describe the specific functionality that an EHR must have if it is to be used to earn MU incentives. There are general criteria as well as criteria specific to inpatient settings and ambulatory settings. Adopted standards address specifications for exchanging health information content, vocabularies for representing health information, and the protection of health information created, maintained, and exchanged by EHR technology.

Figure 1.2.   CEHRT testing and certification process

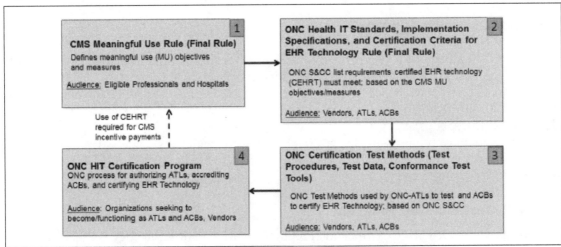

Source: National Institute of Standards and Testing (NIST).

Objectives and Measures for Earning MU Incentives

Objectives and measures for earning MU incentives are defined in CMS regulations (42 CFR 412, 413, 422, and so on). Consistent with the ONC-established standards and criteria, the objectives and measures include those that eligible hospitals (EHs) must meet, those that eligible professionals (EPs)—who are primarily physicians in ambulatory settings—must meet, and those that both EHs and EPs must meet.

Recognizing that it would take time to achieve the objectives of the MU incentive program, the federal government structured the program in three stages, as illustrated in figure 1.3. David Blumenthal, the national coordinator of ONC between 2009 and 2011, likened the stages to an escalator "that moves the health system upward toward improved quality and effectiveness in health care" (Blumenthal and Tavenner 2010). The HealthIT.gov Policy Committee describes the stages of the MU incentives as bending the curve towards transformed health (see figure 6.1 in chapter 6).

The incentives initially provided a maximum of $44,000 for Medicare EPs over the course of the five-year period 2011 through 2015 and a maximum of $63,750 for Medicaid EPs through 2021. For EHs, the incentives are based on a formula that includes a base of $2 million plus $200 per certain number of Medicare (or Medicaid) discharges during the same five-year period. In 2012, stage 2 measures were finalized and one additional year was added for providers to implement EHRs before a downward adjustment in Medicare reimbursement would be applied to those who did not adopt an EHR. There was no downward adjustment for Medicaid incentives.

As providers started implementing MU stage 2, a number of challenges were identified and the industry started calling for a delay of stage 3. On December 6, 2013, CMS announced a delay for stage 3 until 2017; however, work continued on drafting stage 3 requirements to give vendors time to develop products. On October 16, 2015, the federal government issued a final rule with a special

Figure 1.3.   Meaningful use of EHR incentive program structure

Stage 1 **2011-2012** Data capture and sharing	Stage 2 **2014** Advance clinical processes	Stage 3 **2016** Improved outcomes
Stage 1: Meaningful use criteria focus on:	**Stage 2: Meaningful use criteria focus on:**	**Stage 3: Meaningful use criteria focus on:**
Electronically capturing health information in a standardized format	More rigorous health information exchange (HIE)	Improving quality, safety, and efficiency, leading to improved health outcomes
Using that information to track key clinical conditions	Increased requirements for e-prescribing and incorporating lab results	Decision support for national high-priority conditions
Communicating that information for care coordination processes	Electronic transmission of patient care summaries across multiple settings	Patient access to self-management tools
Initiating the reporting of clinical quality measures and public health information	More patient-controlled data	Access to comprehensive patient data through patient-centered HIE
Using information to engage patients and their families in their care		Improving population health

Source: https://www.healthit.gov/providers-professionals/how-attain-meaningful-use

comment period for stage 3 measures. The rule gave providers until January 1, 2018, to comply; incorporated greater flexibility; afforded greater alignment between the clinical quality measures required under MU and those required for the Medicare program; and supported use of newer technologies (McCann 2015).

Despite these changes in the MU incentives program, physicians continued to call for further delays and changes. The Medicare Access and CHIP Reauthorization Act of 2015 (MACRA) afforded an opportunity for such changes. In April 2016, a proposed rule was issued that would establish parameters for a new quality payment program (QPP) for physicians. The QPP includes a merit-based incentive payment system (MIPS) and alternative payment models (APMs). Twenty-five percent of the performance requirements to earn an incentive under MIPS include "advancing care information," which is described as the former MU incentives program. Only time will tell how successful MIPS will be in incentivizing future EHR use among physicians (CMS 2016).

Origins and Future Directions of the EHR

The concept of the EHR has existed since the early use of computers in healthcare in the late 1960s and early 1970s. Figure 1.4 illustrates the major milestones in the history of EHR implementation.

The IOM/HMD Vision for EHRs

Since issuing its first study of applying technology to patient records in 1991, the HMD (formerly IOM), an independent, nongovernmental organization that advises policy makers and the public, has been a strong proponent for vision and benefits of an EHR. Development of the MU requirements were structured around the **National Quality Forum (NQF) Health Outcomes Policy Priorities** (HIT Policy Committee 2009, 2011) that grew out of *To Err Is Human* (1999), a landmark IOM publication that propelled the United States into true action. This study, which was the first in what became a series of IOM reports describing the US "healthcare quality chasm," called upon the nation to do the following:

- Improve quality, safety, efficiency, and reduce health disparities.
  - Provide access to comprehensive patient health data for patient's healthcare team.
  - Use evidence-based order sets and computerized provider order entry
  - Apply clinical decision support at the point of care

Figure 1.4.   History of EHR implementation

1970s Pioneers	1980s Early Limitations	1990s Landmark Effort	2000s Wake-up Calls	2010s Incentives & Controversy
Academic Experiments	Feeder Systems	Hype & EDMS	Clinical Components	EHR & HIE

- ○ Generate lists of patients who need care and use list to reach out to patients

- ○ Report information for quality improvement and public reporting

- Engage patients and their families in their healthcare

  - ○ Provide patients and families with timely access to data, knowledge, and tools to make informed decisions and manage their health

- Improve care coordination

  - ○ Exchange meaningful clinical information among professional healthcare team

- Improve population and public health

  - ○ Communicate with public health agencies

- Ensure adequate privacy and security protections for personal health information

  - ○ Ensure privacy and security protection for confidential information through operating policies and procedures and technologies and compliance with applicable law

  - ○ Provide transparency of data sharing to patient

The contributions of the IOM/HMD to the vision of the EHR are significant. They address a specific need for standards development and certification support and define the scope of the transition to the EHR and the need for interoperability early on. The following key quotes from the original IOM report still remain visionary:

- "Merely automating the form, content, and procedures of current patient records will perpetuate their deficiencies and will be insufficient to meet emerging user needs" (IOM 1991, 2).

- The EHR "encompasses a broader view of the patient record than is current today, moving from the notion of a location or device for keeping track of patient care events to a resource with much enhanced utility in patient care (including the ability to provide an accurate longitudinal account of care), in management of the healthcare system, and in extension of knowledge" (IOM 1991, 3).

- The EHR is "the core of healthcare information systems. Such systems must be able to transmit data to other types of clinical and administrative information systems within healthcare institutions; they must also be able to transmit data to and accept data from other healthcare institutions or secondary databases" (IOM 1991, 51).

The early IOM reports and subsequent works of the Computer-Based Patient Record Institute (CPRI), which grew out of the first patient record study, describe specific outcomes for an EHR that remain valid today. An EHR should do the following (CPRI 1997):

- *Improve quality* of healthcare through data availability and links to knowledge sources.

- *Enhance patient safety* with context-sensitive reminders and alerts, clinical decision support, and automated surveillance, chronic disease management, and drug/device recall capability.

- *Support health maintenance,* preventive care, and wellness through patient reminders, health summaries, tailored instructions, educational materials, and home monitoring/tracking capability.

- *Increase productivity* through data capture and reporting formats tailored to the user, streamlined workflow support, and patient-specific care plans, guidelines, and protocols.

- *Reduce hassle factors* and improve satisfaction for clinicians, consumers, and caregivers by managing scheduling, registration, referrals, medication refills, work queues, and by automatically generating administrative data.

- *Support revenue enhancement* through accurate and timely eligibility and benefit information, cost-efficacy analysis, clinical trial recruitment, rules-driven coding assistance, external accountability reporting/outcomes measures, and contract management.

- *Support predictive modeling* and contribute to development of evidence-based healthcare guidance.

- *Maintain patient confidentiality* and exchange data securely among all key stakeholders.

To solidify these outcomes and add more specificity to the EHR definition, HHS sought further guidance from the IOM on key care delivery–related capabilities of an EHR system. The IOM's *Key Capabilities of an Electronic Health System* (2003) describes the EHR as including the following:

- Longitudinal collection of electronic health information for and about persons, where *health information* is defined as information pertaining to the health of an individual or healthcare provided to an individual

- Immediate electronic access to person- and population-level information by authorized, and only authorized, users

- Provision of knowledge and decision-support that enhance the quality, safety, and efficiency of patient care

- Support of efficient processes for healthcare delivery

In 2009, the IOM published *Computational Technology for Effective Health Care* in conjunction with the National Research Council. Whereas the IOM's series of reports on medical errors describe the need to cross the healthcare quality chasm, this report describes the need to cross the healthcare IT chasm. The study included site visits to eight US medical centers that were acknowledged leaders in applying IT to healthcare. Despite finding a number of successes and considerable money spent on IT, the report observes that "today's health care fails to deliver the most effective care and suffers substantially as a result of medical errors. In addition, many medical interventions undertaken today are in fact not necessary" (Stead and Lin 2009, 3). However, the report notes that "these persistent problems do not reflect incompetence on the part of health care professionals—rather, they are a consequence of the inherent intellectual complexity of health care taken as a whole and a medical care environment that is not adequately structured to help clinicians avoid mistakes or to systematically improve their decision making and practice" (Stead and Lin 2009, 3). The report classifies relevant factors into the following three areas (Stead and Lin 2009):

- *Tasks and workflow of healthcare.* "Health care decisions often require reasoning under high degrees of uncertainty about the patient's medical state and the effectiveness of past and future treatments for the particular patient." "Workflows are often complex and characterized by many interruptions, inadequately defined roles and responsibilities, poorly kept and managed schedules, and little documentation of steps, expectations, and outcomes."

- *Institution and economics of healthcare.* The diversity of payer coverage plans complicates administration. "Incentives for payment are often distorted or perverse, leading (for example) to more generous compensation for medical procedures than for communication with patients or for diagnosis or preventive care."

- *Current implementations of healthcare IT.* Many healthcare institutions spend considerable money on IT, but "IT applications appear designed largely to automate tasks or business processes." "They are often designed in ways that simply mimic existing paper-based forms and provide little support for cognitive tasks of clinicians or the workflow of the people who must actually use the system." Many of the applications do not address "human-computer interaction principles," leading to "poor designs that can increase the chance of error, add to rather than reduce work, and compound the frustrations of executing required tasks." The result is often "new forms of error that are difficult to detect."

In conclusion, the report urges the industry to adopt principles for both evolutionary and revolutionary change and identifies research challenges that the government, computer science community, and healthcare institutions should address.

The Evolution of EHR Technology

Despite their 50-year history and significant refinement over time, EHRs are still described as being "very early in the EHR maturity lifecycle" (Halamka 2012). EHRs were originally built on a **platform** (underlying technology that supports various applications) that used mainframe computers. Today, EHRs predominantly use client/server technology, a second-generation platform that relies heavily on personal computers tapping into first-generation platform mainframe databases (Hanover 2015). These types of EHRs can capture and organize patient information within a hospital or physician office environment, but they are not designed to share and/or organize data across many different systems. Even when EHR software vendors offer software as a service (SaaS) in a cloud-computing arrangement, the software is not built on a third-generation platform architecture (Web Services Architecture [WSA]), so it does not operate as a flexible application program interface (API), which can interact with other applications and share data (Boone 2011). In addition, vendors can charge substantial fees to build interfaces (special software written to help exchange data between two or more second-platform systems) as well as steep per-transaction fees for data sharing. Such vendor practices, known as *information blocking,* may contribute to the inability to share data (Lichtenwald 2015; DeSalvo and Daniel 2015).

There is much room for innovation in EHR design. Many physicians and other clinicians seek improvements to address frustrating productivity issues and inflexibility in EHRs, and federal health reform initiatives require the integration of clinical and financial data for new reimbursement structures and for sharing data across the continuum of care and beyond. The prospect of future EHRs that are enhanced with new technology and support for sharing health data in a much broader environment is very exciting. Ideally, the EHRs of tomorrow will contribute great value by fulfilling the vision of the EHR pioneers and addressing many new demands.

Check Your Understanding 1.1

Choose the best answer:

1. The construct that reflects a record about an individual with the ability to share information is:

   a. Electronic health record

   b. Electronic medical record

   c. Health IT

   d. Personal health record

2. According to HIMSS Analytics, what percentage of hospitals have more health IT than what is required for MU?

   a. Less than 1 percent

   b. 10 percent

   c. 30 percent

   d. 50 percent or more

3. According to ONC, what percentage of nonfederal acute care hospitals have implemented an EHR of some kind?

   a. Less than 25 percent

   b. About 50 percent

   c. About 75 percent

   d. Nearly 100 percent

4. EHRs were first conceived in:

   a. 1960s

   b. 1980s

   c. 1991

   d. 2010

5. In the MU incentive program, which body establishes standards for what is required in an EHR?

   a. Centers for Medicare and Medicaid Services (CMS)

   b. Institute of Medicine (IOM)

   c. National Institute of Standards and Technology (NIST)

   d. Office of the National Coordinator for Health Information Technology (ONC)

6. In the MU incentive program, what describes EHR functionality?

   a. Criteria

   b. Measures

   c. Objectives

   d. Standards

7. Which of the following EHR functions supports the goal to improve patient safety?

   a. Context-sensitive reminders and alerts

   b. Predictive modeling

   c. Secure data exchange

   d. Tailored instructions

8. According to an IOM study conducted in 2009, new forms of medical errors are arising from:

   a. Incompetent use of EHR

   b. Not addressing human-computer interactions

   c. Programming errors

   d. Resistance to use by clinicians

EHR and Health IT Framework and Conceptual Model

EHRs and other forms of health IT are systems. In general systems theory, a **system** is a set of interrelated elements that work together to achieve a goal. A fundamental challenge in health IT remains to achieve **interoperability** among disparate systems—that is, to ensure that applications can work together, it must be possible to share data from one application with another application in a meaningful way.

Components of EHR Systems

As healthcare organizations undertake the evolutionary and revolutionary changes in adopting EHRs and other types of health IT, it is important to remember that elements in these systems include not only hardware and software but also people, policy, and process components, as illustrated in figure 1.5.

Of course, an EHR system must provide technical components that people can use, consistent with policy, for the various processes they perform. Figure 1.6 displays a conceptual model that depicts the technical components of EHR. In contrast to the MU standards, criteria, and measures, which describe the functionality that must be present in an EHR in order for eligible professionals and hospitals to become meaningful EHR users and earn incentives, figure 1.6 illustrates how the functionality is deployed in various applications, supporting infrastructure, and connectivity systems.

Categories of Information Systems in the EHR

As figure 1.6 suggests, there are four main categories of information systems that contribute to and comprise an EHR: source systems, supporting infrastructure, core clinical systems, and connectivity systems. Further information about the privacy and security elements that completely wrap around the EHR components is provided in chapter 12. Further information about interoperability in general is provided in chapter 13.

Figure 1.5.   EHR system components

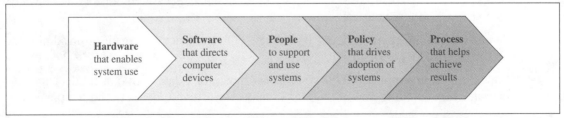

Figure 1.6.   Conceptual model of EHR

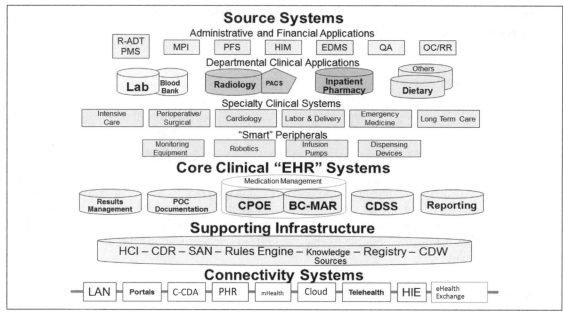

Source Systems

Source systems collect data, including administrative, financial, and clinical data, that contribute to the health record. Examples of basic source systems include laboratory information systems (LISs), pharmacy information systems (PISs), radiology information systems (RISs), nutrition and food service information systems, physical therapy information systems, emergency department information systems, and many other ancillary, or departmental systems. Some source systems distinguish specialized source systems by clinical specialty, such as cardiology or labor and delivery, or by type of services, such as intensive care unit or emergency department. Source systems may also include smart peripherals, such as smart infusion pumps or robotics.

Core Clinical Systems

Core clinical systems enable use of data at the point of care. These applications support specific clinical functionality and are often considered the applications that comprise an EHR and define whether a care delivery organization has an EHR. They include the following:

- **Results management systems** where data from laboratory tests and other diagnostic studies can be trended, potentially with other data such as medication administration, vital signs, and so on

- Point-of-care (POC) charting systems for recording nurse assessment, history and physical examination, progress notes, and so on

- **Medication management systems**, including CPOE and electronic medication administration record (EMAR) or BC-MAR systems

- **Clinical decision support (CDS) systems** for integrating data with clinical decision support rules for supplying reminders, alerts, context-sensitive order sets and templates, and other clinical guidance

- **Reporting systems** to generate visit summaries, referral letters, quality reporting, patient follow-up lists, and other patient care–related reports

Supporting Infrastructure

Supporting infrastructure integrates data from applications internal to a given care-delivery organization. In a hospital, each of the clinical information systems just described may be standalone systems. In an ambulatory care setting, they tend to be less separate. However, for the clinical information systems to be most effective, data should be integrated across the systems and with data from all source systems. Supporting infrastructure, then, may include the following:

- A clinical data repository (CDR) that captures and organizes data in one location

- A **rules engine** (also called **inference engine**) to supply the CDR with programming logic for CDSS

- **Knowledge sources** that supply information from external sources to the rules engine

- **Report writers** or wizards that enable compilation of data into various reports

- **Storage systems,** such as **storage area networks (SANs),** to back up and archive data

- Presentation layer software and **human-computer interfaces (HCI)**, which are various forms of input devices to help capture data at the point of care

- A **clinical data warehouse (CDW)** where sophisticated analysis can be performed on the data

Further information about supporting infrastructure technology is provided in chapter 11.

Connectivity Systems

Connectivity systems support the integration of data across different organizations and with patients or their caregivers. As noted previously in this chapter, it is becoming increasingly important to share data across the continuum of care for a variety of purposes, such as better-coordinated care, quality measurement and reporting, population health, precision/personalized medicine, new reimbursement models, and so on. Examples of connectivity systems include the following:

- *Local area networks (LANs)* support exchange of information within a given organization.

- *Portals* support remote access to the EHR for providers and patients. A patient portal allows patients access to information from their EHR (or to view, but not to alter, their EHR). The Consolidated-Clinical Document architecture (C-CDA) is a standard means with which to exchange documents.

- *Personal health records (PHRs)* enable patients to build their own health records with information obtained from their EHR and information they supply themselves, such as a diabetes management diary or information from another provider.

- *Mobile health (mHealth)* is the use of mobile HCIs as well as physiological monitoring systems (such as activity trackers). Some of these support uploading of data to a PHR and, in some cases, transmission of data to a provider.

- *Cloud computing* refers to using a network of remote servers hosted on the Internet to store, manage, and process data.

- *Telehealth* is the delivery of health-related services and information via telecommunications technologies. Telehealth may support local care to those who are homebound or in difficult-to-access places (such as prisons) as well as remote care around the world. Telehealth technology comes in many forms, from simple telephone connectivity to sophisticated robots.

- *Health information exchange (HIE)* is a term that implies a formal, agreed-upon process of information sharing, typically through a health information organization (HIO) that serves as an intermediary. The eHealth Exchange is a national effort to provide HIE.

As illustrated by this list of examples, connectivity systems refer not only to the hardware to make connections but also to the software that is used with and beyond EHR—making the discussion of connectivity really about EHR *and* health IT. Figure 1.7 superimposes a conceptual model of health IT over the conceptual model of the EHR.

Sequence of EHR and Health IT Systems Implementation

Provider organizations have typically taken an incremental approach to compile the components of an EHR and adopt other types of health IT. Each organization needs to create its own migration path. This path must recognize the existing infrastructure in the organization, its culture and resources, and the goals the organization expects to achieve from an EHR. Migration paths vary depending on whether the organization is a hospital, a clinic, a physician office, an **integrated delivery system (IDS;** a network of hospitals and clinics managed by a parent company), or other type of provider facility as well as the extent to which a suitable HIE is available. The following brief discussion of source systems and core clinical EHR systems is provided in the sequence typically implemented. Further discussion of EHRs in various types of provider settings is found in chapters 14, 15, and 16.

Registration-Admission, Discharge, Transfer and Practice Management Systems

In inpatient settings (hospitals and nursing facilities), the registration-admission, discharge, transfer (R-ADT) system is the most fundamental system needed to register patients, record their demographic and insurance information, and track admission, discharge, and transfer (among different levels of care within the setting) status. In an ambulatory setting (clinic or physician office), the practice management system (PMS) performs these functions as applicable. These systems also include a master person index (MPI), which may serve multiple entities within an integrated delivery system and is then referred to as an **enterprise-wide MPI (EMPI).**

Patient Financial Services and Billing Systems

Another foundational system is one that receives charges and generates claims. These systems, which are known as patient financial services (PFS) in the hospital setting and as billing systems

Figure 1.7.   Conceptual model of health IT

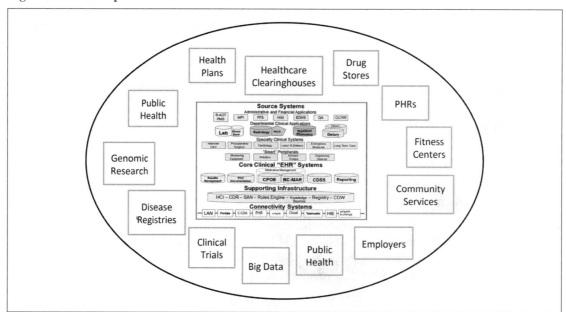

in ambulatory settings, may also support eligibility checking to validate insurance coverage, determine co-payment requirements, and potentially identify deductible amounts. Such systems can also check claims status with an insurance company, receive electronic remittance advice, manage any required prior authorizations, and—in experimental stages now, but expected in the future—process electronic claims attachments. In the ambulatory environment, the PMS often integrates patient registration, scheduling, MPI, and billing.

Administrative Systems

Other systems closely related to financially oriented systems include a number of applications within the health information management (HIM) department, such as chart tracking, incomplete record control, dictation and transcription systems, speech dictation systems, encoders and computer-assisted coding systems, chargemasters, registries, and others. Some of these administration system applications are in transition as EHRs are adopted. For instance, when paper charts become obsolete, organizations will eventually no longer need chart tracking systems (although many organizations continue to maintain older paper charts until the statute of limitations runs out and they can be destroyed). Traditional dictation systems have all but vanished, replaced at least with digital dictation systems and, more recently, with speech dictation. Other applications will likely continue to be used well into adoption of EHRs, including speech commands and discrete reportable transcription (DRT) using speech recognition technology coupled with natural language processing; tools to assign International Classification of Diseases (ICD) codes; and other applications related to revenue cycle management—including those that may be a shared responsibility with the PFS department.

The HIM department may or may not be responsible for other administrative systems, such as physician credentialing systems, which are often managed by the medical staff office; compliance systems managed by a corporate compliance officer; and contract management systems used by procurement officers. In some organizations, HIM departments share responsibility for clinical documentation improvement and clinical quality assurance (QA) with the nursing department, which is responsible for case management and uses various software applications for such services.

Electronic Document Management Systems

A variety of departments may use an EDMS. Most commonly, the HIM department is responsible for the EDMS for the overall health record. However, independent EDMSs (of various types) may commonly be found in the emergency department, radiology, PFS, human resources, and other areas.

There are different types of EDMSs—from simple to sophisticated. **Document imaging systems (DIMS)** merely capture images of forms to be stored in a computer system for later retrieval. Other systems enable electronic feed (formerly referred to as COLD [computer output to laser disk] feed) to store in an automated archive various types of digital documents (for example, typed documents from a transcription system, voice files from a dictation system, electronically generated documents from a speech dictation system, print files such as from a laboratory system, or wave-form files from a monitoring system, e-fax, and e-mail). Most EDMS used in healthcare organizations for managing the health record enable indexing of forms. Some of these systems, known as **electronic document/ content management (ED/CM) systems**, also support management of some data content on forms to aid retrieval of information. Content management systems may also refer to systems designed primarily to support intranets or web pages on the Internet.

An EDMS can be integrated with **workflow technology**, which helps direct work on documents. For example, workflow technology can determine when a record is ready for coding and put it into the appropriate coder's work queue. Simultaneously, the PFS department may access documents in the EDMS for reference or to generate a claims attachment.

An EDMS may have sophisticated functionality to select blocks of text to view or easily distribute work for processing; however, the EDMS primarily affords access to what was originally paper-record content from multiple locations. It is often used as an interim technology or bridge strategy along a migration path to the EHR or as a supplemental technology to achieve a totally paperless environment (Rhodes and Dougherty 2003).

Order Communication/Results Retrieval Systems

Order communication/results retrieval (OC/RR) systems are another type of administrative system. They are not the same as CPOE or results management systems that are part of the core clinical EHR system. OC/RR systems can be used to transmit orders to various ancillary departments and view results of laboratory and other diagnostic studies or the status of orders. OC/RR systems help integrate various source systems for operational purposes. However, they are essentially paper-based because they rely on handwritten orders transcribed into a computer by clerical or nursing staff and diagnostic study results typically generated in a paper or **print file** format.

Staff can use OC/RR systems to automatically transmit orders instead of phoning, using a courier, faxing, or sending orders via pneumatic tube, and these systems provide access to results from multiple locations. OC/RR systems are often among the first information systems acquired in a hospital after the R-ADT and PFS, and their existence is essential for an EHR. If these systems are from different vendors, as they may well be, separate interface programs must be written to permit the systems-wide sharing of patient demographic data.

Ancillary/Clinical Department Applications

OC/RR systems are designed to communicate with systems that receive and process orders and generate results. The three major ancillary or clinical department systems in a hospital include the **laboratory information system (LIS)**, (inpatient/clinical) **pharmacy information system (PIS)**, and **radiology information system (RIS)**. Other systems may include blood bank and imaging (to capture radiology and other clinical images), which are called *picture archiving and communication systems (PACS)*. Other clinical departments may also acquire applications to help them manage their services and workflow. These include dietary/nutrition and food services, central supply, physical therapy, respiratory therapy, speech therapy, occupational therapy, rehabilitation services, and others.

Ancillary systems serve two primary functions. The first is to manage the department. For example, the LIS receives an order for a laboratory test and then provides considerable support for generating specimen collection lists, labels for specimen vials, connectivity with autoanalyzers, calibration of devices, quality checks, and even staff scheduling. A clinical PIS can do similar and equivalent functions, including maintaining the inventory of drugs, tracking drug expiration dates, and so on. The second function of these ancillary applications is to generate the clinical results they have processed (and associated charges). Hence, although the ultimate purpose of an LIS is to generate laboratory test results, it does so with support for many other functions to get to the point that it can generate the results. Similarly, many functions support the dispensing of medication via a clinical PIS or the delivery of a tray of nutritionally appropriate food to a patient on a soft diet via a foodservice ordering system.

Specialty Clinical Applications

Although there may be a fine line between what might be considered a departmental clinical application and a specialty clinical application, the distinction often reflects a matter of priority. Whereas departmental clinical applications serve any patient, specialty clinical applications serve patients with specific disease states or particular levels of required nursing care. Applications for intensive care, perioperative/surgical, and emergency medicine units address the special staffing needs and services of patients who require those types of services. Vendors have also created niche products for cardiology, oncology, labor and delivery, psychiatry, and other highly focused specialties.

There are also applications specific to the various forms of long-term care (LTC): nursing homes, home health, and hospice services. Hospitals and ambulatory settings that support LTC services may acquire these applications as separate products from different vendors or as components within a suite of products from a single vendor (depending on vendor offerings) over a considerable period of time, depending on their patient populations. Dentists, chiropractors, public health professionals, and other specialized healthcare providers may have their own clinical applications.

Smart Peripherals

Smart peripherals are medical devices that can be directly connected to an information system to enable capture of their information into the EHR. For example, monitoring equipment may supply patient-specific information, such as fetal monitoring records, blood pressure data, or blood sugar levels, and may be used in a hospital, other care delivery facility, or the home setting. Robots in laboratories and pharmacies, in particular, can automate, and thus reduce errors, in handling of specimen and drug dispensing. Robots can be programmed to find nursing units or patient rooms and then used as couriers. Again, these systems may be acquired at different times in a migration path, depending on the organization's mission and goals.

Clinical Messaging Systems/Provider-Patient Portals

Clinical messaging systems add to OC/RR and EDMS systems the dimension of real-time access to information through web-based technology. The web-based technology may be applied within the **intranet** (the organization's own internal network) or may entail the exchange of information through a secure web portal from the Internet.

Clinical messaging systems are often used to provide connectivity between a hospital and the offices of its medical staff members, and there is growing interest in using clinical messaging for communications with patients. For example, a patient portal can be used for secure e-mail exchange as well as for other patient applications, such as e-visits. An **e-visit** is a reimbursable evaluation and management service provided by a physician or other qualified health professional to an established patient using an electronic-based communication network. It must be noted that a portal is not the same as a personal health record.

Registries

Registries are systems to which care delivery organizations may contribute specific information for subsequent analysis and comparison. Frequently, registries are disease-, condition-, or procedure-specific, such as cancer registries, diabetes registries, and immunization registries. These registries are often maintained by a medical specialty society or public health department. They support individual patient follow-up as well as aggregation of data for trending and statistical analysis.

An increasing number of EHR vendors, medical specialty societies, and other vendors are developing registries for capturing and reporting quality measurement data. These registries enable hospitals to use a centralized data collection service to contribute quality measurement data to organizations that require such information, including the Joint Commission, Medicare, and MU programs, among others. In addition, providers who contribute to such registry services can receive analyses of their data as well as information about how their data compare to those from other providers.

Results Management Systems

Although OC/RR systems enable viewing and printing of results from laboratory tests and other studies, more sophisticated processing of these results is feasible when they are produced as structured data. For example, if laboratory test results are generated as structured data, they may be graphed or structured into a table. If medication administration and vital signs data are saved as structured data (from BCMAR and POC charting systems), they can be combined with laboratory test results in a structured form to evaluate the impact of the medication on the patient's condition. Because such systems are more sophisticated than results-reporting systems, they are considered an important component of an EHR.

Point-of-Care Charting Systems

Point-of-care (POC) charting systems, also called **clinical documentation systems**, are systems in which clinicians enter data as they care for patients. These data include history and physical exam records, findings from assessments, progress notes, vital signs, and so on. POC charting systems in hospitals initially focused primarily on nursing staff documentation, but these systems increasingly support other clinicians and physicians to a more limited extent. In the ambulatory environment, EHRs are used by all clinicians, especially physicians and nurses. Data entered into POC charting systems may be structured or unstructured.

Structured data, also called **discrete data**, refer to data that have been predefined as a set of limited, standardized options. Structured data enable standardized values to be supplied for specific variables, so the data can be used in clinical decision support systems and provide standardized meaning for reporting purposes. A user selects the data values desired for each variable (such as patient condition or history of present illness) from a drop-down menu or checklist by using a mouse, arrow keys, touch screen, voice command, or other type of human-computer interface. In some cases, the user may be asked to enter a number or numeric score. For example, to record the severity of symptoms, a nurse or physical therapist may select a numeric score from a standard pain scale, as shown in the top portion of figure 1.8. It is important to note that the purpose of structured data entry is to help ensure standardization. Therefore, when setting up structured data entry, it is important to ensure that the appropriate scale, scoring system, or code set is specified in some way. Interestingly, there are several pain scales used in healthcare. Nurses often use a scale scoring pain from 1 to 10 whereas physical therapists typically score pain from 1 to 4.

Unstructured data refers to narrative data or images of information, as is illustrated by the empty box in the section under "Patient Cannot . . ." in figure 1.8. Here, an area is reserved for authorized clinicians to type or dictate anything they want to record. Such unstructured data are more difficult to use in searches or for reporting purposes and generally are not converted into tabular or graphical form; however, they can be essential to ensure complete documentation.

Early in their introduction, POC charting systems required significant changes in workflow. They were often time-consuming and difficult to use. Attempts were made to use computers stationed at the bedside because returning to a small number of computers at a nursing station was inadequate for efficient documentation. Today, POC charting systems are much more sophisticated. Data entry may be performed using handheld devices, such as smartphones, laptop computers, or tablets. Many of these devices are wireless, and some are secured to carts (commonly referred to as **wireless on wheels**, or workstations on wheels, or WOWs).

Structured data may be captured via any of these data-entry devices in a variety of ways. Drop-down menus, check boxes, or radio buttons are commonly used to select data points from templates.

Figure 1.8.   Structured data entry in an EHR

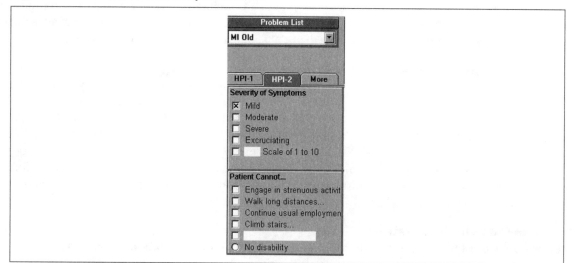

Smart text (or what would be called *macros* in word processing) is a code that, when invoked, represents an entire phrase, sentence, or paragraph. Voice commands, touch screens, a stylus, or the standard keyboard can be used to activate any of these methods. Type-ahead is a function where typing the first few letters in a desired word presents a list of words from which to choose, as illustrated in figure 1.9. Many EHRs may keep track of data frequently entered by a user and automatically build a list of favorites to reduce the time needed to select options from a long, generic list.

To capture unstructured data, users can employ the typical dictation processes (including speech dictation) or simply keyboarding, often using word processing functions such as copy and paste and drag and drop. Unstructured data entry aids can be helpful, but they can lead to errors (for example, copying information into the wrong chart) and compliance issues (for example, notes are not unique to specific patients). The most sophisticated systems will apply **natural language processing** to unstructured data, which permits the narrative text to be converted to structured data for processing by the computer. This last form of data entry is still in the developmental stage.

Computerized Provider Order Entry and E-Prescribing Systems

Computerized provider order entry (CPOE) systems are intended for use by physicians and other authorized providers (for example, physician assistants, nurse practitioners, and nurse midwives, according to their licensure) to enter orders directly into the computer and be given prompts, reminders, or alerts about the order. Because these systems enhance legibility, they reduce the risk of data entry errors, and their decision support capability enhances patient safety and healthcare efficiencies. Decision support might include calculating the appropriate dose of a medication (especially for pediatrics) or alerting the provider that a medication is contraindicated under certain circumstances, such as when the patient has a known allergy to it, is taking another medication that may counteract the effects of the drug being considered, is being prepped for a certain diagnostic study, or has liver or kidney disease. The CPOE system might identify that a specific drug is not covered by the patient's insurance and possibly offer equivalents that are covered or less expensive. CPOE has been heavily promoted for patient safety purposes to avoid medication errors, but it can also be helpful in identifying duplicate orders for services, providing cost comparisons of diagnostic studies, and alerting providers about needed preventive care services. Orders from a CPOE system should be distributed to their respective departmental clinical systems, including tasking nurses to perform specific functions for the patient.

In a clinic or other ambulatory care setting, CPOE systems include the ability to initiate diagnostic studies, order referrals, schedule appointments, and task nursing staff for other functions, such as procedure assistance or identifying when a patient is ready to leave and be given instructions on wound care, medication administration, and so on. In an ambulatory environment, including not only the physician office or clinic but also on discharge from a hospital or emergency department, e-prescribing (e-Rx) systems give the prescriber the ability to write a prescription and

Figure 1.9.   Illustration of the "type-ahead" function

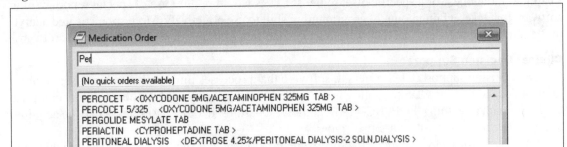

Source: Computerized Patient Record System via US Veterans Health Information Systems and Technology Architecture.

have it transmitted directly to a retail pharmacy system. E-Rx systems may be standalone or a special function of the CPOE system in an ambulatory care EHR system.

Electronic/Bar Code Medication Administration Record

Electronic medication administration record (EMAR) is the automation of many of the processes associated with medication administration in a hospital. In its most basic form, EMAR is a printout generated by the pharmacy system that nurses can use to identify what medications should be administered to a patient and then document the administration. More sophisticated forms of EMAR display the medication administration record on the computer so nurses can perform direct data entry. An EMAR system can have **bar code medication administration records (BC-MARs)**. When an EMAR systems includes bar code or **radio frequency identification (RFID)** technology to add the dimension of positive identification of the patient, the medication being administered, and the nurse administering the drug, the system is referred to as a bar code medication administration record (BC-MAR) system. In addition to identification and documentation, BC-MAR systems provide alerts for medication timing and information about the medication that a nurse can review to better understand potential patient reactions. It also aids workflow by scheduling medication administration. These systems are important for improving patient safety through the **five rights of medication administration**, first promoted through the Institute for Safe Medication Practices (ISMP). These rights are ensuring the right patient, right drug, right time, right dose, and right route (ISMP 1999). Together, CPOE systems and EMAR/BC-MAR systems provide for more accurate medication management.

Reporting

Reporting with respect to EHR may have a variety of meanings. In some cases, reports may be visit summaries, referral letters, or even an electronic copy of the EHR for the patient. Content for these may be standardized using the HL7 Clinical Document Architecture (CDA) standard.

Reporting from an EHR is also the process of querying existing data to search and retrieve data specific to a patient, produce lists (often used for patient follow-up), aggregate data from multiple patients, or perform sophisticated analysis that generates new information. Lists may be in the basic form of a tabulation, but data may also be reported in the form of labels to affix to mailings or even connected to autodial systems to call patients for follow-up or recall purposes. Some EHRs have special report wizards to aggregate data into statistical reports (for example, the number of surgeries each physician performs in a month), whereas others require special report-writing software. To generate new information, special analytical tools may be needed in addition to or in place of report-writing software.

As noted above, an issue with current EHR applications is that they are almost exclusively focused on direct care–delivery functionality because their underlying database structure has been optimized to perform online transaction processing. Consequently, the ability of these applications to develop reports for quality studies or other functions, or even produce a hard copy of the legal health record, is limited. For example, if a provider wants to generate an ad hoc report to compare treatment modalities for a specific disease, most EHRs would require use of special report-writing software that takes a fair amount of programming skill to use effectively. More sophisticated analytics generally require a clinical data warehouse in addition to the sophisticated analytical software.

Clinical Decision Support

Clinical decision support (CDS) refers to software that processes information to help users make a clinical decision. Some CDS capability is embedded within core clinical applications that comprise the EHR, such as within CPOE, BC-MAR, and POC charting. In other cases, CDS may be acquired as separate applications of a variety of types.

Some types of CDS provide active decision support, such as alerts or reminders to which the user must respond. Figure 1.10 is an example of a CDS alert that is called "Order Checks." Other

Figure 1.10.   Example of active CDS

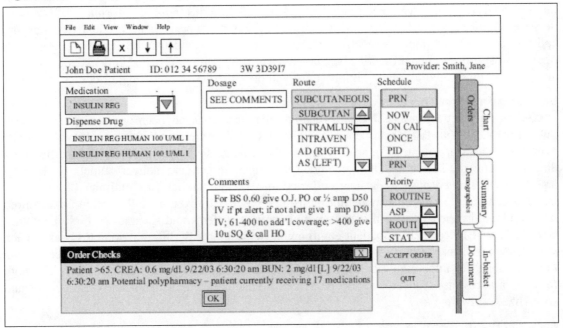

CDS types are considered passive because the user chooses whether to use the support. CDS is generated by preprogrammed logic or rules. For example, if a patient comes to an emergency department with chest pain, a CDS system may remind the physician to check all applicable body systems for the cause of the patient's pain (for example, cardiovascular, gastrointestinal, and pulmonary). Alerts about allergies, contraindications, or a drug being off-formulary are common forms of CDS found in CPOE and e-Rx systems. Other types of CDS support coding in a physician office EHR system, where the complexity of the patient encounter must be reflected in the evaluation and management (E/M) codes from the Current Procedural Terminology (CPT). These codes ultimately contribute to the level of reimbursement for the visit. However, as "Avoiding Fraud Risks Associated with EHRs" by Helton (2010) suggests, "an electronic health record can reduce a healthcare provider's exposure to risk posed by the fraudulent use of healthcare data, but only to the extent that the provider has established proper controls within the system" (2010).

A CDS system also may integrate clinical practice guidelines, protocols, or care pathways into a template used for data entry. The CDS system not only offers the ability to chart against these guidelines or pathways but also makes them **context sensitive**, so that only the parts of the guidelines that are applicable to the given patient are offered for charting. For example, guidelines regarding female anatomy would not be presented as part of CDS for a male patient's physical examination. Moreover, the CDS system may tap external knowledge sources to provide more comprehensive information. For example, if a physician is unfamiliar with a new drug offered as an alternative suggestion, he or she might click a link to access a reference that provides more complete information. A physician faced with an unusual set of symptoms and signs could potentially use the CDS to look for reference material on the Internet to develop a differential diagnosis, or there may be a special form of CDS that provides specific support for differential diagnosis. A pharmacist may need to make suggestions for alternative medications when a patient has an allergy or research the efficacy of various drugs when there is an unusual diagnosis. The CDS system may produce tailored instructions for the patient.

CDS should be contrasted with **executive decision support**, which is typically a standalone system that analyzes a large volume of aggregated data and provides trending information. Executive decision support is typically retrospective, providing quality improvement, productivity, staffing, and marketing information for executives. CDS is concurrent (provided at the time data are entered) or even prospective (when presenting best practices in anticipation of care). Clinical data, however, also may be aggregated for quality improvement studies, predictive modeling, or clinical research.

Clinical Data Repository

A **clinical data repository (CDR)** is a relational database that has been optimized for processing many transactions. Such transactions may be as simple as viewing laboratory test results or as complicated as analyzing data in an HPI against knowledge sources and generating a differential diagnosis. The key is that a CDR is intended to support direct care–delivery functions. In most ambulatory EHRs, because all data are collected into a relational database optimized for processing transactions, the system is by definition using a CDR. However, a CDR is often not acquired in an ambulatory environment that has multiple source systems and separate core clinical components to its EHR or in an inpatient environment with the many different source systems, each with its own database, until such time as many of the core clinical applications are in place. At that time, the need for integrating data from all the different source systems becomes crucial—both for ease of access as well as to support more sophisticated clinical decision support functions and specialized software.

Personal Health Records

Personal health records (PHRs) are systems designed to support patient-entered data. If they are offered to a patient by a provider, they are typically accessed through a patient portal and include a limited amount of data from the patient's EHR—usually as designated by the provider. Provider-offered PHRs are often not very interactive, in that they often do not include the ability for the patient to enter data.

If a patient has multiple providers who are not within a given IDS, the patient could have many different PHRs. These PHRs also generally are not transferable to another provider. It is for this reason that some patients prefer to use a standalone PHR system that is not associated with a provider. In these instances, patients may direct their providers to submit data to the PHR or they may themselves upload the data to the PHR. Many of the standalone PHRs also support structured data entry by the patient. Standalone PHRs may be applications the patient can keep on their own personal devices, or they may be web-based. As noted above, some of these enable connectivity from personal mHealth devices.

Telehealth and Home Monitoring

The terms *telemedicine* and *telehealth* may carry separate connotations or be used synonymously. The "Core Standards for Telemedicine Operations" from the American Telemedicine Association (ATA), defines *telemedicine* as "use of medical information exchanged from one site to another via electronic communications to improve, maintain, or assist patients' health status." In contrast, **telehealth** is "often used to encompass a broader definition of remote health care that does not always involve clinical services" (ATA 2007). Use of this broader term seems to be gaining momentum. Telehealth may include remote monitoring, an actual patient encounter, a consultation, or distance learning. Any use of telehealth for the purpose of care provision requires documentation in the patient's health record. An EHR may facilitate such documentation and may incorporate components of the telehealth encounter that might be considered beyond the scope of the legal health record but useful for other purposes.

Home monitoring may blur the telemedicine/telehealth/mHealth line even further, when it is used for physiological monitoring that is overseen by a healthcare professional. An increasing number of wearable or implantable devices can be used to monitor diabetes, asthma, pacemaker functioning, medication administration, the location of the individual, and so on. Some types of home monitoring even include direct provision of care in the home, such as home-based dialysis. However, in other instances, home monitoring is integrated with a PHR that is accessible to a healthcare professional only on an occasional basis, or home monitoring may simply entail personal use of standalone devices, such as pedometers, scales, thermometers, smart pill boxes, and home pregnancy tests, which are sold directly to consumers. Health plans may use home monitoring as part of a disease management program. For example, text messages to remind adolescents with type 1 diabetes to test their blood sugar could be part of a home monitoring strategy.

Health Information Exchange

Health information exchange (HIE) refers to seamless exchange of health information across disparate organizations, often where the organizations have signed agreements to participate in an **HIE organization (HIO)**. Some HIOs started as local health information organizations (LHIOs) or regional health information organizations (RHIOs). Today, the federal government is promoting statewide HIEs and supports the development of the eHealth Exchange, which is the national **health information network** initiative intended to connect all HIOs. HIOs provide patient identification functionality, record locator services, identity management and security services, and data exchange management. Some HIOs are managing the release of information functionality via patient consent afforded through the service or via their PHRs.

A healthcare clearinghouse is a special type of HIE that receives health data from a source and distributes them to a recipient. Early healthcare clearinghouses provided exchange services for providers who were sending healthcare claims to multiple health plans. Over time, these healthcare clearinghouses also helped the exchange of health plan eligibility information, claims status, and remittance advice information. In some cases, these healthcare clearinghouses also provide additional services, such as claims scrubbing, for the data they transport. More recently, the healthcare industry has been mandated to use electronic funds transfer for the receipt of reimbursement funds, and clearinghouses overseen by the financial services/banking industry provide such services. Healthcare clearinghouses are also used for the distribution of e-prescribing information.

Big Data, Data Warehousing, Analytics, and Population Health

A clinical data warehouse (CDW) is a database that has been optimized for performing sophisticated analysis. A CDW may be used to conduct **data mining**, which is a process that looks for patterns in information. Data mining of EHRs or other health IT is useful for clinical research. **Predictive modeling** has been widely performed by health plans to analyze information that may suggest the likelihood of patients needing health services. Although most hospitals and providers contribute data to external CDWs—most often via claims, although increasingly in the form of quality measures to registries—some hospitals and large clinics may acquire a CDW of their own, especially if they want to perform analytics for quality improvement or conduct clinical or health services research.

Population health also is facilitated through accurate, complete, and timely capture and reporting of public health data, including data relating to homeland security. Population health data collection may be initiated in the provider setting and linked automatically to a state data collection system. Population health may be served by decision support provided to caregivers through alerts from public health departments, such as a notification of a new strain of virus or a reminder to seek certain information from patients who present with particular symptoms. A precursor to population health may be disease management, wherein providers and health plans share data about patients/health plan members who would benefit from certain educational programs or special monitoring.

Check Your Understanding 1.2

Match the terms with the appropriate descriptions:

    A. Bar-code medication administration record

    B. Clinical data repository

    C. Connectivity system

    D. Core clinical system

    E. Laboratory information system

    F. Smart peripheral

    G. Source system

    H. Portal

    1. Automated infusion pump

    2. Form of remote access to EHR

    3. Consolidated-Clinical Document Architecture

    4. Part of medication management

    5. Electronic document management system

    6. Supporting infrastructure

    7. Results management

    8. Departmental clinical application

References and Resources

42 CFR 412, 413, 422, etc. Medicare and Medicaid programs: Electronic Health Record Incentive Program, final rule. 2010.

45 CFR 170(b). Health information technology: Standards, implementation specifications, and certification criteria for electronic health records technology, final rule. 2010.

45 CFR 170(e). Establishment of the permanent certification for health information technology, final rule. 2011

American Telemedicine Association (ATA). 2007. *Core Standards for Telemedicine Operations.* Washington, DC: American Telemedicine Association.

Blumenthal D., and M. Tavenner. 2010. The "meaningful use" regulation for electronic health records. *New England Journal of Medicine.* 363:501–504.

Boone, K.W. 2011 (October 11). The EHR is a platform, not an application. *Healthcare IT News.* http://www.healthcareitnews.com/blog/ehr-platform-not-application.

Centers for Medicare and Medicaid Services (CMS). 2016. Quality Payment Program: Delivery system reform, Medicare payment reform, & MACRA: The merit-based incentive payment system (MIPS) & alternative payment models (APMs). https://www.cms.gov/Medicare/Quality-Initiatives-Patient-Assessment-Instruments/Value-Based-Programs/MACRA-MIPS-and-APMs/MACRA-MIPS-and-APMs.html.

Computer-Based Patient Record Institute (CPRI). 1997. *Valuing CPR Systems—A Business Planning Methodology.* Schaumburg, IL: Computer-based Patient Record Institute.

DeSalvo, K.B. and J.G. Daniel. 2015 (April 10). Blocking of health information undermines health system interoperability and delivery reform. *Health IT Buzz.* http://www.healthit.gov/buzz-blog/from-the-onc-desk/health-information-blocking-undermines-interoperability-delivery-reform.

Halamka, J.D. 2012 (February 14). The perfect EHR. *Life as a Healthcare CIO.* http://geekdoctor.blogspot.com/2012/02/perfect-ehr.html.

Halamka, J.D. 2015 (November 11). The path forward for meaningful use. *Life as a Healthcare CIO.* http://geekdoctor.blogspot.com/2015/11/the-path-forward-for-meaningful-use.html.

Hanover, J. 2015 (April 9). Crossing the innovation gap from 2nd to 3rd platform acute care systems. *IDC Health Insights.* https://idc-community.com/health/healthcare-transformation/crossing_the_innovation_gap_from_2nd_to_3rd_platform_acute_care_syst.

Healthcare Information Management and Systems Society (HIMSS). 2006–2015. *HIMSS Analytics US EMR Adoption Model.* http://app.himssanalytics.org/hc_providers/emr_adoption.asp.

HealthIT.gov Dashboard. n.d. Non-federal acute care hospital electronic health record adoption. Dashboard.healthit.gov/quickstats/quickstats.php.

HealthIT.gov Policy Committee. 2009. Meaningful Use Workgroup Presentation. https://www.healthit.gov/archive/archive_files/HIT%20Policy%20Committee/2009/2009-07-16/Meaningful%20Use_7.16.09.ppt

HealthIT.gov Policy Committee. 2009–2011. *Recommendations to the National Coordinator for Health IT.* https://www.healthit.gov/facas/health-it-policy-committee/health-it-policy-committee-recommendations-national-coordinator-health-it

Health Resources and Services Administration, US Department of Health and Human Services (HRSA) n.d. What is health IT? http://www.hrsa.gov/healthit/toolbox/oralhealthittoolbox/introduction/whatishealthit.html.

Helton, J.R. 2010. Avoiding fraud risks associated with EHRs. *Healthcare Financial Management* 64(7):76–81.

Institute for Safe Medication Practices (ISMP). 1999 (April 7). The "five rights." *ISMP Medication Safety Alert!* https://www.ismp.org/newsletters/acutecare/articles/19990407.asp.

Institute of Medicine (IOM). 1991. *The Computer-based Patient Record: An Essential Technology for Health Care,* edited by R.S. Dick and E.B. Steen. Washington, DC: National Academies Press.

Institute of Medicine (IOM). 1999. *To Err Is Human: Building a Safer Health System,* edited by L.T. Kohn, J.M. Corrigan, and M.S. Donaldson. Washington, DC: National Academies Press.

Institute of Medicine (IOM). 2003. *Key Capabilities of an Electronic Health Record System: Letter Report.* Washington, DC: National Academies Press. http://www.nap.edu/catalog/10781/key-capabilities-of-an-electronic-health-record-system-letter-report.

Lichtenwald, I. 2015. Information blocking in health IT: Myth or reality? *Health IT Consultant.* http://hitconsultant.net/2015/06/15/information-blocking-in-health-it-myth-or-reality.

Markle Foundation. 2009. Achieving the health IT objectives of the American Recovery and Reinvestment Act. http://www.markle.org/publications/403-achieving-health-it-objectives-american-recovery-and-reinvestment-act.

McCann, E. 2015 (October 6). CMS drops final EHR meaningful use rule. *Healthcare IT News.* http://www.healthcareitnews.com/news/cms-onc-release-final-ehr-meaningful-use-rules.

Miliard, M. 2016 (January 12). Meaningful use will likely end in 2016, CMS chief Andy Slavitt says. *HealthcareIT News.* http://www.healthcareitnews.com/news/meaningful-use-will-likely-end-2016-cms-chief-andy-slavitt-says.

National Alliance for Health Information Technology (NAHIT). 2008 (April 28). Report to the Office of the National Coordinator for Health Information Technology on defining key health information technology terms. http://www.himss.org/national-alliance-health-information-technology-report-office-national-coordinator-health?ItemNumber=10884.

National Institute of Standards and Technology (NIST). 2014 (February 12). Framework for improving critical infrastructure cybersecurity. Version 1.0. http://www.nist.gov/cyberframework.

Office of the National Coordinator for Health Information Technology (ONC). 2014. Connecting health and care for the nation: A 10-year vision to achieve an interoperable health IT infrastructure. http://www.healthit.gov/buzz-blog/health-information-exchange-2/call-action-nationwide-interoperable-health-infrastructure.

Office of the National Coordinator for Health Information Technology (ONC). 2015a. Federal health IT strategic plan. https://www.healthit.gov/sites/default/files/9-5-federalhealthitstratplanfinal_0.pdf.

Office of the National Coordinator for Health Information Technology (ONC). 2015b. Connecting health and care for the nation: A shared nationwide interoperability roadmap. Final version 1.0. https://www.healthit.gov/sites/default/files/hie-interoperability/nationwide-interoperability-roadmap-final-version-1.0.pdf.

Office of the National Coordinator for Health Information Technology (ONC). 2015c. About the ONC Health IT Certification Program. https://www.healthit.gov/policy-researchers-implementers/about-onc-health-it-certification-program.

Rhodes, H., and M. Dougherty. 2003. Practice brief: Document imaging as a bridge to the EHR. *Journal of AHIMA*. 74(6):56A–56G.

Snelick, R., and S. Taylor. 2013 (June 3). Understanding meaningful use with a focus on testing the HL7 V2 messaging standards. National Institute of Standards and Testing (NIST). http://healthcare.nist.gov/docs/NIST_MU_Testing_Article.pdf.

Stead, W.W., and H.S. Lin, eds. 2009. *Computational Technology for Effective Health Care: Immediate Steps and Strategic Directions. National Research Council of the National Academies.* Washington, DC: National Academy Press.

Wallace, S. 2014 (December 13). Commentary: Current generation of EHRs impeding volume-to-value transformation. *Modern Healthcare*. http://www.modernhealthcare.com/article/20141213/MAGAZINE/312139978.

Chapter 2
Information Systems Theory and Systems Development Life Cycle

Key Terms

Attributes

Closed system

Cybernetics

Data-information-knowledge-wisdom (DIKW) continuum

Data quality

Electronic systems

Human systems

Human-machine systems

Information systems theory

Inputs

Interoperability

Knowledge

Manual systems

Mechanical systems

Objects

Open source software

Open system

Outputs

Processes

Systems development life cycle

Templates

Learning Objectives

- Understand general systems theory and its relevance to the planning for the components of health IT.

- Understand general information theory as it relates to developing data infrastructure requirements.

- Describe information systems theory and how it can improve the nation's health, cost of healthcare, and experience of care.

- Explain the systems development life cycle within the context of health IT.

An *information system* is a set of components that work together to achieve a common purpose, as illustrated in figure 2.1. In science, *theory* refers to a comprehensive explanation of an important feature of nature that is supported by many facts gathered over time. Theories also allow scientists to make predictions about as yet unobserved phenomena. Thus, **information systems theory** uses facts about information systems to make predictions about how such systems will work. Every information system is described, at a minimum, by its inputs, processes, and outputs. When planning any information system, from the simplest to the most complex, it is necessary to appreciate and anticipate the impact of these system components on the desired outcome of the system. From a practical perspective, the **systems development life cycle**, a model that represents the ongoing process of developing (or purchasing) information systems, is the embodiment of information systems theory. Using this formal methodology will enable the information system to be more valid and reliable.

There are various types of information systems. For example, in healthcare there are laboratory information systems, pharmacy information systems, patient accounting systems, disease registry systems, online purchasing systems, automated instrumentation systems, and many other information systems. Although all these information systems have inputs, processes, and outputs, their purposes are generally limited in scope to either the department's operations in which they exist (for example, laboratory or pharmacy) or their primary function (for example, claims processing, supplies procurement, or vital signs monitoring).

An electronic health record (EHR) is also an information system, and, as such, it has inputs, processes, and outputs. However, an EHR is typically much broader in scope than an application designed for a single department or function. Instead, an EHR depends on many other systems for its input, performs many different types of processes, and generates a wide array of outputs.

Figure 2.1.   Information systems theory

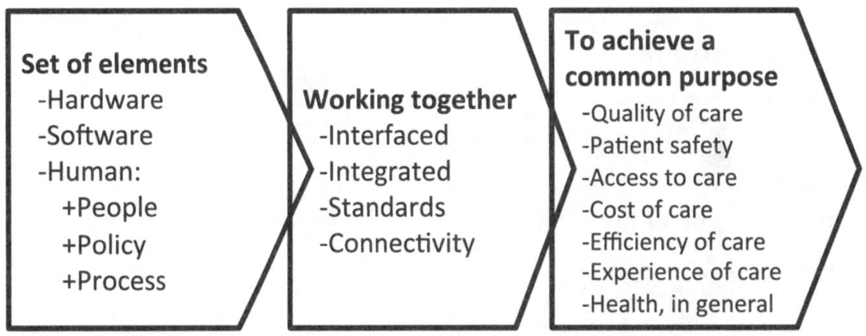

Set of elements
-Hardware
-Software
-Human:
  +People
  +Policy
  +Process

Working together
-Interfaced
-Integrated
-Standards
-Connectivity

To achieve a common purpose
-Quality of care
-Patient safety
-Access to care
-Cost of care
-Efficiency of care
-Experience of care
-Health, in general

Health information technology (health IT) is the broadest focus of health information systems. It incorporates all source systems and core clinical systems used within a healthcare delivery organization, as well as information systems that are external to any given delivery organization and may span multiple health information systems. Examples of health IT include systems that individuals use to monitor their health, systems that support population health, and systems that appropriately connect these components with one another and with research databases, public health systems, and even systems that relate to other determinants of health, such as transportation, housing, or food. These systems and the supporting infrastructure needed for this broadest view of health IT are the next frontier that the federal government wants to address (ONC 2015).

General Systems Theory

Systems theory is an interdisciplinary field of study that analyzes and describes how any group of objects work together to produce a result. Systems theory generally grew out of biology and the notion that systems are open to and can interact with their environments, and they can acquire qualitatively new properties through emergence, resulting in continual evolution.

System Theory Concepts

Rather than reducing an entity (for example, the human body) to the properties of its parts or elements (for example, organs or cells), systems theory focuses on the arrangement of and relations between the parts that connect them into a whole. Thus, the same concepts and principles of theory organization underlie different disciplines. Systems concepts include system–environment boundary, inputs, processes, outputs, and goal-directedness.

Boundaries describe the scope of a system. For example, the boundaries of the EHR system might be defined such that only the core clinical system components are included, or the boundaries could be expanded to incorporate all source systems, supporting infrastructure, and connectivity system components, as described in chapter 1.

In any information system, **inputs** are data entered into the information system, including data from source systems as well as those directly entered by a human. A **process** (a systematic series of actions taken to create a product or perform a service) is used to generate information from inputs. Data processing may also potentially generate new knowledge when experience, such as in the form of knowledge sources, is included in the data contributed to the system. System **outputs** are the outcomes of inputs into a system; output information comes in many forms and formats. Outputs may be laboratory test results, an alert that the patient is allergic to a drug, a visit summary to be given to the patient, a report on how many procedures were performed in the operating room this month, and many other types of information. Finally, for a system to have value, all elements should be directed toward accomplishing something. Systems may have one goal or many, such as to improve documentation, communication, and patient safety.

Examples of Systems

There are many types of familiar systems, including the following:

- **Mechanical systems** are developed by humans but can operate without human intervention. Heating and cooling systems are examples of systems that process external temperature, barometric pressure, humidity, and other inputs to determine adjustments to maintain a constant desired environmental goal.

- **Human systems** are organized relationships among people. The US political system can be described as votes (input) of citizens (boundary) elect (process) officials (output) to govern for the good of all (goal). The healthcare delivery system is a human system. Its boundaries are healthcare services for humans (as opposed to veterinary medicine) defined by reimbursement practices (for example, in the United States, practitioners at massage parlors are not reimbursed by Medicare, Medicaid, or formal insurance programs). Its inputs are individuals seeking healthcare services. The healthcare delivery system's processes are the services performed by providers, payers, oversight agencies, and others who deliver healthcare-related services; its outputs are the health outcomes (such as cures of or improvements in the illnesses and injuries) in the human inputs. Its goals are to keep infants alive, reduce suffering, and so on.

- **Human–machine systems** are any form of supportive operations that assist humans in the performance of their work. **Manual systems** are those that entail humans performing certain processes; **electronic systems** are aided by computing devices. A filing system where paper charts are pulled and filed in accordance with specific policies and procedures is a manual system designed to enable easy retrieval of charts. An *information system* where humans enter data into a computer to be stored and later retrieved to support patient care is an electronic health information system. (Meadows 2008).

Closed Versus Open Systems and Interoperability Challenges

Systems may be characterized as being closed or open (Helms 2006). A **closed system** is one where all parts operate together without external influences. In general systems theory, a closed system may be expected to eventually stop functioning as a system because it does not have the feedback necessary to adjust to changes in the environment. In an **open system**, the parts are affected by the environment. These basic differences are illustrated in figure 2.2.

However, in health IT, the concepts of closed system and open system are used differently than in systems theory. In health IT, a closed system describes health IT that is proprietary and not freely shared with others. Alternatively, information services vendors that apply an open system philosophy do so by adhering to open or readily available standards that enable the software to interconnect with other open source software.

Closed proprietary systems do adhere to standards, but they do so loosely, which makes it difficult for other software to work with them. Although closed health IT systems are influenced by government mandates, they do not necessarily respond to customer demands without such a government mandate. In fact, these vendors' contracts often include provisions that do not permit customers to discuss proprietary information about their products without prior written consent from the company (Advisory Board 2015). The American Medical Association calls these provisions

Figure 2.2.   Closed versus open systems

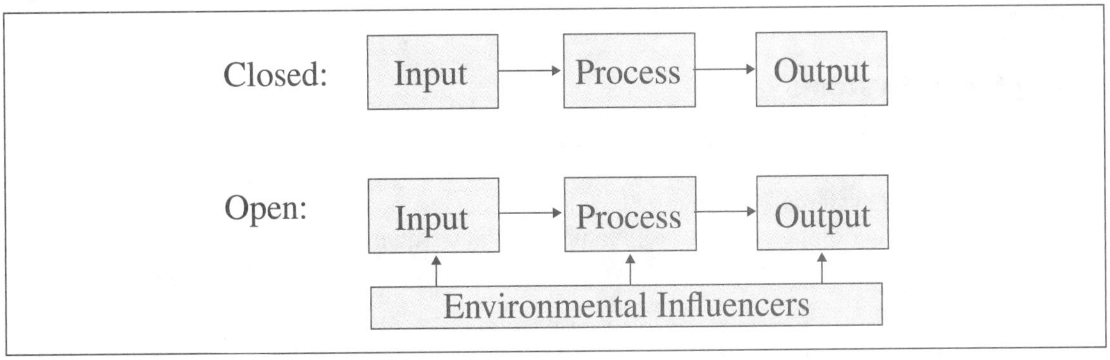

"gag orders" (Friedberg et al. 2013). An Institute of Medicine (IOM) study on the issue noted that "the confidentiality and intellectual property clauses are the biggest barriers to reporting adverse events" (IOM 2011a). The Office of the National Coordinator for Health Information Technology (ONC) and the Centers for Medicare and Medicaid Services (CMS), which jointly oversee the meaningful use (MU) of EHR incentive program, have stated that they oppose these vendor contract clauses but have limited power to ban them. At least one member of Congress (Sen. Bill Cassidy [R-Louisiana]) held hearings on the issue in summer 2015.

One consequence of the proprietary nature of health IT systems has been that healthcare delivery organizations acquire one vendor's software to initiate their use of health IT and then find themselves dependent on the first vendor to meet all of their information system needs. Thus, proprietary systems that essentially force an organization to stay with one vendor have been the norm in the health IT marketplace. Initially, when there was not a lot of interest in exchanging data with other organizations and clinical decision support was in its infancy, this situation worked reasonably well. As time has gone on, however, the proprietary systems have become a huge barrier to exchanging health information among organizations and to reporting patient safety issues with the clinical decision support components. Unfortunately, because the investment in these systems has been so great (in the millions of dollars for most hospitals), it is very difficult to replace the systems with truly open systems, even if such systems were readily available.

It must be noted that, in open-source software in general, readily available does not necessarily mean free. **Open-source software** simply means that the vendor that created an open system is willing to sell the software to others that, because the software is standards-based, may modify it to work with other systems. Once such modifications are made to the open-source software, the modified software may be made freely available or such modifications may become proprietary.

Using open-source EHR software is generally not feasible for hospitals because EHRs must connect with large number of proprietary source systems, but open-source EHRs were initially of interest to physicians whose offices typically had no information systems. Open-source software tends to be relatively inexpensive, or even free, which makes it initially attractive to small practices. However, open-source vendors cannot always provide adequate support or customization. Furthermore, while open-source systems can connect to other open-source systems, they cannot connect with closed systems. Therefore, as the exchange data between the physician office and hospital has become a greater priority, open-source systems have been at a disadvantage because they are not useful for this purpose. For these reasons, open-source EHR vendors struggle to stay in business. The result has been a movement away from open-source systems to closed-systems vendors who sell both inpatient and outpatient products.

One exception to the open-source EHR dilemma has been the open-source EHR developed by the Veterans Health Administration. The Veterans Health Information Systems and Technology Architecture (VistA), is made available to the public through the Freedom of Information Act (FOIA), and this availability has led to a number of distributors that help implement it, especially in small hospitals. Although VistA is available at no cost, the underlying database on which to run the software and other aspects of installation are not free.

The United States is now facing a major challenge to achieve interoperability with closed systems. **Interoperability** refers to the "ability of different information technology systems and software to communicate, exchange data, and use the information that has been exchanged" (HIMSS 2013). In the past, many providers accepted this lack of interoperability for several reasons. Providers adopted information systems slowly, needing to prove the value of such systems. These systems were often limited in scope to the functions of a single department, and sharing data with other systems was not a particular concern. For example, the laboratory did not have a great need to share data with radiology. If a single proprietary vendor was interested in having internal systems communicate with each other, it could often provide almost everything it needed for its basic operations. In a hospital, patient demographic data from an admitting system were shared with other component systems, and the charges captured in each system then were sent to a patient accounting system.

Providers were also slow to adopt EHRs because of the cost and complexity of such systems as well as the need for a fully developed infrastructure. As a result, the information systems typically used by healthcare providers were aids to operations. For example, a pharmacy information system primarily helps the pharmacy maintain an inventory of drugs and dispense them to the nursing unit. These types of systems are not clinical systems because they do not automate clinical information needs. Thus, the pharmacist, not the computer, evaluates the drug's potential efficacy and identifies any contraindications, which the pharmacist communicates (verbally) to the provider.

Providers want to ensure the confidentiality of their patients' health information. Many providers found it easier to manage confidentiality in a paper world than in an electronic world, where sophisticated access and audit controls require added cost and effort, even when they were available in products, which historically was often not the case. Until only recently, standard practice was to print any information from operational systems that was needed for documentation in the health record and from which release of information could be carefully controlled. In the collegial environment of healthcare, physicians wrote referral letters to provide other physicians with information about their patients as needed or permitted copies of documentation to be sent to other providers at no cost to the patient. Although Health Insurance Portability and Accountability Act of 1996 (HIPAA) regulations permit providers to disclose information for treatment purposes without authorization (§164.502[a][1][ii]), many providers still require authorizations because of a lack of trust and to protect themselves against complaints of wrongful disclosures. Providers often viewed the collection of health information about their patients as proprietary. Despite controls that can block attempts to gain access to patient confidential data (which are required under HIPAA, §164.312[a]), many providers are still concerned about the potential for access to information about their practice patterns, which may reveal how much money they earn, errors they have made, or other potentially sensitive information.

Much is changing in the field of healthcare. It is now recognized that readily exchangeable information across the continuum of care is vital to improving the quality of care and patient safety, and such improvements cannot depend on manual system processes. As a result, the need for vendors to achieve interoperability has finally been recognized in the MU incentive program, although MU has not yet resulted in the degree of interoperability that everyone would desire.

Check Your Understanding 2.1

Indicate whether the following statements are true or false (T or F):

1. All information systems must achieve a goal.

2. A system is characterized by having multiple components.

3. In systems theory, a closed system is one with no external feedback.

4. The proprietary nature of closed systems in health IT may discourage providers from working with more than one vendor.

5. All open-source software is free.

6. Closed systems are the norm for health IT.

Information Theory

General information theory can help further the pursuit of health IT in an interoperable environment, where use of EHRs will generate more than merely improved access to information traditionally recorded in paper documents. Ideally, health IT will not only increase availability of records but also supply data that support clinical decision making at the point of care and provide the foundation for real time public health surveillance. Data from health IT can also potentially be used for predictive modeling to develop better treatment protocols and ultimately improve the quality of health and cost of health care. The focus going forward must be on collecting the right data, transforming the data into the right information, sharing the data and information in the right manner, and using the data and information to generate knowledge that improves health and health care.

Data Flow

Basic information theory describes the flow of data from a source to their ultimate destination. (See figure 2.3.) In general, data are input into a system for the purpose of being processed and then output as useful information. From a practical perspective, data flow must be understood to ensure that data needed to create useful information are supplied and do indeed generate the desired information. As a result, data sources and data uses must be considered as key elements in information theory when applied to health data.

Data Sources

Input requires a source, or sources, of data. In the case of health data, the source is generally an observation about a patient or a response to a question asked of the patient.

There must also be a transmitter, which is often a clinician, although the transmitter may be a monitoring device, automated equipment, the patient or patient's caregiver, the patient's health plan, or even a store where the patient obtained healthcare, such as a flu shot or over-the-counter medications. Some data may be strictly objective, such as "The patient is observed to be short of breath" or "The patient complains of shortness of breath for the past 2 days." In some cases, data may be subjective. Some judgment as to the accuracy of the patient's response also may be recorded, such

Figure 2.3.   Information theory

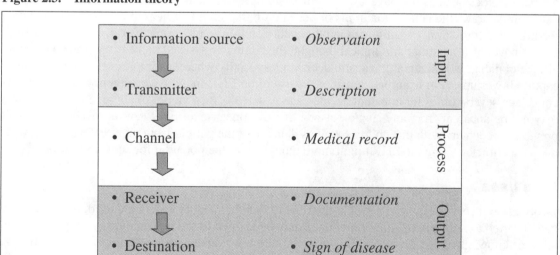

as "The patient states that she has been short of breath for the past 2 days, although she also appears confused about what day of the week today is."

Processing raw data into useful information is performed by a channel. In the manual world, the channel would be paper. Obviously, processing is very limited in this case. At best, there is a process of forms that guide the capture of data. Sometimes, these forms are color coded for ease of retrieval. Some forms may be formatted, which provides direction about where content should be recorded. As EHRs were developed as a channel, considerations had to be made about not only what data to accommodate but also how to guide the transmitter in entering the needed data into the system.

Information theory next recognizes that the channel is not the ultimate goal of the system. To achieve the goals of any information system, there must be a receiver. In the case of the paper health record, the receiver is documentation, the direct output of the process. However, in the case of an EHR, the receiver has enhanced utility beyond documentation—including expanded communication capabilities and knowledge generation. For the broader view of health IT, the receiver is also connectivity and interoperability.

The ultimate destination of the information flow is the goal of the system. There must be value to the information processing. The EHR has many goals. Some are global, such as "Improve quality of care." Others are more specific, such as "Alert the provider to a medication contraindication" or "Provide a differential diagnosis." For health IT in general, the federal government has established the following goals (ONC 2015):

- 2015–2017: Send, receive, find, and use priority data domains to improve health care quality and outcomes.

- 2018–2020: Expand data sources and uses in the interoperable health IT ecosystem to improve health and lower costs.

- 2021–2024: Achieve nationwide interoperability to enable a learning health system, with the person at the center of a system that can continuously improve care, public health, and science through real time data access.

The destination is the information gleaned from processing the data. For instance, the multiple data points captured during the patient history and physical examination relate to a conclusion that the patient does or does not have a certain disease. In the manual world, the clinician records the data points, draws the conclusion in his or her mind based on his or her clinical training, and then records the information, essentially as another data point. In an electronic world, although the EHR should never be a substitute for clinical thought, the computer-assisted processing of the data could aid the clinician in making a diagnostic decision, especially where a complex set of data points is captured over time. For example, consider the use of an EHR in a busy emergency department. A child seen several times for apparent accidents may actually be a victim of abuse, a possibility that may not be apparent from any single episode of care. Because an EHR can retrieve data from all previous encounters with this child as well as data about the patient from other emergency departments, a clinician using the EHR might more quickly spot the potential for such a situation.

Data Uses

Information theory recognizes not only the flow of data but also how data are used, how they may be converted to information, how experience may be applied to the information to support the creation of knowledge, and how multiple iterations of knowledge creation generates best practice. A **data-information-knowledge-wisdom (DIKW) continuum** is often described as part of information theory. (See figure 2.4.)

Figure 2.4.   The data-information-knowledge-wisdom (DIKW) continuum

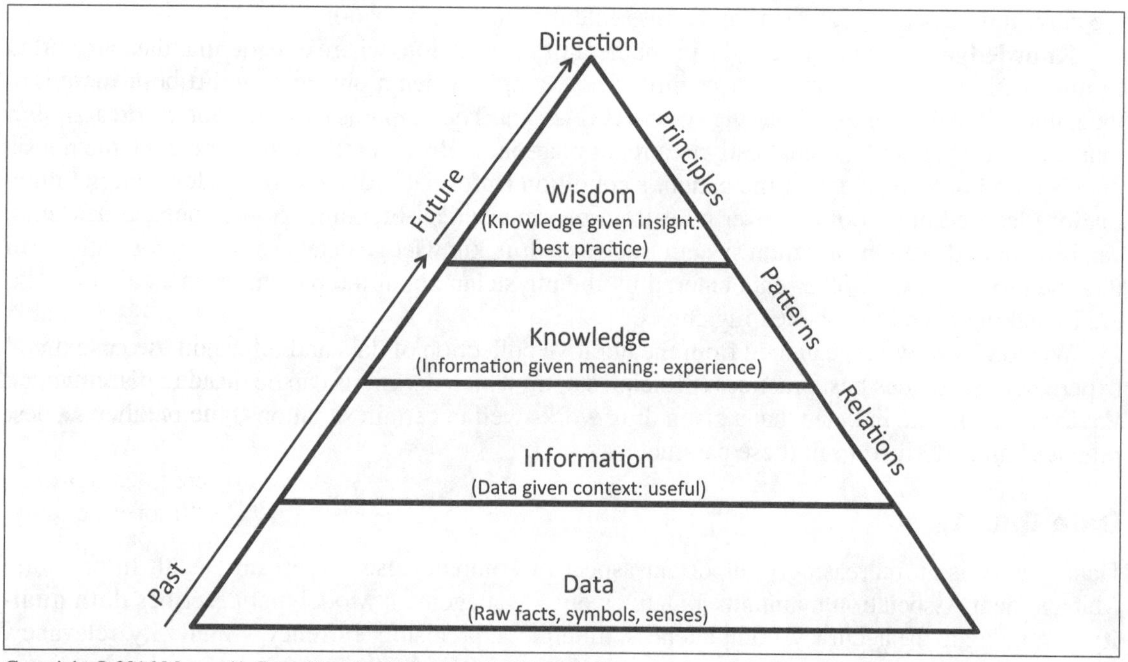

Direction

Future

Principles

Past

Patterns

Relations

Wisdom
(Knowledge given insight: best practice)

Knowledge
(Information given meaning: experience)

Information
(Data given context: useful)

Data
(Raw facts, symbols, senses)

Copyright © 2016 Margret/A Consulting, LLC. Reprinted with permission.

In the DIKW continuum, data are raw facts, symbols, and senses and are generated through research, creation, gathering, and discovery (Baldwin 2014). Data may be structured or unstructured. (See table 2.1.) Structured data are the values or attributes of variables that can be processed by the computer. Unstructured data can be stored in and viewed from a computer, but they cannot be processed by the computer. The distinction between structured and unstructured data is important when planning an EHR and broader health IT system. We may use the term *data* in a generic sense to mean any facts and figures; however, to be processed into information by a computer system, data must be in discrete, or structured, format. Nevertheless, unstructured data are also incorporated into an EHR. (See chapter10 for a much more extensive discussion of structured and unstructured data.)

Information is the result of processing data. This processing forms relationships among data, which gives the data context and makes them useful. For example, when entering a birth date in a

Table 2.1.   Structured vs. unstructured data

Unstructured Data	Structured Data
Definition: Textual objects and images that can be stored in a computer, but not processed by a computer	Definition: Discrete facts and figures that can be encoded and processed by a computer
Examples: • Narrative notes • Print files • Video and voice files • Scanned images of documents • Pictures	Examples: • Data entered into templates • Coded data (for example, ICD, CPT, SNOMED) whether coded by a person or encoded by the computer • Bar codes, radio frequency identification (RFID)

specific field designated to contain birth date, the computer can compare the data in the field with the current date (another element of data) to calculate age (information).

Knowledge is often considered a refinement of information, where experiential data are added to information, forming patterns over time. For example, when a physician writes a prescription, the name of the drug entered into the system is raw data. The output is expected to be a prescription that can be transmitted automatically to a retail pharmacy. However, the drug chosen by the physician is based on knowledge of the patient's condition (information) and properties of drugs (information) learned in school and over time from pharmaceutical literature. Some of this knowledge can be supplied in an information system, such as a drug knowledge database. This information can then be processed with other data entered by the physician about the patient, such as allergies, to aid in making the best possible drug choice.

Wisdom is knowledge gained from the iterative collection of data and informed by context and experience It provides best practices (principles upon which decisions can be made to direct work). For example, if data indicate that a given drug works well in certain situations but not others, a best practice can be formed to fit these parameters.

Data Quality

Data quality is an increasingly important aspect of computer use. American Health Information Management Association maintains a Data Quality Management Model that describes **data quality** as relating to the accuracy, completeness, timeliness, precision, currency, granularity, relevancy, definition, accessibility, and consistency of the input (AHIMA 2015). Attending to data quality is critical in a healthcare environment. For example, if someone entered a patient's admission date in the field designated to contain birth date, the computer will process the date as specified and will thus calculate age incorrectly.

To overcome errors, **templates** designed for data entry often have predefined parameters that are checked as data are entered. However, such edits can address only the most evident logical errors, and too many such checks can be distracting for users. For example, if a medication dose field for a given medication could only logically contain a value between 0.1 and 1.0, the computer can check for any entry outside of these boundaries and alert the user. However, short of comparing previous entries for a birth date field or whether the admission service is newborn, there seem to be few logical ways to check for data entry errors in a birth date field that is used to calculate age.

The potential for data entry errors is a reason that computer systems are designed for fixed data to be entered only once and used in all subsequent processes. For example, when a person's birth date is as positively identified as possible, such as from checking a driver's license, this date is not going to change. Whenever the patient's birth date or age needs to be used elsewhere in the system, it should be derived from the original source, not entered as new data.

Determining whether data are fixed or variable, however, can sometimes be tricky in healthcare. For example, a patient may have a documented allergy to penicillin, but another physician who queries the patient may decide that the patient's reaction is only a hypersensitivity. Although an allergy initially would seem to be a fixed (rather than a variable) data point, the data point could potentially be modified with an addendum that explains what is believed to be currently correct.

Knowledge Creation

Knowledge (the application of experience to information) is an area of health IT that is only just now being explored. A good example of knowledge in health IT is the case of the drug choice described earlier. In addition to applying external knowledge, such as from drug knowledge databases, information systems can also accumulate experience and use it to help with data entry and use. For example, many systems can track which entries are the most common and then present those favorites in subsequent screens.

Although the creation of knowledge is valuable, adding computer-generated knowledge may not be cost effective in cases where human knowledge may be applied more readily and effectively. EHRs should supply appropriate knowledge tools, but not at the expense of preventing clinicians from applying professional judgment or risking that professional judgment will not be applied. In fact, a constant barrage of drug alerts in a medication prescription or administration system can be more annoying than helpful to clinicians. EHR systems that can set the sensitivity of these alerts to the needs of the clinician receiving them are much more successful.

Best Practices

As wisdom is generated from the repeated creation of knowledge over time, it becomes best practice. The Institute of Medicine (IOM; now known as the Health and Medical Division [HMD] of the National Academies of Science, Engineering, and Medicine) defined clinical best practices (referred to as *clinical practice guidelines*) as "statements that include recommendations, intended to optimize patient care, that are informed by a systematic review of evidence and an assessment of the benefits and harms of alternative care options" (IOM 2011b). Clinical decision support afforded through EHRs and other health IT systems should reflect best practices. Best practice guidance, however, is not always available, or it may be considered suspect when it is not supported by the rigor described in the IOM definition. Best practices can (and should) change over time, as new information and new knowledge are generated.

Check Your Understanding 2.2

Choose the best answer:

1. In information theory, the medical record is a:

    a. Channel

    b. Destination

    c. Information source

    d. Receiver

2. In the data-information-knowledge-wisdom (DIKW) continuum, the ultimate goal of processing data is to:

    a. Collect accurate data

    b. Identify best practices

    c. Lend meaning to information

    d. Produce useful information

3. Which of the following are structured data?

    a. Codes representing data

    b. Narrative notes

    c. Print files

    d. Voice files

4. What is a template?

    a. Common entries for documentation

    b. Edit checks for data quality

    c. Format of data

    d. Predefined parameters for data entry

5. To create knowledge, information systems must:

    a. Capture experience

    b. Link to other systems to analyze data

    c. Process unstructured data

    d. Use research databases

Information Systems Theory

Information systems theory explains how information, and ultimately knowledge and wisdom, are generated by data processed in predictable ways to contribute value. An information system does the following (Bryce 2009):

- Uses devices to capture data in multiple formats that are converted to a machine-processable state

- Applies instructions, also converted into a machine-processable state, to index, store, calculate, compare, and perform other functions on the data

- Uses devices to display the original data at another time or place and present the results of calculations, comparisons, and other functions to users in various formats

Just like the human body, which is a system of many components (nervous system, musculoskeletal system, integumentary system, and so on) integrated into the human form that allow people to function (to walk, talk, think, and so on), an information system requires data and instructions for processing to produce results. Unlike the human system, however, information systems are often designed for specific purposes that can—and frequently do—stand alone. The body's musculoskeletal system cannot operate on its own; instead, it must be integrated with the nervous system to detect pulses from the brain that direct movement, with the integumentary system for protection, and so on. In contrast, a laboratory information system (LIS) can manage specimen collection, report results, and generate charges, all based on paper input and output, without ever having any connection to another information system. Of course, it is helpful to connect the LIS to an admitting or practice management system so that patient demographics do not have to be reentered into the LIS. Also, when an organization adopts an order-entry system, that system must be connected to the LIS so that the request for a specific test can be automatically directed to the LIS.

These parallels and distinctions between the human body and information systems are notable because an EHR and other forms of health IT resemble the human system more than other information systems do, because, like the human body, health IT depends on multiple systems. The EHR can capture data from multiple source systems and process the data into many forms for many purposes. As information technology (IT) advances, information systems can be programmed with instructions to perform tirelessly, and sometimes more accurately, many information management functions that the human system can perform.

However, no matter how well the programmatic instructions for an information system are written, they may not fully anticipate changing requirements and changes in the external environment. Information systems have been programmed to simulate learning and prediction through complex pattern analysis. Highly sophisticated information systems may be able to respond to some changes, but most information systems require changes to their instructions to continue to be useful in the face of external change. Information systems also are incapable of heuristic thought or experiencing "gut instincts" that suggest something could be wrong or needs attention.

EHRs represent a clinical transformation that affects many people who have never before been affected by an information system. EHRs are much more integrated than the departmental or operational systems with which they interact. However, EHR systems as well as the ultimate health IT system are only tools and not substitutes for human interaction. Figure 2.5 illustrates the importance of human thought (personal vigilance) as a key element of health IT systems.

Characteristics of Information Systems

As noted previously in this chapter, the fundamental elements of an information system are inputs, processes, and outputs. These fundamental elements are accomplished through the adoption of hardware (equipment) and software (computing instructions), but an information system is more than just these components. One way to describe all the elements of an information system is to consider not only the hardware and software but also people, policy, and process.

People
People are the key reason why information systems exist—and they also determine how information systems exist. Information systems have been characterized as human–machine systems because people design them and people use them. Interestingly, both components of the people equation (design and use) can be troublesome. In the grand scheme of things, people only began to use computers to help process data into information fairly recently. Early computing efforts started about half a century ago. That may seem like a long time to some, but it is very short when one recognizes that the first records of human existence date back thousands of years. The relative youthfulness of computing may help explain why there is often a disconnect between how we can actually design a computer and what we might like it to do. Even today, some people still have never used computers and fear their use. Currently, almost every implementation of an EHR system involves some people who believe they will lose their jobs due to the EHR or who absolutely

Figure 2.5.   The role of technology in healthcare

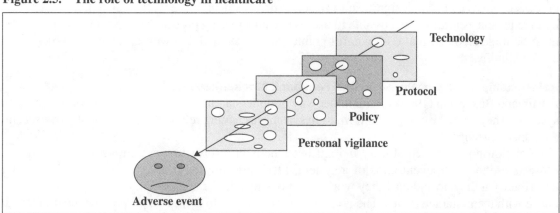

Source: Adapted from Reason, cited in Valusek, 16;1: 34–39.

refuse to use the system. Because computer design is not yet perfect, even those who use computers regularly for some part of their work or leisure may find that computers are not yet suitable for other aspects. Taking people into consideration when designing an information requires attention to detail and management of change.

Policy

Policy refers to directives or principles on which people perform their work or other activities. People's policies may center on their business practices, social interactions, use of drugs, frequency of watching television, or myriad other things that influence how they live their lives. When a person becomes a member of a group, the group may establish policies. In informal groups, these policies may be more likely to be normative behaviors. In communities, policies may be codified by local ordinances, state statutes, and federal or international laws and regulations. In social organizations, bylaws or codes of conduct may be the policy directives that provide guidance. In business organizations, policies may be written or unwritten, formal or informal. For example, businesses may have formal, written policies on who may access what information, as well as informal, unwritten policies on acceptable attire for the workplace.

In a health IT environment, where so many intended users are new to computers and where the EHR itself is a relatively new construct, there are often few formal written policies, but that does not diminish the importance of such policies. For example, policies on what information should or should not be entered into the EHR may seem unnecessary when data entry is highly structured, but many healthcare organizations are struggling to decide whether to require a rationale for overriding a clinical decision support alert. Policies also may be needed to direct whether organizations will continue to provide printed records to some users, whether some users will be permitted to continue dictating instead of directly entering data, and so on. Such policies may have huge economic and safety consequences for a healthcare organization, because multiple and parallel processes always add operational costs and are frequently prone to error.

Process

Process is the manner in which a task is performed. A simple example is the process a provider uses to write an order for medication. In the past, the provider may have handwritten an order on an order sheet or called an individual qualified to accept a verbal order, possibly without referencing the patient's chart. When a computerized provider order entry (CPOE) system is available, the provider is expected to look up the patient, key in the various components that comprise an order, and respond to any alerts or reminders for contraindications. These are very different processes for performing essentially the same task.

Process change is one of the most significant factors in the success or failure of EHR adoption. Even where people may be willing to use a computer or where policy dictates that they must use it, process changes can have a significant impact. Processes need to be well designed, accurate, kept up to date, and as intuitive as possible to use. When considering process changes, current processes must be understood so that both control points can be retained and workarounds and bottlenecks can be eliminated.

Relationships, Unity of Purpose, and Feedback Mechanisms

Austin and Boxerman (1998) offer another way of understanding the characteristics of information systems. They describe complex information systems as having relationships, unity of purpose, and a feedback mechanism.

Relationships between objects and attributes help an information system achieve its purpose. **Objects** are the component parts of a system; **attributes** are the properties of those objects that describe what they do and how they work. Relationships tie the component parts together in accordance with their characteristics. The goal of a relationship is to achieve a purpose or function equal to or better than what any individual object could achieve alone. Relationships may be planned or unplanned, formal or informal, but they must exist if the collection of components is to constitute a system. A key lesson for designing an EHR system is that many disparate systems and their respectively disparate stakeholders must come together to form new relationships.

Unity of purpose causes the collective parts of an information system to have integrity. A system must have an identity and describable boundaries. Interestingly, information systems are becoming so vast in scope, with so many potential relationships, that unity of purpose is becoming less clearly defined—or at least less proscriptive. One only needs to consider the Internet as a vast information system. Although the Internet's purpose is to exchange information globally, its integrity is subject to many factors. Closer to home, the EHR system must be designed around well-established policies that set the boundaries not just for where the system starts and ends but also for the adoption and realization of benefits. Too often, such systems are implemented but not fully adopted, which results in less-than-expected value.

Feedback mechanisms provide information about environmental factors that interact with the functioning of the system. An EHR system can transform clinical practice. This level of change can be neither created nor maintained without a constant feedback mechanism that both celebrates success and identifies where course correction is needed. Feedback includes a number of social, economic, and political factors.

Social factors (characteristics of individuals and groups of people involved in use of the information system) may dictate how a system is designed, what input devices are used, and how users are trained to use the system. They are important determinants of EHR adoption, requiring significant human-factor engineering of the information system as well as change management for the intended users.

Economic factors are well-known determinants of whether and what information systems are acquired. Unfortunately, economic factors are often directly in conflict with social factors—highly sophisticated, intuitive systems are easier to use than more basic options, but they are also much more expensive.

Political factors are the competing demands that influence both the social and economic factors. Political factors may promote incentives for use of an information system over disincentives, or they may discourage use. For example, a physician who is required to adopt an EHR to continue practicing may decide to retire rather than invest in the technology.

Cybernetics Applied to Information Systems Theory

Early information system theorists described a special case in which information systems incorporate self-regulation. Wiener (in Austin and Boxerman 1998) uses the term *cybernetics* to label this special case. **Cybernetics**, which is derived from the Greek word for "pilot" (as in "autopilot" or "pilot light"), is a theory of control systems based on communication (transfer of information) between components of systems with respect to their environment. The following is an example of how cybernetics might be applied to a clinical laboratory system (Austin and Boxerman 1998):

- *Inputs* are the scheduled laboratory tests, stat orders, and various professional, technical, and material resources.

- *Processes* are the specimen collection, testing, and results reporting.

- *Outputs* are the test reports, patient charges, and statistical reports.

- *Sensors* are the number of tests by category, quality control data, and resources consumed. The outputs are used to capture these data.

- *Standards monitoring* is performed by comparing the sensor data to various standards and cost/efficiency goals.

Figure 2.6.   Cybernetics feedback loop

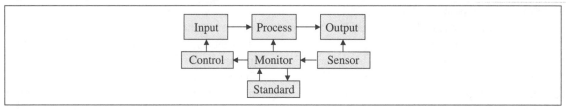

- *Control processes* are then instituted when standards monitoring detects variation in the sensor data from the standard data. Control processes may include continuing education, retraining, revised policies and procedures, staffing changes, recalibration of equipment, and so on.

Applying cybernetics to information systems is probably more important than ever before. Although organizations have implemented EHR systems, many clinicians are not comfortable using them, and some chief executive officers (CEOs) do not see a return on their investment (Monegain 2015). The control processes in cybernetics creates a feedback loop that ensures integrity among the basic elements that have relationships comprising an information system. This feedback loop is an important element in creating value from today's EHRs, as shown in figure 2.6. All too often, EHR systems are treated as yet another standalone system, assuming that another part of the overall healthcare delivery system will sense a potential error and take corrective action. However, people, policy, and process often converge in the EHR system with the result that there is no other feedback mechanism—an issue that is being seen in unintended consequences from using an EHR and especially its clinical decision support mechanisms. For example, allergy data previously entered may lead the system to issue an alert that a patient is allergic to a drug being ordered. However, if the purported allergy is actually a hypersensitivity that should not have been entered in the allergy field of the record, an ordering provider may follow the alert and unnecessarily change the order to a less-effective drug. Alternatively, if the provider knows the issue is hypersensitivity not allergy, he or she may conclude that the system's alerts are unreliable, even though the underlying error involves data entry, not how the alert is programmed.

Check Your Understanding 2.3

Choose the best answer:

1. Which key element of health IT systems must be present for their success?

    a.   Organizational policy on use

    b.   Personal vigilance

    c.   Quality software

    d.   Reliable protocols

2. Which characteristic of an information system describes how a task is performed?

    a.   Policy

    b.   Process

    c.   Relationships

    d.   Software

3. Cybernetics is a mechanism that ensures:

    a.   Accurate software development

    b.   Adherence to standards

    c.   Data quality

    d.   Feedback mechanism

4. Complex information systems must have unity of purpose in order to have:

    a.   Data quality

    b.   Feedback mechanisms

    c.   Integrity

    d.   Interoperability

Systems Development Life Cycle

By reflecting on general systems theory and general information systems theory, one comes to appreciate the steps necessary to develop, or at least plan for implementing, an EHR system. The systems development life cycle (SDLC) is often cited as the primary resource for managing complex information system projects. The primary purpose of the SDLC is to ensure that a project is developed correctly and within time and budget constraints. As a conceptual model for project management, the SDLC has been around for as long as computerized applications have been built, and it continues to be applied in new software development projects (Woodward et al. 2010), information system vendor selection, workflow and process redesigns, strategic planning, and many other types of projects.

Traditional SDLC Methodology

The traditional SDLC methodology (figure 2.7) includes the following steps:

1. *Feasibility* (also called *the planning step*): The existing (manual) system is evaluated and deficiencies are identified to determine whether it makes sense to proceed with the project.

Figure 2.7.   Traditional SDLC

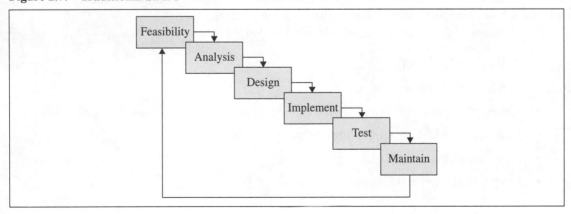

2. *Analysis:* New (automated) system requirements are defined. In particular, deficiencies in the existing system are addressed with specific proposals for improvement.

3. *Design:* Plans to address the physical construction, hardware, operating systems, programming, communications, and security issues of the proposed system are laid out.

4. *Implement:* The new system is developed. The new components and programs are obtained and installed. Users are trained in its use, and all aspects of performance are tested. If necessary, adjustments are made at this stage.

5. *Test:* The system is put into use. This can be done in various ways. The new system can be phased in, according to application or location, and the old system gradually replaced. In some cases, it may be more cost-effective to shut down the old system and implement the new system at the same time.

6. *Maintain:* When the new system is up and running for a while, it should be exhaustively evaluated. Maintenance must be kept up rigorously at all times. System users should be kept up to date about the latest modifications and procedures.

Some discussions of the SDLC include either a seventh step or replace the sixth step (maintain) with a disposition or disposal step, sometimes also referred to as a *sunset step* or *retirement step* (Radack 2008). This step is particularly relevant when SDLC is being used in development of commercial software where the version or release is being retired.

SDLC for Health IT

The traditional SDLC methodology has been called a waterfall methodology because it describes a linear set of phases. This traditional model does not emphasize a feedback mechanism. However, feedback is especially important for complex systems projects, including health IT systems, that require change over time. Therefore, the more modern SDLC is modified to include a feedback mechanism and is often referred to as a spiral methodology. (See figure 2.8.)

The basic tenets of the SDLC are frequently adapted for project management of any type of project, including replacement of an old EHR, adding new components to create a broader health IT infrastructure, or gaining value from the information system that is currently in use. In general, when the SDLC is applied to project management where software is being acquired, the following phases are included: identification of need, specification of requirements, acquisition, implementation, maintenance, and monitoring of results.

Identification of Need

Identification of need often addresses both the feasibility and analysis aspects of the traditional SDLC. In fact, because health IT is now viewed as an ongoing cost of doing business, rather than a one-time endeavor, "feasibility" may be transformed into "readiness assessment" and be associated with each new component or new step in the adoption process.

Components of this phase often include the following:

- Setting strategic business goals

- Defining expected benefits

- Anticipating potential organizational changes regarding facilities, staffing, and so on

- Identifying budgeting, scheduling, and personnel constraints

- Assessing attitudes and beliefs

- Assessing computer skills

Figure 2.8. Modern (spiral) methodology for the SDLC

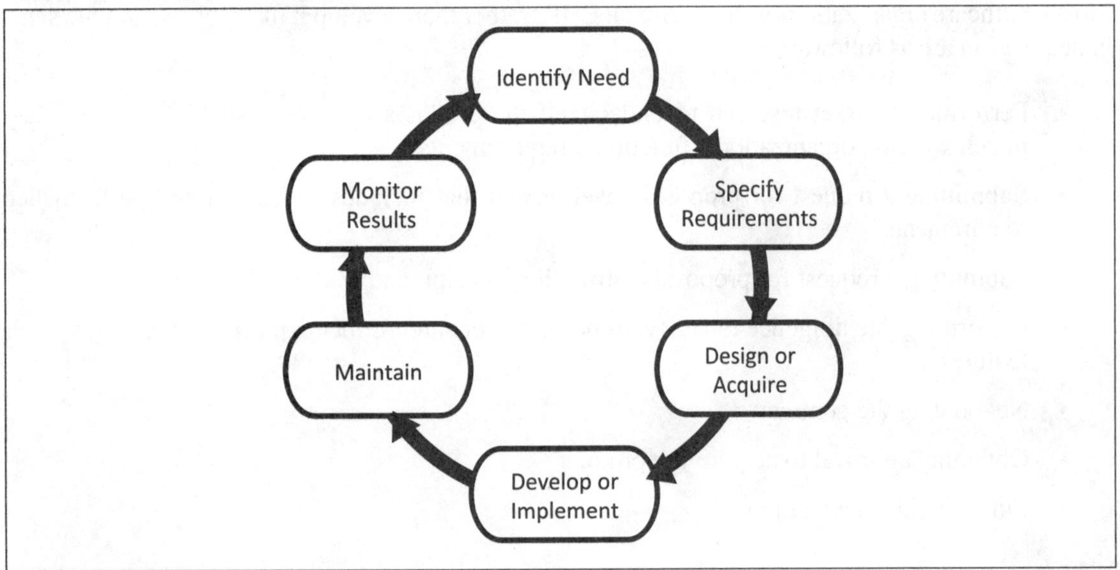

- Performing communication planning, including what messages should be provided to whom, by whom, and when
- Performing change management to address the human factor elements
- Doing a cost-benefit analysis and assessing the financial feasibility

Specification of Requirements

Specification of requirements is potentially the most important, but most often shortchanged, phase. It entails the following:

- Executing a project overview for all stakeholders, including creating a migration path for the various components of EHR system implementation
- Delineating staff roles and responsibilities and appointment/acquisition
- Performing process mapping and specifying functional requirements that specifically link to the business goals and expected benefits
- Specifying technical requirements
- Identifying project- and risk-management methodologies
- Defining deliverables, based on the migration path
- Identifying control requirements and standards
- Charting a conversion strategy and implementing any bridge technologies
- Documenting the planning for everything from requirement specifications to a code of conduct for vendor selection to project issues, job descriptions, and policies and procedures for use of the new system
- Performing staff development, from education to skills building to training

Acquisition

Most healthcare organizations will acquire an EHR, rather than develop it themselves, and the steps in acquisition are as follows:

- Performing market research to understand the products that are available and how they match with the organization's functional requirements

- Submitting a request for proposal development that includes functional and performance requirements

- Submitting a request for proposal distribution, receipt, and analysis

- Performing due diligence to verify proposal content and further explore product and vendor features

- Negotiating the contract

- Obtaining approval to acquire the product

- Financing the acquisition

Implementation

Implementation of acquired health IT includes product installation, customization of the system to meet the organization's requirements, and turning the system over to users. It is important to recognize that implementation is more than just installation. A common misconception relating to EHR implementations is that software can be installed and used directly thereafter. Even the simplest EHR for a small clinic or solo practitioner requires some system configuration, training, and testing. Steps for implementation include the following:

- Establishing an issues management and change control process

- Scheduling project tasks, milestones, and resources, including budgeting project expenditures over the life of the project

- Developing a turnover strategy

- Planning for training

- Planning for testing

- Installing hardware and software, including storage components

- Reconfiguring communications and network components, as needed

- Configuring the system, including data modeling, tables and files creation, clinical content and template design, report development, and associated workflows

- Implementing security controls

- Unit and system testing

- Training "super" users who assist other end users in learning the system

- Developing an interface and testing integration

- Converting data

- Performing stress testing

- Performing end-user training

- Providing documentation

- Providing go-live management and support

- Performing acceptance testing

Maintenance

Maintenance relates to the ongoing support needed to keep the system current and accurate. All software requires ongoing support, if only to ensure that errors in development are corrected and patches to continually enhance security protection are applied. Most health IT systems, however, must also be kept current with new information, continually refined best practices, updated drug data, reimbursement codes, and many other changes and enhancements.

Borrowing from the traditional SDLC methodology, maintenance also includes the orderly disposal of surplus or obsolete hardware, software, and data. This aspect of maintenance may involve a change in vendor control or software obsolescence. Many providers look to replace EHRs because the vendor is retiring them, because the vendor has gone out of business, or because the system is not keeping current with the MU incentive program stage requirements. In addition, some providers replace EHRs that to live up to their expectations.

In general, maintenance includes the following:

- Software maintenance, including patches, routine modifications, major upgrades, emergency changes, and renewal of subscriptions

- Hardware upgrades and maintenance

- Hardware and software inventories and license agreement maintenance

- User preference changes

- Disposal of out-of-date system components

Monitoring of Results

Monitoring of results provides the feedback mechanism needed to assess whether the intended goals and benefits of a project are being met and what changes need to be made to either the components of the project or the goals and expected benefits (which may have been set too aggressively, or not aggressively enough). Because the monitoring of results is such an important step in health IT, it is separated from maintenance to ensure that it is actually performed. Monitoring involves the following:

- Performance measurement

- Benefits realization: Return on investment, provider and patient satisfaction, outcomes assessment, celebration, and course correction

Meaningful Use Incentives and SDLC

The stages of the federal MU incentive program for EHRs were built around a SDLC perspective:

- Stage 1: Implementation, where basic functionality is put into place and users use the minimum functions of the EHR to earn incentives

- Stage 2: Adoption, where intended users manage the majority of their basic information needs

- Stage 3: Optimization, where value is realized from mastery of the EHR for all aspects of knowledge management

Check Your Understanding 2.4

Match the terms with the appropriate descriptions:

A. Identification of need

B. Stage 3 meaningful use of EHR incentives

C. Maintenance

D. Testing

E. Spiral model of systems development life cycle

1. Disposal of software

2. Monitoring of results

3. Implementation

4. Goal setting

5. Optimization

References and Resources

Advisory Board. 2015. When doctors have EHR safety concerns, "gag clauses" may stop them from speaking out. https://www.advisory.com/daily-briefing/2015/09/14/ehr-gag-clauses.

American Health Information Management Association (AHIMA). 2015. Data quality management model (2015 update). *Journal of AHIMA* 86(10).

Austin, C.J., and S.B. Boxerman. 1998. *Information Systems for Health Services Administration,* 5th ed. Chicago: Health Administration Press.

Baldwin, D.A. 2014. The continuum of understanding. Dave Baldwin Consulting http://www .davebaldwinconsulting.com/UnderstandingContinuum.html.

Bryce, T. 2009. Information systems theory 101. EZine@rticles. http://ezinearticles .com/?Information-Systems-Theory-101&id=2756189.

Friedberg, M.W., P.G. Chen, K.R. Van Busum, F.M. Aunon Chau Pham, J.P. Caloyeras, S. Mattke, E. Pitchforth, D.D. Quigley, R.H. Brook, F.J. Crosson, and M. Tutty. 2013. *Factors Affecting Physician Professional Satisfaction and Their Implications for Patient Care, Health Systems, and Health Policy. Joint Research Report of the RAND Corporation and American Medical Association.* Washington, DC: RAND Corporation. http://www.rand.org/content/dam/rand/pubs/ research_reports/RR400/RR439/RAND_RR439.pdf

Helms, M.M ed. 2006. Open and closed systems. *Encyclopedia of Management.* Detroit: Gale Cengage.

Healthcare Information and Management Systems Society (HIMSS). 2013. Definition of interoperability. http://www. himss.org/library/interoperability-standards/what-is-interoperability.

Institute of Medicine. 2011a. *Health IT and Patient Safety: Building Safer Systems for Better Care.* Washington, DC: National Academies Press. http://www.nap.edu/catalog/13269/ health-it-and-patient-safety-building-safer-systems-for-better.

Institute of Medicine. 2011b. *Clinical Practice Guidelines We Can Trust.* Washington, DC: National Academies Press. http://nationalacademies.org/hmd/Reports/2011/Clinical-Practice-Guidelines-We-Can-Trust.aspx.

Marcinko, D.E., and H.R. Hetico, eds. 2007. *Dictionary of Health Information Technology and Security*. New York: Springer.

Meadows, D.H. 2008. *Thinking in Systems: A Primer*. White River Junction, VT: Chelsea Green.

Monegain, B. 2015. Pressure on CIOs to pull value from EHRs. *Healthcare IT News*. http://www.healthcareitnews.com/news/pressure-cios-pull-value-ehrs.

Office of the National Coordinator for Health Information Technology (ONC). 2015. Connecting health and care for the nation: A shared nationwide interoperability roadmap, final version 1.0. https://www.healthit.gov/policy-researchers-implementers/interoperability.

Radack, S., ed. 2008. The system development life cycle (SDLC). Computer Security Division, Information Technology Laboratory, National Institute of Standards and Technology. http://www.nist.gov/customcf/get_pdf.cfm?pub_id=902622.

Woodward, E., S. Surdek, and M. Ganis. 2010. *The Agile System Development Life Cycle (SDLC)*. IBM.

Chapter 3
Strategic Planning for Health IT

Key Terms

Acquisition strategy

Best-of-breed strategy

Best-of-fit strategy

Chief information officer (CIO)

Chief medical informatics officer (CMIO)

Chief technology officer (CTO)

Clinical data analyst

Data administrator

Database administrator

Data governance

Dependency

Dual core

Enterprise health information management professional

Environmental scan

Governance

Health informatics professional

Implementation plan

Information governance

Information security analyst

Maturity model

Medical director of information systems

Migration path

Patient safety

Project plan
Strategic planning
SWOT analysis

Learning Objectives

- Define the purpose, scope, and governance of strategic planning for health IT.

- Describe the strategic planning process.

- Explain how to construct and document a migration path to describe the strategic plan for health IT.

- Identify critical success factors in health IT strategic planning, including the importance of and procedure for conducting a functional needs assessment.

Strategic planning is a process typically conducted by senior management that describes the organization's future state. Strategic planning typically covers a period of at least three to five years and, ideally, ten years; considers past successes and failures; analyzes the current and future environment; and then maps out the directions the organization needs to follow to accomplish its mission. In other words, strategic planning determines where an organization is going over the next several years, how it is going to get there, and how it will know whether it got there (McNamara 2007). The strategic plan is the documentation of the process and resultant directions.

Strategic planning for health information technology (health IT) can be a frustrating and time-consuming endeavor because plans are frequently threatened with obsolescence by technology changes and revised government mandates before the plans are even fully drafted. In this context, the process of strategic planning may seem to be a distraction from (rather than a contribution to) the real work of building and maintaining an adequate technology infrastructure. However, many believe that a health IT strategic plan is needed. For example, Glaser observes that "developing a sound IT strategy can be very important for one simple reason—[if] an organization defines the IT agenda incorrectly or partially correctly, it runs the risk that significant organizational resources will be misdirected." In fact, "being on time, on budget, and on specification is of diminished utility if the wrong thing is being done" (Glaser 2006).

Because the federal meaningful use (MU) of electronic health record (EHR) incentive program laid out a specific plan for hospitals and physician practices, some people concluded that health IT strategic planning at the organizational level was unnecessary. However, Knickrehm contends that the MU incentives are "often wrongly characterized as a check-the-box qualification for stimulus monies" (2011). Effective health IT strategic planning uses the systems development life cycle (SDLC) model and involves monitoring results of existing health IT, understanding the likelihood of changes in the industry and technology, and setting appropriate goals and expectations as systems are maintained and new systems acquired. (See chapter 2 for more information on SDLC.)

As the federal government moves beyond MU incentives for the EHR to defining the broader scope of health IT, the importance of strategic planning increases. To determine the right health IT path, each healthcare provider will need to consider the environment in which it operates, the actual value it gets from its current information systems, and its goals under health reform.

Purpose of Strategic Planning for Health IT

Strategic planning for health IT is ideally an inherent part of the organization's overall strategic plan, although that frequently is not the case. In the past, planning for health IT was usually tactical (short term) and focused on one component or project at a time, such as MU. However, when strategic planning for health IT adopts a systems perspective, the strategic planning process can accomplish the following:

- Consider how well the existing health IT is working and whether it is meeting the needs of the organization. Evaluate whether the existing health IT needs to be improved or optimized, or if it should be replaced.

- Identify what types of health IT are needed to support the broader organizational goals. This aspect of strategic planning involves both an understanding of the general directions in which health IT is trending and an appreciation of the broader strategic plan for the organization.

- Document needs and directions, using a feedback mechanism for continuous systems analysis and improvement.

Scope of Strategic Planning for Health IT

Strategic planning that takes a systems perspective and follows the SDLC will ensure that the scope of strategic planning addresses all components of the health IT system. Strategic plans for health IT at the national, vendor, and local organizational levels all require a sufficiently long life cycle so that IT needs and resources can be proactively anticipated. Plans that are merely reactive put the healthcare delivery system at risk.

Historically, strategic planning for health IT has focused almost exclusively on technology and rarely considered the people, policies, and processes that ensure users will actually use and benefit from the technology. For example, many physicians contend that EHRs increase their clerical responsibilities and do not improve patient care (Russell 2015). While the vision for EHRs was laudable and many physicians do find value in health IT, many of the people charged with implementation lost sight of the human factors as they rushed to earn MU incentives for technology that met federal certification requirements.

Because the scope of health IT has been focused almost exclusively on the EHR and preparing for the transition to the *International Classification of Diseases, Tenth Revision, Clinical Modification (ICD-10-CM);* and *International Classification of Diseases, Tenth Revision, Procedure Coding System (ICD-10-PCS),* strategic responses to other aspects of health IT—such as cyberthreats, wearable devices used outside of the traditional health IT domain, shifting reimbursement models, mergers and acquisitions, and principles of accountable care—have been lacking. It can plausibly be argued that such a specific focus was necessary due to the size and complexity of the new EHR systems and that a broader focus would have overwhelmed health IT organizations. However, the lack of strategic planning both by the federal government prior to implementing the MU program and at the organizational level has resulted in technology that is insufficient to address the additional needs of health reform that have emerged before the MU incentive program has even concluded. The EHR originated from a system that is transactional and not analytical, and it was originally intended to be mostly used within one organization, not across disparate organizations. Therefore, EHRs may not be capable of supporting data sharing and data analytics, patient engagement, and population health required for health reform (Eastwood 2014).

Health IT strategic planning must be as broad in scope as possible, encompassing all components of a health IT system, including human and computer elements (Cole 2015). Health IT strategic planning should also enable flexibility and adaptability. If an organization's plan is too detailed and rigid, the organization will not be able to nimbly respond to unanticipated environmental changes. The plan must balance a focus on external factors that may ultimately affect health IT with an internal (organizational) focus on whether existing technology works, needs improvement, or should be abandoned or augmented.

Governance of Health IT Strategic Planning

Governance refers to the establishment of policies for the effective and efficient management of an organization's assets and the continual monitoring of how well those policies are working to achieve their stated ends (Johns 2015, xxii). Good governance of health IT strategic planning significantly improves the effectiveness of the strategic plan. Good governance results from inter-actions among key stakeholders in which the stakeholders are held accountable for following a transparent, responsive, equitable, and inclusive process to make decisions about how an organiza-tion will use its assets to achieve a specific goal or set of goals (Good Governance Guide 2012).

Governance for health IT strategic planning is performed by representatives of an organiza-tion's leadership in finance, operations, and clinical areas as well as the leadership of information technology and enterprise health information management. The chief financial officer (CFO), or a deputy, imparts information on healthcare financing. Participation in the health IT strategic plan-ning also affords the CFO a better understanding of IT resource needs. The chief operations offi-cer (COO), or a deputy, ensures that the human element of the information system is recognized. The COO also anticipates change management needs. Senior clinical officers, including the chief medical officer (CMO) and chief nursing/patient care officer (CNO), represent the primary users of health IT. Their input into the health IT strategic planning process ensures that user needs are met and also garners trust from their constituents in the new technology being planned. The **chief information officer (CIO)** is a member of executive leadership and is responsible for the overall management, implementation, and usability of information (Rouse 2015). The **chief technology officer (CTO)** reports to the CIO and is responsible for management, implementation, and mainte-nance of computer technologies (Rouse 2013).

Staff members in IT are generally represented in the health IT strategic planning process by the CIO, but additional IT staff may be called to participate in parts of health IT strategic planning based on special needs relative to their domain expertise. Key IT staff include the following:

- **Clinical data analysts**, who configure information systems specific to organizational needs (Darling 2011)

- **Database administrators**, who design and manage the technical implementation and main-tenance of databases (Gillenson, et al. 2008)

- **Data administrators**, who apply domain expertise to the design of databases, establish policies for their creation and use, maintain data dictionaries, and manage the quality of data (Gillenson et al. 2008, 302)

- **Information security analysts**, who plan and carry out information security measures to protect an organization's computer networks and systems (BLS 2014–2015)

- **Enterprise health information management professionals**, who provide perspectives on **information governance** (addressing system outputs and uses) and **data governance** (addressing system inputs), and ensure that the business processes, compliance, legal pur-poses, privacy protections, retention policies, and preservation of evidence are addressed in health IT strategic planning (Johns 2015; Washington 2015)

Health informatics professionals also play a role in strategic planning and governance in health IT. These professionals are enlightened advocates of health IT and strong proponents of sys-tem usability (the efficiency, effectiveness, and satisfaction with which users achieve results from health IT) as well as **patient safety** (that is, preventing harm to patients, learning from errors, and building a culture of safety) (Pfister and Ingargiola 2014; Hughes 2008). Among the participating informatics professionals may be the **chief medical informatics officer (CMIO)**, who is typically a practicing physician who volunteers to serve as the bridge between the medical staff and administration of a healthcare organization implementing health IT, as well as equivalent professionals in nursing, pharmacy, applied health, and public health.

Some organizations hire a **medical director of information systems (MDIS),** who is a physician who provides clinical support for EHR configuration and training. Organizations may also hire other health informatics professionals to provide clinical expertise regarding how data and information are analyzed, transformed, used in decision support, and disseminated within a learning health system (AMIA/AHIMA 2012).

Check Your Understanding 3.1

Match the term with the appropriate description:

    A.   Chief information officer

    B.   Chief technology officer

    C.   Chief medical informatics officer

    D.   Database administrator

    E.   Enterprise health information management professional

    F.   Health informatics professional

    G.   Medical director of information systems

1. Physician who serves as liaison between administration and the clinical community.

2. Individual responsible for implementing and maintaining computer technologies.

3. Physician responsible for providing clinical support for EHR configuration and training.

4. Member of the executive team responsible for overall management, implementation, and usability of information.

5. Individual who designs and manages the technical implementation and maintenance of databases.

6. Individual responsible for how data and information are analyzed, transformed, used in decision support, and disseminated within a learning health system.

7. Individual responsible for data and information governance across the entire organization.

The Strategic Planning Process and Documentation

Health IT strategic planning represents congruence between information system and organizational planning. Both organizational and health IT strategic planning establish an overall purpose, set of goals to be accomplished, and define the benefits to be achieved by its outcome. Although the strategic plan for health IT should identify specific milestones to help executive management monitor progress, it is not supposed to focus on task-level detail.

Choosing a Strategic Planning Model

There is no one perfect planning model for strategic planning. Often, organizations try various models for a period of time and then settle on one model or a hybrid. Models also can be integrated, using one form to creatively identify strategic issues and goals and another to determine how issues will be addressed and goals reached. Table 3.1 offers a set of strategic planning models from a *Field Guide to Nonprofit Strategic Planning and Facilitation* (McNamara 2007). Note that the terminology in the table is not universally used; consultants or strategic planning facilitators use various sets of terms to describe different types of strategic planning models.

Table 3.1.   Strategic planning models

Basic *Typically for small organizations or those with minimal planning experience*	1. Identify purpose. 2. Determine goals to accomplish mission. 3. Identify strategies or approaches to implement each goal. 4. Identify action plans to implement each strategy. 5. Monitor and update the plan.
Issue-based *Suitable for experienced planners and large organizations updating current plans*	1. Update vision, mission, and values if necessary. 2. Conduct external and internal SWOT assessment. 3. Identify and prioritize major issues. 4. Design major strategies (or programs) to address issues. 5. Establish action plans. 6. Record in a strategic plan document. 7. Develop yearly operating plan. 8. Develop and authorize budget. 9. Conduct organization's operations. 10. Monitor, review, evaluate, and update strategic plan.
Alignment *Helpful for organizations experiencing a large number of internal inefficiencies*	1. Outline mission, programs, resources, and needed support. 2. Identify what is working and what needs adjustment. 3. Identify how adjustments should be made. 4. Include adjustments as strategies in plan.
Scenario *Appropriate for ensuring strategic thinking in the face of potential major change in direction*	1. Select several external forces (such as recently identified in news headlines) and imagine related changes that might influence the organization. 2. For each change in a force, discuss best-case, worst-case, and most likely case scenarios as a result of the change. 3. Suggest potential strategies in response to each of the three scenarios. 4. Identify common strategies among the scenarios. 5. Select the most likely changes to affect the organization and identify the common strategies to respond to the change.
Organic *A self-organizing approach (as opposed to the typical linear plan); may be more suitable for certain cultures or when senior management changes*	1. Clarify organization's values using dialogue techniques. 2. Articulate group's vision for the organization, also using dialogue techniques. 3. Regularly dialogue about processes needed to arrive at vision. 4. Continually reinforce value of dialogue and patience. Focus on learning rather than method. 5. Agree on how to portray the results of this planning to key stakeholders.

Source: Adapted from McNamara 2007.

Conducting the Strategic Planning Process

Whatever strategic planning model is chosen, the most important elements of strategic planning entail adequate preparation, strategic analysis, strategic direction, and evaluation, as illustrated in table 3.2.

Health IT strategic planning is often conducted by the governance leaders in a retreat environment. A facilitator may be used to overcome bias and other group-process pressures as well as to prepare perspectives or conduct an environmental scan or SWOT analysis in advance. An **environmental scan** focuses on factors that are external to, and often not under the control of, the organization conducting the strategic planning. It is an analysis of what others are doing and, to the extent possible, what others are planning to do in the future. Industry future needs are anticipated from a study of trends in the industry. For health IT strategic planning, the environmental scan can use data from vendors as well as other healthcare organizations to evaluate the maturity of the EHR and health IT in general. A **SWOT analysis** focuses on the organization and its strengths, weaknesses, opportunities, and threats. It is an honest appraisal of how well the organization achieves its objectives and where it is struggling to perform well. The maturity of the industry's EHR and health IT in general can be used for comparison purposes in the SWOT analysis. To conduct such a comparative analysis, the individuals involved in strategic planning must also have ready access to information about the outcomes of the organization's programs. The SWOT analysis also postulates where the organization may capitalize on its strengths and how it can minimize or overcome its weaknesses.

At the conclusion of the strategic planning activity, a written plan is produced that summarizes the planning activity and records goals, strategic initiatives, general action plans, responsibilities and accountabilities, timelines, and milestones. Executive management may plan regular meetings to review the strategic plan, discuss reports, analyze deviations from the plan, and generally monitor progress. As with any evaluation process, feedback is essential so participants can appreciate and celebrate accomplishments and find the root cause of issues and take corrective action.

Legal and Ethical Issues in Strategic Planning for Health IT

An organization's executive leadership (and board of directors or managing partners to whom the chief executive reports) is responsible for ensuring that the organization is well managed. Strategic

Table 3.2.   Components of strategic planning process

Planning Stage	Components
Preparation	1. Who 2. When 3. Where 4. Why 5. How (see strategic planning models in table 3.1)
Strategic analysis	1. Environmental scan 2. Organization's strengths, weaknesses, opportunities, and threats (SWOT) 3. Comparative analysis of environment and organization's SWOT
Strategic direction	1. Review and reaffirmation of mission, vision, and values (unless a significant change in organization would lead to creation of new statements) 2. Strategic goals 3. Strategic initiatives 4. Action plans (with timelines and milestones) and designation of responsibilities and accountability
Evaluation and feedback	1. Evaluation of planning process and plan 2. Acknowledgment of completion and celebration of results

planning is an integral part of good management. During the strategic planning process, the focus should be fully on the organization's mission and vision (or changes to them) and how the environment may affect the organization. Everyone needs to be open and honest about the organization's strengths and weaknesses so that the strategic plan can be as successful as possible. However, executives (and board members or partners) can have personal biases that can interfere with what is best for the organization in comparison to what is best for them personally. In this respect, a facilitator can help ensure that all participants' views are heard without judgment or bias and that self-interests are put aside. In fact, bylaws for board members include the requirement that any board members who may have conflicts of interest with a subject upon which a vote must recuse themselves from the vote, if not also the discussion. Such a process is not as common in executive leadership discussions, but it can be used in the event of a particularly obvious or risky situation arises.

As the strategic plan is put into place, executive leadership should monitor progress to ensure the plan is being carried out and results are as expected. It is the responsibility of executive leadership to both report to the board of directors on the outcomes of the organization's strategic planning and take steps to correct course if outcomes are not as expected.

Maturity Models for Health IT

Historically, several descriptions of how the United States might implement an EHR, and health IT in general, have had a profound effect on health IT efforts. These descriptions go by different names, but all depict essentially how EHR and health IT might mature over time, and the term **maturity model** has therefore been commonly applied to such descriptions. The generic maturity models continue to be referenced today as a way to describe trends in EHR, specifically, and health IT in general. The following sections offer some examples of these models.

Gartner Generations Criteria for EHR Adoption

Gartner Generations Criteria for EHR Adoption is one of the most widely recognized descriptions of a pathway to an EHR, even as Gartner Healthcare Research has replaced it with its Magic Quadrant for Global Enterprise EHR Systems (Handler and Hieb 2007; Handler 2013). The generations and their levels of functionality are illustrated in figure 3.1, along with the implementation timeline that was forecast in 2007. In this model, the *collector generation* refers to basic access to health data. The *documenter generation* is where clinicians begin to use technology at the point of care for objectives beyond merely accessing clinical data, such as performing results management. The *helper generation* is characterized by rudimentary clinical decision support, with the *colleague generation* providing more enhanced clinical decision support. Finally, the *mentor generation* is the most complex and sophisticated phase of EHR implementation, where the EHR is fully integrated across the continuum of care and guides clinicians through highly advanced knowledge management, decision support,

Figure 3.1.   Gartner EHR Generation Criteria

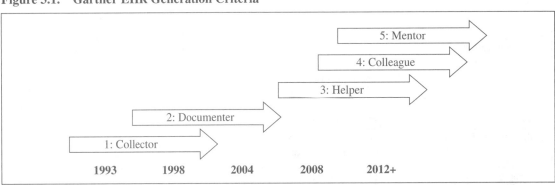

Source: Compiled from information described in Handler and Hieb 2007.

and predictive modeling. Since the Gartner EHR Generation Criteria were originally proposed, the MU incentive program extended and supplanted this maturity model.

US EMR Adoption Model from HIMSS Analytics

Healthcare Information Management and Systems Society (HIMSS) Analytics provide another widely referenced description of EHR maturity, the US EMR Adoption Model. In addition to describing stages of EHR adoption, HIMSS Analytics has developed a methodology and algorithms to automatically score more than 5,000 hospitals in its database relative to where they are on the model. The US EMR Adoption Model describes the following eight stages of applications for hospitals (HIMSS 2015):

- Stage 0: Not all three key ancillary systems (that is, laboratory, pharmacy, radiology) are installed.

- Stage 1: All three key ancillary systems are installed.

- Stage 2: Major ancillary clinical systems feed data to a central data repository (CDR) that provides access for retrieving and viewing results. The repository contains a controlled medical vocabulary and clinical decision support (CDS)/rules engine for rudimentary conflict checking. Information from document imaging systems may be linked to the CDR. The hospital has the capability of performing health information exchange (HIE) with other patient-care stakeholders.

- Stage 3: Nursing/clinical documentation is used, including an electronic medication administration record (eMAR). The first level of CDS is implemented to conduct error checking with order entry. Some level of medical image access from picture archival and communication systems (PACSs) is available outside of the radiology department.

- Stage 4: Computerized practitioner order entry (CPOE) has been added to at least one patient service area, and a second level of CDS related to evidence-based medicine protocols is used.

- Stage 5: Closed-loop medication administration (bar code electronic medication administration records [BC-MARs]) is fully implemented and integrated with CPOE and the pharmacy information system.

- Stage 6: Full physician documentation/charting using structured templates is implemented for at least one patient service area. Level 3 of CDS provides guidance for all clinician activities related to protocols and outcomes in the form of variance and compliance alerts. PACS fully replaces film-based images.

- Stage 7: The hospital no longer uses paper charts to deliver and manage patient care and has a mixture of discrete data, document images, and medical images within its EHR environment. Clinical data warehouses (CDWs) are used to analyze patterns of clinical data. Clinical information can be readily shared via standardized electronic transactions (that is, continuity of care documents [CCDs]). The hospital demonstrates summary data continuity for all hospital services (for example, inpatient, outpatient, emergency department, and any owned or managed ambulatory clinics).

HIMSS Analytics provides the following, similar model for ambulatory products (HIMSS 2015):

- Stage 0: The practice is paper-chart based.

- Stage 1: The practices uses some intraoffice/informal messaging and desktop access to clinical information, often in unstructured form.

- Stage 2: The practice has the beginning of a clinical data repository in which orders and results are placed. The practices can also access laboratory test results from outside facilities.

- Stage 3: Computers have replaced paper in the practice. The practice uses electronic messaging, clinical documentation at the point of care, and clinical decision support.

- Stage 4: The practice uses CPOE and structured data are accessible from the EHR for internal and external sharing.

- Stage 5: The practice has a personal health record and/or online tethered patient portal.

- Stage 6: The practice uses advanced clinical decision support; the system supports proactive care management and structured messaging.

- Stage 7: The practice is HIE-capable and shares data between its EHR and a community-based EHR; the practice generates business and clinical intelligence.

Federal Meaningful Use Maturity Models

The federal incentive program for MU of the EHR has included three stages of maturity, with each stage providing criteria intended to support more rigorous and robust quality measurement and improvement over time, with the ultimate goal being improved health outcomes and reduced cost growth (HealthIT.gov Policy Committee 2009). Figure 1.3 in chapter 1 provides an illustration depicting the MU stages. As of the publication of this edition, Stage 3 regulations were not yet finalized, with many professional associations and medical societies urging that their implementation be put off at least until 2019. On January 12, 2016, the Centers for Medicare and Medicaid Services (CMS) acting administrator told a conference that the MU program will likely end in 2016 as new regulations aimed at value-based payment models demand a more streamlined regulatory approach (Miliard 2016).

Connecting Health and Care for the Nation: A Shared Nationwide Interoperability Roadmap is another federal depiction of strategic directions for the United States with respect to health IT. Issued by the Office of the National Coordinator for Health Information Technology (ONC), this roadmap focuses broadly on interoperability (ONC 2015). Figure 3.2 describes how the roadmap is organized. The publication also has an appendix that provides complete milestones, calls to action for the industry to participate, and commitments from the federal government for the three time frames covered: 2015–2017, 2018–2020, and 2021–2024.

Figure 3.2   Shared nationwide interoperability roadmap

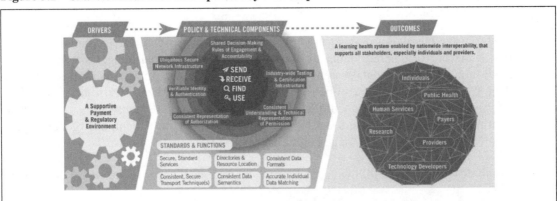

Source: Office of the National Coordinator for Health IT (ONC) (2015). Connecting Health and Care for the Nation: A Shared Nationwide Interoperability Roadmap Final Version 1.0. How the Roadmap is Organized (p. xv). https://www.healthit.gov/policy-researchers-implementers/interoperability.

Check Your Understanding 3.2

1. In which of the Gartner generations is clinical decision support initiated in the EHR?

   a. Collector

   b. Documenter

   c. Helper

   d. Mentor

2. Which stage in the HIMSS US EMR Adoption Model is roughly equivalent to the Gartner colleague generation?

   a. Stage 3

   b. Stage 4

   c. Stage 6

   d. Stage 7

3. In which stage of the meaningful use of EHR incentive program is computerized provider order entry (CPOE) required?

   a. Stage 0

   b. Stage 1

   c. Stage 2

   d. Stage 3

4. What stage of the HIMSS US EMR Adoption Model would be consistent with the ONC Shared Nationwide Interoperability Roadmap timeframes?

   a. Stage 2

   b. Stage 4

   c. Stage 6

   d. Stage 7

Construction of a Health IT Migration Path

Generic maturity models as described in this chapter provide an overarching framework for how the EHR and health IT should mature over time. However, each organization's strategic plan must reflect its own specific organizational needs and timelines. As is true for all naming conventions, documentation of such specifics may go by a variety of names. This book uses the term **migration path** to reflect the milestones in the strategic plan for EHR and health IT implementation, adoption, and optimization. Although a migration path documents issues related to hardware and software, it also addresses operational elements that involve people, policy, and process.

A migration path is distinct from an **implementation plan** (also called a **project plan**) in three important ways First, a migration path recognizes that EHR and health IT are systems with many components that must work together to achieve a purpose. An implementation plan generally focuses on one component at a time. Second, a migration path describes the overall picture of all components of the system—some would describe this as the 30,000-foot view of the roadmap or journey to EHR and health IT. In contrast, an implementation plan is a ground-level view that describes every specific detail of how any one of the given components described in the migration path will be selected, installed, customized, tested, and rolled out to end users. Third, as the documentation of health IT strategic planning, the migration path represents a long-term vision whereas an implementation plan is generally short-term for the duration of time required to complete one component's implementation.

Most organizations appreciate the need to gain an overview of how the EHR and health IT will be developed. A tool illustrating the various applications, supporting structures, and sequencing can provide such an overall picture and help establish milestones. Figure 3.3 depicts a sample matrix diagram of a migration path to describe the milestones toward the EHR and health IT. This example is drawn from a community-based integrated delivery network (IDN), with a hospital, owned physician practices, and a home health agency in a heavily managed care environment. The migration path matrix describes where the organization began its journey and where it anticipated it would be after a period of time that it divided into five phases.

When constructing a migration path, it is not necessary to use the particular format shown in figure 3.3. Different organizations may use a set of building blocks, a step diagram, a table, a narrative description, or other pictorials rather than the matrix diagram. Figures 3.4 and 3.5 illustrate two pictorial formats. Note that the format is less important than content and there is no single path that is right for all organizations. Each format, however, does have strengths and weaknesses for planning purposes.

A building-block approach (figure 3.4) typically focuses exclusively on applications. As a result, it does not identify where other elements, such as operations and technology, are needed. These elements might include such issues as when an EHR or health IT steering committee will be formed, when a CMIO or MDIS will be identified, what interfaces are needed to connect applications, network upgrades, storage additions, and so on. This approach also does not definitely describe the timeline; instead, it only identifies the sequence of implementations. Still, the building-block approach emphasizes that the EHR and health IT are a system of components, a concept sometimes lost on stakeholders.

A step diagram (figure 3.5) is similar to the building block approach, although the time frame is a bit clearer in the step diagram and a step diagram can generally include more elements, such as technical and operational aspects needed to support the applications. Although the goal for each phase and even dates or other timeline elements are not included in figure 3.5, it would be easy to add this information to this sort of illustration.

A flow chart is another option for reporting the migration path. The flowchart in figure 3.6 uses various line designations to illustrate current and proposed applications and some technology. It clearly illustrates the flow of information throughout systems, but it lacks a timeline.

The matrix-format migration path template in figure 3.7 covers all the components that are typically desired to depict a strategic plan for EHR and health IT. This type of matrix gives an elevated view of goals, applications, technology, and operations across a series of phases, or major milestones, such as the stages of the MU incentive program or the Shared Nationwide Interoperability Roadmap. It helps identify what applications will be implemented, when, and which supporting technology and operational elements are needed. Such a matrix migration path allows for easier understanding of dependencies. For instance, if a pharmacy information system needs to be upgraded prior to implementing a BC-MAR system, one can look across from one phase to another to check that such a dependency is illustrated. One can also look down to determine whether nurses are being engaged as the BC-MAR is implemented in defining policies associated with use of the BC-MAR application.

As the migration path is planned, it also can highlight issues of appropriate sequencing and help strategic planners overcome a "stovepipe" mentality (that is, decision-making in an isolated

Figure 3.3.   Sample matrix diagram of migration path toward the EHR

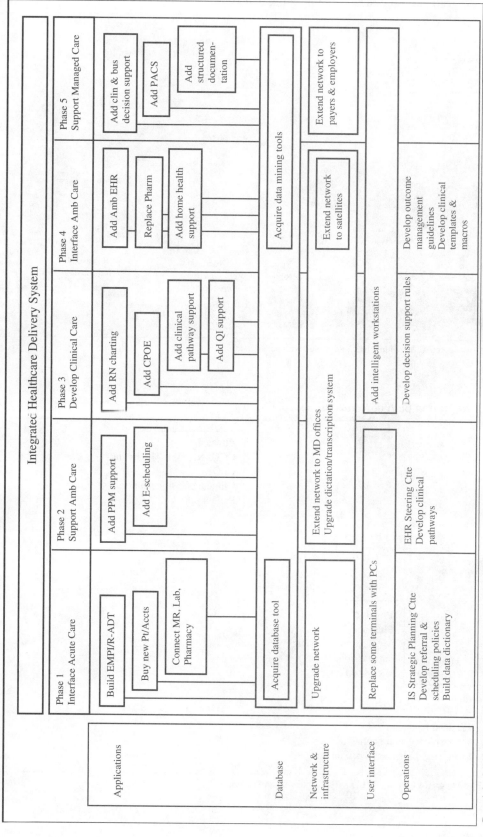

Figure 3.4. Migration path described by building blocks

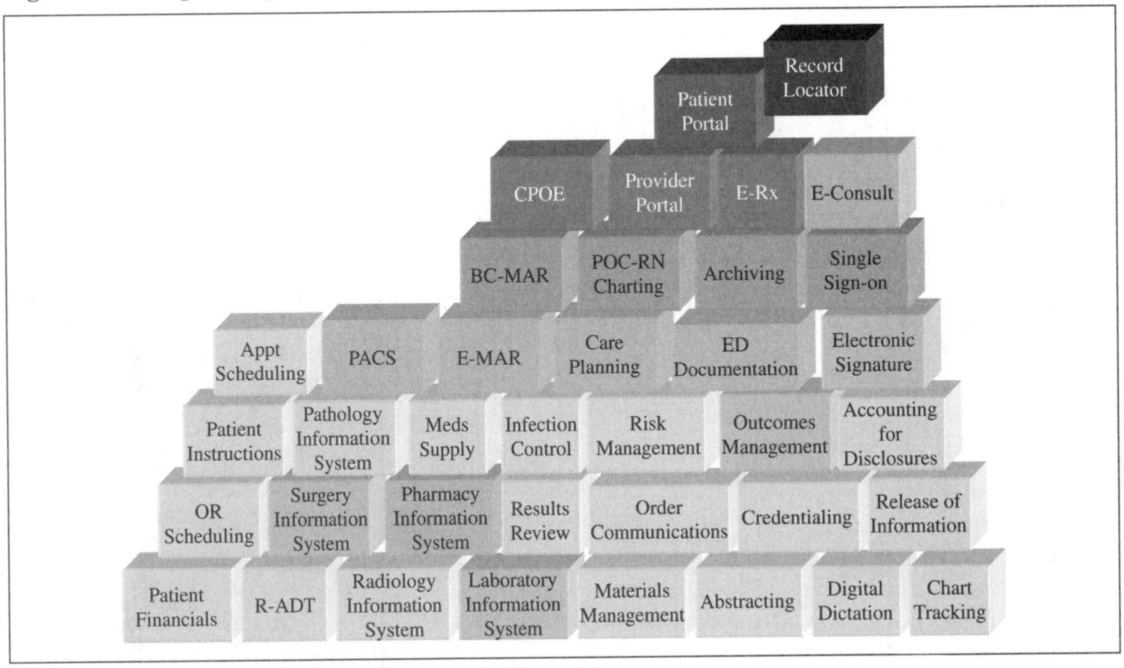
Record Locator
Patient Portal
CPOE
Provider Portal
E-Rx
E-Consult
BC-MAR
POC-RN Charting
Archiving
Single Sign-on
Appt Scheduling
PACS
E-MAR
Care Planning
ED Documentation
Electronic Signature
Patient Instructions
Pathology Information System
Meds Supply
Infection Control
Risk Management
Outcomes Management
Accounting for Disclosures
OR Scheduling
Surgery Information System
Pharmacy Information System
Results Review
Order Communications
Credentialing
Release of Information
Patient Financials
R-ADT
Radiology Information System
Laboratory Information System
Materials Management
Abstracting
Digital Dictation
Chart Tracking

Figure 3.5. Migration path described as a step diagram

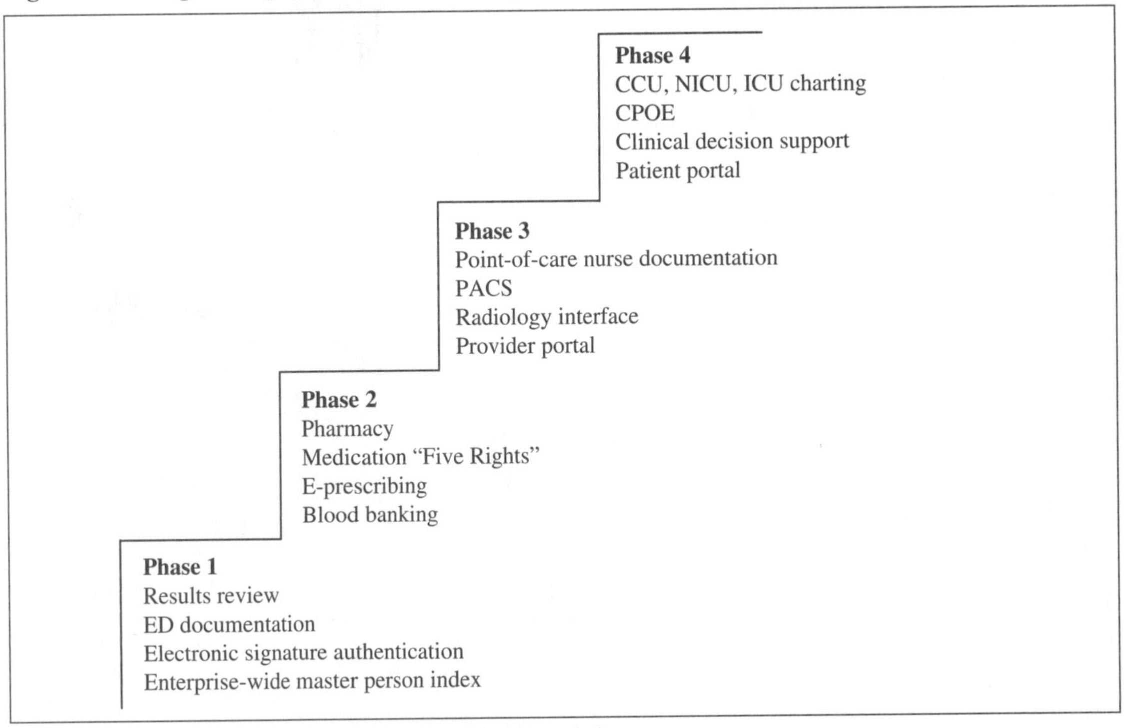
Phase 4
CCU, NICU, ICU charting
CPOE
Clinical decision support
Patient portal
Phase 3
Point-of-care nurse documentation
PACS
Radiology interface
Provider portal
Phase 2
Pharmacy
Medication "Five Rights"
E-prescribing
Blood banking
Phase 1
Results review
ED documentation
Electronic signature authentication
Enterprise-wide master person index

Figure 3.6.   Migration path as a flowchart

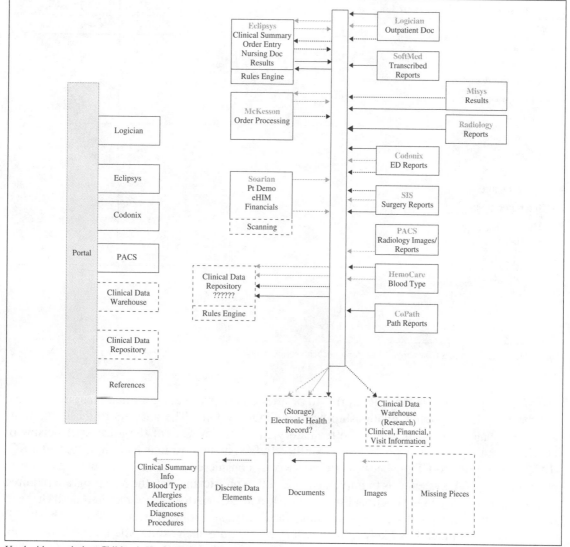

Used with permission, Children's Health System, Birmingham, AL.

context without regard for the bigger picture). For example, in one case, a hospital found itself planning a comprehensive electronic document management system for use by its health information management department. Another, separate document imaging system was being planned by its contracted emergency department physicians. Finally, a vendor was trying to sell a third document imaging system to the radiology department, which had just acquired a PACS and no longer had a pocket in the film jackets to store copies of radiology orders and reports. Although differences in electronic data management systems based on workflow needs may preclude one system being used for all three purposes, the acquisition of three similar systems should be evaluated. Ideally, a solution would emerge that would either address all three needs or enable interoperability among the disparate applications.

A migration path also will help resolve issues of sequencing: Should a CPOE system be implemented in the hospital before or after a nursing documentation system? Should an e-prescribing system for the physicians be acquired before, simultaneously with, or after a CPOE system? Should

Figure 3.7.   Matrix format for migration path template

Timeline	Current	Phase I	Phase II	Phase n
Goals				
Applications: • Financial/ administrative • Operational • Clinical				
Technology • Database • Network & infrastructure • Interoperability • Human-computer interfaces • Storage				
Operations • People • Policy • Process				

a BC-MAR system be implemented prior to or after a new pharmacy information system? What will the BC-MAR system's relationship be to a CPOE system? The answers to these questions depend on many factors, including the regulatory environment. One of the greatest criticisms of the MU incentive program is its lack of flexibility. In fact, many hospitals had implemented a BC-MAR system prior to CPOE because BC-MAR was considered easier to implement and sell to nurses than a CPOE system was to implement and sell to physicians. Yet, the MU program required at least rudimentary CPOE functionality in Stage 1, and BC-MAR was not required until Stage 2. Stage 3 was, in fact, revised to incorporate some flexibility, and, going forward with other health IT, the government is much less likely to require a rigid structure such as the MU incentive program. Of course, future health IT initiatives are also unlikely to include the federal incentives. Organizations will have to find return on investment in interoperability in their ability to be successful in an era of health reform that reimburses on value rather than volume.

The construction of a migration path for the EHR might best include the following components, as illustrated in the template shown in figure 3.7:

- Time frame
- Goals
- Applications
- Technology
- Operations
- Dependencies

Time Frame and Goals

Time frame refers to the overall period of time in which the strategic plan for health IT is expected to be accomplished. Although strategic planners have traditionally preferred to plan for only two to three years, most healthcare organizations recognize that the planning horizon for an EHR has been much longer, and the federal government has recognized that achieving interoperability may take up to ten years. When drafting a strategic plan for health IT, it may be appropriate to start with phases and add dates later. The phases can be described across the top of the migration path. Organizations typically like to describe the current state of their information systems, using the first column in the migration path to do so.

It is generally desirable to have a place to record the primary goal or goals for each phase. Although goal setting should be explicit, detailed goals can be provided in an addendum. (See also chapter 4.)

Applications

Applications are the most commonly described component of a migration path and are identified following the time frame and goals. Organizations that are currently focused on clinical information systems may try to simplify their migration path by listing only the applications related to clinical information. This tactic is generally not advisable because clinical systems need information from financial/administrative and operational systems, and clinical systems must feed financial/administrative systems with charge information. The interdependence among all of these components is increasing as health reform focuses on value, which is the intersection of clinical quality and cost of healthcare services. In an IDN, some effort may be given to grouping the applications by type of organization, such as hospital, clinic, and so on, especially if they follow a best-of-fit acquisition strategy where most of their applications are from a single vendor. (Best-of-fit acquisition strategy is explained in greater detail later in this chapter.)

In the migration plan, the applications are best described by their function and not by vendor name. Some stakeholders may not know what a particular product is when it is identified only by vendor name. Also, vendors can merge or be sold, so the name of the vendor can change. If the organization wants to illustrate that it has been using a best-of-breed acquisition strategy (that is, acquiring applications from different vendors, as explained later in this chapter), the vendor name can be listed parenthetically after the functional description (for example, radiology information system [GE]; laboratory information system [Siemens]; pharmacy information system [McKesson]; registration-admission, discharge, transfer or R-ADT [Cerner]; medication supply [Pyxis]; and so on).

Technology

In the past, technology was fairly consistent because of IT strategies and vendor recommendations. As organizations looked to EHR systems and different technologies became available, the selection of technology that could support EHR applications became a more important consideration in the migration plan. Now, in an era in which mobile and personal technology have become the norm among consumers, healthcare organizations must not only consider whether technology supports their own applications but also how their applications will interact with their patients' devices. The focus must also shift to enhanced security and data quality. In fact, keeping up-to-date with technology is a key decision factor for many providers—can they, indeed, keep up with the changes? Technology changes include those in database structures, network and infrastructure, interoperability, human–computer interfaces (input/output devices), and storage (see chapters 10, 11, 12, and 13).

Operations

The final category of information captured in a migration path addresses the operational elements that need to support health IT as each application and technology is implemented. Operational elements address the people, policies, and processes needed to achieve successful implementation, adoption, and benefits realization from an EHR or other type of health IT. Some examples of operational elements include hiring specialized staff; establishing benefits metrics and measurement processes (see chapter 4); workflow and process redesign (see chapter 5); change management strategies (see chapter 6); and policies on how various applications and their functionality will be used (see chapters 14–20). What is not included under operations are those things that would normally be part of any project plan, such as hiring a project manager, selecting a vendor, implementing software, and so on. These issues are not considered part of a strategic plan; rather, they belong as part of the implementation plan for each new application, hardware, or other system component being implemented.

Dependencies

Once all applications, technologies, and operational elements are identified, the organization should review the migration path and ensure that all dependencies are addressed. A **dependency** is a relationship between two elements. In strategic planning, a dependency exists if elements directly rely on one another in order for the overall system to produce the desired result. In implementation planning, dependency is often more pronounced, where one element must be completed for another element to be started. For instance, a laboratory information system may need to be updated to provide structured data for clinical decision support of drug-laboratory checking. A pharmacy information system may need updating to provide unit dose medications and bar codes on IV bags for BC-MAR applications. Broadband availability may need to be enhanced if the organization is opening a provider or patient portal, especially in inner-city and rural communities where broadband service continues to be less than desirable. Basic computer training may be needed to support workers who have not previously used a computer in front of a patient; and workflow changes certainly need to be supported.

Dependencies are not listed on the migration path. Rather, they are illustrated by aligning components on the migration path, both across the phases and down through the various planning components. For example, a laboratory information system upgrade may be listed in Phase II under Applications and the drug-laboratory decision support listed in Phase III across from the laboratory information system upgrade. As another example, when a BC-MAR application is being adopted, policies on what constitutes a medication administration error may need to be reviewed.

Check Your Understanding 3.3

1. Write a brief description of the difference between a migration path and an implementation, or project, plan:

2. Provide two examples of each of the following as might be documented on a migration path (Answers may include anything listed in chapter 1 or new components as shown below as examples):

Critical Success Factors for Health IT Strategic Planning

A final step in all strategic planning is to describe the critical success factors that define how plans are evaluated. Critical success factors for health IT strategic planning include the following:

- Creating the vision
- Identifying the planning horizon
- Gaining agreement

- Developing a financing and acquisition strategy
- Mapping workflows and processes
- Developing functional, data, and technical strategies
- Carrying out a vendor selection process
- Planning the implementation
- Conducting benefits realization

Creating the Vision

A vision for health IT may be articulated by experts in the industry, such as was done by Gartner, HIMSS, the federal government, and others for the EHR and by the federal government for interoperability. However, each organization developing a strategic plan for health IT must create its own vision that reflects how health IT specifically applies to the organization.

A visioning exercise during strategic planning can help put participants in the right frame of mind with respect to what the future might look like, and hence what the organization needs to put into place to accommodate the future. Strategic planning facilitators use various exercises for this purpose, including the following three common examples:

- Ask participants to envision themselves receiving an award for being the most successful in implementing health IT in healthcare organizations. Participants are asked to annotate what specifically the award would be for and how that accomplishment contributed to the organization's overall success. For example, if such an award was given today, it might recognize the implementation of health IT to support health reform, including the ability to integrate quality and cost data, present quality and cost data to providers at the point of care, coordinate care among disparate provider organizations, and allow providers to share in savings accrued from fewer admissions and fewer emergency department visits.

- Give participants a scenario and then ask them to describe a typical day in that scenario. For example, the scenario might be health reform is in full force with much more information about cost and quality of care being available to providers, much more care coordination occurring, and all providers participating in shared savings. For this scenario, participants might note that they start their day by looking at a dashboard that tells them where they stand in terms of care-delivery savings that come from up-to-date financial information; next they go to a meeting with their major health plan in which they have all the information at their fingertips about what their actual costs and savings are (including quality data for specific metrics), and they conclude their day at the local Chamber of Commerce meeting with community and business leaders who are pleased with lowered cost of supplying health insurance to their employees and improved productivity because of a healthier workforce.

- Ask participants, especially physicians, to describe one of the worst days of their lives in their practice and note what improvements they would like to see. Very likely, they will want more time with their patients, fewer lost laboratory test results, fewer scheduling snafus, and so on. From this starting point, the discussion can focus on whether health IT offers any solutions. For example, would having patients enter their health history before the time of the examination reduce the amount of data entry required of physicians, thereby freeing up time to examine patients, engage in their personal health agendas, and help them understand their treatment regimen?

Identifying the Planning Horizon

Once the vision is articulated, the components identified by the participants set the stage for identifying the planning horizon. The planning horizon must consider the external environment as well as the capacity for the organization to respond to external factors. The most successful organizations in strategic planning can match external factors with internal capacity. For example, if the scenario about living in a health reform environment is the current vision, the fact that Medicare anticipates reimbursing on value (cost and quality of care, not just services provided) over a timeline that includes milestones at 2016 and 2018 (CMS 2015) could help participants realize that a data warehouse is needed or improvements to an existing warehouse must be made sooner rather than later.

No single environmental factor determines the planning horizon. For example, the ONC Shared Nationwide Interoperability Roadmap in figure 3.2 establishes a ten-year timeline with three milestones for achieving the degree of interoperability believed to be necessary for the future.

Gaining Agreement on the Strategic Plan

To finalize and gain agreement on its strategic plan, an organization must have the capacity to carry out the elements that need to be included in the plan. Gaining agreement on the strategic plan is critical because participants must have a stake in its success. A strategic plan will not succeed if there is dissent or if the plan is viewed as belonging to the CEO or the CIO. As part of the broader organization's strategic plan, the health IT strategic plan needs to be constructed in a manner that demonstrates clear support for each of the elements on the organization's plan. This approach is generally the only way that additional resources can be allocated. A return on investment analysis where benefits equal or exceed costs is important, but it is not always feasible for some of the needed initiatives. Sometimes, it is necessary to weigh what penalties or disincentives may result in not doing something against the costs of doing something. In certain circumstances, healthcare organizations may decide they cannot undertake a given health IT project (or other project) at a certain time and will need to suffer the consequences. Ideally, however, a sufficient business case is made and the strategic planning participants can agree about what is needed to carry out each of the elements of the strategic plan.

Financing and Acquisition Strategy

The financing and acquisition strategy refers to how health IT is paid for and acquired. This strategy often part of a strategic plan because decisions about the acquisitions are a significant factor in the overall cost and ability to finance health IT.

With respect to health IT, **acquisition strategy** refers to how an organization attains the health IT that it uses. As shown in table 3.3, there are three general types of acquisition strategy: best of breed, best of fit, and dual core.

A **best-of-breed strategy** uses several different vendors to supply various applications because each vendor is believed to provide the best application in its class. When using a best-of-breed health IT strategy, the organization is challenged to get the various systems to exchange data and requires interfaces to do so.

The opposite of a best-of-breed strategy is a best-of-fit strategy. Using a **best-of-fit strategy**, a single vendor provides virtually (although not absolutely) all applications. With this strategy, it is easier to add new applications from that vendor; however, this strategy makes adding products from other vendors potentially more difficult.

Some organizations find that their best-of-fit financial, administrative, and operational system vendor is not as strong in EHR components as they would desire. At the same time, best-of-breed organizations find sustaining that type of acquisition strategy to be difficult and costly. In both types of organizations, there is recent movement toward a rip-and-replace acquisition strategy, wherein

Table 3.3.   IT acquisition strategy

Best of Fit	Dual Core	Best of Breed
One primary vendor	Two primary vendors: • Financial/administrative • Operational or clinical	Many vendors
Generally found in small hospitals or corporate organizations seeking standardization	Both best of fit and best of breed moving to this strategy	Generally found in large, stand-alone or academic medical centers
Generally simpler to implement and maintain	Viewed as either a consolidation strategy or a means to achieve a comprehensive EHR	Generally more difficult to implement and maintain due to interface requirements for exchange of data

the organization replaces all of its disparate applications over a relatively short period of time (a few years) with a comprehensive, integrated, best-of-class suite of products from a best-of-fit vendor.

Some organizations that are not financially able to rip and replace are migrating to a **dual-core strategy**, where one primary vendor supports financial or administrative applications and possibly the operational applications, and another vendor supports the operational and clinical applications or just the clinical applications. The primary advantage to the dual-core strategy is the organization can retain any legacy systems that are working well. The biggest disadvantage is that interfaces between the applications from each of the vendors are still required.

Another aspect of the acquisition strategy is whether the organization designs and builds its own applications or acquires them from either a single vendor (best-of-fit strategy) or a set of vendors (best-of-breed strategy). Some organizations believe that developing their own applications saves them money or enables them to get better results. Most healthcare organization today, however, find neither of these potential reasons for self-development to be compelling. In fact, self-development generally has increased costs and does not support interoperability with other applications.

An acquisition strategy is considered a matter for strategic planning because changing to a different strategy is difficult and costly (although not unheard of). Choosing an acquisition strategy, therefore, is critical to successful achievement of a health IT strategic plan.

Financing options are also considered strategic matters and a critical success factor for the strategic plan because they influence the overall cost of expenditures. Financing options include purchase, lease, or various partnering/codevelopment options. Many organizations must finance at least some of their health IT investment through bank loans or more directly in capital markets. Some vendors offer financing or discounts, and some vendors have partnered with pharmaceutical companies, medical device suppliers, hardware vendors, and other suppliers to provide reduced prices in exchange for using their products, obtaining data, or even allowing pop-up advertisements in an EHR. Major employers and some health plans in the area may be a source of funding if they are interested in negotiating reduced costs of care. The MU incentives were a factor to consider in seeking loans or other external financing options; however, because the MU program was frontloaded, the amount of the incentives in the later stages may not be sufficient to cover the organization's costs of adding applications or enhancements. Although some of these options may provide significant benefits to the healthcare organization, strategic planners must take care to fully understand what the organization must do to obtain the funding support and what that support costs.

Other policies considered in the financing and acquisition strategy include the purchasing requirements that stipulate the stability of the vendor business, the number of other installations it must have, the size and type of clients, and so forth. Some organizations are more willing to assume risk than others. The financing and acquisition strategy must reflect the degree of risk-taking a healthcare organization is willing to accept.

Although the financing and acquisition strategies are first addressed in strategic planning, they are further developed until the time an acquisition is actually made. Further information on financing and acquisition options is discussed in chapter 7.

Workflow and Process Mapping

Maps of workflows and processes show how current work is performed. Understanding work performance is necessary to begin the change management process and support the success of any health IT project. While workflow and process mapping is tactical in nature, strategic planning must ensure that the mapping will be performed first as an integral part of functional requirements specification (see next section of this chapter), again at the time of health IT implementation, and at any time when monitoring of the new application reveals less than the desired degree of success. Of all the operational elements needed for success with health IT, workflow and process mapping is probably the most critical and the least well performed. See chapter 5 for complete coverage of this critical success factor.

Functional Strategy

When the need for a type of health IT system is identified, the functional strategy describes how the system will perform with respect to its users and in relationship to its boundaries with other systems. There are essentially two levels of functional strategy. The first supports the overall strategic plan and its documentation in a migration path. Executive management approves this functional strategy.

The second, more detailed level of functional strategy defines the specific, detailed functions to be performed by any given application and generally serves as a set of functional specifications for vendor selection. An organization may require process mapping to identify this level of functional detail. A process map documents operations and workflows to identify process improvements needed prior to implementation of an application and establishes the functional requirements necessary to support improvements in processes through an EHR. Process mapping and functional specification is discussed fully in chapter 5.

Functional needs assessment entails studying the various groups of processes and translating that discussion into a statement of functional needs that can be taken to a vendor or information system designer for development. Functional needs assessment is discussed fully in chapter 7.

One way to distinguish processes from functions is to consider that functionality is what is "bought" in an EHR; processes must be built into the functions of an EHR. Processes are unique to the organization; functions are provided by a vendor.

Data Strategy

Data strategy refers to the overall manner in which the organization plans to use data standards and build its data infrastructure. Strategic-level decisions must be made about the infrastructure, adoption of standards, and the degree to which unstructured versus structured data will flow throughout the migration path for health IT. The detailed execution of the strategic directions is discussed in chapter 10.

Technical Strategy

Technical strategy describes what technology will support various health IT applications. At the highest level, technical strategy indicates, for example, whether an EHR will run in a client/server environment, use web-enabled technology, include a wireless network, and so on. The health IT strategic plan should establish standards for best practices with regard to technology that will be used. For example, the plan might indicate that a specific operating system environment will be used for all applications and that specific technical standards must be used. However, the identification of the specific operating system and standards are generally tactical decisions.

The health IT strategic plan should support a technical strategy that is flexible enough to accommodate the rapid pace of technological change. Technology infrastructure is discussed in chapter 11.

Vendor Selection Strategy

Many hospitals and clinics are well on the path toward achieving success with an EHR and other health IT. However, the most successful organizations are also the ones most likely to acknowledge that they still have a long way to go. There are always some health IT components to add, upgrade, enhance, decommission, or change. Consequently, while vendor selection for a comprehensive health IT strategy is probably not necessary for most healthcare organizations today, organizations still need to select vendors for niche products or replacements.

A thoughtfully constructed process to obtain information about products, perform thorough due diligence in selecting the right vendor for the organization, and negotiate favorable terms in a contract is, indeed, a critical success factor for health IT strategic planning. The vendor selection process for any component can take some organizations as long as 6 to 18 months to accomplish. Vendor selection processes are more fully described in chapter 7.

Implementation Strategy

The implementation strategy describes the sequence in which an organization undertakes discrete project tasks, such as infrastructure building, new application system implementation, and organizational change. These tasks are prioritized based on the organization's clinical and strategic needs.

Strategic planners also consider issues of dependency and precedence when developing an implementation strategy. For example, some organizations believe that all elements of the technical infrastructure should be built or acquired at once and the applications phased in over time. Although this approach may seem ideal, the rapidly changing pace of IT and system upgrades may lead an organization using this strategy to install out-of-date applications or retrofit new applications to an older platform. Other organizations believe all aspects of health IT should be phased in, where pieces of infrastructure are implemented in accordance with a particular application requirement. Although this approach offers distinct advantages, it can result in a piecemeal approach in which no application is fully implemented. Each organization must weigh the risks associated with each implementation approach and select the one with which it is most comfortable.

The implementation strategy also addresses the philosophy of how rapidly users are trained and expected to be fully operational when using new applications. There are costs and benefits to both a slower-paced implementation, where all system functionality is fully tested and users fully trained, and a more rapid implementation, in which some system issues are addressed while users are still learning. Yet another approach is to fully implement a system but allow users to learn various parts of the applications on their own, which could extend full adoption for a fairly long period of time.

Another aspect of the implementation strategy is the approach to cutover. Will everyone be required to use the new system at a certain date, or will people be allowed to phase in use over time? Providers have different philosophies about this and also change their philosophies based on economic factors.

Chapter 9 describes the components of health IT implementation and provides more detail on various implementation options.

Benefits Realization

Formal benefits realization studies have not been the norm and are often difficult to conduct. Nevertheless, a critical success factor in health IT strategic planning is a process to establish whether goals are being met. At a minimum, an organization needs to monitor systems are being used as anticipated, especially if there are incentives involved, such as earning the MU incentives. Finally, benefits realization is necessary for ongoing operations, system maintenance, and staging future enhancements. Chapter 4 covers the basic construct of a benefits realization study and relates this process to return on investment.

Check Your Understanding 3.4

Choose the best answer:

1. The way in which health IT performs with respect to its users and in relationship to its boundaries with other systems is a consideration of which critical success factor?

    a. Data strategy

    b. Functional strategy

    c. Technical strategy

    d. Workflow and process mapping

2. Which of the following critical success factors in health IT strategic planning is most often not performed well?

    a. Creating a vision

    b. Gaining agreement

    c. Identifying the planning horizon

    d. Workflow and process mapping

3. Determining the organization's acquisition strategy for health IT has direct bearing on:

    a. Acceptance of health IT by users

    b. Benefits realization of health IT

    c. Cost of health IT

    d. Implementation of health IT

4. Which of the following visioning exercises is often effective when working with physicians?

    a. Receiving an award

    b. Typical day in a future state

    c. Visits to organizations with health IT already in place

    d. Worst-day improvements

5. Which of the following statements is *true*? A formal health IT vendor selection process is:

   a. Continually needed for upgrades, replacements, enhancements, and so on

   b. No longer needed if an organization already has an EHR

   c. Only needed when replacing a bad system

   d. Rarely needed because one vendor will cover all health IT needs

Current Status of Health IT Strategic Planning

In a healthcare organization, the "tipping point" for health IT is when strategic planning recognizes the supporting role the EHR and other health IT plays in every planning component (Gladwell 2000). Such a position requires the combined efforts of all stakeholders: executive management, users, technology experts, and support staff. Some have suggested that most organizations have not yet reached this tipping point, in part because the MU stage 2 and stage 3 challenges have been much greater than anticipated (Hirsch 2014; Monegain 2015).

In fact, most organizations with exemplary implementations of EHRs and health IT indicate that, although lack of physician support is the single point of failure, executive management support is the most critical success factor. If the EHR and health IT are not passions of the CEO, their chance for success is far less than if the CEO is a strong supporter (Baldwin 2003). The CEO's degree of passion is felt throughout the organization, and especially by physicians who can be turned around by a supportive CEO; on the other hand, a CEO whose EHR fails, may have to resign (Dunn 2014).

Strategic planning in which a clearly defined migration path is established sets the stage for the more focused planning and detailed tactical plans necessary to carry out the organization's vision of the EHR and health IT. A migration path also should be sufficiently flexible to permit new factors to be addressed. Whether these factors are new technology, changes in the organizational structure, regulations, or something else, the migration path must be flexible enough to accommodate—and stable enough to withstand—the various external and internal influences.

There are several critical success factors that health IT strategic planning should address. While each critical success factor has tactical components that do not belong in a strategic plan, strategic planning must provide general directions for each factor and ensure that each factor is carried out at the appropriate time. These directions include envisioning the future state; having a planning horizon, gaining agreement on the plan; developing a financing and acquisition strategy; ensuring that workflows and processes are mapped; developing functional, data, and technical strategies; carrying out a formal vendor selection process when applicable; implementation planning; and conducting benefits realization.

References and Resources

American Medical Informatics Association and American Health Information Management Association (AMIA/AHIMA). 2012 (January 16). Joint AMIA/AHIMA summary of their relationship and links to the informatics field. https://www.amia.org/joint-amia-ahima-summary.

Baldwin, F.D. 2003. CPRs in the winner's circle. *Healthcare Informatics,* 33–36. http://www.healthcare-informatics.com/issues/2003/05_03/cover.htm.

Bureau of Labor Statistics, US Department of Labor (BLS). 2014–2015. Informational security analysts. Occupational Outlook Handbook. http://www.bls.gov/ooh/computer-and-information-technology/information-security-analysts.htm.

Centers for Medicare and Medicaid Services (CMS). 2015 (January 26). Better care. Smarter spending. Healthier people: Paying providers for value, not volume. https://www.cms.gov/Newsroom/MediaReleaseDatabase/Fact-sheets/2015-Fact-sheets-items/2015-01-26-3.html.

Cole, B. 2015 (May 19). Fresh look at governance required to maximize information as an asset. SearchCompliance website. http://searchcompliance.techtarget.com/feature/Fresh-look-at-governance-required-to-maximize-information-as-an-asset.

Connecting for Health Steering Group. 2009. Bending the curve towards transformed health: achieving meaningful use of health data. *Achieving the Health IT Objectives of the American Recovery and Reinvestment Act.* New York, NY: Markle Foundation.

Darling, G. 2011. What does a clinical informatics data analyst do, exactly? Healthcare IT Today blog. http://healthcareittoday.com/2011/11/08/clinical-informatics-data-analyst.

Dunn, L. 2014 (May 28). CEO resigns over EHR fail—is your job at risk? *Becker's Hospital Review.* http://www.beckershospitalreview.com/healthcare-blog/ceo-resigns-over-ehr-fail-is-your-job-at-risk.html.

Eastwood, B. 2014 (November 3). Predicting the role of healthcare CIOs in 2020. *CIO.* http://www.cio.com/article/2842376/healthcare/predicting-the-role-of-the-healthcare-cio-role-in-2020.html.

Gillenson, M., P. Ponniah, A. Kriegel, B. Grukhnov, A. Taylor, and G. Powell. 2008. *Introduction to Database Management.* Hoboken, NJ: John Wiley & Sons.

Gladwell, M. 2000. *The Tipping Point: How Little Things Can Make a Big Difference.* New York, NY: Back Bay Books/Little, Brown.

Glaser, J.P. 2006. Information technology strategy: Three misconceptions. *Journal of Health Information Management.* 20:69–73.

Good Governance Guide. 2012. What is Good Governance? http://www.goodgovernance.org.au/about-good-governance/what-is-good-governance.

Handler, T.J. 2013. Magic quadrant for global enterprise EHR systems. Gartner Healthcare Research. https://www.gartner.com/doc/2586552/magic-quadrant-global-enterprise-ehr.

Handler, T., and B. Hieb. 2007. *The Updated Gartner CPR Generation Criteria.* Stamford, CT: Gartner, Inc.

Healthcare Information Management and Systems Society (HIMSS). 2015. HIMSS Analytics US EMR adoption model. http://app.himssanalytics.org/hc_providers/emr_adoption.asp.

HealthIT.gov Policy Committee. 2009. Meaningful Use Workgroup Presentation. https://www.healthit.gov/archive/archive_files/HIT%20Policy%20Committee/2009/2009-07-16/Meaningful%20Use_7.16.09.ppt

Hirsch, MD. 2014 (December 24). EHRs in 2014: Nearing a tipping point. *FierceEMR.* http://www.fierceemr.com/story/ehrs-2014-nearing-tipping-point/2014-12-24.

Hughes, RG., ed. 2008. *Patient Safety and Quality: An Evidence-Based Handbook for Nurses.* Rockville, MD: Agency for Healthcare Research and Quality.

Johns, ML. 2015. *Enterprise Health Information Management and Data Governance.* Chicago: AHIMA.

Knickrehm, M. 2011 (January 20). Many health systems unprepared to meet meaningful use federal guidelines by 2015. Accenture news release. http://newsroom.accenture.com/article_display.cfm?article_id=5132.

McNamara, C. 2007. *Field Guide to Nonprofit Strategic Planning and Facilitation,* 3rd ed. Minneapolis, MN: Authenticity Consulting.

Miliard, M. 2016 (January 12). Meaningful use will likely end in 2016, CMS chief Andy Slavitt says. *HealthcareIT News.* http://www.healthcareitnews.com/news/meaningful-use-will-likely-end-2016-cms-chief-andy-slavitt-says.

Monegain, B 2015 (October 15). CIOs share meaningful use concerns at CHIME. *Health IT News.* http://www.healthcareitnews.com/news/chime-meaningful-use-deconstructed.

Office of the National Coordinator for Health Information Technology (ONC). 2015. Connecting health and care for the nation: A shared nationwide interoperability roadmap. Final version 1.0. https://www.healthit.gov/sites/default/files/hie-interoperability/nationwide-interoperability-roadmap-final-version-1.0.pdf.

Pfister, H.R., and S.R. Ingargiola. 2014 (February 20). ONC: Staying focused on EHR usability. iHealthBeat. http://www.ihealthbeat.org/insight/2014/onc-staying-focused-on-ehr-usability.

Rouse, M. 2013. Chief technology officer (CTO) definition. TechTarget website. http://searchcio.techtarget.com/definition/Chief-Technology-Officer-CTO.

Rouse, M. 2015. Chief information officer (CIO) definition. TechTarget website. http://searchcio.techtarget.com/definition/CIO.

Russell, J. 2015 (December 12). Beleaguered by electronic record mandates, some doctors burning out. *Chicago Tribune*. http://www.chicagotribune.com/business/ct-doctors-hate-records-mandate-1213-biz-20151211-story.html.

Washington, L. 2015 (November 12). Information governance provides the framework for data governance. Journal of AHIMA blog. http://journal.ahima.org/2015/11/12/information-governance-provides-the-framework-for-data-governance.

Chapter 4
Health IT Goal Setting and Measuring the Impact on Healthcare Value

Key Terms

Accountable care organization (ACO)

Anecdotal benefits

Automated history taking

Benefits realization study

Business case

Care coordination

Care management

Case management

Clinically integrated network (CIN)

Clinical quality measures (CQMs)

Clinical trials

Confounding variables

Cost–benefit analysis

Discharge planning

Disease management

Electronic CQMs (eCQMs)

Electronic visits (e-visits)

Evidence-based guidance

Fee for service (FFS)

Goal

Implementation

Installation

Internal rate of return (IRR)

Just culture

Maintenance costs

Measure

Meta-analysis

Metric

Net present value (NPV)

Patient-centered medical home (PCMH)

Patient engagement

Payback period

Population health

Precision/personalized medicine

Pro forma

Quantifiable benefits

(ROI) analysis

Scribe

Service level agreement (SLA)

Shared decision making

SMART goals

STRETCH goals

Support costs

System build

Total cost of ownership (TCO)

Transitions of care (ToC)

Utilization management

Value

Value-based payment (VPB)

Learning Objectives

- Recognize the concept of healthcare value and the US focus on the Triple Aim goals for the EHR and health IT.

- Describe the importance of establishing goals and benefits expectations for the EHR and health IT as supporting mechanisms for the US learning health system.

- Demonstrate use of a template for constructing SMART and STRETCH goals and creating a tool to monitor goal achievement.

- Distinguish among types of benefits.

- Describe how to measure benefits, including specific examples of clinical and financial benefits that can be achieved with an EHR and health IT in general.

- Describe when various forms of financial impact studies, including total cost of ownership/cost–benefit feasibility, benefits realization, and return on investment are performed.

- Explain how to compile a total cost of ownership and return on investment analysis for the EHR and other types of health IT.

Many people believe that widespread adoption of electronic health records (EHRs) and other health information technology (health IT) will result in increased efficiencies in the healthcare delivery system and improved patient care. The federal government certainly banked on getting value from its investment in the meaningful use (MU) of EHR incentive program, and a study conducted by the Medical Group Management Association found that more than 60 percent of practices increased revenues (MGMA 2011). The following case studies further illustrate the worth of EHR and other health IT in diverse healthcare organizations:

- Mount Sinai Medical Center in New York City found that its EHR improved continuity of care. Providers also reported new efficiencies in refilling medications, receiving patient messages, and releasing test results. Readmissions decreased (for example, the readmission rate for congestive heart failure patients decreased by 60 percent). Finally, average monthly collections increased by $27 million over the 4-year period of EHR implementation.

- Jeremy L. Bradley, MD, FAAFP, found that the EHR used in his family practice clinic in Owensboro, KY, increased his time spent with patients by 20 percent; increased patient volume by 28 percent; reduced patient wait times by 80%; yielded a 15% reduction in medical malpractice insurance costs; reduced a variety of administrative costs by $32,400; saved $18,000 in overtime costs; and ultimately led to 45% increase in revenue (Wise 2013).

Randomized controlled studies have demonstrated benefits of health IT in patient safety and quality of care. As just one of many examples, there was a significantly lower instance of antibiotic use when following an integrated clinical prediction rule in their EHR (McGinn, et al 2013).

Patients have also been found to appreciate online EHR access and even to trust technology over paper. A 2014 survey conducted by the National Partnership for Women and Families found that the more frequently individuals access their health information online, the more motivated they are to do something to improve their health (Savage 2014). As compared to the 2011 survey by the same group, privacy and security were less of a concern of respondents in 2014, and patients with online access were found to have a higher level of trust in their doctors than those without online access.

However, an increasing number of commentators are expressing concerns about EHRs. Some question the financial return on investment (ROI) from EHRs (Mace 2014); others worry about potential unintended consequences from their use (Toll 2012), reduced time for patient-clinician interaction (Oxentenko et al. 2010), and reports of patient complaints that "my doctor pays more attention to the computer than to me" (Payne et al. 2015).

A critical step in both demonstrating and ensuring the worth of the EHR and health IT is to understand what benefits are feasible along the migration path to the EHR and health IT, and to establish specific goals and processes to achieve them. Goals help set expectations for their achievement. Impact analyses, such as benefits realization and ROI studies, recognize achievements to be celebrated or bring attention to areas where lack of achievement needs correction. Kraus (2008) identified that Minnesota mandated EHR implementation earlier than the federal MU program, and he observed that "you have to [learn how to] get your investment back." As an example, he estimated that he could save $2,400 per year by cutting out the hours spent by front desk staff in locating and moving paper, and he asserted that this savings was one of many financial benefits that provided a strong incentive to move forward with an EHR. Interestingly, he seemed satisfied that these savings without taking what could be the next step—establishing what front desk staff can do with the time savings.

Each organization needs to determine how to get the most from its EHR and health IT. Organizations also need to learn how to set the expectation that such value will happen, monitor that it does happen, and use feedback from monitoring to make further improvements, not only for the EHR and health IT, but the healthcare delivery system overall.

Value and the Triple Aim Goals

Value, in general, refers to "the fair return in goods, services, or money for something exchanged" (Merriam Webster n.d.). Terms frequently associated with value include worth, usefulness, or importance in comparison with something else. For the US healthcare system, the concept of value grew out of the Institute of Medicine (IOM; now known as Health and Medical Division [HMD] of the National Academies of Science, Engineering, and Medicine) 2001 report *Crossing the Quality Chasm: A New Health System for the 21st Century*. This report described the need for the healthcare system to strive for care that is safe, effective, patient-centered, timely, efficient, and equitable. However, since its publication, healthcare costs have continued to rise, with increasing costs associated with medical errors, inability to share health information across the continuum of care, and duplication of services/redundant costs (Foster 2012). Health reform, representing a significant shift in healthcare policy relating to how care is delivered and paid for, has been the impetus for even greater attention on value. The Health Information Technology for Economic and Clinical Health Act (HITECH) of 2009 and the Affordable Care Act of 2010 set in motion many programs that have focused on the improvements called for in the 2001 IOM report as well as in the seminal work conducted by the Institute for Healthcare Improvement (IHI), which was reported in "The Triple Aim: Care, health, and cost" (Berwick et al. 2008). The IHI proposed the following three priorities (that is, the Triple Aim) for healthcare reform:

- Improve the experience of care—provide care that is effective, safe, and reliable—to every patient, every time.

- Improve the health of a population, reach out to communities, manage chronic conditions, and so forth.

- Decrease per capita costs of healthcare.

Berwick introduced the framework to the Centers for Medicare and Medicaid Services (CMS) when he was temporarily the administrator of CMS, and in 2015 CMS released a National Impact Assessment of Quality Measures Report indicating that delivery system transformation across the United States has made progress in achieving the Triple Aim of providing better care, lowering costs, and improving health (Buechner 2015).

The Triple Aim has broader objectives than pursuing value from the EHR and health IT. However, EHRs and other types of health IT contribute to what the IOM/HMD calls the *learning health system*, which "aligns science, informatics, incentives, and culture for continuous improvement and innovation" (IOM 2012). The result of the learning health system is best practices that are "seamlessly embedded in the delivery process and new knowledge captured as an integral by-product of the delivery experience" (IOM 2012). From 2009 to 2012, the IOM produced a series of informative works on the learning health system that contributed to the federal MU of EHR incentive program and to CMS creating its Center for Medicare and Medicaid Innovation (CMMI) (Berenson and Cafarella 2012). Figure 4.1 describes the relationship between the Triple Aim and the learning health system from a systems development life cycle (SDLC) perspective.

Figure 4.1.   The learning health system

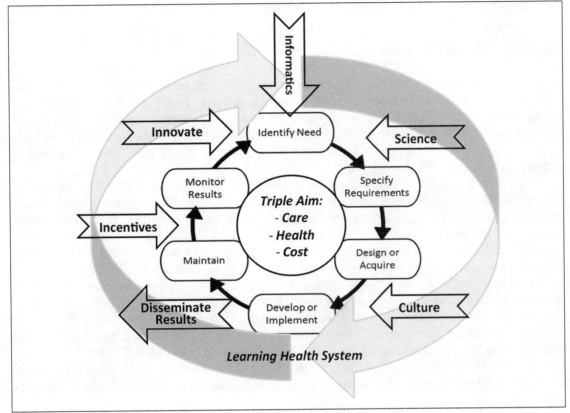

Setting Goals and Expectations for Achievement of Value

A **goal** is a specific, intended result of a strategy (such as a strategy to achieve value). To be useful, goals must be "SMART," which stands for *specific, measurable, achievable, realistic,* and *time-based.* The concept of **SMART goals** has been recognized for many years, and no one has identified a specific individual or entity who first coined the acronym. However, these traditional attributes, or ones that enhance their meaning further, are believed to be critical to achieving fast-paced results for any major project. Vishwasrao (2012) has suggested variations on the acronym that may be useful to consider when constructing goal statements: *S* may stand for stretching, systematic, synergistic, and significant; *M* for meaningful, motivating, and magical; *A* for accountability, acumen, and agreed-on; *R* for realistic, resonating, results-oriented, rewarding, rooted in facts, and remarkable; and *T* for tangible and thoughtful.

When considering SMART goals, particular attention should be paid to the concept of **STRETCH goals.** STRETCH stands for *SMART* goals that *teach* an organization how to *reach* higher levels of performance by *engaging* everyone in *testing* hypotheses through *cross-functional cooperation* in a *human* fashion. Miller (2009) distinguishes SMART goals, which tend to be narrow in scope and individually and discretely attainable, from STRETCH goals, which are meant to be ambitious, challenging, and out-of-reach according to the current ways of working. In Miller's view, there is a positive tension between SMART and STRETCH goals. Sheehan (2014) believes that STRETCH goals that are SMART are the most provocative for strategic planning because they serve to set expectations for something more than the status quo.

Writing SMART Goals

Goals are not always easy to write. Typically, organizations start out with overarching platitudes, such as "save money" or "improve quality." Although outlining such general objectives is helpful, moving to SMART goals helps an organization establish expectations for their achievement. Figure 4.2 provides a template to guide the writing of SMART goals. As the figure suggests, a key element in setting a SMART goal is identifying "who," "what," "why," "how," and "when" will be considered in the process.

The SMART goal set in figure 4.2 may be inspired by broad objectives such as "saving money" and "contributing to profitability." Because there are potentially a number of ways to achieve such overarching objectives, organizations need to specify those approaches that are most relevant to the focus of the project (such as EHR and health IT). One common goal for an EHR is to save money by reducing transcription expense. However, an organization needs to think critically about this goal. For example, the organization could conceivably save money in transcription expense in other ways—including paying transcriptionists less money. In addition, the organization would want to analyze the impact of the goal on its providers and whether they will support it. Although it may seem inconceivable that providers would not see their role in this goal without it being made explicit, weaning providers off dictation to reduce transcription expense is a major undertaking. Finally, when defining the value of the EHR, the organization may find that reducing transcription costs is not the only benefit of the goal; the potential to earn the MU incentives has been an additional justification for implementing an EHR, as these incentives require structured data to be captured in the EHR in support of quality measurement and reporting.

After considering all these factors, the final statement of the goal focuses on who (providers) will do what (reduce dictation) and why (to reduce transcription expense and earn MU incentives). In some organizations, the sequence of reasons why providers should undertake such an enormous change would be more politically acceptable if earning MU incentives were listed first and reducing transcription expense were second. How goals are stated can be important in determining how well they are received by stakeholders, and hence how likely the stakeholders will work toward their achievement.

A SMART goal, furthermore, calls for a statement that demonstrates the goal is realistic—how will the goal be achieved or what support will be provided? In this case, templates in the EHR will substitute for dictation or transcription and aid in capturing structured data. To ensure the goal is

Figure 4.2. Writing SMART goals

		Sample Scenario	
	Goal Elements	*The EHR will*	
Who	**S**pecific	Reduce provider dictation	
What	**M**easurable	by 50 percent	by 85 percent
Why	**A**chievable	To reduce transcription expense and earn M.U. incentives	
How	**R**ealistic	Using EHR templates for capturing structured data	
When	**T**ime-based	by Yr 1	by Yr 2

measurable and time-based, realistic milestones are included: figure 4.2 shows that providers are expected to reduce dictation by 50 percent in the first year and 85 percent in the second year. In summary, the goal statement could be stated as follows:

> To reduce transcription expense and earn MU incentives, providers will reduce dictation by 50 percent within one year and by 85 percent within two years of using EHR templates for capturing structured data.

Setting Expectations for Goals Accomplishment

As EHRs and health IT are increasingly accepted as a necessary cost of doing business, and not an optional capital investment, some people may question the need to establish goals up front for EHR and health IT systems. However, as figure 4.3 summarizes, there are many reasons to set goals and anticipate the benefits of the EHR and health IT.

Goal Setting and Education

When goal setting is performed during the planning stages for an EHR or other health IT, it helps stakeholders understand the scope, complexity, and what it means to actually achieve the desired benefits. A simple example is illustrative:

> A small physician office considering an EHR brought in a consultant to assist with the selection process. When the consultant asked what they hoped to accomplish, the physicians noted cost savings as one of the benefits they anticipated. This goal was not very specific, so the consultant asked them to quantify what cost savings meant to them. The physicians said that they believed that EHRs could reduce their transcription expense, perhaps by 50 percent or 75 percent. This was a broad range, so the consultant asked them what function they thought could be eliminated by using an EHR. The physicians suggested that note dictation could be

Figure 4.3. Impact of goal setting

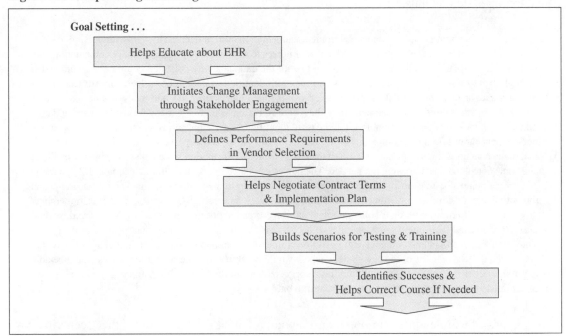

eliminated, which they estimated accounted for about 75 percent of the office's transcription expense. When the consultant asked how the EHR would help reduce the expense of transcribing notes, the physicians literally had to stop and think a moment before they realized that they would no longer be dictating notes. When the consultant asked how they expected their notes would be entered into the EHR if not through dictation, the physicians were taken aback as they realized that they would have to type all the content themselves, and they expressed fear that they would become transcriptionists. Finally, the consultant arranged for some product demonstrations, which reassured the physicians that templates with point-and-click data-entry options, drop-down menus, and perhaps even a structured patient self-assessment or personal health record would be available so that they would be doing very little typing. Furthermore, the demonstration showed that, as the information was being entered into the EHR, the template could be context-sensitive, recognizing, for instance, that the patient has diabetes and providing guidance on what diabetes-related information the physicians should collect. Even though use of templates would reduce typing, the physicians learned that they would have to review the vendor-provided templates to be sure they met the physicians' expectations. Moreover, the practice would likely have to modify the templates to conform to the practice's standards and the physicians would have to achieve some level of standardization of documentation across the practice, in addition to keeping the templates up to date.

The entire process of establishing this goal explained a lot to these physicians. Even though they had seen some product demonstrations and discussed the benefits of EHR, they had done so only from a 30,000-foot-level, so to speak. They had not yet internalized what the EHR would mean to them directly as they performed their work. Interestingly, the physicians in this practice went on to set several additional goals, finding that the exercise pushed them to understand how an EHR worked and helped them realize the changes it would bring about. They also felt better prepared to evaluate vendor offerings.

Goal Setting and Change Management

Going through a process of identifying goals for an EHR also can help potential users "buy into" the results, but the goals must be clear and complete. Generally, people who set their own goals are more inclined to commit to achieving them than if they are told what to do. However, clear articulation of the intent of the goals and how they should be achieved is another critical element of getting all stakeholders to adopt the goals. An example from a hospital considering acquiring a point-of-care charting system is illustrative:

> A large hospital about to embark on an electronic documentation system decided to start with nursing. As part of the planning process, the hospital created teams of nurses to review the various types of documentation they performed. The planners' purpose was to ensure that all the data currently collected could be accommodated through the electronic system, eliminated as unimportant, identified as data to be collected by someone other than a nurse, or identified as data to be obtained from some other source. As one team of nurses started to review their patient admission documentation, they were surprised to find how many forms they used and how much time it took to complete them. In total, the team identified 11 different forms and found that, on average, nurses spent about 1.75 hours completing them. The nurses then analyzed the data on each form and recognized that many contained duplicate data, some contained data from an information system elsewhere in the hospital, and some contained data that were not needed. The nurses estimated they could eliminate almost 1.25 hours by adopting a point-of-care charting system integrated with other systems in the hospital. They set as their goal the completion of admission documentation within 30 minutes. Interestingly, however, as the team members discussed their findings with their colleagues and as word spread about the time that would be saved, several nurses approached their union representative with concerns that the new system would cost them their jobs. Thus, although the planning and goal setting had been fine, the team had failed to state the goal in a way that articulated the true benefits of the new system, which would be to free up time so that the nurses would be able to provide better information to patient families, support patients in following care instructions, take more care in administering medications to reduce errors, and so on.

This scenario illustrates just one potential outcome of goal setting. Many other scenarios have played out with respect to the time it takes to complete the nursing assessment—in some cases, use of an EHR increases documentation time whereas EHR documentation in other situations takes less or equal time than traditional methods. When reviewing studies of the effects of an EHR, it is important to recognize that they typically measure EHR benefits in isolation without analyzing the root cause that explains why results are what they are. For example, Moody et al. (2004) studied documentation by 100 nurses at a Florida hospital and found that one-third of nurses perceived that using EHRs decreased their workload, and two-thirds of nurses preferred bedside documentation but reported that environmental and system barriers often prevented EHR charting at the bedside. This study then took the next step to look at usability issues—finding, for example, that computer access was not available 20 percent of the time; 50 percent of nurses reported that nurse colleagues continued to chart on paper, resulting in a hybrid environment that was difficult to manage; 60 percent of participants reported they used multiple documentation systems and consequently had to learn how to use more than one system (which might affect the nurses' efficiency); and half of the nurses believed that interruptions when documenting were more difficult to manage when they used an EHR that timed out or had multiple screens to follow.

The important lesson here is to establish goals that set the parameters within which the outcomes are expected to result. A goal that documentation time for nursing assessments will be reduced by half is specific and measurable. However, the goal is unachievable if the organization does not establish that nurses will have sufficient access to workstations.

Another important element of goal setting is buy-in. Goal setting is important to the change management process. People who set their own goals and understand what the goals mean will be enlightened and will likely have a strong desire to see them accomplished. These stakeholders can anticipate the change and be more accepting of it. However, in most healthcare organizations, not everyone can be involved in every planning and goal-setting process, so care must be taken to state goals in a manner that describes their actual benefit (for example, not to reduce nurses' hours but to make better use of their time).

Goal Setting and Vendor Selection/Contract Negotiation and Implementation Planning

Not every EHR component is selected separately. To the contrary, organizations will implement some components as part of a larger EHR project. Beyond the EHR, healthcare organizations will also implement other types of health IT. Regardless of the scope of the project, goal setting can help describe more fully what functions are desired and establish performance metrics the vendor should demonstrate. For instance, as the United States moves to expand quality reporting as part of the reimbursement mechanism, providers want to be able to collect the relevant quality data in their EHR to avoid costly and error-prone abstraction. They also want to be able to evaluate the data being submitted and perform their own analysis, and they are therefore increasingly seeking other types of health IT to perform such functionality. If, for example, a clinic sets a goal of improving its childhood immunization rates by a certain percentage, it will want to evaluate products that can collect immunization data, embed clinical decision support to remind providers to collect the data, and provide monthly or quarterly reports on progress toward the goal.

Part of any contract negotiation with a health IT vendor will be to establish the implementation plan. Although ultimately there will be a very detailed project plan to guide the many steps in system configuration, testing, and training, the overall implementation plan should be guided by the project goals.

Goal Setting and System Configuration, Testing, and Training

When goals include clear metrics and explicit descriptions of how health IT will realistically help achieve the specific objectives, a healthcare organization can use these goals to help focus its health IT implementations. For instance, a bar code medication administration record (BC-MAR) system involves more than scanning a patient's identification band and then administering medication. Rather, it is a complex system that requires connectivity with other information systems and substantially alters workflow in ways that can affect the flexibility of patient care and the clinician's application of professional judgment; furthermore, the system must be configured to ensure that its templates aid in capturing the appropriate information and guide the practice of care (Guite et al. 2006). If medications are normally distributed early in the morning but a particular patient takes them at night, the BC-MAR system must allow the nurse to make appropriate adjustments in the schedule. If medications are to be administered on a certain schedule but the patient is in surgery at the scheduled time, the system should be sufficiently flexible to allow for this variation without treating it as a medication administration error. The system must permit clinicians to override alerts and reminders where professional judgment indicates a reason to do so. Although there is some controversy over whether these overrides should be documented, many systems have such functionality as a means to reduce questions during the patient care event and after, including during quality reviews and potential litigation (Rollins 2005).

At the conclusion of workflow redesign and system configuration, the same goals that supported the implementation steps should be used to construct test scenarios and training tools. As users anticipate all potential scenarios in which they will use the system during their workflow analysis and redesign, the documentation should serve to be a test script to ensure that the system works as intended. If not, obviously more system configuration or attention to workflow will be needed; or the organization may determine that the system does not have the hoped-for capabilities and sanctioned workarounds need to be planned. Once a system is fully tested and new workflows are documented, these test scenarios are used to train all new users. Test scenario development and training are vital for all users—including physicians who may think they can intuitively learn the system. In fact, one industry observer notes that organizations should run away from any EHR vendor who claims that minimal training is needed because the system can be learned as you go. This observer further argues, "Trying to master sophisticated EHR software is roughly akin to having been handed a 747 [plane] and told to fly it" (Aita 2008).

One of the major reasons that systems are not used effectively is lack of training—not just on the system features but also regarding new workflows. According to Newman (2010), the best training starts "early and trains to workflows—not [just] how to 'push buttons.'"

Monitoring Goal Achievement

Writing SMART goals that carry appropriate expectations is an exercise in futility if goal setting is not followed by measuring the goals' results, identifying successes, and providing support for making progress or course corrections where needed (Amabile and Kramer 2010). Figure 4.4 provides a description of a process that may be useful to reassure individuals engaged in writing goals that their goal activity is important, that goal accomplishments will be measured, and that lack of success for any reason is not subject to punishment.

Check Your Understanding 4.1

Using the template in figure 4.2, write a SMART goal for a healthcare organization to support patient use of a personal health record.

Types of Benefits

Healthcare organizations rarely find it easy to determine whether expected benefits have been achieved. When conducting benefits studies, it is important to understand the nature of the benefits, which may be quantitative or qualitative, and quantifiable or anecdotal. In healthcare, benefits of initiatives such as the EHR and health IT may also be clinical or financial.

Figure 4.4. Monitoring SMART goal achievement

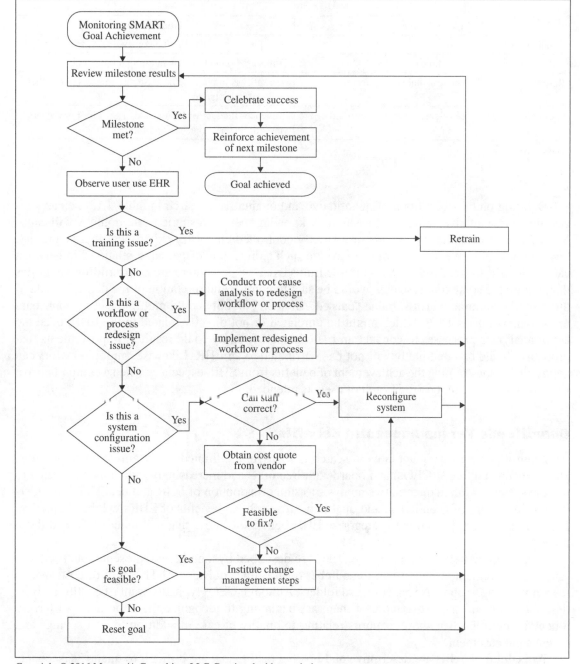

Quantitative Versus Qualitative Benefits

A research methodology perspective is a good source for understanding the difference between the terms *quantitative* and *qualitative*. A benefits study is actually quite similar to a research study in many respects. In her chapter on research methods in *Health Information Management: Concepts, Principles, and Practice*, Forrestal distinguishes between quantitative and qualitative research, as described in table 4.1 (2016).

Table 4.1.   Comparison of assumptions in quantitative and qualitative research approaches

Quantitative	Qualitative
Single truth exists	Multiple truths exist simultaneously
Single truth applies across time and place	Truths are bound to place and time (contextual)
Researchers can adopt neutral, unbiased stances	Neutrality is impossible because researchers choose their topics of investigation
Chronological sequence of causes can be identified	Influences interact with one another to color researchers' views of the past, present, and future

Source: Forrestal 2016

Building on the description of quantitative and qualitative research in table 4.1, one can suggest that a quantitative benefit is measured by knowing there is a single truth: doing X will cause Y to happen. Unfortunately, outside of a strictly controlled chemistry experiment in a laboratory, few things in life have a single truth or involve such a direct and discernable relationship between cause and effect. More frequently, multiple truths exist—that is, there are **confounding variables** that, within the context of research, would be said to confuse interpretation of the data and make it difficult to determine which variable "caused" another. Not only could multiple factors contribute to the benefits of an EHR, which might be unrelated or not directly related to the EHR, even the act of analyzing processes to conduct an EHR feasibility study could result in improvements that probably should be—but likely will not be—attributed to an EHR. Likewise, multiple factors can contribute to constraining the achievement of benefits from EHR, especially when a comprehensive EHR system and other health IT are not used as intended.

Quantifiable Versus Anecdotal Benefits

Although it is clear that quantitative research is focused and limited to certain domains of study, chief executive officers (CEOs) and boards of directors—and increasingly individuals expected to use the system—want a quantitative analysis to support adoption of EHR and health IT. Considering the definitions of quantitative and qualitative research, all benefits of EHRs will be qualitative. Probably a better approach is to categorize EHR benefits as those that are quantifiable and those that are anecdotal.

Quantifiable benefits are tangible. They are described by a numeric representation, such as a rate of improvement, a decrease in the number of full-time equivalent (FTE) staff, or cost savings from not having to purchase paper record folders. Although CEOs typically want a benefits analysis described in monetary terms, more of them are beginning to recognize the importance of having a benefits portfolio that shows benefits relating to quality of care in addition to cost savings and revenue enhancement.

Anecdotal benefits are descriptive and involve factors that are difficult to quantify. Accounts of events that occurred or were avoided when the EHR was used may be examples of anecdotal benefits. For example, the fact that a talented nurse turned down an employment offer because she would not work for an organization that did not have an EHR might be persuasive anecdotal evidence to support the case for EHR implementation. Another example may be that an EHR improves care of patients with diabetes by more closely monitoring their compliance with their treatment regimen. Anecdotal evidence of benefits can be strengthened in several ways. One way is to gather and report anecdotes from other organizations, taking care to select relevant stories from similar situations (an anecdote from an academic medical center might not seem convincing to the CEO of a community hospital). Another way to strengthen anecdotal evidence is to combine it with evidence from **meta-analysis**, which integrates research findings from many similar organizations that use similar systems so that all evidence is consistent and substantiates the benefit statement. Important distinctions between quantifiable and anecdotal evidence are shown in table 4.2.

Quantifying benefits is both an art and a science. Not everything can be studied in depth, but what is to be studied should be decided by not only how easy it is to study but also how meaningful the study is to the organization. For example, if an organization is exploring whether to eliminate dictation and have clinicians enter data directly into an EHR, it is easy and important to study lines and cost of transcription. However, it is difficult to study the amount of time that use of the EHR saves a clinician in a day. A stopwatch time study could be done, but it probably would be of little value. Even if the study were designed so it would not interrupt workflow (which is one of the biggest challenges in such research), clinicians who were not included in the study would probably still discredit the findings. All clinicians believe they are unique or different or that their patients are sicker than anyone else's patients.

Time savings may be achieved in downstream processes or by eliminating wasted time, even if these savings are difficult to measure. For instance, the physician may find that entering a prescription into an e-prescribing (e-Rx) system takes as much time or more than scribbling a prescription on a pad of paper. However, the system saves time later in the prescribing process because the pharmacist does not have to call the physician to interpret a scribbled prescription or review contraindications to which the prescriber could have been alerted through the clinical decision support associated with the e-Rx system. In addition to not tracking such downstream time savings, physicians may not think about the time they spend by searching a paper record for information about the patient's allergies, other medications being taken, or laboratory test results that may reveal contraindications. Several studies have found that a significant number of questions arise during the course of patient care that could benefit from using a reference to find an answer, but 45 percent to 70 percent of those questions go unanswered because few physicians are willing to take the time to find an answer, or because they believe they could not find an answer (Ketchell et al. 2005; Ely et al. 2007; Graber et al. 2008). Not only is time wasted, but the impact on patient care is unknown.

Benefits Measurement, Reporting, and Improvement

To assess whether goals are achieved, an organization must establish metrics with which to measure benefits. Measurement alone, however, rarely results in continual improvement. Measurement findings must be reported to the appropriate stakeholders so they have feedback on whether desired benefits are being realized or if improvements are needed.

Table 4.2.   Quantifiable versus anecdotal evidence

Quantifiable/Tangible	Anecdotal/Intangible
Numeric representation (preferably in monetary terms)	Scenario-based case description
Requires establishment of metrics and baseline data for comparison	May reflect quantifiable data from other sources if organization is unwilling or unable to conduct its own study
Provides opportunity for course correction	Requires leadership faith in others' experiences; does not provide direct opportunity for course correction
Example: Today, organization spends Y dollars on transcription. EHR will reduce transcription by X percent, resulting in cost savings of Y − X dollars.	Example: EHR has contributed to attracting qualified nursing staff as evidenced by consistent comments in staff evaluations and applicant interviews.

Measurement

A **metric** is a standardized description of what will be measured. For example, to measure the height of something, one can use a ruler that references a standardized way (such as the metric system) to measure units of length (for example, centimeters). When measuring benefits, one also chooses standards against which the measurement will be taken. The more precise and standardized the metric is, the more accurate the measurement can be. (Note that **measure** is often used, incorrectly, as a noun in place of the term "metric." For example, it is often common to hear or read that "**clinical quality measures [CQM]** are used to measure results." In keeping with common usage and to avoid confusion, this book will use the term "measure" when referring to both the metric [noun] and the process of measurement [verb], but readers should be aware that *metric* is the more correct noun and may be encountered in scientific publications.) There are two primary types of measures: process and outcomes.

Process Measures

Process measures are those that "capture the rate of use of specific processes" (Janssen Pharmaceuticals, 2014). Process measures can be used to measure any type of process, including revenue cycle processes (such as the rate at which patient insurance eligibility is checked), administrative processes (such as the rate at which patient identification is verified before procedures are performed), and clinical processes (for example, the rate at which smokers are enrolled in smoking cessation programs). Process measures contribute to patient satisfaction and the quality of the care experience.

Outcomes Measures

Outcomes measures report a change in a condition (Janssen Pharmaceuticals 2014). They are critical to ensuring that processes are working and improvements are actually occurring.

Just as with process measures, outcomes measures can be financial (for example, eligibility checking decreases bad debt by 30 percent), administrative (for example, patient identification verification has resulted in 75 percent fewer medication errors), or clinical (for example, Mary's hemoglobin A1c improved from 9 percent before she quit smoking to 8.2 percent after 6 months in the smoking cessation program). Improvement in processes should yield improvement in outcomes; however, process improvement does not always guarantee improvement in outcomes; therefore, it is important to measure outcomes as well as processes.

Reporting

Reporting systems collect data consistent with the metrics or measures set forth, offer comparisons and trending information between baseline data and current state, and may provide recommendations for further improvement. Reports of measures should be directed to those individuals who can make changes that result in improvement. However, a culture of shame and blame in healthcare may lead healthcare employees to hide rather than report errors; this culture has been cited as the antithesis of a culture of safety (Wiseman and Kaprielian 2014). The Joint Commission has called for a framework to create a culture of safety in healthcare, which has been coined a "just culture" (Wyatt 2013). A **just culture** ensures a balanced approach to error, recognizing that a "trust, report, and improve" cycle promotes proactive and reactive risk reduction because staff are willing to report errors, close calls, and unsafe situations and solve problems before patients are harmed. The just culture model recognizes two key concepts. First, it is the nature of humans to make mistakes. No one wants to make mistakes, but they happen. Second, accountability must be shared. Individuals are accountable for the quality of their choices; however, organizations are accountable for the systems they have designed, and caregivers should be held blameless when a system or process allows an error to happen (Panten and Torrance 2014). The American Nurses

Association (ANA 2010) has adopted a position statement that interprets the just culture concept and encourages classifying human errors as inadvertent, risky where risk is not recognized or is mistakenly believed to be justified, and reckless behavior.

Reports of measures must be accurate, trustworthy, timely, equitable, and transparent. Inaccurate or dated metrics, sloppy data collection, out-of-date reports, and other issues can derail the use of quality reporting for improvement.

Reports must also be easy to understand. Graphics can be very effective, but they must be simple and to the point. Many clinicians do not study statistics in school, and complex scatter diagrams, three-dimensional views of data, and other types of sophisticated graphics may only frustrate them. Using the distinction between individual versus organizational accountability and the ANA classification of errors can help ensure that reporting is equitable and transparent.

Improvement

Reports that allow individuals to recognize a specific opportunity for improvement help generate improvement. EHRs and other types of health IT that provide data specific for the case at hand and at the point of care can be effective—if the data are right for the context. For example, a physician's ratings for diabetes care may help a patient select a doctor, but reporting the ratings is not helpful during the actual visit. In contrast, real-time analysis can be effective when it relates to care of a specific patient, such as pointing out that a particular patient with diabetes is not an appropriate candidate for a hemoglobin A1c goal of less than 7 percent. Reports do not have to relate solely to clinical benefits. A physician who is aware that the patient is worried about medical expenses may value information about the cost of a specific drug. Integrated clinical and financial data available at the point of care have the potential to help providers select appropriate drugs, make referrals, avoid duplicative and unnecessary diagnostic studies, and coordinate care.

In some settings, reporting may encourage healthy competition that can effectively lead to change. Where clinicians have easy access to trend data for themselves and others, as well as information that supports the need for improvement, they may be inclined to do better. Seeing scores go up for both individuals and the group as a whole is gratifying and encourages continual improvement. In fact, in Minnesota, where a community measurement program has been in place since 2005, healthy competition across all clinics in the state has resulted in several of the measures being retired because they are at a Six Sigma point from 100 percent (Minnesota Community Measurement 2014).

Check Your Understanding 4.2

Indicate whether the following statements are true or false (T or F):

1. All anecdotal benefits are quantifiable.

2. Quantitative benefits of EHR and health IT are almost impossible to determine because of confounding variables.

3. Meta-analysis refers to conducting a research project to achieve a single point of truth.

4. The terms "metric" and "measure" have the same meaning.

5. A good way to determine outcomes is to infer them from process measurement.

6. A balanced approach to reporting errors is termed a "just culture."

7. Healthy competition can be an effective means to achieve improvement.

Clinical Benefits

Clinical quality measures (CQM) have been established to measure outcomes for many common disease conditions. For example, the hemoglobin A1C test is a standard metric used to measure whether a patient's diabetes is "under control." The results of this test for any given patient may be compared to the generally recognized desired outcome. However, in reality, measuring health status and treatment outcomes is not this simple. The hemoglobin A1C test result is a good measure, but it has been modified over time by new research findings. Prior to 2008, a hemoglobin A1C result of less than 7 percent was understood to indicate that a patient's diabetes was controlled. Then, new findings suggested that the 7 percent benchmark was not necessarily appropriate for all patients, and the metric was adjusted to less than 8 percent for most people with diabetes—although hemoglobin A1C less than 7 percent is still appropriate for selected patients (Janssen Pharmaceuticals 2014). Hemoglobin A1C is also not the only factor used to determine the health status of a patient with diabetes. Recognizing that factors relating to comorbidities also affect the health status of people with diabetes, the Minnesota Community Measurement program (2014) describes "The D5" (measures of blood pressure, cholesterol, blood sugar, tobacco usage, and aspirin regimen) as treatment goals for people with diabetes. Notably, not all healthcare conditions have even as "good" measures as those for diabetes.

Considerable work is being conducted on creating measures and establishing methods for how to use them to measure healthcare quality (processes and outcomes). The National Quality Forum (NQF) is one organization that CMS turns to for quality measure definition and tools for performance measurement, especially in the MU program (NQF n.d.). Other organizations are also devoted to establishing CQMs—in fact, an issue with CQMs today is that there are too many of these measures. Both the health insurance industry and providers are coming to recognize this issue. America's Health Insurance Plans (AHIP 2013) studied 23 different commercial health plans (Aetna, Cigna, UnitedHealthcare, and others) and found 546 distinctly different measures in use. In addition, AHIP found variation in measures intended to measure essentially the same thing. Furthermore, many of the measures in place were not necessarily contributing to actual quality improvement. Eisenberg and colleagues studied the impact of the MU CQMs and found a lack of clarity in the measure specifications as well as technology challenges where EHRs could not draw relevant data from other systems. Additionally, the **electronic CQM (eCQM)** reporting tools were not aligned with clinical workflow; many of the eCQMs were out of date; and the MU measures were not aligned with measures required by other payers and organizations—often requiring slight but necessary variations in data collection (Einsenberg et al. 2013). The result of these studies and other efforts has been the development of a Core Quality Measures Collaborative between AHIP, CMS, NQF, and national physician organizations (Caramenico 2015).

Measuring the Clinical Impact of the EHR and Health IT

The EHR and other types of health IT offer many potential benefits. Many of the CQMs in the MU program are intended to measure how well the EHR can support clinical benefits. Some specific examples of additional other considerations are as follows (AMGA and JHD Group 2009):

- Access to clinical information
- Patient follow-up/recalls
- Reduced errors/patient safety
- More tailored patient education
- Enhanced documentation

- Physician-patient communication/more time to spend with patients
- Clinical decision making with guidelines and protocols
- New models of care

Access to Clinical Information

Better access to clinical information not only supports provider productivity but also contributes directly to better diagnosis and treatment. Patient records that are immediately accessible in the emergency department can ensure that a patient's chronic conditions and current medications are taken into account during his or her evaluation and treatment. Answering phone inquiries and triaging patients in real time may prevent utilization issues and ensure that proper treatment is provided when necessary. Clinical information that is always available can provide a much fuller picture of a patient's health history. For example, in a busy inner-city outpatient department, the ability to have a single problem list that was always the first screen presented led to identification of an unusual syndrome in a patient that might otherwise have gone years without being recognized.

Patient Follow-Up/Recalls

The ability to generate patient lists that can be used to create materials to contact patients (including labels, letters, and even automated messages) is an easy benefit to achieve from an EHR. Such materials may be used not only to remind patients about their appointments but also to schedule visits for chronic care patients, remind patients about their preventive service needs (for example, immunizations or mammograms), check on patients after visits to determine whether they understand their instructions and are following their treatment regimen, and ensure that all patients who need follow-up after diagnostic studies are contacted. Organizations can also promptly notify patients of Food and Drug Administration drug and device recalls by generating a list of patients on the specific drug or using the specific device.

Reduced Errors/Patient Safety

Error reduction and improved patient safety are accomplished primarily through alerts and reminders—such as drug allergy and drug–drug contraindication alerts that are embedded in computerized provider order entry (CPOE) or e-Rx systems and BC-MAR systems. Dmyterko (2010) describes a number of additional technological tools that can help minimize human error. In addition to alerts and reminders, such technology can contribute to medication reconciliation, notify the practitioner when a redundant test is ordered (which if performed could cause patient harm or discomfort), help appropriately schedule diagnostic testing, provide alerts when a patient's vital signs are deteriorating, and supply other information to reduce error. Dmyterko, however, also states that organizations may need to customize the technology to suit the nature of their staff and patient population. For instance, a teaching hospital may require more alerts to be embedded in technology than would a community hospital. Dmyterko also raises the important point that the human habit of relying on technology to solve problems can be hard to break. Individuals from the studies cited by Dmyterko were quick to point out that "certain critical thinking skills lapse after the implementation of new technology," but these skills are essential and must be emphasized in the training and reinforcement of use of the technology.

More Tailored Patient Education

Although many providers keep a supply of instructional handouts available to give their patients, the EHR not only can generate handouts as needed but can also incorporate into patient education a patient's specific medications and other information that may be unique to his or her situation.

The MU incentives require that providers give each patient an after-visit summary that includes patient instructions as well as an entire description of the details of the encounter, as suitable for the patient. Boast and Potts (2010) report on several examples of improved patient comprehension and follow through with use of automating discharge instructions. In addition, such instructions significantly reduced calls and readmissions to a medical center where patients were given written information, including pictures, about what to expect after surgery (Kelly 2010).

Enhanced Documentation

Although enhanced documentation may generally be regarded as an administrative issue, the legibility, accuracy, and completeness of documentation all contribute significantly to reduced errors and improved quality of care. When clinical decision support is integrated with documentation applications, these applications also support accuracy and completeness of data and address quality of care beyond patient safety.

The benefits of CPOE and other components of EHRs are not new. Teich and colleagues began publishing extensive studies on the impact of clinical decision support on medication errors and adverse drug events in 1996. Table 4.3 provides a sample of some of the results they identified at Brigham and Women's Hospital (Teich et al. 1996). Interestingly, these researchers attempted to estimate the monetary value of the patient safety and quality effects by estimating the costs of an average day of hospital care and how many more days a patient would have to use hospital services if the adverse drug event or medication error had occurred. Teich and colleagues did not evaluate costs associated with hospital liability, which could be impressive. They also did not estimate any postdischarge costs associated with the detrimental effects to the patient. Historically, costs of longer lengths of stay and readmissions have generally been reimbursed; however, the Affordable Care Act (ACA) of 2010 directs Medicare to penalize hospitals with higher than expected readmission rates for certain specified conditions.

A final consideration with respect to documentation benefits, however, is that many physicians see data entry into a computer as a clerical function. Historically, physicians dictated notes, discharge summaries, and so on, and the transition to data entry into EHRs has been challenging for physicians. Many physicians find data entry into CPOE systems particularly cumbersome. In the paper environment, the physician would handwrite an order and someone else would key it into the

Table 4.3. Examples of medication errors reduced through CPOE

Intervention	Description	Means of Benefit	Potential #/Year	Effect	Savings $/Year
Ondansetron guidance	Changed default frequency for IV administration	Guided toward effective, but less expensive dose	3,000 displays per year	92% switch to new dose	$500,000 in charges
Vancomycin guidance	Prompt to guide initial use of drug and to consider stopping after 3 days	Reduce overutilization; decrease spread of vancomycin-resistant *Enterococcus*	5,000 orders per year	Under study	Under study
Nephros/ Gerios	Changes recommended dosing based on patient's renal function and age	Prevent adverse events due to failure to reduce drug dosing	106 adverse events per year	Not measured yet	$640,000 in costs*

Source: Teich et al. 1996.

*Estimated hospital cost savings based on prior analysis that shows that each adverse event costs $6,000 to the hospital. These costs are primarily due to extended length of stay and to additional testing and therapeutic measures needed because of the adverse event. This figure excludes cost and detrimental effect to the patient, as well as any liability the hospital may incur.

computer to be communicated to the various ancillary departments required to carry out the orders. With a CPOE system, the physician must go through a lengthy checklist to place orders and must respond to various alerts and reminders from the clinical decision support embedded in the system.

Recently, physicians have started hiring **scribes**, individuals who document in the EHR as the physician is examining the patient. The intended benefit from this practice is to free up physician time, presumably to improve patient communications. Some physicians, however, may use scribes to improve their personal productivity in order to see hospitalized patients more quickly or to see more clinic patients. There are risks in using scribes, especially for order entry into CPOE systems. *Kaiser Health News* reports that many scribes do not have the qualifications to make sure they put the right information into the CPOE system (Gillespie 2015). There are also concerns that patients may not fully disclose information with a scribe present in the examining room. With the number of scribes expected to increase significantly in the coming years, some believe improved regulation and training is needed. The Joint Commission does not endorse or prohibit the use of scribes, but it does not permit delegation of authentication and does not support scribes being used to enter orders due to the additional risk added to the process (Joint Commission 2016). American Health Information Management Association has provided guidance on use of scribes that should be a critical starting point for any policy on their use (AHIMA 2012).

Physician–Patient Communication/More Time to Spend with Patients

Many of the benefits (and challenges) of health IT converge to affect workflow. Ideally, having information at their fingertips would make practitioners more efficient and allow them to spend more time to spend with patients, improve care, and contribute to the improved quality of life for both patients and caregivers. Although the changes in documentation have not as yet resulted in more time for clinicians to spend with each individual patient, there have been breakthrough strategies that demonstrate that process redesign can achieve such results.

For example, at Wisconsin Hospital and Clinics, intake data did not have to be collected numerous times, and, consequently, nurse time was reduced from 35 to 20 minutes for initial office visits and from 35 to 15 minutes for return visits. Moreover, patients were considerably less frustrated because they no longer had to fill out forms with the same information for every part of the clinic they visited (Dassenko and Slowinski 1995). Other studies have reported even more dramatic results in settings where patients used **automated history taking** tools to enter information in advance of a visit (Bachman 2003; Adamson and Bachman 2010). In 2007 Allen Wenner, a family practitioner and vice president for clinical applications design for Primetime Medical Software, told a reporter that his software company's Instant Medical History system reallocated time during a visit away from subjective history taking to treatment planning and patient education (Conn 2007). (These results are summarized in figure 4.5.)

Wenner also notes that such software improves identification of depression by family physicians, where more patients tend to be more open with the computer, particularly with highly sensitive information such as feelings of depression.

Even in an emergency department (ED), where one would not necessarily expect to find people taking the time to use a computer, Porter and colleagues found that electronic information about medication allergies and history of present illness provided by the parents of pediatric patients in two EDs met or exceeded the quality of data documented by ED nurses and physicians (Porter et al. 2010). In a pilot study at the Mayo Clinic Department of Family Medicine, Adamson and Bachman (2010) found that online office visits (often referred to as **e-visits**) allowed the clinic to document and bill for "processes previously given as a free service or from nurse triage and subject to malpractice (protocols)." While there are pros and cons of e-visits, some researchers predict that their use will markedly increase with improvements in health IT and pressures to reduce health care costs while improving the quality of care (Porter 2013). An increasing number of payers are

Figure 4.5.   12-Minute patient visit without and with patient history-taking software (S/W)

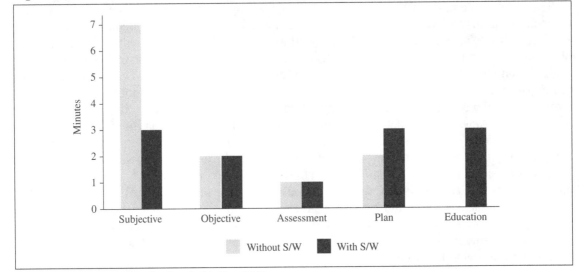

Source: Compiled from information described in Conn 2007.

reimbursing for e-visits (Joseph and Stuhan 2015), and the American Academy of Family Physicians (AAFP) provides basic guidelines to help ensure that quality of care during e-visits is high (AAFP 2015). However, some physicians may shy away from the use of e-visits, perhaps because they fear adopting this innovation will be disruptive to their workflow.

Clinical Decision Making with Guidelines and Protocols

According to many published reports, adding reminders at the point of care that are **evidence-based** (resulting from a research study or expert panel consensus process) can lead to specific clinical improvements. Not all of these reminders have been in the form of alerts. Other types have included protocols for adjusting hypertensive drugs (Goldstein et al. 2002), queries to registries that improve compliance with diabetes care guidelines (Stevens 2010), standardized order sets that support management of complications such as pneumonia (Peitzman 2009), and calculators that provide more appropriate dosing of renally cleared medications (Fields et al. 2008).

Two other factors are important to consider when adopting evidence-based clinical guidance into EHR systems. First, data from EHRs can make an important contribution to strengthening the guidance. Such "rapid learning" can create a much larger research base of patient experience (Manos 2007), which is important because evidence-based guidance is often based on **clinical trials** (research studies on human subjects to determine the efficacy of a treatment regimen) that use small groups of participants (Tonelli 2006). Second, as Tonelli observes, "application of (evidence-based medicine) EBM to individual cases requires clinicians to ask whether the patient at-hand differs in a meaningful way from the 'average' patient of the clinical trial."

New Models of Care

New models of care that rely heavily on the EHR and other types of health IT are being designed to improve the quality, cost, and experience of care. Some of them focus on payment for care and others focus on the delivery of care. Together they support the Triple Aim goals.

Some of the new models of care originate from payers and attempt to better coordinate care among providers. These models include **care coordination, care management, case management, disease management, utilization management**, and **discharge planning**. (See table 4.4 for definitions of these terms.) Many of these new models of care either analyze claims data stored in

Table 4.4. Definitions of models of care, payment models, and organizational models[1]

Concept	Definition
Models of Care	
Care coordination	Deliberate organization of patient care activities between two or more participants (including the patient) involved in a patient's care to facilitate the appropriate delivery of healthcare services. Care coordination may include facilitation among providers as well as social services (AHRQ 2007).
Care management	Program that supplies systems, science, incentives, and information to improve medical practice and help consumers become engaged in a collaborative process designed to manage medical, social, or mental health conditions more effectively and hence improve wellness (CHCS 2007).
Case management	A collaborative process of assessment, planning, facilitation, and advocacy for options and services to meet a consumer's health needs through communication and available resources to promote high-quality, cost-effective outcomes (CMSA n.d.).
Disease management	A system of coordinated healthcare interventions and communications for populations with conditions in which patient self-care efforts are significant. Also called *integrated care* (URAC 2005).
Utilization management	The evaluation of the medical necessity, appropriateness, and efficiency of the use of healthcare services, procedures, facilities under the provision of the applicable health benefits plan. Also called *medical management* (URAC 2005).
Discharge planning	Case management that focuses specifically on addressing consumers' health needs once discharged from a hospital or other inpatient setting (CMSA n.d.).
Payment Models	
Fee for service (FFS)	A method of payment for healthcare in which doctors and other healthcare providers are paid for each service performed (CHPQR n.d.).
Shared savings	An arrangement in which providers are reimbursed based on FFS but are also eligible to receive shared savings payments after they meet quality performance and risk-adjusted standards. Also called *gain sharing* (CHPQR n.d.).
Shared risk	An arrangement in which providers are reimbursed based on FFS but also are at risk for the same portion of spending over the target as the health plan. If the spending is less than the target, providers share the savings; if spending exceeds the target, the providers share the expense (CHPQR n.d.).
Bundled payments	A method in which payments to providers are based on the expected costs for a clinically defined episode or bundle of related healthcare services, including costs associated with preventable complications (CHPQR n.d.).
Capitation	A fixed payment amount given to providers for the care that patients may receive in a given time period, such as a month or a year. Capitation may be implemented globally for all services or partially for specific services only, and it may be implemented with or without payment adjustments based on measured performance and/or patient acuity or level of risk. Also known as full risk (CHPQR n.d.).
Organizational Models	
Accountable care organization	An organization that includes doctors, hospitals, and other healthcare providers who are not commonly owned or operated as a single unit but who come together voluntarily to participate in one of the new, risk-based payment models (CMS n.d.).
Clinically integrated networks	A legal arrangement, often but not always including restructuring of an integrated delivery network with a single ownership, to improve and maintain the health of the people in their communities (Koppenheffer 2013).

(continued)

---

[1]The definitions in this table are largely from organizations that represent the concept in some official capacity. However, use of the terms in actual practice may vary considerably.

Table 4.4.   Definitions of models of care, payment models, and organizational models (Continued)

Concept	Definition
Models of Care	
Organizational Models	
Patient-centered medical home	A physician practice and patient partnership that provides accessible, interactive, family-focused, coordinated, and comprehensive care and is reimbursed under FFS with reimbursement for care coordination and sometimes pay for performance bonuses. Also known as healthcare home (NCQA n.d.).
Care Delivery Models	
Population health	A cohesive, integrated, and comprehensive approach to health that considers the distribution of health outcomes in a population, the health determinants that influence the distribution of care, and polices and interventions that impact and are impacted by the determinants (Jacobson and Teutsch 2012).
Transitions of care	A continuous process in which a patient's care shifts from being provided in one setting of care to another (Health Affairs 2012).
Patient engagement	The combination of patient activation ("a patient's knowledge, skills, ability, and willingness to manage his or her own health and care") with interventions designed to promote positive patient behavior (Health Affairs 2013).
Shared decision making	A collaborative process that allows patients and their providers to make health care decisions together, taking into account the best scientific evidence available, as well as the patient's values and preferences (Informed Medical Decision Making Foundation n.d.).
Precision/personalized medicine	A medical practice that aims to customize health care, with decisions and treatments tailored to each individual patient in every way possible, often including pharmacogenomics in which drugs are targeted to specific genomes (Mayo Clinic 2015).

payer databases to determine which patients need enhanced management or use payer's contractual requirements to improve the quality and/or cost of care.

New payment models have also been introduced to further relate quality of care to cost of care. Ultimately, these models aim to improve the quality of care so that a healthier populace will not require as much care; it is hoped that this strategy will lower the overall cost of care, which currently represents the largest proportion of the US gross domestic product. The new payment models move away from **fee-for-service (FFS)**—payment that reimburses solely on volume of services performed—to models that shift financial risk for healthcare to providers, thus increasing their incentives to improve quality and hence reduce cost. These models, collectively referred to as **value-based payment (VBP)**, include shared savings, shared risk, bundled payments, and capitation. In these models, providers assume some degree of financial risk as a stimulus to improving care. For example, in a FFS environment, a primary care provider who is not reimbursed for patient follow-up calls may not conduct such calls to determine whether the patient is taking a prescribed medication; however, a provider who receives a VBP may be more likely to follow-up to increase the likelihood that the patient complies with the medication regimen and will experience improved health. Some of these new payment models include the creation of new organizational models that further emphasize the roles of all players in keeping people healthy—even to the point of ensuring that the patient has transportation to a doctor's office for follow-up care or is eating a proper diet. Examples of these new organizational models include the **accountable care organization (ACO]), clinically integrated network (CIN)**, and **patient-centered medical home (PCMH)**. (See table 4.4 for definitions of these models.) All of these payment models require integration of clinical data from EHRs as well as financial data from other health IT systems, such as data warehouses, that support new forms of data analysis.

New care delivery models are also emerging that complement the new payment models in order to further improve the quality, cost, and experience of care. These models include **population health, transitions of care (ToC), patient engagement, shared decision making**, and **precision/personalized medicine**. (See table 4.4 for definitions of these models.) Most EHRs support the collection of data only during the care delivery process for each patient; therefore, these new care delivery models need the support of new types of health IT systems achieve results. For example, in shared decision making, patients must be able to see the impact of various potential treatment regimens on their personal health situation in order to contribute to decisions about their care. This evaluation of treatment options requires access not only to the patient's data in the EHR but also data from a population of patients and modeling tools.

Most coordination of care is focused on patients with high-cost, high-risk conditions and is typically performed by a third party representing either a provider or a payer. Although both payers and providers assert that they want to ensure quality of care, their perspectives on care coordination differ. For many providers, the aim is to get appropriate reimbursement and reduce the potential for claims adjustments and denial; in contrast, payers focus primarily on reducing reimbursement costs. Obviously, ensuring quality of care is of primary interest to patients, and a healthier person will consume fewer resources. An EHR could play a role in quality of care by providing a longitudinal view of the patient's health history that would improve the provider's response to that specific patient's service needs. Furthermore, EHRs could contribute data to a pool of knowledge that would support systematic reviews to improve patient outcomes and healthcare costs (AHRQ 2007). Unfortunately, today's EHRs are not longitudinal, and data warehouses are largely made up of only claims data. Despite these current constraints, technology has the potential for improving the coordination of care even more (Thompson 2010).

Check Your Understanding 4.3

Choose the best answer:

1. Which of the following would be a clinical measure focused on outcomes?

   a. 50% of patients with diabetes see the doctor every six months

   b. 75% of patients with diabetes have hemoglobin A1C below 8%

   c. 80% of patients with diabetes follow the D5 treatment regimen

   d. 95% of patients with diabetes are measuring their own blood sugar

2. Alerts and reminders should be an integral part of EHRs:

   a. As appropriate for the setting of care

   b. In all clinics

   c. In all teaching hospitals

   d. In emergency departments only

3. A way to improve physician time for patient communication is:

   a. Automated history taking performed by patients

   b. Hiring of scribes

   c. Reducing the amount of data collected

   d. Use of nurses to interview patients

4. Which of the following is an example of an evidence-based guideline that is not an alert?

   a. Drug-drug contraindication notification

   b. Pop-up notification that the patient is allergic to penicillin

   c. Reminder to check for influenza vaccination

   d. Standardized order set

5. The focus on health IT needs beyond EHR is *especially* evident from the need to:

   a. Access clinical information

   b. Engage with new care delivery models

   c. Enhance documentation

   d. Improve patient safety

Financial Benefits of Health IT

Determining total cost of ownership, cost-benefit feasibility studies, ROI analysis, and benefits realization studies are critical tools for any new program and are important for monitoring cost-reduction efforts in virtually all existing programs, including the EHR and other types of health IT. Types of financial benefits that can accrue from EHRs and health IT are identified in figure 4.6.

Value from EHR and health IT, however, has become an increasingly important focus. Previously cited in this book was the theme of the 2015 annual conference of the College of Healthcare Information Management Executives (Monegain 2015) where it was observed that there is increasing pressure on chief information officers (CIOs) to "pull value from EHRs" (Monegain 2015). In the past, EHRs came to be considered a cost of doing business. While at least stage 1 of the MU program did essentially require providers to adopt EHR, the cost of meeting the requirements of subsequent stages, concerns by clinicians about their value, and the growing list of other health IT needed to keep pace with other industries and patient expectations has a very high price tag.

Forms of Financial Impact Analysis

Three basic types of financial impact analysis may be performed for an EHR or health IT project. These include cost-benefit feasibility analysis, ROI analysis, and benefits realization studies.

Cost-Benefit Feasibility Analysis

A **cost-benefit analysis** is an estimate of costs and benefits conducted before vendor selection to determine the budget for and feasibility of a given project. The cost-benefit feasibility analysis relies on two other important tools: a total cost of ownership and a pro forma.

A **total cost of ownership (TCO)** estimates all anticipated costs for the project. These costs can be based on rough estimates that are later fine-tuned as actual bids are received from vendors. The costs include both one-time and ongoing costs for hardware, software, physical/environmental changes to the organization, and staff.

Pro forma means "provided in advance," and this tool is used to analyze what an organization's assets, liabilities, and fund balance would be for some period of time into the future if the organization incurred the costs described in the TCO. Thus, the pro forma helps the organization determine whether it can afford the TCO of the new project. Strategic planners need this information, and it

Figure 4.6.   Types of financial benefits associated with EHRs and health IT

Cost Savings
- Eliminate paper chart supplies and associated clerical costs of processing and storing paper charts.
- Reduce transcription and transcription processing costs.
- Reduce copy services through patient access to online information.
- Reduce courier costs through enterprise-wide access to the EHR.
- Reduce malpractice insurance premiums or premium increases by better measuring outcomes, improving outcomes, and increasing patient satisfaction via shared decision making.

Cost Avoidance
- Eliminate need to expand paper chart filing space or warehousing.
- Reduce need to hire more staff when patient volume increases, because current employees work more efficiently.
- Hire fewer specialty staff because existing employees are working at the level of their credentials
- Avoid 30-day readmission penalties from Medicare through improved care coordination in an enterprise-wide health IT environment.
- Reduce the incidence of unnecessary emergency department visits.
- Avoid excessive specialty care referrals.
- Avoid repetitive/unnecessary diagnostic studies.
- Select expensive medications less frequently.

Revenue Increases
- Attract more business.
- Retain patients, due to better follow-up, shorter wait times, and greater patient satisfaction.
- Receive appropriate reimbursement for the level of service provided.
- Earn incentives.
- Reduce lost charges.
- Reduce bad debt.

Contributions to Profit
- Improve cash flow.
- Launch or expand e-visits and telehealth.
- Reduce risk of exceeding expenses in a bundled payment or capitation payment model.
- Reduce lengths of stay or numbers of visits.

Productivity Improvements
- Increase number of patients seen by providers in a day.
- Use physician extenders to see more patients in a day.
- Use time savings in nursing to improve patient instruction, care coordination, and follow-up.
- Use time savings in the front office to increase patient appointment follow-up and improve verification of eligibility for benefits to reduce denial of coverage.
- Use time savings in the back office to negotiate improved contracts and more aggressively perform collections.
- Automate tasks for patients or their caregivers such as appointment scheduling, bill paying, and retrieval of diagnostic study results.

helps the organization respond when a bank or bonding commission that may provide a loan or bond asks: "Can you pay for this initiative (including the cost of the debt) and still keep the organization running?"

ROI Analysis

ROI analysis is used to evaluate the TCO after fairly firm cost and benefits estimates from finalist vendor candidates are available. The comparison of costs and financial benefits given the specific product's functionality is evaluated against the organization's required **payback period** or **internal rate of return (IRR)** threshold criteria. ROI analysis is one of the final steps in vendor selection, and its purpose is to determine which product has the most value—considering that value is a factor of both cost and quality. The result of an ROI analysis is frequently a time-phased budget to ensure the project's expenditures are within the organization's ability to manage its cash flow.

Benefits Realization Study

A **benefits realization study** is an evaluation of the financial benefits that have accrued from the investment made in the project. It may be performed at specific milestones in the life of the project and is used to help in future systems planning, design, and implementation. If either cost-benefit or ROI analysis (or both) is performed, a benefits realization study also can identify any deviations from projected benefits so that corrective measures can be taken.

Data Collection for Financial Impact Analysis

Certain basic data must be collected for any type of impact analysis. Essentially, these are cost data and benefits data.

Cost Data

Collecting cost data for an EHR or other health IT project involves both psychology and financial skill. Organizations may try to attribute only those costs directly associated with the EHR or other type of health IT to the project because these organizations want to keep those costs within some preconceived notion of a budget. However, with this approach, organizations run the risk that they will not anticipate acquisition costs for less-direct but still necessary components and those costs may therefore not be approved. In the end, the failure to anticipate such costs can put the project over budget or diminish success because the additional expenditures could not be made. For example, organizations that do not initially invest in sufficient disaster recovery or other security services could increase their future risk of problems with downtime and data breaches. Alternatively, organizations that attribute all costs to the EHR or other health IT project to ensure its success must plan for greater expenditures from the beginning. This "sticker shock" may delay the project or stretch out the migration path.

Many organizations underestimate the cost of the EHR or health IT project. They often underestimate the costs associated with the level of effort needed to configure the system to their needs, maintain it, and properly train and support users. Furthermore, the impact of the EHR on other systems and associated operations may not be fully anticipated or represented in the cost-benefit feasibility or ROI analysis. That is why it is so critical to develop a migration plan that clearly lays out the various associated strategies for the success of the project. A migration path also contributes to the psychology of budgeting for the project, as executive management and the board of directors understand how the pieces tie together and how ongoing commitment is necessary to keep the project up to date.

The following descriptions help identify all the costs associated with an EHR or other type of health IT. How costs are categorized is not as important as ensuring that all costs are considered. However, care should be taken not to include the same costs more than once.

Hardware Costs

Hardware costs include the cost of computers, network devices, workstations (of all forms), printers, scanners, and any other equipment associated with the project. Sometimes, hardware costs also include special furniture or remodeling. Hardware is usually a one-time, fixed cost unless the equipment is leased, in which case the cost of the lease is spread over time. Even though hardware is generally considered a one-time cost, planning for obsolescence and additions should be identified across the entire budget period.

Software Costs

Software may or may not be a onetime cost. Some vendors price EHR software as a onetime cost that is essentially a license through perpetuity; others sell a software license that must be renewed periodically, at which time the cost will likely increase. Some vendors license EHR software for a given number of users (which may need to be updated as staffing levels fluctuate) or according to some other pricing structure. For physician offices, many vendors price the license per provider and include a ratio of support staff to the provider (for example, four or five support staff to every physician). Thus, software pricing varies considerably.

Software includes not only the software licensed from the EHR or other health IT vendor but any other software that the organization may need to make it work, such as the operating system, database management system, interfaces from other systems, an interface engine, a data repository, rules engines, and so on. Another common software expense is a license fee for access to special utilities, such as report-writing software, Common Procedural Terminology (CPT) codes, drug knowledge databases, pharmaceutical formulary information, and benchmarking data. Additional fees may be associated with using network transmission media. Some vendors include these sorts of additional licenses in their overall licensing agreement. Others price them separately or do not include them at all—in the latter case, the organization must conduct separate negotiations for such licenses.

Implementation Costs

Sometimes, *implementation* and *installation* are used synonymously. However, according to most EHR vendor contracts, **implementation** means that the system has been configured as applicable to the organization, it has been tested, users have been trained, and the system has been readied for go live. In contrast, **installation** refers only to the process of loading software onto applicable servers.

Implementation costs are primarily onetime costs, but because an EHR is often a series of health IT components, these costs can extend over a long period of time. Implementation costs generally include those for project management, installation, system build, workflow redesign, testing, training, go-live and ongoing support, and system maintenance. An EHR vendor may supply these services; an organization may seek consultants to perform such services; or a mix of resources may be used. Implementation costs vary significantly depending on the organization's acquisition strategy (see chapter 7).

Project Management Costs

Project management costs vary depending on the nature of the acquisition strategy and size of the organization. However, organizations rarely find that they can manage an EHR project without incurring costs for some form of project management expertise. Project management costs can also include hiring, contracting, or compensating an informatics specialist, chief medical informatics officer, systems integrator, web administrator, data administrator, IT operations manager, application specialist, and others as applicable.

Installation Costs

In addition to the costs of installing software onto servers, organizations must budget for the installation of hardware by the EHR vendor, a third party, organization staff, or a combination thereof. Some organizations use a third-party hosting company for the bulk of their hardware, whereas others maintain a data center within their organization and manage all of their own equipment. Other hardware requirements depend on what the organization already has in place, but most EHRs and other types of health IT require additional network devices, cabling, human–computer interfaces, printers, scanners, and so on.

Implementation/System Build Costs

Although some set-up is required for any EHR or other type of health IT application, most implementation costs are for the **system build**, which is the configuration of the system to meet the organization's specific needs. It includes creation of master tables with the organization's information, such as its physician list, employee list, names of departments, formulary, guidelines and protocols, and many other types of organization-specific information. It also includes the design and documentation of screens and their drop-down menus, pick lists, and customization of other data-capture tools. Additionally, it includes construction of rules logic, clinical protocols, incorporation of knowledge bases, and other decision-support factors. Most EHR products come with a default set of such system characteristics, and customization increases implementation costs. Interfaces and data conversions may also be considered components of system build.

Workflow and Process Improvement Costs

Workflow and process improvement can either be considered to be part of implementation or treated separately. The latter perspective helps emphasize that workflow and process improvement is more than an aspect of implementation—it is also a consideration during vendor selection as well as a part of the optimization of the EHR or other type of health IT for value achievement.

Workflow and process improvement has not received nearly enough attention—but it is often at the top of the list of things organizations wish they had done earlier and better for EHR implementation (CHCF 2011). Ideally, individuals who currently do the work to be redesigned participate in workflow and process improvement; additionally, organizations can benefit from using consultants to help them. A few EHR vendors include workflow and process improvement in their implementations, but most do not or charge an additional fee.

Testing Costs

Budgets for testing and its associated costs are often inadequate. A test environment and testing processes are used for the initial component development and to test fixes, patches, upgrades, and their associated interfaces without affecting the production systems. Not all organizations create test environments, and some vendors do not support test environments.

Training Costs

Although training is listed toward the end of this discussion of costs, it is performed throughout the entire implementation process, from the initial training for super users through just-in-time training for end users. The importance of training cannot be overemphasized. Training costs include one-time and ongoing costs, as well as direct and indirect costs. Training may be conducted in a variety of ways, but, typically, a set of super users are trained first, often by the vendor and at a direct cost. These individuals then train trainers who train end users. The cost of training super users includes vendor fees and may also include the expense of travel to a vendor training site. If staff must be replaced during their training experience, overtime or replacement staff costs may be incurred. If training can be performed directly on the job, the costs may be minimized but not altogether eliminated.

Other training expenses may include costs associated with outfitting a training room, buying training materials, or establishing a training or demonstration system. An organization could choose to hire temporary staff to train and support users during their initial work with the system. However, if temporary staff are used, the organization will need a plan (and budget) to train newcomers in the future. Most EHR products come with online help, but some organizations prepare a basic set of EHR training materials for all new users, customized to the organization's requirements. The initial training effort will be large, but the organization must remember to also budget for ongoing training of new members of the workforce as well as reinforcement of training.

Another consideration when budgeting for training is reimbursement of physicians for their training time. Physician offices may lose revenue if the physicians' schedules are altered to accommodate the learning curve, and such organizations must be prepared to reimburse (or at least account for) such losses.

Go-live and Ongoing Support Costs

Go-live and ongoing support costs are expenses associated with helping users use the EHR. They begin with the go-live stage and extend through the life of the EHR or other type of health IT. **Support costs** include ongoing training costs for new users, reinforcement training for users not meeting goals, and training on system modifications and upgrades; they may also include the costs of workflow and process improvement activities associated with optimizing value from the EHR and or other health IT. Clinicians need to continually review clinical decision support (CDS) systems and keep CDS tables current with the latest medical knowledge, vocabularies, drugs, and so on. Organizations must regularly audit data quality and take any resulting quality concerns to committees tasked with approving ongoing modifications. In this context, support costs are internal costs incurred by the organization.

Maintenance Costs

Vendors frequently use the terms *support* and *maintenance* synonymously because costs to supply support to troubleshoot software issues are typically included with maintenance costs. In this context, **maintenance costs** refer to the fees paid to vendors to respond to software issues that arise during use as well as to keep the software up to date and supply certain enhancements. Most vendors charge a flat maintenance fee, which can initially be anywhere from 15 percent to 20 percent of the software licensure, subject to annual increases. Other vendors have a fee schedule based on usage, which may be described as a **service-level agreement (SLA)**. Such SLAs may be based on the nature of the service to be provided, the time during which service may be available (for example, 24/7 or only certain hours of operation), or the volume of service calls. Organizations can also purchase a maintenance program for hardware.

Sources of Cost Data

The sources of various cost data and cost estimates depend partly on the timing of the impact analysis. During a feasibility study, the organization will have fairly broad cost estimates but no firm cost data. At this point, the organization may have invited a few vendors to provide a rough cost estimate. However, because the vendor has not yet done a comprehensive evaluation of the organization's present systems, and because the organization may not yet have a comprehensive set of functional requirements, both parties are somewhat "blind." Moreover, at this time, the vendor does not provide any discount or incentive pricing. However, these rough estimates can provide a good budget estimate for the hardware required for the kind of system being considered and a range of prices for the software. The fact that the estimates are not discounted probably is in the organization's favor because discounted costs might contribute to an underestimation of the true cost.

On the other hand, if the organization is conducting an ROI analysis, it will want to obtain a firm quote from the vendor or vendors of choice for the specific configuration desired. At this time, the organization may have already begun to negotiate some form of discount, incentive, or financing and can factor these costs in as well.

In both scenarios, it is important to ensure that as many of the costs as can be identified have been covered adequately. The organization should be realistic in its estimates for potential unplanned costs. Because an EHR or other health IT project is truly a strategic investment—on par with bricks-and-mortar projects with which it regularly competes—contingency costs are common and should be anticipated by the individuals with final authority to approve them. It is not unusual in a building or renovation project to include the costs of dealing with labor issues, unexpected shortages of materials, and so on, and similar contingency costs also should be included in the budget for an EHR or other health IT project. Some organizations budget as much as 30 percent for contingencies, especially when they are new to implementing clinical systems and are planning implementation of a large array of components.

Benefits Data

As described earlier in this chapter, there are five ways to achieve financial benefits: cost savings, cost avoidance, revenue increases, contribution to profit, and productivity improvements.

Cost Savings

The cost savings associated with moving from paper to electronic record keeping can be considerable. The first step to estimate how much will be saved is to determine current paper-processing costs.

The EHR and other types of health IT may also help providers save on malpractice premium insurance. The amount saved will depend on the carrier and the degree to which the provider has baseline data and can demonstrate that risk associated with patient safety issues is reduced and patient outcomes are improved.

Cost Avoidance

Organizations can avoid costs by taking steps to reduce the use of expensive, repetitive, and unnecessary services and procedures. Under the FFS model, payers generally reimbursed these types of services and procedures without question, so they were actually a source of revenue for healthcare organizations. In an era of health reform, however, where profit depends on keeping costs low while ensuring quality of care, healthcare organizations focus on finding ways to simultaneously improve quality and lower costs. For example, care coordination and other programs to keep patients out of the hospital or emergency department or reduce their hospital length of stay can lower the risk of medical errors, the risk of infections that are more prevalent in hospitals than in a patient's home, and the costs associated with those risks (Adamopoulos 2014). Another example of cost avoidance involves improving medication compliance by informing providers and patients about the cost and efficacy of medications. When patients can better afford the cost of their medications, they are more likely to fill prescriptions and take their medications (Iuga and McGuire 2014). In an accountable care organization or other value-based payment model, referring patients only to specialists who have been identified as those with high quality and low cost (dubbed a "narrow network") is a means to reduce overall costs (Herman 2015).

Revenue Increases

The potential for revenue increases from the EHR and other types of health IT has been hotly debated, and the widespread effects of the EHR on revenues in the healthcare industry are not yet known. Although it may seem that every healthcare provider now has an EHR as a result of the MU program, that is not entirely true, especially for small physician practices. Furthermore, some practices and even some hospitals may have an EHR but do not fully utilize it or explain its value to patients. However, when an EHR is used effectively, revenue can increase as a result of patient retention, payer incentives, and reductions in lost charges and bad debt. Patient follow-up after an episode of care as well as for preventive services can also attract more business.

Contribution to Profit

Net profit is the amount of money left after expenses have been paid from revenues. Even though nonprofit organizations are prevalent in healthcare and physician practices are not permitted under Internal Revenue Service rules to build reserves, all organizations must be profitable to stay in business. Profitability in healthcare has generally entailed improving cash flow and generating more revenue than expenses. EHRs and other health IT, however, can significantly improve revenue cycle management and reduce costs such that profits can accrue.

Productivity Improvements

EHRs and other types of health IT can improve productivity, but these improvements may or may not result in actual financial savings and are often not recognized as financial benefits. Most productivity improvement benefits must be projected through process redesign efforts. Each area affected by the EHR or another form of health IT for which an impact analysis is being performed should identify specific goals and the functionality that will assist in achieving those goals, and then commit to seeing the goals realized.

Several sources of data may be used to anticipate productivity improvements. The primary resource should be the workflow and process improvement performed by the organization (see also chapter 5). Vendors with implementation experiences at similar institutions may also have useful insights for the organization regarding where to look for additional benefits. Moreover, the body of literature on EHR and other health IT benefits is solid and fairly extensive and can be invaluable in benchmarking how realistic an organization's forecasts may be. The federal government's website on health IT lists a number of benefits and features statistics on how frequently physicians identify each benefit (HealthIT.gov 2015).

Figure 4.7 illustrates an example of how workflow and process improvement may reduce costs in a variety of ways and how to calculate the cost of a medication error. The figure provides the process redesign tool a clinic used to compare the workflows of processing a prescription refill request from a patient in a manual versus an automated environment.

Figure 4.7.   Achieving value from productivity improvements

Process: Prescription Refill   Department: Nursing   Date: _____

T = Time in number of days   U = Number of units   ? = Potential for error, see explanation below

Current Process	Description	T	U	?	Proposed Process	Description	T	U	?
	Pt calls for refill		10			Pt calls for refill		10	
	Clerk takes message		10	a		Clerk enters message		10	a
	Clerk puts in MD slot	½	10			Routed to RN or MD		10	
	RN reviews message		10			RN/MD rev & rec	½	10	
	Calls pt if incomplete	1	2			To pharmacy		10	
	Requests record	1	5	b					
	RN follow protocol?		10	c					
	Puts in MD slot	½	8						
	RN/MD record		10	d					
	To pharmacy		10						

Summary (Current): 4, 3, 2, 5, 1

Summary (Proposed): 2, 2, 2, 1, 1   ½

Quantitative Benefits:

	# Units /Day	# Min. /Unit	Tot # FTEs	Tot $ FTE/Yr	Material $/Unit	Tot $ Mat/Yr	# Errors /Yr	Ave $ /Error	Tot $ Error/Yr
Present					$0.02	$50	75	$60	$4,500
Clerk	10	5	0.125	$2,600					
RN	10	15	0.313	$11,719					
Total		20		$14,319					
Proposed					$0	$0	0	0	0
Clerk	10	10	0.25	$5,200					
RN	10	5	0.10	$4,773					
Total		15		$9,973					
Savings					$0.02	$50	75	$60	$4,500
Clerk		(5)		($2,600)					
RN		10		$6,946					
Total		5		$4,346					

Assumptions

There are 250 days that the clinic is open in which calls for prescription refills are received from patients. All employees work 8 hours per day and are paid for 2,080 hours per year. The clerk makes $10 per hour, and the RN makes $18 per hour.

Summary of Quantitative Benefits

Although there are fewer steps to the process and less of the RN time reviewing message and medical records, this did not equate to one actual staff person. The $4,346 savings therefore cannot be realized in impact analysis.

Cost savings in materials come about through not recording on a form sent to the medical record. While this is a real cost savings, most organizations do not track cost savings this small.

There is potential for reduced errors. The organization previously did a quality assurance study that demonstrated that there were 75 errors out of 2,500 refills (3%) due to information not being available or other operational considerations. It was estimated that each error resulted, on average, in one additional visit to the clinic, priced at $60 per visit, for a total of $4,500 in loss to profit in a capitated environment.

This $4,500 is the quantitative benefit in contribution to profit.

(continued)

Figure 4.7.   Achieving value from productivity improvements (Continued)

Description of Potential for Error and EHR Improvement
a. Clerk may get the patient's name wrong, in which case there is a delay in waiting for patient to call back and potential for patient to be dissatisfied. Using an EHR, the clerk calls up the patient while on the phone and verifies accuracy of patient name and phone number. The frequency with which this happens is minimal. Clerk may get patient name correct, but wrong telephone number, requiring check that delays processing with MPI if patient must be contacted. The frequency with which this happens is moderate. Clerk may not get complete information necessitating RN review of message and call to patient, constituting a delay and potential for patient to be dissatisfied. The frequency with which this happens is moderate to often. With an EHR that calls up the current medications and prompts the clerk to check off requested refill, opportunity for error is greatly reduced (although still possible for clerk to check off wrong medication). b. In half of the instances, the medical record is required for checking other medications the patient is currently taking, resulting in a significant delay. It is possible, however, that the medical record does not have the desired information or is not requested due to oversight. c. The RN may not follow protocol for whatever reason. The frequency with which this happens is minimal. The EHR will automatically check that there is an RN protocol and route the request to the RN if so, or the MD if not. There is still some delay in that the RN or the MD probably does not clear the in-basket constantly. d. The RN or the MD may err in writing the refill, although there is the potential for error in the EHR. The frequency with which an error in writing happens is minimal; the potential for error through the EHR is considered even less. The record of the refill may also not make it to the applicable medical record. The frequency with which this happens is minimal to moderate. This would be totally avoided in the case of the EHR.

The following metrics quantify the steps in the process described in figure 4.7:

- *Number of units performed:* Generally, this information is captured per day, week, or month, depending on the number of units performed. The goal is to summarize the data on an annual basis.

- *Number of minutes it takes to perform the step:* Generally, the average number of minutes is recorded. If the step takes a highly variable amount of time, the minimum, maximum, and most common times can be recorded. Also, if certain tasks are performed only on certain days of the week or month, care should be taken in performing subsequent calculations. In addition to actual minutes to perform the step, some process redesign analysts may include the number of minutes of elapsed time between steps. This type of data helps illustrate the delay factor.

- *Number of full-time equivalents (FTEs) to perform the step:* Generally, this field identifies the percentage of each FTE's time. The calculation is done in the following manner:

  - Assume it takes 5 minutes to handle a refill call from a patient (the first task) and there are 10 calls per day; thus, 50 minutes are spent on this process per day. If an FTE is 8 hours (480 minutes), the total number of FTEs for this task is 10 percent (50 minutes divided by 480 minutes). However, many process redesign analysts account for staff breaks and therefore use a percentage of the workday rather than the full workday as the basis for the calculation. This percentage is called a person's productivity rate. This productivity rate could be calculated for each worker or class of worker through an observational study, or an industry average could be used. Typically, a productivity rate of 86 percent (or 413 minutes per 8-hour day) is used in healthcare (Dunham-Taylor and

Pinczuk 2005). If that rate is used, the number of FTEs would be 12 percent (50 divided by 413).

  ○ It should be noted that the figure shows multiple tasks the same line, as if they were performed simultaneously. If tasks are truly performed simultaneously by the same person, this approach is acceptable. However, because the goal of process redesign is to reduce the total number of tasks or to shift tasks to lower-paid workers, it may be best to separate the tasks.

- *Cost of FTE per year:* This cost is the salary plus benefits earned by the person performing the task multiplied by the percentage of time spent on the task. If a full-time nurse earning $45,000 per year (salary and benefits) answers the refill calls, the cost of the FTE performing that task per year is 10 (or 12) percent of $45,000, which is $4,500 (or $5,400).

- *Percentage of times a particular decision must be made* (represented in the systems flowchart in figure 4.7 by a diamond shape): The percentage of time that a particular decision must be made can represent a potential for error. Although not always having a monetary amount associated with it, it is a metric to investigate further to describe the potential financial impact. In the example, one of the decisions to be made with respect to prescription refills may be to recall from memory the patient and his or her prescription in the event the chart cannot be found immediately. The risk, of course, is that memory is not perfect, and the chart may reveal a reason for the patient to be seen prior to refill or that the refill dosage or amount needs to be changed. The metric will likely be reported as "number of times refill decisions are made because the chart cannot be found."

- *Number of errors per year:* The number of errors is the actual number of errors. It is unlikely that every task will have a figure in this column. But it should be possible to attribute any errors to a specific task that was performed incorrectly or could not be performed. For example, if a clinic knows three medication errors occurred last year because charts were not reviewed, this number of errors should be posted on the same line as the decision task described earlier. After all metrics are quantified, it may be appropriate to review the task list to determine whether all known errors have been accounted for. If they have not, the task associated with the error should be incorporated into the chart and the metrics.

- *Cost of errors:* Many factors contribute to the cost of an error of any kind. If the organization has kept risk management data, the total cost of all actual errors (of each type) can be recorded here. However, this should be carefully studied, as previous experience is not always an indicator of future events. In the case of medication errors, the following consequences could occur:

  ○ Revisit(s) to clinic

  ○ Additional or repeat diagnostic test(s)

  ○ Loss of revenue if patient chooses to get healthcare elsewhere

  ○ Cost of consultation/specialist visit(s)

  ○ Cost of hospitalization(s)

  ○ Impact on malpractice insurance

  ○ Cost of lawsuit

  ○ Settlement amount of lawsuit

Caution must be exercised when identifying productivity improvements as financial benefits of the EHR project. This example illustrates how to calculate potential financial benefits in staff time. However, unless the staff time can actually be reduced or staff members eliminated, this time savings is still a "soft" benefit, not a financial benefit. Most organizations attempt to redeploy staff where they can, and where there are fractional gains, establish expectations for how the time should be spent. For example, the 10 percent or 12 percent of nurse time could be redeployed to perform patient call-back. This redeployment may result in increased patient satisfaction, which is a good outcome but not a financial benefit. On the other hand, if more time spent on call-backs increases the number of patient visits per day, the result *is* a revenue increase.

Conducting Financial Impact Analysis

Total Cost of Ownership

As described previously, TCO entails detailing every potential cost and financial value of benefits for a project being evaluated. Costs include both initial (one-time) costs and ongoing costs. Benefits include those with a financial component. Figure 4.8 provides a template for the cost component of a TCO as documented in a spreadsheet. It includes some examples of cost elements and their assumptions (but without dollar amounts assigned). Figure 4.9 provides a template for the financial benefits component of a TCO.

Cost-Benefit Analysis

Once all costs and benefits are quantified, they can be compiled into a cost-benefit analysis, such as in the example in figure 4.10. A *net impact* is then determined by subtracting costs from benefits. In

Figure 4.8.   Total cost of ownership template for costs

Figure 4.9.   Total cost of ownership template for benefits

	Benefits	Current Cost Calculation	Goal % Δ	Year 0	Year 1	Year 2	Year 3	Year 4	Year 5
73									
74	Paper Chart Supplies								
75	Assumptions: Annual cost of file folders, forms printing, etc.								
76	Paper Chart Storage								
77	Assumptions: Warehousing fees								
78	Assumptions: Revenue from chart room conversion (be careful to count only once)								
79	Clerical Chart Costs								
	Assumptions: Clerical hours spent								
110	Other, specify:								
111	Assumptions:								
112	**Total Benefits**			0	0	0	0	0	0
113	Impact (Benefits – Costs)			0	0	0	0	0	0
114	Payback Period (Year in which benefits exceed costs)				0	0	0	0	0

Figure 4.10.   Cost–benefit analysis

$M	Year 1	Year 2	Year 3	Year 4	Year 5	Total
Costs						
Hardware	1.30	0.50	0.25	0.00	0.00	2.05
Software	1.20	0.00	0.10	0.00	0.00	1.30
Installation and training	0.50	0.10	0.00	0.00	0.00	0.60
Maintenance	0.00	0.75	0.75	0.75	0.75	3.00
Support	2.60	2.15	1.80	1.80	1.80	10.15
Total	5.60	3.50	2.90	2.55	2.55	17.10
Benefits						
Charge capture	0.00	0.22	0.58	1.20	1.45	3.45
Clinical trials	0.00	0.00	0.10	0.50	0.75	1.35
Decision support	0.00	0.10	0.50	0.75	1.00	2.35
Diagnostic studies	0.00	0.20	0.75	1.10	1.50	3.55
Financial management	0.00	1.10	0.20	0.20	0.20	0.70
Med record operations	0.00	1.50	4.00	4.50	4.50	14.50
Nursing department	0.00	0.00	0.30	0.50	0.60	1.40
Referral management	0.00	0.20	0.50	0.70	0.80	2.20
Total	0.00	2.32	6.93	9.45	10.80	29.50
Net impact	–5.60	–1.18	4.03	6.90	8.25	12.40

this example, the first year's net impact is the total cost of the EHR and its implementation, or $5.6 million. Over the five-year period for which the cost-benefit analysis is constructed, some benefits are realized in the year following implementation, but most do not begin to be realized until the next year. After the second year, most benefits become fairly stable. In this example, there is a positive net impact projected of $12.4 million over a five-year period.

Some practical considerations in presenting a cost-benefit analysis, as shown in figure 4.10, include simple issues, such as naming the years. Some organizations prefer to consider the year of implementation to be year 0, with the first year of benefits being year 1. Obviously, an EHR implementation may take more or less than a year. It may take less time in a small- or medium-sized physician office but will generally take more time in small hospitals and certainly requires more time in medium to large hospitals.

Another consideration is that the benefits are described by type. This is often not how a provider's financial statements look. Income statements and balance sheets are based on revenues and expenses, and assets and liabilities, respectively. As previously noted, some providers would like to see pro forma income statements and balance sheets to determine the impact the EHR or another health IT project has on them. Generally, the accounting staff or finance officer incorporates the cost-benefit analysis data into a pro forma income statement and balance sheet.

Return on Investment Models

In addition to the TCO, cost-benefit analysis, and pro forma financial statements, specific financial measures can be calculated based on the net impact identified from the cost-benefit analysis. The most common financial measures are the payback period, the internal rate of return, and net present value. It should always be remembered, however, that the numeric variables used to compute any of these ROI measures are imprecise. They are based on estimates.

Payback Period

Payback period is the number of years it takes to recoup expenditure. It is typically calculated by dividing the total cost of the project by the annual incremental cash inflows. However, if the annual cash inflows are variable, as in the example in figure 4.10, the payback period is more readily calculated by dividing the total net impact by the total cost. For the example, $12.4 million is divided by $5.6 million to calculate a payback period of 2.2 years. Although the data in figure 4.10, when presented as a table, are intuitive to some, it is often helpful to plot some of this information on graphs for visual effect. Such graphics are useful for presentations to executive management and especially boards of directors. Some of the major pitfalls of the payback period analysis are that it ignores the costs and benefits that occur after the breakeven point as well as the time value of money. By ignoring future costs, this analysis may reflect an accelerated payback period. Figure 4.11 illustrates this concept; it considers the cumulative impact of the EHR, where the cumulative effect of both the project costs and the ongoing costs are not offset until year 4. Some financial analysts prefer to use this alternate timeline as the payback period. By ignoring benefits beyond the payback period, the payback period analysis does not show potential profitability over the longer term. By ignoring the time value of money, the analysis does not address the issue of how funds that make the expenditure are paid for or what the difference would be if the funds were invested another way.

Internal Rate of Return

Internal rate of return (IRR) is a financial measure that considers the time value of money. Its strict definition is the interest rate that makes the net present value calculation equal zero—in other words, the interest rate at which the present value of the projected cash inflows equals the initial investment. To calculate the IRR, a financial calculator, a table of present values for an annuity, or a spreadsheet with an IRR function should be used. For the example in figure 4.10, the IRR is 42 percent. Financial analysts would compare this rate with the rate they could earn on other investments.

Figure 4.11.   Cumulative impact of the EHR

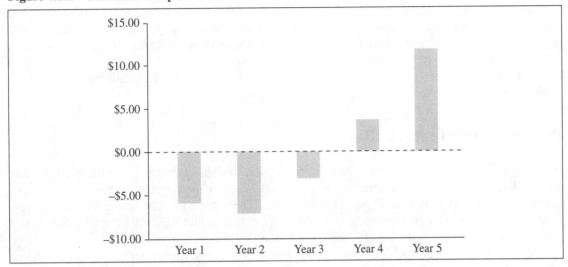

If the project's IRR is higher, investment in the project is good. If it is lower, the investment is not good. Some describe the IRR as the "hurdle rate," because the IRR of the project being proposed has to pass the IRR of alternative investments. It should be noted that an IRR of 42 percent is not only "good" but probably unrealistic, especially given the discussion earlier in this chapter of concerns about not achieving expected value from EHR and health IT. Such an IRR is definitively a STRETCH goal. It may be desirable and even feasible with very strong systems and motivating factors in place. However, in most cases, such a high IRR should trigger a review and modification of the benefits assumptions.

Net Present Value

Net present value (NPV), which is often considered the most precise method of cash flow analysis, is typically reserved for investments of long term, continual value. It uses the organization's cost of financing to determine the present value of incremental cash inflows and compares the present value with the cost of the project. The project is considered favorable if the NPV is positive. Again, a financial calculator or other tools are needed to perform the calculation. For the example in figure 4.10, the NPV at 12 percent cost of financing is $13.92 million, which is favorable. NPV is not often used for EHR projects because the EHR is a set of components that change and are upgraded over time.

Business Case

After a cost-benefit analysis is compiled and ROI calculated, it is possible to create a business case. In some contexts, **business case** for a project simply means that the ROI projections are positive. In the more formal sense, a business case is a comprehensive document that compiles all elements of a project's scope, context, goals, anticipated outcomes, value proposition, description of resource capabilities, and commitments to a project charter, plan, controls, budget, and deliverables (Hut 2009). The business case is often developed by a project manager, in consultation with the project's steering committee. It may be used to present to the capital budget committee for approval to go forward with acquiring the project. A business case may also be required when seeking a bank loan, selling bonds, floating debt in tax-exempt equity markets, or using some other sources of funding. In that scenario, the chief financial officer works with the project manager to compile the content prescribed by the funding organization.

An important element of the business case for the EHR and other types of health IT is that its formality can motivate an organization to be more diligent in its efforts to achieve real results. Ward and Daniel (2006) link the business case closely to organizational change. They describe a benefits dependency network wherein benefits depend on stakeholder ownership of the project. To date, stakeholder ownership has often been missing in EHR and other health IT projects, especially in hospitals. When the project is viewed solely as an IT project and physicians and nurses are unengaged, the projects goals can prove difficult to accomplish.

Benefits Realization Studies

As described earlier in this chapter, a benefits realization study is conducted after the EHR or other health IT project has been implemented to determine whether the benefits described in the cost-benefit analysis and/or ROI analyses have been met. The same tools and metrics used to assess value from productivity improvements should be used to conduct the benefits realization study. This methodology is both the benefits realization study's strength and weakness.

A benefits realization study performed after a project has been implemented without a baseline set of values relies on guesswork and is often influenced by satisfaction or dissatisfaction with the project. However, if a baseline set of values exists, comparison should be relatively straightforward. Unfortunately, the timeline for EHR and other health IT selection and implementation is frequently anywhere from 2 to 5 years, and sometimes as long as 10 years, depending on the migration path. Proponents of benefits realization studies suggest conducting the studies at designated milestones if the migration path is expected to be lengthy. If this milestone approach is used, interim ROI analyses also should be calculated as baselines. Even so, the biggest drawback to the accuracy of the benefits realization is the presence of confounding variables. Anything from a new physician leader to a new disease and everything in between—including changes in reimbursement structures, different accreditation processes, new legislation, and so on—can intervene and interfere with the accuracy of the calculations.

If an organization is not interested in a benefits realization study, it may be appropriate to consider conducting EHR or other health IT benefits surveys that assess user satisfaction, overall financial performance, productivity improvements, quality improvements, and patient satisfaction. Such surveys do not depend on time-consuming quantification processes but can reveal successes and problems to be addressed.

Healthcare organizations that do not conduct benefits realization studies may cite a lack of time or skills to do so, or the many intervening variables that may play a role in results. For example, when implementing a CPOE system, the implementation strategy may be to gradually introduce alerts, so as to avoid alert fatigue in users of the system. In this example, intervening variables associated with benefits realization for CPOE may be the nature of the alerts and how many physicians pay attention to them. Still, Classen and colleagues stress the importance of continual evaluation of such systems. CPOE systems, in particular, have invited considerable scrutiny after some notable failures and unintended consequences. Benefits realization studies, if nothing else, can ensure that appropriate utilization of these systems is monitored (Classen et al. 2007). Others also observed that if systems are "left unmanaged, financial benefits realization will never occur" (Staren and Eckes 2009). Behkami and colleagues (2010) found that "effective use of health IT approaches breakeven point faster . . . than average or poor use of health IT" in clinics, with a business case serving as a dynamic policy intervention to improve adoption.

Healthcare is not the only industry challenged to perform benefits realization. Several studies of IT managers conducting benefits realization studies in all industries have found that, although quantifiably measuring and reporting the benefits of IT projects is considered important, evaluating project benefits after completion is seldom performed (Planview 2007) and too hard (Curran 2010). The evaluation of IT investments "requires multidimensional measures and is a complex tangle of financial, organizational, social, procedural, and technical threads" (Lin et al. 2005). Mello (2001) has pointed out that internal benefit realization studies can be made to show any desired outcome. Another consideration for healthcare relates to the fact that under the current reimbursement process, the benefits of IT investment accrue to many beneficiaries, not just to the entity making the investments (Vogel 2003).

New cost analysis and savings measures are needed to address the complex nature of healthcare today. Impact analyses are often time-consuming, and most benefits realizations studies are completed retrospectively. These approximate values suggest new metrics are needed. Classen et al. (2007) describe several approaches for evaluating CPOE systems, including internal organizational studies, vendor studies, certification of products, and the Leapfrog Group and NQF.

In healthcare, the bottom line is measured by improvements in quality, cost, and access to care. Quality matters, and improved quality can reduce costs—even though such improvements cannot always be directly quantified. In fact, Mello (2001) suggests that ROI analysis should not be used for projected intangible benefits or broad or necessary strategic initiatives. Whether or not your organization agrees, no EHR or health IT impact analysis would be complete without recognizing the nonquantifiable results.

Check Your Understanding 4.4

Match the terms with the appropriate descriptions:

    A.   Benefits realization

    B.   Cost-benefit feasibility analysis

    C.   Internal rate of return (IRR)

    D.   Net present value (NPV)

    E.   Payback period

    F.   Pro forma financial statement

    G.   Total cost of ownership (TCO)

    1.   Reserved for determining return on investment for long term projects

    2.   Enumeration of all potential costs and benefits for a proposed project

    3.   Tool to assess the impact of an investment on the organization's ability to continue operations

    4.   Tool to determine whether the net impact of an investment enables the organization to proceed with the project

    5.   An assessment of the results of an investment decision

    6.   Financial measure that determines the potential return on investment of a project over time

    7.   The number of years it will take to recoup the cost of a potential project

References and Resources

Adamopoulos, H. 2014 (August 7). Does more value mean less profit? How to keep pay-for-performance from hurting hospital income. *Becker's Hospital Review.* http://www.beckershospitalreview.com/finance/does-more-value-mean-less-profit-how-to-keep-pay-for-performance-from-hurting-hospital-income.html.

Adamson, S.C., and J.W. Bachman. 2010. Pilot study of providing online care in a primary care setting. *Mayo Clinic Proceedings.* 85(8):704–710.

Agency for Healthcare Research and Quality (AHRQ). 2007. *Closing the Quality Gap: A Critical Analysis of Quality Improvement Strategies: Volume 7—Care Coordination.* Rockville, MD: AHRQ. http://www.ncbi.nlm.nih.gov/books/NBK44015.

Aita, S. 2008. Implementing an EHR with ROI in mind. *Journal of Medical Practice Management.* 23(4):244–246.

Amabile, T.M., and S.J. Kramer. 2010. What really motivates workers. *Harvard Business Review.* 88(1):43–45.

American Academy of Family Physicians (AAFP). 2013. e-visits. http://www.aafp.org/about/policies/all/e-visits.html.

American Health Information Management Association (AHIMA). 2012. Using medical scribes in a physician practice. *Journal of AHIMA.* 83(11): 64–69.

American Medical Group Association (AMGA) and JHD Group. 2009 (November/December). Exploring meaningful use: Results of an EHR survey by AMGA and JDH Group. *Group Practice Journal.* pp. 12–17.

American Nurses Association (ANA) 2010 (January 28). Just culture: Position statement. Congress on Nursing Practices and Economics, ANA Board of Directors. http://nursingworld.org/psjustculture.

America's Health Insurance Plans (AHIP). 2013 (August 6). New analysis in health affairs assesses performance measures across public, private sectors. AHIP coverage. http://www.ahipcoverage.com/2013/08/06/new-analysis-in-health-affairs-assesses-performance-measures-across-public-private-sectors.

Bachman, J.W. 2003. The patient-computer interview: A neglected tool that can aid the clinician. *Mayo Clinic Proceedings.* 78:67–78.

Behkami, N.A., D.A. Dorr, and S. Morrice. 2010. A business case for HIT adoption: Effects of "meaningful use" EHR financial incentives on clinic revenue. *Studies in Health Technology and Informatics.* 160(1): 779–783.

Berenson, R.A. and N. Cafarella. 2012. The Center for Medicare and Medicaid Innovation activity on many fronts: a timely analysis of immediate health policy issues. Robert Wood Johnson Foundation Urban Institute. http://www.urban.org/sites/default/files/alfresco/publication-pdfs/412499-The-Center-for-Medicare-and-Medicaid-Innovation-Activity-on-Many-Fronts.pdf

Berwick, D.M. T.W. Nolan, and J. Whittington. 2008. The Triple Aim: Care, health, and cost. *Health Affairs.* 27(3):759–769.

Boast, P., and C. Potts. 2010. Enhancing patient safety by automating discharge instructions. *Patient Safety and Quality Healthcare.* 7(1):14–16.

Buechner, M. 2015 (March 10). CMS reports progress toward Triple Aim. *America's Essential Hospitals Newsline.* http://essentialhospitals.org/policy/cms-reports-progress-toward-triple-aim.

California Healthcare Foundation (CHCF). 2011 (January). Workflow analysis: EHR deployment techniques. http://www.chcf.org/~/media/MEDIA%20LIBRARY%20Files/PDF/PDF%20W/PDF%20WorkflowAnalysisEHRDeploymentTechniques.pdf.

Caramenico, A. 2015 (August 3). Making quality measures work. America's Health Insurance Plans. http://www.ahipcoverage.com/?p=16137.

Case Management Society of America (CMSA). n.d. What is a case manager? http://www.cmsa.org/HOme/CMSA/WhatisaCaseManager/tabid/224/Default.aspx.

Center for Healthcare Quality and Payment Reform (CHQPR). n.d. The payment reform glossary, first edition. http://www.chqpr.org/downloads/paymentreformglossary.pdf.

Center for Health Care Strategies (CHCS). 2007. Care management definition and framework. http://www.chcs.org/media/Care_Management_Framework.pdf.

Centers for Medicare and Medicaid Services (CMS). n.d. Accountable care organizations. https://www.cms.gov/Medicare/Medicare-Fee-for-Service-Payment/ACO/index.html?redirect=/Aco.

Classen, D.C., A.J. Avery, and D.W. Bates. 2007. Evaluation and certification for computerized provider order entry systems. *Journal of the American Medical Informatics Association.* 14(1):48–55. http://jamia.oxfordjournals.org/content/14/1/48.

Conn, J. 2007 (May 24). Software helps docs ID depression. *Modern Healthcare.* http://www.modernhealthcare.com/article/20070524/INFO/70524004/1029/FREE.

Curran, C. 2010 (May 20). Why don't we track project benefits? *CIO Dashboard. h*ttp://www.ciodashboard.com/metrics-and-measurement/we-dont-track-project-benefits.

Dassenko, D., and T. Slowinski. 1995. Using the CPR to benefit a business office. *Healthcare Financial Management.* 49:68–73.

Dmyterko, K. 2010 (June 22). Medication management: Can IT systems minimize human error? CMIO. http://cmio.net/index.php?option=com_articles&article=22839.

Dunham-Taylor, J., and J.Z. Pinczuk. 2005. *Health Care Financial Management for Nurse Managers.* Burlington, MA: Jones & Bartlett.

Eisenberg, F., C. Lasome, A. Advani, R. Martins, P.A. Craig, and S. Sprenger. 2013. A study of the impact of meaningful use clinical quality measures. American Hospital Association. http://www.aha.org/content/13/13ehrchallenges-report.pdf.

Ely, J.W., J.A. Osheroff, S.M. Maviglia, and M.E. Rosenbaum.. 2007. Patient care questions that physicians are unable to answer. Journal of the American Medical Informatics Association. 12(4):407–414.

Fields, W., C. Tedeschi, J. Foltz, T. Myers, K. Heaney, K. Bosak, A. Rizos, R. Snyder. 2008. Reducing preventable medication safety events by recognizing renal risk. *Clinical Nurse Specialist.* 22(2):73–78.

Forrestal, E. 2016. Research methods. In *Health Information Management: Concepts, Principles, and Practice,* 5th ed. Oachs, P. and A. Watters, eds.. Chicago: AHIMA.

Foster, R. 2012 (May 29). How the big data tools ACA, HITECH enable willmprove care. *Healthcare IT News.* http://www.healthcareitnews.com/news/how-big-data-tools-aca-hitech-enable-will-improve-care.

Gillespie, L. 2015 (December 7). Jobs for medical scribes are rising rapidly but standards lag. *Kaiser Health News.* http://khn.org/news/jobs-for-medical-scribes-are-rising-rapidly-but-standards-lag.

Goldstein, M.K., B.B. Hoffman, R.W. Coleman, S.W. Tu, R.D. Shankar, M. O'Connor, S. Martins, A. Advani, and M.A. Musen. 2002. Patient safety in guideline-based decision support for hypertension management: ATHENA DSS. *Journal of the American Medical Informatics Association.* 9(6 Suppl 1):S11–S16.

Graber, M.A., B.D. Randles, J.W. Ely, and J. Monnahan.. 2008. Answering clinical questions in the ED. *American Journal of Emergency Medicine.* 26(2):144–147.

Guite, J., M. Lang, P. McCartan, and J. Miller.. 2006. Nursing admissions process redesigned to leverage EHR. *Journal of Healthcare Information Management.* 20(2):55–64.

Health Affairs. 2012 (September 13). Improving care transitions. Health policy brief. http://www.healthaffairs.org/healthpolicybriefs/brief.php?brief_id=76.

Health Affairs. 2013 (February 14). Patient engagement. Health policy brief. http://www.healthaffairs.org/healthpolicybriefs/brief.php?brief_id=86.

HealthIT.gov. 2015 (July 30). Benefits of electronic health records (EHRs). https://www.healthit.gov/providers-professionals/benefits-electronic-health-records-ehrs.

Herman, B. 2015 (March 28). Network squeeze: Controversies continue over narrow health plans. *Modern Healthcare*. http://www.modernhealthcare.com/article/20150328/MAGAZINE/303289988.

Hut, P.M. 2009 (January 8). Building a project's business case. *Project Management Best Practices*. http://www.pmhut.com/building-a-projects-business-case.

Informed Medical Decisions Foundation. n.d. What is shared decision making? http://www .informedmedicaldecisions.org/what-is-shared-decision-making.

Institute of Medicine (IOM), Committee on Quality of Health Care in America. 2001. *Crossing the Quality Chasm: A New Health System for the 21st Century*. Washington, DC: National Academies Press. http://www.nap.edu/catalog/10027/crossing-the-quality-chasm-a-new-health-system-for-the.

Institute of Medicine (IOM). 2012. *The Learning Health System Series*. http://www.nap.edu/catalog/13301/the-learning-health-system-series.

Iuga, A.O., and M.J. McGuire. 2014. Adherence and healthcare costs. *Risk Management and Healthcare Policy*. 7:35–44. https://www.dovepress.com/adherence-and-health-care-costs-peer-reviewed-fulltext-article-RMHP.

Jacobson, D.M., and S. Teutsch. 2012. An environmental scan of integrated approaches for defining and measuring total population health by the clinical care system, the government public health system, and stakeholder organizations. National Quality Forum. http://www.qualityforum.org/Publications/2012/06/An_Environmental_Scan_of_Integrated_Approaches_for_Defining_and_Measuring_Total_Population_Health.aspx.

Janssen Pharmaceuticals. 2014 (August). Trends in diabetes quality measurement. http://www .janssenpharmaceuticalsinc.com/sites/default/files/pdf/Diabetes-quality-measurement-trends.pdf.

Joint Commission. 2016. Standards FAQ details: What is a scribe? https://www.jointcommission.org/standards_information/jcfaqdetails.aspx?StandardsFaqId=1206&ProgramId=46.

Joseph, A., and C. Stuhan. 2015 (February 18). The reimbursement outlook for virtual visits. *Advisory Board Company Practice Notes*. https://www.advisory.com/research/medical-group-strategy-council/practice-notes/2015/february/virtual-visits.

Kelly, T. 2010 (September 2). Employing a strategic approach to implementing meaningful use objectives. *Healthcare IT News*. http://www.healthcareitnews.com/blog/employing-strategic-approach-implementing-meaningful-use-objectives.

Ketchell, D.S., L. St. Anna, D. Kauff, B. Gaster, and D. Timberlake. 2005. PrimeAnswers: A practical interface for answering primary care questions. *Journal of the American Medical Informatics Association*. 12(5):537–545.

Koppenheffer, M. 2013 (April 15). Clinical integration, demystified. Advisory Board Company Care Center Transformation Blog. https://www.advisory.com/research/care-transformation-center/care-transformation-center-blog/2013/04/clinical-integration-defined.

Kraus, S. 2008 (April 22). The return on the digital investment: Why the EHR ROI is making digital inevitable. *Dynamic Chiropractic*. 26(9). http://www.dynamicchiropractic.com/mpacms/dc/article.php?id=53181.

Lin, C., G. Pervan, and D. McDermid. 2005. IS/IT investment evaluation and benefits realization issues in Australia. *Journal of Research and Practice in Information Technology*. 37(3):235–251.

Mace, S. 2014 (February 13). In search of EHR's ROI. *Health Leaders Media Magazine*. http://www.healthleadersmagazine-digital.com/healthleadersmagazine/january_february_2014?pg=12#pg12.

Manos, D. 2007 (January 29). Study: Rapid learning through EHRs advances evidence-based medicine. *Healthcare IT News*. http://www.healthcareitnews.com/news/studyrapid-learning-through-ehrs-advances-evidence-based-medicine.

Mayo Clinic. 2015 (January 5). Personalized medicine and pharmacogenomics. http://www .mayoclinic.org/healthy-lifestyle/consumer-health/in-depth/personalized-medicine/art-20044300.

McGinn, T.G., L. McCullagh, J. Kannry, M. Knaus, A. Sofianou, J.P. Wisnivesky, and D.M. Mann. 2013. Efficacy of an evidence-based clinical decision support in primary care practices: a randomized clinical trial. *JAMA Internal Medicine*. 173(17):1584–1591.

Medical Group Management Association (MGMA). 2011. Electronic health records: status, needs, and lessons. http://www.mgma.com/Libraries/Assets/Practice%20Resources/Topics/EHR2010-Report-PNC-2011-04-05-1120---Final-with-cover.pdf.pdf.

Mello, A. 2001 (October 3). Why ROI can sometimes lie. *TechUpdate*. http://www.zdnet.com/article/why-roi-can-sometimes-lie.

Merriam-Webster. N.d. Value. http://www.merriam-webster.com/dictionary/value

Miller, J. 2009 (December 14). The positive tension between SMART and Stretch goals. Gemba Panta Rei blog. http://gembapantarei.com/2009/12/the_positive_tension_between_smart_and_stretch_goa.html.

Minnesota Community Measurement. 2014. The D5 and the V4. http://mncm.org/reports-and-websites/the-d5.

Monegain, B. 2015 (September 11). Pressure on CIOs to Pull Value from EHRs. *Healthcare IT News*.

Monegain, B. 2015 (October 15). CIOs share meaningful use concerns at CHIME. *Health IT News*. http://www.healthcareitnews.com/news/chime-meaningful-use-deconstructed.

Moody, L.E., E. Slocumb, B. Berg, and D. Jackson. 2004. Electronic health records documentation in nursing. *Computers, Informatics, Nursing*. 22(6):337–344.

National Committee for Quality Assurance (NCQA). n.d. Patient-centered medical home. http://www.ncqa.org/home/patient-centered-medical-home.

National Quality Forum (NQF). n.d. Improving healthcare quality. http://www.qualityforum.org/Setting_Priorities/Improving_Healthcare_Quality.aspx.

Newman, M. 2010 (May 7). Implementing an EHR: Top 10 lessons learned. *Physicians News Digest*. https://physiciansnews.com/2010/05/07/implementing-an-ehr-top-10-lessons-learned.

Oxentenko, A.S., C.P. West, C. Popkave, S.E. Weinberger, and J.C. Kolars. 2010. Time spent on clinical documentation: A survey of internal medicine residents and program directors. *Archives of Internal Medicine*. 170(7): 639.

Panten, N., and A. Torrance. 2014 (January 13). Just culture. The missing ingredient in patient safety. *Healthcare Executive Insight*. http://healthcare-executive-insight.advanceweb.com/Features/Articles/Just-Culture-The-Missing-Ingredient-in-Patient-Safety.aspx.

Payne, T.H., S. Corley, T.A. Cullen, T.K. Gandhi, L. Harrington, G.J. Kuperman, J.E. Mattison, D.P. McCallie, C.J. McDonald, P.C. Tang, W.M. Tierney, C. Weaver, C.R. Weir, and M.H. Zaroukia. 2015 (May 28). Report of the AMIA EHR 2020 Task Force on the status and future direction of EHRs. *Journal of the American Medical Informatics Association*. http://jamia.oxfordjournals.org/content/early/2015/05/22/jamia.ocv066.

Peitzman, L.R. 2009 (November/December). Advancing the practice of evidence-based medicine with standardized order sets. *Patient Safety and Quality Healthcare*. http://psqh.com/advancing-the-practice-of-evidence-based-medicine-with-standardized-order-sets.

Positive NPV. 2007 (October 17). Benefits realization a key IT challenge for *Fortune* 1000 companies. http://www.benefitsrealization.blogspot.com/2007/10.

Porter, S. 2013 (March 13). E-visits versus office visits: Researchers compare care. *AAFP News*. http://www.aafp.org/news/practice-professional-issues/20130313researchevisits.html.

Porter, S.C., P. Forbes, S. Manzi, L.A. Kalish. 2010. Patients providing the answers: Narrowing the gap in data quality for emergency care. *Quality and Safety in Health Care*. 19: e34). doi:10.1136/qshc.2009.032540.

Rollins, G. 2005. The prompt, the alert, and the legal record: Documenting clinical decision support systems. *Journal of AHIMA* 76(2):24–28.

Savage, M. 2014 (December 10). Engaging patients and families: how consumers value and use health IT. National Partnership for Women and Families. http://www.nationalpartnership.org/research-library/health-care/HIT/presentation-patients-speak.pdf.

Sheehan, R. 2014 (March 11). The power of goals. Presentation at Executive MBA Council Southeast Regional Meeting, New Orleans, LA. http://www.emba.org/pdf/regionals/embac-goals-slides-rob-sheehan.pdf.

Staren, E.D.. 2009 (May 14). Building the financial case for electronic health records. *Healthcare IT News*. http://www .healthcareitnews.com/blog/building-financial-case-electronic-health-records.

Stevens, M. 2010 Beyond alerts: Linking CDS to evidence-based medicine. *CMIO*, http://www .cmio.net/index.php?option=com_articles&views=article&id=23404.

Teich, J.M., J.P. Glaser, R.F. Beckley, M. Aranow, D.W. Bates, G.J. Kuperman, M.A. Ward, C.D. Spurr. 1996. Toward cost-effective quality care: The Brigham integrated computing system, Brigham and Women's Hospital. *Second Annual Nicholas E. Davies Award Proceedings of the CPR Recognition Symposium.* Schaumburg, IL: CPRI.

Thompson, D.I., J. Osheroff, D. Classen, and E.F. Sittig. 2007. A review of methods to estimate the benefits of electronic medical records in hospitals and the need for a national benefits database. *Journal of Healthcare Information Management.* 21(1):62–68.

Thompson, J. 2010 (May 10). EHR boosts care coordination, but better access is needed. *Healthcare IT News.* http:// www.healthcareitnews.com/print/12631.

Toll, E. 2012 (June 20). A piece of my mind. The cost of technology. *Journal of the American Medical Association.* 307(23):2497–2499.

Tonelli, M. 2006 (February). Evidence-based medicine and clinical expertise. *Virtual Mentor.* 8(2):71–74.

URAC. 2005. Trends and practices in medical management: 2005 industry profile. http://www.urac .org/resources/careManagement.aspx.

Vishwasrao, P. 2012 SMART GOALS. http://www.self-help-and-self-development.com/smart-goals.html.

Vogel, L.H. 2003. Finding value from IT investments: Exploring the elusive ROI in healthcare. *Journal of Healthcare Information Management.* 17(4):20–28.

Ward, J.L., and E. Daniel. 2006. *Benefits Management: Delivering Value from IS and IT Investments.* West Sussex: John Wiley & Sons.

Wise, P. 2013 (February 26). The EHR: Providing exceptional value. Healthcare Information and Management Systems Society. http://www.himss.org/ResourceLibrary/ResourceDetail.aspx?ItemNumber=17246.

Wiseman, B., and V.S. Kaprielian. 2014. Culture of safety: the culture of healthcare organizations. Duke University School of Medicine Department of Community and Family Medicine. http://patientsafetyed.duhs.duke.edu/module_c/ culture_healthcare.html.

Wyatt, R.M. 2013 (December 18). Blameless or blameworthy errors—does your organization make a distinction? The Joint Commission Leadership Blog. http://www.jointcommission.org/jc_physician_blog/ blameless_or_blameworthy_errors.

Chapter 5
Healthcare Workflow and Process Improvement

Key Terms

Agile scrum
Baseline data
Benchmarking
Benefits realization
Continuous quality improvement
Cycle time
Essential use case
Flow process chart
Information flow
Process
Process boundaries
Process decisions
Process diagram
Process improvement
Process mapping
Process operations
Process redesign
Process reengineering
Role ambiguity
Root cause
Swim lane chart
System flowchart
Team empowerment

Thoughtflow

Unintended consequences

Use case

Workflow

Workflow and process analysis

Learning Objectives

- Identify the importance and scope of workflow and process improvement.

- Describe the purpose and timing of the workflow and process improvement efforts.

- Identify the steps in workflow and process improvement.

- Describe workflow and process mapping tools and the skills needed to use them.

- Articulate how to ensure solid process improvement through managing team empowerment, group facilitation, and adopting process improvement techniques.

- Understand the role of HIM and IT professionals in process mapping.

When an organization has determined its vision, goals, and a strategic plan for an electronic health record (EHR) or other health information technology (health IT) initiative, planning for changes in workflow and processes must be initiated. Many organizations have discovered that paying insufficient attention to workflow and process improvement in the EHR planning stages can lead to serious negative outcomes—from not fully understanding what functional requirements are needed for an EHR to loss of productivity during go-live, costly rework of the implementation, and potential unintended consequences of poorly designed EHRs. **Unintended consequences** are outcomes of a purposeful action that are not expected to occur. Although unintended consequences can be positive, the term usually suggests a negative outcome. Unintended consequences are a considerable concern as EHRs are becoming more widely used and as new forms of health IT are being implemented. New types of errors with deleterious results are likely when an EHR or health IT system is not designed properly, not implemented with consideration for changes likely to occur in processes and workflows, or not well integrated with other systems. Errors can also happen when users do not apply professional judgment in their use of EHRs and health IT. *Process improvement* describes how workflows and processes are analyzed and improved upon. Many terms are used as synonyms for process improvement, but, whatever it is called, the objective of process improvement is a clear understanding of current workflows and processes and how an EHR or other type of health IT will affect them to minimize to the extent possible unintended consequences and contribute to improvement.

Importance and Scope of Workflow and Process Improvement

Understanding how current work is performed and the sequence of steps involved in order to make improvements is the general purpose of what this book terms **workflow and process improvement**.

Terminology and Methodologies

Workflow and process improvement (or just *process improvement*) is not new—neither in general nor to healthcare. It has been a longstanding technique, adopted in multiple different settings, with many different approaches, and sometimes with similar approaches going by different names. In general, **workflow** refers to the sequence of steps in a process. **Process** refers to the manner in which work is performed to achieve a particular result. A workflow and process map (or just *process map*) is the depiction of the workflow and process that is being studied, and the act of making the map is called **process mapping**. Finally, workflow and process mapping must be coupled with **workflow and process analysis** of the current process to determine ways to make improvements. Process improvement may also be referred to as **process redesign** or **process reengineering** (generally, these latter terms are not well liked in healthcare because they connote a manufacturing perspective). A variety of statistical and analytical methods may aid workflow and process improvement. Still other techniques may be needed to implement the improvement. When process mapping is performed to describe a desired process or functionality that a system should have, *use case modeling* may be used to define a scenario that is the ideal state for incorporating process improvement.

Approaches to identifying and implementing improvements include Lean, Six Sigma, TQM, ISO 9000, Kaizen, and others. These methodologies have similarities and differences, and they are often combined to achieve the most value of each. For example, Lean, Six Sigma, and Kaizen are often used together. Lean is "a methodology that is used to accelerate the velocity and reduce the cost of any process . . . by removing waste" (George 2008). Six Sigma is most closely associated with identifying and eliminating defects and improving quality. Kaizen is a philosophy of continuous improvement throughout all aspect of life. When these methodologies are combined into a Lean Kaizen methodology complemented with Six Sigma, there can be a significant impact on the systems development life cycle not only of information systems, but any process that should be continuously monitored for improvement. More recently, Lean has been coupled with Agile methodology for software development, also known as **Agile Scrum**, which is a technique where system-wide workflows are evaluated for the purpose of improving project management, software development, and managing value (Agilean 2010).

Purpose of Process Improvement

What should become apparent in considering the number of techniques and methodologies for workflow and process improvement is that there has been a continual quest for improvement in work, and, over time, many have attempted to find better ways to make such improvements. However, it should also be observed that almost all of the formal methodologies that have emerged are grounded in manufacturing, sales, and other non-healthcare fields and are frequently focused on people and materials rather than the data-information-knowledge-wisdom continuum. Therefore, although much can be learned from these techniques, they may not necessarily apply without some modification to EHRs and other types of health IT. As a result, the process mapping techniques described in this chapter combine many of the principles of **continuous quality improvement (CQI)**—a management philosophy that emphasizes the importance of knowing and meeting customer expectations, reducing variation within processes, and relying on data to build knowledge for process improvement—but these techniques are also focused on the information payload that is the EHR or other type of health IT. In fact, the following is a good mantra to keep in mind:

> EHR is not about automating charts ("material") and you can't automate people ("man"), but about automating data collection and using information to generate knowledge that improves the care delivery process, empowers consumers, and transforms the health services industry. (Amatayakul 2007)

Put another way by Dr. David Smith of Riverton Family Health Center in Utah, "The single area that requires the highest level of attention during the planning and deployment of an electronic medical record is practice workflow" (Smith and Newell 2002).

Process Improvement Case Studies

A practice was anxious to acquire and implement an EHR in order to take advantage of the federal government's meaningful use (MU) incentive program. In the practice's haste, it did not map most of its EHR workflows before going live. As a result, the employees had to figure out a lot of how to improve upon their workflows as they started using the system, which frustrated new users who had anticipated the system would be easy to use. Of primary concern were workflows associated with non-interfaced laboratory test results that came back on paper (often via fax), not electronically, and had to be figured out via trial and error in the middle of office visits. The workflow problems created long waits for patients and office bottlenecks that lasted for weeks. In addition, in this practice's quest to figure out how to enter results for in-house laboratory tests, some nursing staff at the site entered the data in one part of the EHR, the so-called workflow module, whereas others entered data directly into individual patient EHR visit notes, creating more confusion and delays for physicians looking for laboratory test results. While this case study may seem like ancient history today, organizations that have implemented EHRs more recently have faced, and continue to face, similar problems.

Another example relates to integrating preventive services workflows into an EHR, which presents several workflow challenges. First, EHRs from other providers, the patient's personal health record, information from public health departments (where patients may been vaccinated), and pharmacies generally do not have the ability to automatically share data with a primary care provider's EHR. As a result, even with a preventive services reminder system, the primary care provider frequently does not have the most complete or current information. In addition, providers themselves have personal preferences for when they want to discuss preventive services with patients, and who in an office or clinic might be the best person to do so. Nurses might best be suited for discussions about routine vaccinations, mammograms, and routine laboratory tests, such as blood tests for diabetes, but a primary care provider may prefer to talk with patients about more invasive preventive services, such as colonoscopies. Also, some providers will want to have these conversations at the start of a visit, whereas others approach preventive care topics during a history and physical, and still others wait until the end of a visit.

Process mapping is critical in solving these sorts of issues. However, because many organizations, including physician practices in particular, did not map processes when they implemented the EHR, many are now considering whether to replace their original EHRs with newer EHRs—both to acquire EHRs that are easier to tailor and to start fresh with process mapping. A survey conducted in 2014 found that 25 percent of both large and small physician practices were considering replacing their EHR and that another 12 percent wanted to replace their system but could not do so for financial or organizational reasons (Leventhal 2014). In addition, this survey found that about 20 percent of midsized practices were planning to add other types of health IT, such as patient portals, kiosks, health information exchange capability, and population health tools. While the underlying need for replacement may reflect an inherent flaw in the EHR itself, many believe that starting over again from scratch will enable them to "do it right this time" (Wietecha 2013).

Workflow and process improvements are critical success factors in an ambulatory or inpatient setting, although ambulatory organizations may be less likely to recognize the need for or be willing to take the time to perform a concerted workflow and process improvement activity. Guite and colleagues (2006) offer a good example of a redesigned process in the inpatient environment, where the nursing admission process was studied in depth prior to EHR implementation. Challenges faced by the nurses included considerable duplication of documentation, complex rules for coordinating care, and pressure to accelerate patient admission. Stakeholders from the admissions department, nursing, and other departments that would potentially be a part of the future process were convened, and the hospital decided to adopt an electronic admission referral process (EARP) that simplified the nursing work and led to more appropriate referrals to the ancillary departments. After implementation of the EARP, information for more than 25 percent of the patients could be imported from a previous encounter, and the elimination of duplicate documentation also improved patient satisfaction. More accurate and complete admission information is also used to monitor and support a variety of quality initiatives, including the MU incentive program.

There is great need to ensure that processes and workflow changes brought about by an EHR are understood and adopted so clinicians can take full advantage of the system and inefficient and ineffective processes can be corrected. However, it is also essential to understand that some EHR processes and workflows do not fit a given situation, and organizations should not force clinicians to change how they work only to fit a computerized system. Instead, organizations need workflow and process improvements to make the *right* changes for the *right* EHR (see figure 5.1 and table 5.1).

The following three examples of lack of attention to process improvement have become classic in the industry:

> At Cedars-Sinai Medical Center in Los Angeles, a physician "revolt" required them to remove part of their CPOE system. While no one intends to set themselves up as an example, the Cedars-Sinai experience provided significant lessons learned for the industry. They have attributed much of their CPOE implementation problem to inadequate education and physician involvement, lack of consideration for human factors, inadequate study of workflow, functionality issues in the software, weak pilot testing (in OB only), and a too aggressive rollout (two weeks per floor). (Polaschek et al. 2003)

Another experience was reported in *Pediatrics*, the journal of the American Academy of Pediatrics (Han et al. 2005). In this case, a computerized provider order entry (CPOE) system primarily used in general hospitals (with a large percentage of adult patients) did not have incorporated control points for pediatric cases, which often require weight-based dose adjustments and have many more precautions than for adults. The academy offered an opportunity for readers of its journal to post comments on its website, under the heading "Post-publication Peer Review (P3R)." Don Levick, president of the Medical Staff Physician Liaison Information Services at Lehigh Valley Hospital, posted this telling comment:

> The issue with CPOE is usually not in the software, but in the *process change* that is required to successfully implement such a complex system. These challenges were well documented in the article. . . . But *rather than conclude that work process and infrastructure issues must be completely understood, investigated, and resolved prior to implementation*, the authors conclude that hospitals should monitor mortality rates after CPOE implementation.

Figure 5.1.   The right way to implement an EHR is not necessarily the new way, my way, your way, or the old way—but likely a combination that achieves the five rights for EHR

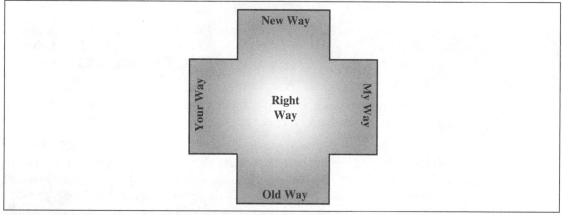

Table 5.1. Five rights for EHR

- *Right clinical data:* The EHR enables complete and accurate data capture in the manner that is most meaningful for all users and uses—be it structured, standardized, and encoded data; narrative information; or clinical images
- *Right presentation:* The EHR provides a human–computer interface that enables the most efficient and effective means of capturing (such as via context-sensitive templates or self-administered questionnaires) and displaying data (facts, findings, observations, plans, rationales, and conclusions recorded by clinicians, consumers, and others about patient care), information (narrative and graphical displays), and knowledge (alerts and reminders)
- *Right decision:* The EHR supplies clinical decision support that is context-sensitive, tailored to the user, and based on scientific evidence, which is kept current at all times, and which provides a means to document legitimate reasons when professional judgment calls for overriding the proposed support
- *Right work processes:* The EHR supports processes and workflows that are most efficient and effective for all users and uses
- *Right outcomes:* The EHR supports value-driven healthcare, with the right quality and cost results

A similar study was reported in the *Journal of the American Medical Association* (Koppel et al. 2005). This article describes 22 discrete ways in which a CPOE contributed to medication errors at a teaching hospital. Even though the system was reportedly replaced with a newer product, Koppel and coauthors note that it still has "oodles of problems." Despite this observation, Koppel and colleagues conclude CPOE deployments can offer "extraordinary advantages" in reducing many mistakes as long as the hospital provides "vigilance and self-examination" to ensure proper functioning.

Additional examples continue to be found. For example, a 2011 *Chicago Tribune* article reported on errors caused by computerized systems in hospitals, including the misadministration of an intravenous (IV) solution to an infant, Genesis, that caused her death (and for which the hospital settled at $8.25M in 2012) (Graham and Dizikes). Although the *Tribune* headline stated, "Baby's Death Spotlights Safety Risks Linked to Computerized Systems," the debacle that caused the death of baby Genesis, born prematurely to parents who had been trying to conceive for several years, had much more to do with human errors and potentially unethical decision-making than unintended consequences of the technology itself. The hospital had MU-certified EHR technology and more—including CPOE, barcode medication administration record (BC-MAR) system, an automated intravenous (IV) compounding machine, laboratory auto-analyzers, vital signs monitoring systems, and nursing information systems. However, the scenario (which diagrams the broken links in the process in figure 5.2) played out as follows:

1. The physician entered a correct order for an admixture of compounds specifically tailored to the baby and to be administered intravenously.

2. The pharmacy technician transcribed the order from the CPOE into the IV compounding machine and entered a dosage that was 60 times the correct dose of sodium chloride. (Notably, an interface between the CPOE and IV compounding machine, but this had not been done because the interface was deemed too expensive.)

3. Alerts on the IV compounding machine that could have detected that the incorrect manual entry was the wrong dose for a baby were not activated.

4. Labels produced by the IV compounding machine were stacked on the IV bag on top of each other, with the top label listing only the patient identification. This practice is a common one because "accordion" style labels are more expensive and it is time-consuming for nurses to "wand" every label. However, wanding the complete set of labels containing the actual amounts of the admixture could have triggered an alert that the admixture

Figure 5.2.   Example of unintended consequences of health IT

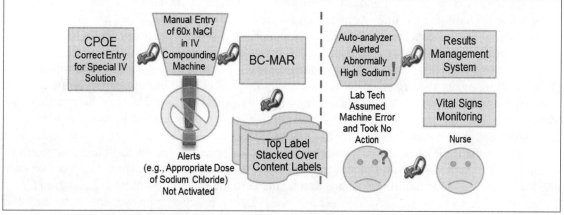

was inconsistent with the order because orders flow from the CPOE system through the pharmacy information system and then to the BC-MAR, even though the IV compounding machine continued to require manual entry.

5.   Continuous blood work performed on the baby quickly showed abnormally high sodium levels, but the laboratory technician who read the results assumed the machine was producing an error and took no action.

The article reporting the incident did not describe the relationship between the laboratory results management system that would have displayed the alert and any vital signs monitoring equipment or other nursing information system that could have resulted in pulling the IV, or whether the baby's response was so rapid that any such alert at the bedside would have been too late.

Despite both early findings and continuing concerns about the safety and efficacy of EHR systems, US healthcare may be reaching a turning point. In 2010, *Pediatrics* published an article that reported on significant reductions in mortality rates in an academic children's hospital after implementation of a CPOE system (Longhurst et al. 2010). In a *Guide to Reducing Unintended Consequences of Electronic Health Records* prepared for the Agency for Healthcare Quality and Research (AHRQ), Jones and colleagues (2011) note the following:

> The management expert, Peter Drucker, called health care workplaces "the most complex human organization[s] ever devised." Interactions between these complex environments and increasingly complex EHRs can spawn subtle unintended consequences of EHR implementation. These consequences do not result from malfunctions within the EHR, but from the interactions between the EHR and the work environment or between the EHR and the technical and physical infrastructure.

Increasingly, this interaction between the EHR and the environment is being recognized, and workflow and process improvement is being applied (Dooley 2016).

Purpose and Timing of Process Improvement

The EHR and other types of health IT are not just technology or products—these systems also involve people, policy, and process. However, workflow and process mapping, if performed at all, is often postponed until the EHR or health IT implementation stage. Even then, many EHR vendors do not support workflow and process improvement, which means the hospital or physician office must recognize the need and do it themselves (Kudyba 2010; HealthIT.gov 2013). This is unfortunate because process improvement that begins early in the EHR project can offer a number of benefits. Table 5.2 lists the key benefits associated with process mapping and when it should be performed.

Conducting workflow and process mapping in the early planning stages of EHR or other health IT not only prepares the organization for the technological change but also often helps identify process changes that can take place immediately. This proactive approach can help achieve an early payback for the work effort and also ease change into an organization in which resistance to innovation is a major impediment. Process mapping also can help an organization determine the feasibility of the EHR or health IT project and assess its potential results to obtain management or clinical leadership approval. Process mapping should identify where changes in processes are needed, as well as what modifications need to be made to the system to reflect organizational processes that need to remain intact. Identification of potential process improvements with the EHR or other type of health IT also helps change management. Finally, early process mapping can help produce cost projections. When an organization requires a thorough cost-benefit justification for an EHR or other health IT project, what and how processes will be redesigned must be understood to identify potential cost savings. (See chapter 4 for information on cost-benefit analysis.) When an organization intends to do a comprehensive benefits realization study after EHR or health IT implementation, the analysis phase of process improvement can produce data for the baseline, and the final, improved process documentation helps focus the study on the impact of the EHR or other form of health IT.

Table 5.2.   Multiple benefits of process assessment performed over time

When	What	Why
Planning	Current process mapping	Initiates change management by highlighting processes that need improvement
Assessment	Process improvement	Addresses processes that need to be improved prior to EHR implementation so bad processes are not carried forward into the EHR Acclimates users to potential changes, such as standardized templates and order sets
Selection	Use case scenarios	Describes the desired functionality for process improvements Enables cost–benefit analysis to determine potential return on investment
System build	Proposed process mapping	Enables the EHR to be configured in a way that will help achieve process improvements for right outcomes
Testing	Use case models	Ensures integrated system testing, not just unit testing of each system part
Training	Improved process map	Serves as training tool and documented procedure for ongoing reference
Benefits realization	Process assessment	Utilizing all components of the previous steps validates that new processes are working, helps celebrate success, and identifies course correction where necessary

Check Your Understanding 5.1

Choose the best answer:

1. An advantage of conducting workflow and process improvement before implementing a new system is:

   a. Changes to be made with a new system are clearer.

   b. Management is more supportive of workflow and process improvement prior to, rather than after, system implementation.

   c. Some improvements do not depend on implementing a new system.

   d. Workflow and process improvement will take less time.

2. Process mapping conducted prior to vendor selection:

   a. Ensures system-wide testing of new systems

   b. Helps identify whether changes are successful

   c. Identifies desired functionality

   d. Serves as a training tool to learn the new system

3. A risk of implementing a system without workflow and process improvement is:

   a. Achieving education about a system prior to acquiring the system

   b. Improved staff ownership of the system

   c. Increased price of the system

   d. System is configured to precisely match existing processes

4. At which point in the systems development life cycle should workflow and process improvement be initiated?

   a. Identification of need

   b. Design of system

   c. Implementation

   d. Monitoring results

Steps in Process Improvement

Although the purpose of the process improvement may vary with the timing of its performance, the steps in performing process improvement are similar at whatever time they occur. Table 5.3 summarizes the steps that are typically performed in process mapping. Subsequent sections of this chapter discuss these steps in greater depth and note variations related to timing and purpose.

Table 5.3.   Steps in process improvement for EHR (or other health IT)

1. Identify processes to be assessed; that is, those that will be impacted by the EHR being acquired.
2. Create process assessment teams of individuals who perform the process today and those who will be impacted in the future.
3. Select process assessment tools suitable to the process assessment purpose, and learn how to use the tools.
4. Map the process as actually performed. Avoid identifying opportunities for improvement now, or critical controls built into current processes may be overlooked.
5. Validate maps to ensure they reflect current processes, all variations, and the information payload.
6. Collect all forms and reports that are part of the process to be automated.
7. Obtain baseline data to define expectations for change and for use in benchmarking for benefits realization studies.
8. Identify potential problems and determine their root cause (not just symptoms).
9. Identify changes that would address root cause of problems: Some may be addressed now; others will require EHR.
10. Identify other desired improvements from use of an EHR.
11. Document proposed changes by creating a proposed map.
12. Use new processes to create use case scenarios to identify EHR functional specifications, and later to build out the EHR application to achieve improvements. (This may require a second "improved" with EHR map.)
13. Test new workflows and processes.
14. Train all on new workflows and processes.
15. Incorporate changes in workflows and processes into policy and procedure.
16. Conduct benefits realization and celebrate successful change/correct course as necessary.

Processes to Be Mapped

The first step in process improvement is to identify processes to be mapped. For organizations evaluating the EHR or another health IT project, the processes to be assessed should follow the specific project's migration path, because not every process needs to be assessed for any given component implemented. However, if the organization plans a comprehensive EHR rollout, then a comprehensive set of processes should be mapped. Table 5.4 identifies potential processes for hospitals and

Table 5.4.   Processes to be assessed for an EHR project

Hospitals	Clinics
• Admission/discharge/transfer	• Scheduling and registration/check-in and check-out
• Patient assessment	• Patient intake
• Medications reconciliation	• Results review
• H&P/differential diagnosis	• H&P/encounter notes
• Care planning	• Care plan/guidelines
• Provider order entry	• Medication management: medication list maintenance/prescribing/refills/compliance
• Procedures	• Order entry
• Medication administration	• E/M coding
• Patient monitoring	• Charge capture
• Patient care charting	• Patient instructions
• Care coordination	
• Charge capture/coding	
• Reporting	

clinics that would be mapped during an EHR project. This approach to mapping may be modified for any specific organization and its migration path and for other forms of health IT.

Process Mapping Teams

Although a single management team, consultant, or vendor can provide leadership, education, direction, and assistance, process mapping will be much more successful when it is done by teams made up of the people who will actually implement the redesigned processes and use the EHR or other type of health IT. Teams should be responsible for the actual workflow and process mapping, analysis, redesign, and feasibility testing. Effective EHR or health IT process improvement teams are interdepartmental and interdisciplinary. The EHR and other types of health IT will cut across all departments and have multiple potential users. Teams should solicit the input of all users in their respective areas and keep them abreast of progress made. Teams that include individuals at the lowest applicable levels of the organization heighten the staff's sense of ownership of and responsibility for the process improvement activity. Finally, teams should be encouraged to accurately map workflows and processes as they are actually performed—not how a policy or procedure says they should be performed. If actual processes are not mapped, the process mapping effort will not identify workarounds, delays, and other factors that contribute to current issues. Furthermore, mapping only formal policies and procedures may not identify control points in processes that must carry forward to the EHR or other type of health IT. Mapping current processes should find all the issues. As a result, process improvement is not the time to lay blame for problems that have arisen in the current processes.

A special case must be considered for mapping workflows and processes conducted primarily by physicians. Ball and Bierstock (2007) coined the term **thoughtflow**, defining it as the process by which physicians obtain, assess, prioritize, and act on information. They observe that "vendors long have developed systems based on presumptions about the way clinicians work, but without a clear understanding of how clinicians think. Developers must understand how physicians think and then work." Interestingly, Bierstock, himself a physician and developer of information systems, further notes that "such knowledge can come only from physicians who have been in the trenches" (Ball and Bierstock 2007). Therein lies the dilemma—getting physicians to map their workflows and processes, or even their thoughtflows, is a daunting task (Poggio 2010).

Despite the challenges of engaging physicians in key elements of important programs, it is feasible to engage them in process mapping when it is performed in a way that delivers direct value to them (Amatayakul 2007). Physicians may not be willing to participate directly in the actual construction of a map—someone will have to document a best guess—but those conducting process mapping can get valuable feedback by asking physicians to review the map before implementing changes. An industry insider suggests focusing on the clinical aspects, not the automation aspects, of the change (Essin 2011). However, physicians typically are not technophobic and may enjoy trying out new technology. For example, one can learn about their documentation preferences by asking them to try something like a digital pen and supply feedback that links to the workflow (McGee 2011).

When engaging physicians and other clinicians, it may help to be firm about the fact that change is forthcoming (Van Dijk and Van Dick 2009). Many hospitals have feared mandating use of EHR technology by physicians, and yet hospitals are told to "make change stick by nurturing a new culture" (Cohn et al. 2009). Finally, clinicians may be more willing participants in process improvement if they can maintain their self-esteem (Fillingham 2008). Physicians can be particularly sensitive to the suggestion that they may be doing something wrong, even though workflow and process mapping is about making something better, not necessarily correcting something wrong. When asked for *input* rather than ways to *improve* a process map, individuals may be less likely to personalize the activity.

Process Mapping Training

Many organizations select people to participate on process mapping teams because they are intimately familiar with current processes. However, the organization cannot assume these people have the skills to do process mapping, fully understand the features and functions of an EHR or other type of health IT, or even know how to function as a team. Thus, orientation and training in these areas are essential.

Orientation to an EHR or other health IT system must be comprehensive, with a fair amount of coaching. A single product demonstration will not suffice. Ideally, introductory reading materials are distributed first and then seminars, actual demonstrations, or websites with demonstrations are provided. As processes are analyzed and redesign work begins, at least one expert in the EHR or other health IT system should be available to answer questions, coach, and work with the teams to help them understand what is feasible.

Process Mapping Validation

Once a current process has been mapped, it is important to validate that the map is complete and accurate. Process mapping must also reflect **information flow**—bearing in mind that the EHR or other type of health IT automates the collection and processing of data into useful information; it does not automate the chart, processes, or people. This step is often challenging. Although it is easy to see where a paper chart and people are at all times, it can be difficult to understand what data are being processed mentally. For this reason, the people who actually perform the processes should map them.

It can be helpful for an unbiased observer (who may be a consultant or simply someone in the organization not engaged in performing the process) to ask key questions about the maps. Such questioning will help ensure that the process has been thoroughly described. Table 5.5 provides a set of questions that may be helpful in validating the completeness and accuracy of current process maps.

Table 5.5.   Key questions to validate current process maps

- Is the scope of the process appropriate for EHR mapping?
- Are these all the tasks performed in this process?
- Does the map focus on information flow or only the chart or the person? Are all sources of input and uses of information identified?
- Are clinical decision-making tasks performed mentally included?
- Are some tasks performed only occasionally? Are they included? What triggers their performance?
- Are there tasks performed differently by different people or for different people? If so, are the variations included or more than one map made?
- Are some tasks performed outside of this process but impact its boundary?
- Are there some tasks identified that really are not a part of this process and could be dropped or placed at the boundary?
- What tasks are critical? That is, if not performed, the process is meaningless; or must be included in any new HIT adopted? Highlight these.
- Are there tasks not performed today that would improve efficiency, patient safety, and outcomes?
- Were all associated forms, reports, job descriptions, policies, and procedures collected?
- Did you collect baseline data if desired? Do you have benchmark data for comparison? Do you have plans to acquire such?

Process Changes

Once it is time to begin analyzing the current workflows and processes, the process improvement team should focus on what changes are appropriate and when they can be implemented. The following are key strategies for evaluating processes for improvement.

- *Liberate team members to make appropriate changes.* Too often, management is taught to control processes rather than change them. Changes proposed by nonmanagement staff are often regarded as situations out of managerial control. The process mapping teams must understand that they are free to make appropriate changes. The result may be a modification of the technology rather than a change in the process, and the decision will have been made within the appropriate context. For example, when evaluating the process of nursing documentation, the technology may accommodate point-of-care charting and adopting the new method would be a significant change from charting at the nursing station. Neither the current process or the potential change is right or wrong, and nursing personnel should be open to understanding the ramifications of each. They may initially think point-of-care charting is too intrusive for their patients and decide to keep charting at the nursing station. However, that choice would possibly not alter the process sufficiently to improve documentation or productivity. An alternative then may be identified, such as charting at kiosks placed strategically throughout the nursing unit.

- *Solve problems rather than symptoms.* The hardest part of any problem-solving situation is defining the exact problem. Symptoms are often obvious, but it is imperative to dig deep to find the **root cause** of (or underlying reason for) the problem. This endeavor is analogous to pulling a weed out of a garden. If the root is left in the soil, the weed grows back. Similarly, if only the symptoms of a problem are solved, the problem will most likely recur. A healthcare example that is currently a major issue relates to patient safety and medication errors. Many assume that CPOE and BC-MAR are the solution. However, a study of the flow of the entire process and quantifying where errors are occurring at each step in a given organization may reveal that errors are occurring not in the ordering process but in different locations, such as around formulary access, pharmacy processes, or medication administration. Each environment may be different.

- *Stay focused on the ultimate goal.* Automation can speed up or compound ineffectiveness. The goal of the EHR or other health IT project should not just be to go paperless but to improve the organization's use of health information to achieve its strategic initiatives. Although achieving a paperless environment is ultimately appropriate, project improvement efforts cannot succeed by focusing exclusively on going paperless. Teams should also understand that islands of information systems have long characterized healthcare computing. The lack of system integration within organizations is due in part to the nature of systems development over time, how organizations have historically functioned, the often insular nature of various medical specialties, and backlogs in information technology (IT) departments that have led to acquisition of departmental systems. For whatever reason, each of these information systems has had its own database. An EHR and other health IT environment ideally must be able to tap into all of these databases and have them communicate with each other. Current technology has approached this problem by creating a central repository of information to which each user (person and system) has specified access. Newer technology shares data across disparate databases through application of browser-based technology and cloud computing. Because departments typically are reluctant to give up the perceived power associated with having their own database, the benefits of sharing data must be made clear. Departments should be advised that sharing data enhances everyone's access and that data translated into information is the achievement of real power for the organization as a whole.

- *Focus on the primary customer.* The first step in an EHR or health IT project may be to determine who the customers are. There are actually several types of customers. Ultimately, the most important customer may be the patient or the individual about whom the EHR or health IT provides information. Many view the clinician users as primary customers, and, indeed, they probably are the users most affected by the process changes brought about by EHR and some other health IT implementations.

- *Study existing systems only enough to understand them without limiting breakthrough thinking.* Sometimes processes can be studied at such a level of detail that the overall impact on the organization becomes unclear. Just as an initial reaction to an event or intuition about something can sometimes be the best guide, so, too, should teams rely on their experience and expertise when evaluating whether a process is right or when a redesign makes sense.

- *Look at the big picture.* The scope of the EHR as well as some other health IT projects is to improve results throughout the organization. Process changes will necessarily affect many people, from the physician (who learns the value of clinical decision support as part of the medication ordering process) to the coder in the health information management (HIM) department (whose challenge in an EHR may be to find the data needed to perform coding), to the materials manager (whose inventory records are automated), and even the chief executive officer (who has the ability to produce executive reports at the desktop). Process teams must solicit all these areas for input and ensure that all affected areas are covered in any assessment. The goal of EHR and health IT process mapping is not simply to change processes for the sake of change but to improve outcomes.

Check Your Understanding 5.2

Match the following steps in workflow and process improvement with its purpose:

   A.   Identify processes to be assessed.

   B.   Create process assessment teams of individuals who perform process today.

   C.   Select process assessment tools.

   D.   Map process as actually performed.

   E.   Validate process maps.

   F.   Identify problems and desired changes.

   G.   Determine root cause of problems.

   H.   Document proposed changes.

   I.   Test new workflows and processes.

   J.   Conduct benefits realization.

1. Maintains a record of before and after to use as each step of the systems development life cycle is carried out

2. Chooses the most appropriate tool to assess a process

3. Ensures that all steps in a process, their variations, and their information have been identified

4. Ascertains whether process redesign has yielded improvements

5. Constrains the workflow and process improvement work to those processes that will be affected by a change

6. Provides opportunities for staff to understand how impending changes will improve work performed today

7. Ensures that the process as performed today (and now how it should be performed or will be performed) is described

8. Enables changes to focus on process components that need improvement

9. Addresses underlying issues with current processes rather than only their symptoms

10. Ensures that redesigned workflows and processes work as intended and can produce improvements

Workflow and Process Mapping Tools

A variety of workflow and process mapping tools is available. Table 5.6 identifies some of the process mapping tools and their advantages and disadvantages.

Process Diagramming Tools

Process mapping can be kept at a simple level. For example, the team could use sticky notes to record tasks, place the notes on a large sheet of paper or a wall to illustrate the flow, and then analyze opportunities for improvement. One advantage of using this form of mapping is that workers can map process while they perform their work tasks. Staff members can stash a stack of sticky notes in their pocket and make a record of each task as they do it. This method usually means the process mapping team spends less time formalizing the overall diagram and gets an accurate representation of what is actually happening. However, a simple sticky note map is not an easily transferable document, and the method lacks some mapping integrity because the various symbols or other aids available in more sophisticated tools are often not incorporated. Still, this approach could be a good way to start the mapping process or to ensure a map's accuracy.

Process Diagrams

Process diagrams are free-form illustrations using special symbols and are most commonly used to illustrate the movement of humans, materials, and machinery when mapping an engineering or manufacturing process. Table 5.7 provides often-used flow process chart symbols, their interpretation, and examples of how they might be used to map information flows in a traditional HIM department.

Swim Lane Chart

A swim lane chart is so named because it illustrates processes performed simultaneously (like multiple swimmers in a swimming pool). Figure 5.3 provides an example of a swim lane process

Table 5.6.   Process mapping and system flowchart tools

Tool	Illustration	Advantages	Disadvantages
Process Diagram		Using standard symbols, process diagrams can map both the tasks and their sequence of current or improved processes easily.	Process diagrams do not lend themselves to extensive annotation, so may be difficult to translate into EHR system requirements.
Swim Lane Chart		Swim lane charts add the dimension of clearly identifying the different roles people play in a process. They may simply use boxes, colored boxes, or the process diagram symbols.	Because the focus of EHR process mapping should be on the information flow, the swim lane chart can put too much emphasis on the person or chart.
Flow Process Chart		This chart uses symbols from the process diagram to characterize narrative descriptions of tasks. These charts add the ability to record time a task takes and quantity of work performed.	The flow process chart is an older tool and often focuses on person or chart rather than information flow. They are more difficult to use in illustrating branching logic or decision points, which are often illustrated by indention of the narrative.
System Flow Chart		System flow charts are universally recognized. Although they use a different set of symbols than the process diagram or flow process chart, they are still standardized. These are ideal charts for illustrating decision points.	As with most charts, the amount of narrative that can be accommodated in a system flow chart is limited. Many overcome this by keying narrative descriptions to the symbols where necessary.

map for the referral management process in a clinic. This map uses the same symbols as the process diagram but depicts flow across department boundaries. Swim lanes can be vertical, as illustrated in figure 5.3, or horizontal, as illustrated in table 5.6, which illustrates a swim lane chart created only with colored boxes as opposed to process diagramming symbols.

Flow Process Chart

A **flow process chart** is an older process mapping tool that uses a list structure with accompanying symbols to illustrate the flow of a process. When attempting to map processes performed by clinicians (especially physicians), use of charting symbols may seem too technical. Flow process charts can be a way to incorporate the narrative a physician may be willing to document for a clinical process with symbols that may be applied to a chart form later, if desired. Figure 5.4 is a blown-up version of the flow process chart included in table 5.6.

Table 5.7.   Flow process chart symbols

Symbol	Process	Example
◯	Operation make-ready	Sorting
⬤	Operation do	Coding
⇨	Transportation	Faxing
▽	Storage	Permanent file
▢	Inspection	Proofreading
D	Delay	Awaiting signature

Copyright © 2016, Margret\A Consulting, LLC. Reprinted with permission.

System Flowcharts

System flowcharts are tools used to illustrate the flow of data and information as it is input, processed, and output. They are the most often used tools for workflow and process mapping associated with adopting information technology. They are familiar to most people who would perform this work and are relatively easy to explain to others. System flowchart symbols are provided in table 5.8. Although there are a number of special symbols that can be used to elaborate on components in the flowcharts (some of these are used in figure 5.4), basic symbols depicting boundaries, operations, and decisions can be very effective.

Process boundaries depict where a process begins and ends. Ideally, all maps of associated processes can be linked by way of these boundaries. Ensuring that boundaries are well defined

Figure 5.3.   Sample swim lane process map

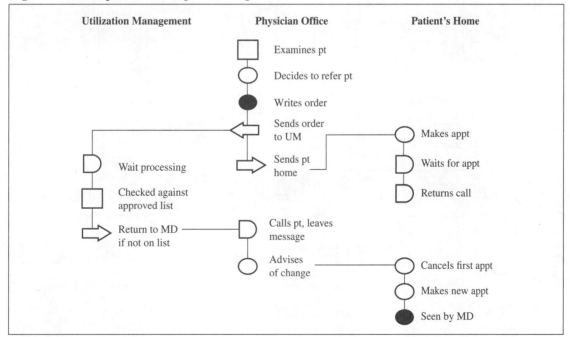

Copyright © 2016 Margret\A Consulting, LLC. Reprinted with permission.

Figure 5.4. Flow process chart

Flow Process Chart

Performed by:

Date:

Process:
- ☐ Present
- ☐ Person
- ☐ Proposed
- ☐ Material

Analysis (✓):
- Why is it done this way?
- Why is it done by this person?
- Why is it done at this time?
- Why is it done at this location?
- Why is it done—is it necessary?

Columns: Operation | Transportation | Inspection | Delay | Storage | Distance in feet | Quantity | Time

Details of Present/Proposed Process:	Operation	Transportation	Inspection	Delay	Storage	Notes
1.	○	⇧	☐	D	▷	
2.	○	⇧	☐	D	▷	
3.	○	⇧	☐	D	▷	
4.	○	⇧	☐	D	▷	
5.	○	⇧	☐	D	▷	
6.	○	⇧	☐	D	▷	
7.	○	⇧	☐	D	▷	
8.	○	⇧	☐	D	▷	
9.	○	⇧	☐	D	▷	
10.	○	⇧	☐	D	▷	

Totals:

Summary:	Present		Proposed	
	No.	Time	No.	Time
Operations				
Transportations				
Inspections				
Delays				
Storages				
Totals:				

Table 5.8. Basic flowchart symbols

Basic Symbols	Purpose
	Terminator—designates where a process begins and ends
	Process—performance of an operation
	Decision—directs flow to two or more branches depending on the alternatives available. If there are more than three options a circle with multiple branches may be used instead. If there are many options, a decision table may be referenced (see figure 7.4)
	On-page and off-page connectors—designates when the flowchart extends to another location on a page or to one or more pages
Special Symbols	**Purpose**
	Manual operation—indicates where a manual operation must occur in a largely electronic workflow
	Document/s—indicates where a paper-based form or document is used, potentially an external document to be scanned
	Magnetic storage/direct access storage—often used to designate a database as well as storage
	Display—terminal or workstation monitor Manual input—keyboard

Copyright © 2016 Margret\A Consulting, LLC. Reprinted with permission.

keeps the mapping process on target. Processes selected for mapping should not be too small or too large. For example, an entire clinic visit, from the time the patient is greeted in reception to the time the patient is sent home with a visit summary, is too large a process to document in one map. On the other hand, the process to take and record a patient's blood pressure is probably too small for an EHR process mapping (Amatayakul 2012).

Process operations are the work performed on data to convert those data to information and, ideally, knowledge. As noted previously, workflow and process mapping should reflect not only visible operations but also operations that are thought processes. As such, the scope of a map may seem small at first, but it can be quite extensive when all decision-making processes are considered. For example, a physician treating a patient whose medication is not working will think about many different factors and seek information from a variety of sources.

Process decisions are the choices or alternatives made in relationship to how data are processed. The key to mapping a "selection of a drug" process, for example, is the decision symbol.

Decisions always reflect a question or choice and always have at least two branches. Branches may signify yes/true and no/false; positive or greater than, negative or less than, and neutral or equal to; or even multiple choices, potentially depicted as a, b, c, d, and so forth. Sometimes, the decision making process is so complex that it is difficult to map by drawing it in a system flowchart. A decision table may be needed to illustrate all the decision points. A sample is shown in figure 5.5.

Workflow is then illustrated by arrows. Typically, arrows are applied from top to bottom and left to right, with the potential exception of an arrow coming from a decision symbol where there are more than two choices, one of which would go right and the other down. Connector symbols are also available if it is necessary to continue a workflow onto a second column of a page or onto another page.

Workflow and Process Mapping Skills

Although process mapping is not difficult, it does take some skill to map processes with the desired level of precision and ensure that what is mapped reflects actual work, including workarounds. When people are new to process mapping, they often map at a very high level. But the particular issues associated with redesigning workflows and processes for adopting an EHR are much more specific. Redesigning workflows and processes for the EHR involves decisions about where in a template a specific type of data should be captured, what specific types of alerts should or should not be generated, and so on. Documenting decisions is perhaps the most difficult task for new process mappers, because most decision making is not observable. However, decision making drives clinical decision support in EHR systems. Clinical decision support is probably the least mature component of the technology and the root cause of many of the unintended consequences frequently described in use of EHRs. As such, it is very important that process mappers make thought processes visible by mapping them carefully and thoroughly. If a consultant or other person is guiding the process mapping, that person must be skilled in interviewing the people who perform processes so that such thought processes are revealed.

Once a current process is mapped, the map should be set aside for a day or so and then validated by those who documented the map and others who also perform the work. This review ensures not only that all steps are actually documented but also that variations are reflected. The mapper must be capable of stepping back and viewing the map from a fresh perspective. The mapper must question every step: Does the map show how this step is performed all the time? Are there variations? When do they occur? What are the paths and outcomes that occur as a result of each difference?

Figure 5.5.   Sample decision table

Conditions	Condition Alternatives							
	Printer does not print	Y	Y	Y	Y	N	N	N	N
	Red light is flashing	Y	Y	N	N	Y	Y	N	N
	Printer is unrecognized	Y	N	Y	N	Y	N	Y	N
Actions	Action Entries							
	Check power cable			X					
	Check printer-computer cable	X		X					
	Ensure printer software is installed	X		X		X		X	
	Check/replace ink	X	X			X	X		
	Check for paper jam		X		X				

Similarly, does this operation have a decision component? What is the decision? What are the choices? What are the paths and outcomes that occur as a result of each choice? For instance, if three nurses perform a refill process in a clinic and each uses a slightly different process, these variations should be illustrated in the map. What may seem to be a slight difference in one nurse's approach may actually be a great idea that should be incorporated into the improved process for all. Alternatively, the difference may be a poor workaround. In this case, the variation should not be punished but assessed for whether it can be corrected prior to EHR deployment or something that requires special functionality in an EHR. Either way, the identification of a suboptimal workaround is extremely important.

Once current processes have been mapped and validated, the next step is to construct a map reflecting an "improved" version of the process. Several versions of this improved map may be created. An initial version may simply reflect what issues the mappers would like to see overcome with an EHR or other type of health IT. Once more is learned about the EHR or other health IT, the improved version can be refined to reflect more specific points about the functionality desired. A version may also be constructed during implementation that reflects the actual improved process—which may reflect some concessions based on product limitations or illustrate further improvements as mappers learn more about product capabilities. Sample before-and-after system flowcharts are illustrated in figure 5.6.

Figure 5.6.   Sample before-and-after workflow charts

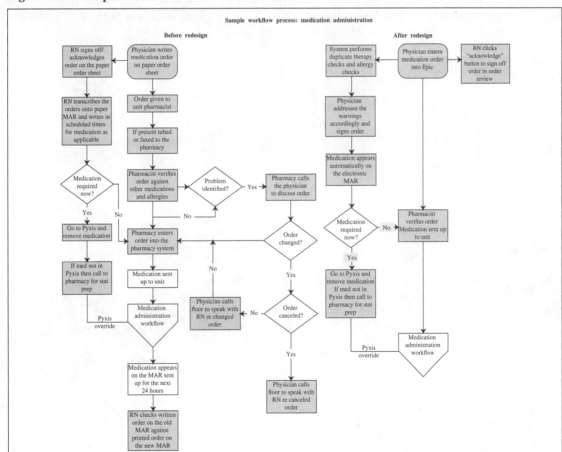

Source: NorthShore University HealthSystem. Used with permission.

The case of NorthShore University HealthSystem (formerly Evanston Northwestern Healthcare [ENH]) gives some sense of the scope of a process improvement project to implement an EHR. The process improvement teams initially developed 500 high-level workflow charts similar to those illustrated in figure 5.6 for medication administration, and these initial documents were eventually developed into 2,000 detailed workflow charts (Smith et al. 2005). As the NorthShore teams proceeded with the redesign of the workflows, they simultaneously gathered all paper documentation tools and order sets. Working with the clinicians, the teams analyzed and classified the data elements to enable them to redesign the clinical information gathering by units. They then worked with information system staff to build the documentation in their system so that users would enter data only once. From there, the data could be shared, retrieved, and reused by any clinician in the care and outcomes management of the patient across the continuum of care (Smith et al. 2005). As of press time for this book, the NorthShore HealthSystem continues to do well with its implementation.

Use Case

Use cases are another tool for describing workflows and processes. A **use case** is a description of the steps between a user and computer software to accomplish a process. Where a systems flowchart illustrates workflow (or thoughtflow) throughout a current or revised process, a use case specifically focuses on the interactions between the user and an information system. Use case methodology was originally developed as a software modeling technique that would help developers understand their customers' needs (Wiegers 1997). It is currently in use in several forms. One form uses the standard Unified Modeling Language (UML) graphic notations, as illustrated in figure 5.7. Microsoft Visual Studio 2015 supports drawing of such use case diagrams. Because many end users

Figure 5.7.   Example high-level use case for clinic visit

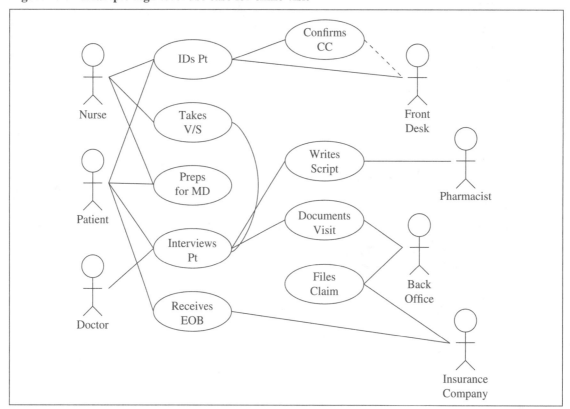

prefer narrative over pictures, the stick figures in the UML diagrams can be converted to boxes. The *essential use case*, also referred to as a *use case scenario*, is another form of use case that is perhaps even easier to construct and more narrative in form. It is essentially a table wherein one column identifies each step in a process that a user would perform, and the other column identifies how the information system would react. An example is provided in figure 5.8.

There are four key elements in the construction of any use case, regardless of its format. First, the use case should be user-focused, not system-focused; in other words, it should depict how the user uses IT to achieve a particular goal. Second, the use case should not include any technical language (a risk when software engineers are using the tool). Third, use cases should be constructed at the appropriate level of detail for the progress of the project. Finally, even though some use cases are more detailed than others, the level of detail should describe the business (clinical) rules, not detailed screen design or data-level information. In other words, a use case should not get to the level of being a data model. Although use cases can easily be used in process mapping at all stages

Figure 5.8.   Example of use case scenario

Provider	System
Primary Success Scenario: Receive appropriate D-D, D-L, D-A, D-W, and D-Dose	CPOE with interface from ADT, Problem List, Medication List, Allergy Documentation, Laboratory, Pharmacy, and Referral systems
Secondary Success Scenario: Retrieve list of patients who may be pregnant, become pregnant, or nursing to advise them of birth defect warning	Data mining capability
Basic Flow: 1. Provider enters order for Paxil 2. D-D contraindication *alert* if patient taking MAOIs or thioridazine 3. D-L *alert* if patient has severe renal or hepatic impairment 4. D-A *alert* if patient has a hypersensitivity to paroxetine (active ingredient in Paxil) or any inactive ingredients 5. D-W (obtain psych consult *reminder*) if patient is at risk for suicide 6. D-dose *recalculation* for starting dose in pediatric patients	1. System finds structured product label (SPL) information from drug knowledge base 2. System compares D-D contraindications from SPL to active medication list 3. System compares most recent creatinine clearance with SPL warning of <30 mL/min 4. System compares ingredients in Paxil to drug allergy information on SPL 5. System checks patient problem list for suicide risk 6. System recalculates starting dose for patients under specified age, height, and weight

Extensions (or alternative flows):
2-a: Alert with respect to MAOIs or thioridazine fires
    1. Cancels order
    2. Requests to see detailed SPL
    3. Selects alternative antidepressant
    4. Overrides alert and retains for Paxil
 	
2-b: Overrides presents list of potential rationales required for order to be accepted
    1. Selects rationale
    2. Cancels order
	1. System deletes order for Paxil
	2. System supplies content of SPL
	3. System performs checks as above on alternative order
	4. System accept override request and supplies rationale requirement per organizational policy

Secondary Flow: 1. Request system to search for all patients for whom Paxil was ordered AND who are women between 12 and 50 years old. . . 2. Produce mailing labels of all patients on report	

in the EHR or other health IT project, they typically have been more closely aligned with defining functional requirements (Shrivathsan 2012) and as a training tool. This is because use cases relate a scenario that focuses more on the desired state rather than current state. Use cases are described from the perspective of functional needs assessment for vendor selection in chapter 7.

Check Your Understanding 5.3

Match the tool to the process for which it is most suited:

   A. Process diagram

   B. Swim lane chart

   C. Flow process chart

   D. System flow chart

   E. Use case

   F. Decision table

   1. Process that entails multiple people performing steps in the process

   2. Documentation of process for health IT

   3. Process with a well-defined sequence of steps that will not be automated

   4. Situation where users need to understand impact of automation

   5. Situation where there are multiple, and often nested, choices to be illustrated

   6. Documentation that produces an easy-to-understand narrative

Document Analysis

In addition to documenting the sequence of steps and decision points in a process, workflow and process mapping should be accompanied by collection of all associated documents and a document analysis. The purpose of this step is to begin the process of defining data requirements associated with each process (although, as already noted, data modeling is not performed at this stage or by process mappers). Such a document analysis can be conducted using vendor-supplied worksheets or a set of spreadsheets, such as those illustrated in figures 5.9 and 5.10. In the first spreadsheet, every document is analyzed. In the second, a database is created of all data elements appearing in all the documents.

Mapping processes across nursing units, clinic sites, or other organizational units helps standardize processes. An interdisciplinary/cross-location approach makes it easier for staff to float among the units as necessary and provides for enhanced adherence to clinical practice guidelines. The process maps themselves can be compared for this purpose, or a spreadsheet can be created to illustrate differences, such as is shown in figure 5.11.

Baseline Data Collection

Another aspect of workflow and process mapping is collection of baseline data. **Baseline data** are data about how a process currently performs that later serve as a comparison to evaluate how a process performs after a change (for example, implementation of EHR or another type of health IT) occurs. Baseline data might include volume of work, time to complete steps, and number of errors or near misses identified. Baseline data collection helps identify opportunities for improvement. It

Figure 5.9. Document analysis: Document review

	Form #	Form Title	Current Version	Data Elements	Entry Responsibility	Frequency of Use	Validation Responsibility	Frequency of Validation	Purpose	Disposition: Medical Record Communication Reference	Omissions	Analysis
	A	B	C	D	E	F	G	H	I	J	K	L
1	EHR Forms Inventory											
4	C12	Chart Note	12/1998	Med Rec No.	Reception	98%	None		Identification	Medical Record		
5				Pt Name	Reception	100%	MD	?	Identification			
6				Date of Visit	?	97%	MA and MD	?	Documentation			
7				Temperature	MA	98%	None		Care Plan		Signature of MA	
8				Pulse	MA	99%	None		Care Plan			
9				Respiration Rate	MA	97%	None		Care Plan			
10				Blood Pressure	MA	85%	MD	75%	Care Plan			Often repeated by MD
11				Reason for Visit	MD	98%	None		Care Plan			Asked by MA but not documented
12				HPI	MD	96%	None		Care Plan			Parts asked by MA but not documented
13				Findings	MD	98%	None		Care Plan			
14				Procedures	MD	63%	Coder	Audit	Documentation			
15				Plan	MD	89%	Coder	Audit	Documentation			Includes Drug Name and Dose if prescription
16				Diagnosis	MD	97%	Coder	Audit	Care Plan Documentation			
17				Signature of MD	MD	98%	Coder	Audit	Documentation			
18				Date of Signature of MD	MD	76%	Coder	Audit	Documentation			
19		Prescription	9/2002	Pt Name	MD	100%	Pharmacist	?	Prescription	Communication	Med Rec No.	Would be helpful for reference & refills
20				Pt Address	MD	75%	Pharmacist	?	Prescription			
21				Pt Phone No.	MD	78%	Pharmacist	?	Prescription			
22				Diagnosis	MD	83%	Pharmacist	?				
23				Drug Name	MD	100%	Pharmacist	?	Prescription		Allergy	Generates 12 calls per week.
24				Dose	MD	100%	Pharmacist	?	Prescription		Contraindications	
25				Refills permitted	MD	97%	Pharmacist	?				Would be helpful to have in MR for reference & refills
26				Generic permitted	MD	96%	Pharmacist	?				Would be helpful to have in MR for reference & refills
27				SIG	MD	96%	Pharmacist	?	Prescription			
28				Signature of MD	MD	100%	Pharmacist	?	Prescription			
29				Date of Signature of MD	MD	97%	Pharmacist	?	Prescription			

also helps organizations set goals and expectations for what can be accomplished with the EHR or other health IT, and it can inform those who conduct benefits realization studies on how well the EHR or other type of health IT is performing in comparison to paper-based or previous electronic processes. Furthermore, baseline data can be used in benchmarking the organization's EHR or health IT performance against best practices.

Some organizations find the process of baseline data collection tedious and time-consuming, especially when they have faith that the EHR or other type of health IT is needed and will achieve intended results. However, an objective assessment of the results of EHR or other health IT implementation is critical to progress. Nevertheless, it is true that baseline data collection must be performed in a manner that is useful, not simply as an exercise that may detract from patient care or be viewed as disciplinary.

Figure 5.10. Document analysis: Data element database

	Current Data Elements	Current Definition (& Reference)	Occurs in Chart Note Y/N	Occurs in Prescription Y/N				Required for:	Data Origination Screen #	Primary Source: Entry ID Reference Pt Portal	Validation Required by	Required in Rule #	Lexicon
	A	B	C	D	E	F	G	H	I	J	K	L	M
1	EHR Forms Database												
4	Allergy to Drugs		N					MR	103	MA	MD	4.32	
5	Allergy to Food		N					MR	103	MA		4.32	
6	Blood Pressure		Y						201	MD			LOINC
7	Date of Signature of MD		Y	Y									
8	Date of Visit		Y							Reception			
9	Diagnosis	Narrative & ICD Code	Y	Y						MD			ICD
10	Dose		Y	Y				Rx					
11	Drug Name	Narrative	Y	Y				Rx				4.32	RxNorm
12	Findings		Y										
13	Generic permitted		N	Y									
14	HPI		Y							Pt Portal	MD		Medcin
15	Med Rec No.		Y	N									
16	Plan		Y										
17	Procedures	Narrative & CPT Code	Y					Bill					CPT
18	Pt Address			Y									
19	Pt Name		Y	Y									
20	Pt Phone No.			Y									
21	Pulse		Y										
22	Reason for Visit		Y										
23	Refills permitted		N	Y									
24	Respiration Rate		Y										
25	SIG	State Bd of Pharmacy		Y									
26	Signature of MD		Y	Y									
27	Temperature		Y										

Figure 5.11.   Sample comparison of processes across sites

Name Box	A	B	C	D	E	F	G
1	Medication Refill Process Mapping						
2		Site 1	Site 2	Site 3	Site 4	Site 5	Site 6
3	Contact Person						
4	1. Refill request faxed/called from pharmacy to clinic	X	X	X	X	X	X
5	2. Fax retrieved by medical records staff	X	X	X	5% of refills are faxed	X	X
6	3. If request called into clinic, Registrars will leave a message (in IDEAL) to have medical records pull the chart	If request is called into clinic, Registrars will contact Pharmacy to have refill faxed request faxed to clinic	If called, phone room leaves a message for medical records to pull chart	X	If called, message left with either Registrars or Triage. If Triage, RN will create a message (via IDEAL) for MR to pull chart	X	If request called into clinic, call is directed to the CMA, who handles all refill requests
7	4. Medical Records pulls the chart and delivers it to the Medical Assistant's inbox	X	MR pulls the chart and places it in the prescribing provider's "in-box"	MR pulls the chart and places it in the triage "in-box" for review	MR pulls the chart and delivers it to the "in basket" at Peds nursing station	MR pulls the chart and delivers it to the "in basket" at nursing station	If the request is for an antibiotic, narcotic, sedative, or migraine medication, the CMA requests the chart from MR. For all "routine medications, patient info. is looked up in IDEAL.

Considerations for baseline data collection include determining what data will be collected (for example, all data or only a sample), how frequently data will be collected, how they will be collected (for example, manually, as a byproduct of another task, or via an automated tool), how they will be summarized (for example, individualized or aggregated), and how they will ultimately be used.

When baseline data are then used in benefits realization, the team must take steps to ensure that apples-to-apples comparisons are being made. **Benefits realization** is the process of collecting the same type of data about process performance for the new process that was collected for the old one. In fact, the challenge of making valid comparisons is often give as a reason for not doing benefits realization. A classic example is medication errors in a hospital. In almost every case of BC-MAR system implementation, the number of documented medication errors increases—not because the system contributes to making errors but because capturing data for medication errors is much easier than before. With better reporting capability, errors seem to increase when the actual number may have decreased. The definition of *medication error* also needs to be considered. For example, many BCMAR systems have tight windows of time in which medications can be administered without calling out an error state; therefore, what might not have been considered an error in the manual environment may now be considered an error by the system. Hence, it is important to make sure benefits realization is performed by knowledgeable individuals, that those who are performing the processes have contributed to their design (including the benefits realization study), and that all such studies are followed up with appropriate celebration and course correction.

If an organization has not collected baseline data, an alternative to a benefits realization study may be a benchmarking study. **Benchmarking** is the process of comparing process performance against an industry best practice or industry standard. Data would still need to be collected about how well the EHR or other health IT is performing, but benchmarking would not require data about performance before the EHR or other type of health IT was implemented.

Process Redesign

The final steps in process mapping relate to process redesign in order to achieve improvement. While it is important to recognize the types of changes that may be feasible now and appropriate for the future, process redesign is not solely about change but also about empowering people to transform their practices to achieve best outcomes. When implementing an EHR, this empowerment has been described as clinical transformation. Process improvement, then, empowers teams to recognize opportunities for improvement and gives them the latitude, within the constraints of the EHR technology, to effect the necessary changes.

Team Empowerment

Team empowerment allows people to make decisions about their work. Although this decision-making capacity is a typical trait of physicians, it is not always embodied by other clinicians—and even physicians may feel constrained in making decisions where an EHR or other health type of IT is involved. Workflow and process mapping should support and encourage such empowerment. This endeavor is a comprehensive undertaking, with many people and even different types of teams coming together at different points within the EHR or other health IT initiative. Checks and balances within an EHR or other health IT project stop any one group from being a significant outlier. Each set of people and teams should be given not only responsibility for the work of process mapping but also appropriate authority to carry out the work and responsibility for seeing to it that redesigned processes are carried out. If a process mapping team believes that its recommendations will not be carried out, it will not succeed.

Process mapping teams may include individuals who have not previously participated in the type of team required for process mapping. Team building is extensively discussed in chapter 8. With respect to process mapping teams, it is important to recognize that people tend to differ according to their preferences for working at a certain level of detail, making decisions, acting as overseers or finishers, and so on. The most desirable process assessment team brings together different types of people who can each contribute in their unique way to the common good.

After the group is formed, it needs a leader. The leader's role is not to direct the group to a specific conclusion but to facilitate the proceedings, keep the group on track, and encourage everyone to participate.

Group Facilitation

Specific techniques are used to facilitate the type of thinking required to conduct process redesign (Terry 2015; Lundblad and O'Neill 2014). These techniques include the following:

- *Brainstorming:* In this technique, as many ideas for the redesign of a process as possible are suggested without any critique. In fact, the most unusual, wild, or crazy ideas are typically the ones that spark creativity among group members. When all the ideas are on the table, the group returns to each one to seek clarification or enhancement. Still, no criticism of any idea is permitted. As clarification is provided, new ideas may be identified. Over the course of this process, people may withdraw ideas that are clearly out of scope or unworkable. Usually, one idea emerges that is the most creative and yet the most manageable.

- *Round robin:* This technique is sometimes referred to as *silent brainstorming* because there is a period of idea generation before each person is asked in turn to either offer ideas or pass. The round robin technique provides an opportunity for everyone in a group to participate.

- *Double reversal:* This technique is a type of brainstorming that helps overcome a lack of ideas. Members of the group are asked to describe the worst way a process could be redesigned. Team members then sort through the ideas generated to determine whether any of them could, if reversed, improve or even totally redesign the system.

- *Nominal group process:* This technique is similar to brainstorming, except that ideas are generated outside the group and then brought to it for consideration. Group members first discuss the meaning and implications of the ideas and then rank-order them to reach consensus on one.

- *Probing:* Probing is often used when individuals find it difficult to break out of their usual ways of thinking. In probing, a facilitator uses various questioning techniques. Probing questions such as "What do you mean by that?" elicit greater detail about an idea just mentioned. A similar type of questioning technique is to ask a series of why questions to uncover personal concerns, political realities, and cultural issues. Mirroring questions, which are basically restatements of what has been said, can be at technique to prevent misunderstanding. For example, a question might start, "If I hear what you are saying . . ." and be followed by a reiteration of the original speaker's comment. Mirroring also tends to elicit further description without appearing to be accusatory, as other probing questions can sometimes seem to be. Many people believe that the best type of question for eliciting detail is an open-ended question. Although open-ended questions are critical in brainstorming, a series of closed questions (with yes-or-no answers) or questions that provide only specific facts can be equally effective in some situations. A trained facilitator knows when to use each type of question to maximize results in a minimum period of time. Figure 5.12 describes facilitator competencies.

Process Redesign Techniques

As the process mapping team starts to redesign workflows and processes for improvement there are some specific things to look for that may signal areas for improvement or where redesign is necessary. These are identified in figure 5.13.

Caution should be applied in process redesign not to strip away processes that may seem like a human–computer interaction problem but that actually mitigate risk (Campbell et al. 2008). For example, taking a blood pressure reading two or three times during a clinic visit may seem to be duplicative or unnecessary, but the process may be clinically relevant. In healthcare, licensure requirements also contribute greatly to determining what person may perform what task, so apparent **role ambiguity** (confusion with respect to tasks a given professional may perform in accordance with education, certification, and/or professional licensure) may be the result of such regulations. For example, in some states, only physicians or registered nurses are permitted to approve prescription renewals for most drugs, whereas in other states medical assistants can also do so.

Cycle time (the time a process takes from start to finish) is often a factor to explore in implementing an EHR or other type of health IT. For example, physicians may believe e-prescribing takes

Figure 5.12. Facilitator competencies

A facilitator . . .	
• Is effective in distinguishing process from content	• Orchestrates the event drama
• Carefully manages the scope of the project	• Releases blocks to the process
• Uses time and space intentionally	• Is adroit in adapting to the changing situation
• Is skillful in evoking participation and creativity	• Assumes responsibility for the group journey
• Is practiced in honoring the group and affirming its wisdom	• Can produce powerful documentation
• Is capable of maintaining objectivity	• Demonstrates professionalism, self-confidence, and authenticity
• Is skilled in reading the underlying dynamics of the group	• Maintains personal integrity

Source: Schuman 2004. Reprinted with permission from the Institute of Cultural Affairs, ICSUSA, Chicago, IL.

Figure 5.13. Opportunities for improvement

• Bottlenecks	• Long cycle time
• Sources of delay	• Lack of adherence to standards
• Rework due to errors	• Lack of information
• Role ambiguity	• Lack of quality controls
• Unnecessary duplications	

longer than writing a prescription on a prescription pad. However, in a paper-based system, more time may be wasted downstream because prescription information is incomplete or illegible. Thus, contrary to the physician's perspective, the automated process could reduce the cycle time.

Ensuring that quality controls are sufficient is an absolutely critical component of process improvement. Such controls need to be in the form of both automated controls and the application of professional judgment. Many of the unintended consequences associated with EHRs or other types of health IT are due to a lack of quality controls, or the failure to apply quality controls (consider the case described in figure 5.2).

Effecting Change

Change management is the process by which an organization gets to its future state—the vision for improvement (Lorenzi and Riley 2000). Much has been said about the need for change management to facilitate adoption of the EHR and other types of health IT. See chapter 6 for more information on this topic.

Role of HIM and IT Professionals in Process Mapping

HIM and IT professionals have a vested interest in the EHR and other health IT, and both kinds of professionals play valuable roles in process improvement. Many HIM and IT professionals are trained in the mapping techniques described in this chapter. However, other members of process improvement teams may be unfamiliar with these techniques. Thus, it may be appropriate to give some just-in-time training to the novices on the various techniques, rather than bombard everyone with all they have to learn up front. If process mapping is not the primary job of team members and they are expected to apply the various techniques over time, it is best to provide training as required.

The appropriate role of the HIM and IT professionals in process improvement should also be noted. The purpose of process improvement is to make the organization's processes compatible with the EHR and other health IT and ensure that these systems do not replicate but improve current processes. Because HIM and IT professionals know how to use the tools, an obvious role for these professionals is that of trainer or facilitator.

However, facilitators are supposed to remain neutral and unbiased. If the HIM or IT professional has strong ideas about what an EHR or other health IT should be and how it should function, the facilitator role would be the wrong choice for that person. The individual in the facilitator role is excluded from the decision-making process and without influence. Each situation is different, however. The HIM or IT professional may be suited to provide training but leave the actual facilitation to someone else. In another situation, the position of trainer may be considered to be outside of the primary decision making group, in which case the HIM or IT professional may prefer to be a member of the assessment team.

References and Resources

Agilean. 2010. Agile & Lean Glossary. http://www.agilean.com/resources/faqs/agile_lean_glossary/agile_lean_glossary.htm.

Amatayakul, M. 2007. To achieve clinical quality improvement through IT, engage clinicians. *Healthcare Financial Management.* 61(2):122–124.

Amatayakul, M. 2012. *Process Improvement with Electronic Health Records: A Stepwise Approach to Workflow and Process Management.* Boca Raton, FL: CRC Press.

Ball, M.J., and S. Bierstock. 2007. Clinician use of enabling technology. *Journal of Health Information Management.* 27(3):68–71.

Campbell, E.M., K.P. Guappone, D.F. Sittig, R.H. Dykstra, and J.S. Ash. 2008. Computerized provider order entry adoption: Implications for clinical workflow. *Journal of General Internal Medicine.* 24(1):21–26.

Cohn, K.H., J. Berman, B. Chaiken, D. Green, M. Green, D. Morrison, and J.E. Scherger. 2009. Engaging physicians to adopt healthcare information technology. *Journal of Healthcare Management.* 54(5):291–300.

Dooley, S. 2016 (January 7). Avoid EHR unintended consequences with good follow through. The Coding Institute. http://blog.supercoder.com/emrehr/avoid-ehr-unintended-consequences-with-good-follow-through.

Essin, D. 2011 (January 24). EHRs: Think clinical process, not automation. CancerNetwork.com. http://www.cancernetwork.com/oncology-ehr/content/article/1462168/1781523.

Fillingham, J. 2008. Getting the change process right using the human needs model. ChangingMinds.org. http://changingminds.org/articles/articles08/the_philosophy_of_change.htm.

George, M. 2008, Integrating Lean and Six Sigma. http://www.isixsigma.com/library/content/ask-02.asp.

Graham, J., and C. Dizikes. 2011 (June 27). Baby's death spotlights safety risks linked to computerized systems. *Chicago Tribune.* http://articles.chicagotribune.com/2011-06-27/news/ct-met-technology-errors-20110627_1_electronic-medical-records-physicians-systems.

Guite, J., M. Lang, P. McCartan, and J. Miller. 2006. Nursing admissions process redesigned to leverage EHR. *Journal of Healthcare Information Management.* 20(2):55–64.

Han, Y.Y., J.A. Carcillo, S.T. Venkataraman, R.S. Clark, R.S. Watson, T.C. Nguyen, H. Bayir, and R.A. Orr. 2005. Unexpected increased mortality after implementation of a commercially sold computerized physician order entry system. *Pediatrics.* 116(6):1506–1512.

HealthIT.gov. 2013 (June 10). What is workflow redesign? Why is it important? https://www.healthit.gov/providers-professionals/faqs/ehr-workflow-redesign.

Jones, S.S., R. Koppel, M.S. Ridgely, T.E. Palen, S. Wu, and M.I. Harrison. 2011. *Guide to Reducing Unintended Consequences of Electronic Health Records.* Rockville, MD: Agency for Healthcare Research and Quality. http://www.healthit.gov/unintended-consequences.

Koppel, R., J.P. Metlay, A. Cohen, B. Abaluck, A.R. Localio, S.E. Kimmel, and B.L. Strom. 2005. Role of computerized physician order entry systems in facilitating medication errors. *Journal of the American Medical Association.* 293(10):1197–1203.

Kudyba, S.P., ed. 2010. *Healthcare Informatics: Improving Efficiency and Productivity.* Boca Raton, FL: CRC Press.

Leventhal, R. 2014 (August 26). KLAS: One quarter of ambulatory EHRs could be replaced. *Healthcare Informatics.* http://www.healthcare-informatics.com/news-item/klas-25-percent-ambulatory-ehrs-could-be-replaced.

Longhurst, C.A., L. Parast, C.I. Sandborg, E. Widen, J. Sullivan, J.S. Hahn, C.G. Dawes, and P.J. Sharek. 2010. Decrease in hospital-wide mortality rate after implementation of a commercially sold computerized physician order entry system. *Pediatrics.* 126(1):14–21.

Lorenzi, N.M., and R.T. Riley. 2000. Managing change: An overview. *Journal of the American Medical Informatics Association.* 7(2):116–124.

Lundblad, J.P., and K.M. O'Neill. 2014 (July). Effective QI meeting management and facilitation for nursing homes. Stratis Health. https://www.stratishealth.org/documents/Effective-QI-Mtg-Mgmt-Facilitation-Slides-2014-07-09.pdf.

McGee, M.K. 2011 (January 11). HealthEssentials' clinicians to use digital pens. *Information Week*. http://www .informationweek.com/story/showArticle.jhtml?articleID=229000424.

Microsoft Developer Network. 2015. UML use case diagrams: Guidelines. Visual Studio 2015. https://msdn.microsoft .com/en-us/library/dd409432.aspx.

Poggio, F. 2010 (February 24). CPOE and the doc dilemma. *Health Informatics*. http://www .healthcare-informatics.com/article/cpoe-and-doc-dilemma.

Polaschek, J., et al. 2003. (November 10). Lessons from the front line—The good, bad, and ugly: The Cedars-Sinai CPOE experience. *Proceedings of the American Medical Informatics Association*.

Shrivathsan, M. 2012 (June 13). Features vs. use cases vs. requirements. http://rmblog.accompa .com/2012/06/features-vs-use-cases-vs-requirements.Smith, D., and Newell, L.M. 2002. A physician's perspective: Deploying the EMR. *Journal of Healthcare Information Management*. 16(2):71–79.

Smith, T., N. Semerdjian, P. King, B. DeMartin, S. Levi, K. Reynolds, RN, J. Ryan, and J. Dowd. 2005 (December). Transforming healthcare with a patient-centric electronic health record system. Evanston Northwestern Healthcare, Nicholas E. Davies Award of Excellence. Chicago: Healthcare Information and Management Systems Society.

Terry, B.D. 2015. Working in groups: Facilitating positive group interactions. University of Florida Institute of Food and Agricultural Sciences (IFAS) Extension. https://edis.ifas.ufl.edu/fy1377.

Van Dijk, R., and R. Van Dick. 2009. Navigating organizational change: Change leaders, employee resistance and work-based incentives. *Journal of Change Management*. 9(2):143–163.

Wiegers, K.E. 1997. Listening to the customer's voice. *Process Impact*. http://www.processimpact.com/articles/usecase .html.

Wietecha G. 2013. An eBook guide to EHR replacement, NextGen Healthcare. https://bridge.nextgen.com/media/815/ nextgen-healthcare-ehr-replacement-edu15.pdf.

Chapter 6
Change Management for Health IT

Key Terms

ADKAR model of communication
Agile
Change agent
Change leader
Clinical transformation
Communication
Communication plan
Culture
Groupware
Influencer
Knowledge worker
Motivational interviewing
Patient empowerment
Patient engagement
Refreezing
Shared decision making
Stages of change

Learning Objectives

- Discuss the nature of health IT change and the need for making change management a priority in a knowledge worker environment.

- Recognize the primary role that change leaders play in EHR and health IT adoption.

- Describe the importance of and how to plan communications for change.

- Identify and describe uses of tools to manage change in order to effect the clinical and cost transformation expected from EHR and health IT.

The scope of change that the electronic health record (EHR) and other types of health information technology (health IT) brings to healthcare is immense. But the enormity of the change is actually not so much in the use of a computer (many clinicians use other technology that is equally or more sophisticated). Rather, the change is in how clinicians perceive the EHR and health IT, which requires them to work differently. Clinicians' questions can sometimes seem repetitive, but they do not ask them just because they do not have access to previously collected data, or because they do not trust the reliability of those data. Instead, each clinician tends to ask patients the same questions as other clinicians because asking questions and listening to the answers helps the clinician process information. Most clinicians have not adapted to process information by merely reviewing patient data collected by someone else. In fact, mental processes are very physical for clinicians. Like other knowledge workers, they find the questioning process, where they ask for information in the sequence in which they prefer to think about it, gives them the logical ability to make appropriate connections needed to diagnose and treat. For change to occur, then, different strategies for change management must be used, and they must be purposeful.

The process, then, of managing the change brought about by the EHR and other health IT begins with defining the true nature of the change, recognizing barriers to change that may be different than the obstacles that were first anticipated or even understood by those individuals who are expected to change, and identifying and using change strategies that would best achieve the clinical transformation that is desired with the EHR and health IT. Change leaders must manage the change through effective communications, change processes, monitoring reactions to change, and providing meaningful feedback.

The Nature of EHR and Health IT Change for Knowledge Workers

Change is a constant in any environment, but, for healthcare, it seems that changes are greater and more rapidly paced change than ever before. Between 2011 and 2016, major changes in healthcare regulations and policy requirements have included the meaningful use (MU) of EHR incentive program, breach notification regulation, conversion from ICD-9-CM to ICD-10-CM, health reform requiring new models of care and reimbursement, and ever greater emphasis on quality and cost improvement (National Learning Consortium 2013). At the same time, the healthcare industry is also experiencing significantly more mergers and acquisitions in provider organizations, health plans, and EHR vendors.

Change is stressful for most people, but it can be especially difficult for **knowledge workers** (people whose life work is developing or using knowledge), including most people working in healthcare, and certainly all clinicians. Although the term *knowledge worker* was first described by Peter Drucker in 1959, a recent article in *Harvard Business Review* suggests that Drucker (who died in 2005) knew more about the environment of 2020 than most leaders managing organizations today (Wartzman 2014). Studies of knowledge workers spanning several decades have found that such workers are characterized by the following:

- Ability to work on many projects at the same time

- Ability to multiply the results of their efforts through soft factors such as emotional intelligence and trust

- Creative learning style, in an inquiry-driven and self-controlled manner

- Autonomy of decision making, where a traditional command-and-control management style is not effective for them to contribute to the achievement of organizational interests (Malhotra 1997; Robins and Webster 2003; Holsapple 2013)

Despite knowledge workers' focus on contributing their experience to create knowledge from information, the following have also been observed about them:

- They need to be empowered to make the most of their deepest skills.

- They often possess inadequate skills in using productivity software and get distracted in their core focus when attempting to use such software.

- They lack training in following a systematic approach in the development of knowledge that would support application of technology to such knowledge generation.

- They lack the ability to effectively structure and communicate newly created knowledge.

Superimposed upon the distinctive characteristics of knowledge workers are the more universal concerns around change as well as reactions that often intensify resistance to change. Change creates uncertainty. Some people are uncertain whether they can learn the new technology well enough to keep their job. Others feel a loss of self-esteem when they believe they appear inadequate to others. In a clinical environment, uncertainty also translates into fear of doing harm to patients as well as the ever-present fear of the potential for a malpractice lawsuit.

Change prompted or coerced by external forces can frustrate individuals and provoke feelings of uncertainty, and the immaturity of products can compound these reactions. EHRs were first conceived in the mid-1960s, but their use for the first 40 years was largely restricted to academic medical centers and those providers who developed their own EHR. It was not until the MU program was instituted under the Health Information Technology for Economic and Clinical Health Act (HITECH) of 2009 that most clinicians were expected to use EHRs. This forcing mechanism also came with very high expectations (as illustrated in figure 6.1). Under MU milestones, clinicians were expected to go from data capture and sharing to using advanced clinical processes via technology by 2013, and they were expected to demonstrate improved outcomes through the use of EHRs by 2016. The result was a rush by vendors to create products suitable for mass adoption. These products were largely untested, and when clinicians' early experiences with EHRs did not live up to expectations, they began to resist using the systems. In fact, the EHR technology itself did not to

Figure 6.1.   Expectations for MU program

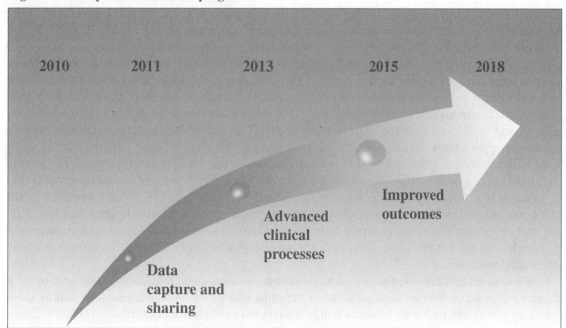

Source: HIT Policy Committee

lead to failure—research on EHR failures shows that failure occurred because the MU initiative did not deal with changes in how people and organizations work(Kaplan and Harris-Salamone 2009).

Collective pressures to resist change are powerful. As some individuals expressed concerns about the EHR, many others followed suit. Even published research papers that describe positive results from EHRs, and their clinical decision support in particular, often frame the results in terms that seem negative or ambivalent at best. For example, in an article titled "Effect of clinical decision-support systems," Bright and colleagues report positive findings that "clinical decision support systems improved health care process measures" in preventive services, clinical studies, and the prescription of therapies. However, the authors set this research in a negative context, stating "despite increasing emphasis on the role of clinical decision support systems for improving care and reducing costs, evidence to support widespread use is lacking," and "evidence for clinical, economic, workload, and efficiency outcomes remains sparse" (Bright et al. 2012). The fact that studies have not been performed and there is therefore not a lot of evidence should not be interpreted that clinical decision support systems are bad, or that they do not have opportunities for improvement, but, unfortunately, it is human nature to view things negatively.

Change Management Leadership

A recently published book on change management, titled *Influencer,* describes a new science of leading change through influence (Grenny et al. 2013). According to Grenny and colleagues, **influencers** are those who attempt to influence behavior (encourage) rather than change behavior (force). Influencers can create rapid, profound, and sustainable behavior change. They are clear about the results they want to achieve and how they will measure them, and they focus on a small number of vital behaviors that will help them achieve the desired results. This method of change succeeds because influencers help people love what they hate and master new skills; provide encouragement and assistance; reward early successes; and change physical surroundings to make good behavior easier and bad behavior harder. Interestingly, in addressing reward systems, the authors encourage a strategy of modest and intelligent rewards, punishments only when necessary, and using incentives last.

Identifying Change Leaders

Change leaders (also known as **change agents**) are individuals who act as catalyst for change. They have a clear vision and can articulate it to others. Change leaders are patient, recognizing that change does not occur rapidly; however, they also are persistent in taking opportunities to move closer to a change. They ask tough questions—not to be naysayers, but to ensure that participants in the change have an emotional connection for the change. Change leaders are considered knowledgeable and able to lead by example. For this reason, many chief medical informatics officers (CMIOs) do not want to give up practice to take on an informatics role. They want to be able to have at least as much knowledge of and experience with the EHR or other health IT as any of their colleagues. Finally, change agents are approachable and reliable. People trust them. When change leaders in the health IT arena need to have tough conversations with someone resistant to use the EHR or other health IT, the trust they have already built enables them to do the right thing even if it is uncomfortable (Couros 2013).

People in a formal leadership position, such as the CMIO, the EHR project manager, or the chief executive officer of the organization, are often considered to be change leaders. But John Kotter, one of the world's most recognized experts in change management, argues that management and leadership are not the same—and both are needed (Kotter 2012). Table 6.1 compares management and leadership.

While managers are often expected to be change leaders, change leaders do not have to be in formal leadership positions. In fact, some of the most successful change leaders are simply those who can effectively influence others. Change leaders have the skill set described in figure 6.2.

Table 6.1.   Management versus leadership

Management	Leadership
Functions	
Planning and budgeting	Establishing direction
Organizing and staffing	Aligning people
Controlling and problem solving	Motivating and inspiring
Outcomes	
Predictable order that produces consistent short-term results expected by various stakeholders	Change that has the potential to transform

Recognizing and Responding to Resistance to Change

Recognizing people's concerns and feelings about change and preparing to respond to them is an important task of change leaders. As illustrated in table 6.2, people react to change in different ways—from threatening to leave to actively supporting the change (Amatayakul 2012). Change leaders should interpret reactions from and respond appropriately to all people in the organization. Although EHR and health IT represent a huge change for clinicians, all employees within an organization who are affected by these changes must be engaged (Brown 2012). Particular attention should be give to informal leaders or opinion leaders who are naysayers, so they can become supporters of the change and not sabotage it.

Change Leaders Becoming Influencers

Personal motivation is probably the most powerful way for someone to change. But personal motivation needs to be stimulated when there is an external factor causing change. As noted earlier in this chapter, knowledge workers need to be empowered to make the most of their skills. Likewise, they need to be empowered to accept change. **Motivational interviewing** is a counseling approach first made popular by clinical psychologists Rollnick and Miller in the treatment of individuals who abuse or misuse alcohol; it is now recommended as a supportive communication technique to engage patients in important lifestyle changes and as a technique that can be used for eliciting behavior change in other contexts (Rollnick and Miller 1995; Stratis Health 2014a).

Motivational interviewing is typically performed in a one-on-one environment with individuals who are negative about or actively resistant to a change. Change leaders who wish to use the

Figure 6.2.   Skills of change leaders

Change leaders have:
- *People skills:* They are able to understand the diversity among all individuals, skill sets, and positions that are affected by EHR and health IT. Effective change leaders are able to listen, restate, reflect, clarify without interrogating, draw out the quiet, quiet the verbose, channel discussion, plant ideas, and develop trust and confidence among users.
- *Political skills:* They need to understand the various viewpoints and counterpoints that may arise during discussions about EHR and other types of health IT.
- *System skills:* They help organize and manage technology while translating this into language that users will understand and respect.
- *Analytical skills:* These skills ensure that members of the organization not only understand and appropriately improve upon workflow and processes but also use workflow and processes to assess and manage the financial impact of change.
- *Business skills:* These skills are needed to understand the underlying way the health care organization works and the underlying clinical processes. Change leaders need be able to "talk the talk and walk the walk" related to their roles.

Table 6.2.   Reactions to change and potential responses

Reaction	Response
Leaving	Some people indicate that they will go to another facility or retire before adopting the EHR or other form of health IT. Some can be convinced to stay and serve the organization well if their active resistance can be channeled into representing a resister's viewpoint for the good of the project. However, if this is not possible, simply acknowledge these individuals' accomplishments and let them make their own decisions. Threats to go elsewhere are generally no longer effective, as most facilities have adopted or are in the process of adopting an EHR and other types of health IT.
Active resistance	In active resistance, the facility has an advantage because the individuals are clear about how they feel. Such individuals can be a benefit to an EHR or health IT project if, as described above, the active resistance can be channeled into representing a resister's viewpoint for the good of the project. Once active resisters are turned around, they can be equally active in their support. Active resisters often do not threaten to leave, either because they are not old enough to retire or because they know other facilities are also adopting EHR and health IT. As a result, they are easier to influence than those who are simply threatening to leave. It is important to turn around active resisters because their resistance can be infectious.
Opposition	A person who opposes the EHR and health IT but is not overtly resistant or threatening to leave can be the most difficult to identify and to turn around. Often, this is a person who is negative about everything. Offering counseling to such individuals may be necessary (see information on motivational interviewing later in the chapter). The benefits can be substantial, not only for the EHR and health IT projects but also for the individual.
Acquiescence	An individual who grudgingly accepts the EHR or other type of health IT is someone who needs to be monitored closely. This individual could swing to either (active or passive) opposition or acceptance. Involving this individual with specific tasks and recognition for work well done will help ensure acceptance.
Acceptance or modification	An individual who claims to accept the project but continually offers modifications to the system can put a project at risk for delay or going over budget. Often, a person with such a reaction actually opposes the project and is trying to avoid using the system or any change it may be designed to impose. This exuberance for modifying the new system back to old ways absolutely needs to be managed immediately.
Acceptance	A person who quietly accepts the change is certainly one to be appreciated. However, such individuals can contribute more to the process of turning others around if they are more actively supportive of the project. They should be encouraged to describe their support and help them become "gentle" change leaders themselves.
Active support	Some people will be genuinely active supporters and should be greatly appreciated. Their energy and enthusiasm should be channeled into constructive help.

Source: Amatayakul 2012

technique with those who are resistant to using the EHR or health IT should be provided additional information and training to hone their skills.

Sobell and Sobell (2008) provide rationales and examples for steps to be taken in motivational interviewing of those persons who are struggling to change. Steps and rationales with examples tailored for a discussion about EHR are summarized in table 6.3.

Change Leaders Empowering Others

When positive change occurs, change leaders should reinforce it to further empower workers to continuously learn and improve. Another supportive communication technique to engage patients in important lifestyle changes is **patient engagement** (also called **patient empowerment**), a technique used to assess a patient's knowledge, skills, ability, and willingness to manage his or her own

Table 6.3. Motivational interviewing steps: Rationales and examples

Steps	Rationale	Examples
Ask permission to talk about a change	Communicates respect	Do you mind if we talk about how you are using the EHR?
Elicit change talk	Allows person to give voice to the need for change	What would you like to see different about use of the EHR? What would be the good things that would result from using the EHR? How can I help you get past some of the difficulties you are experiencing?
Rate importance and confidence	Helps the interviewer understand how close to, or far from, making a change an individual is	How would you rate the importance of the EHR? How would you rate your confidence in using the EHR? Why did you describe (each answer in turn) as X? What would need to happen to make you consider the EHR as more important or your confidence in it to increase?
Open-ended questions	Allows for deeper conversation and builds empathy with the individual	What happens when you attempt to use the EHR?
Reflective listening	Encourages persons to state arguments for change	It sounds like… What I hear you saying is…
Normalizing	Communicates that change is not uncommon	A lot of people are concerned about using the EHR. Many EHR users report good things and not so good things about their use.
Decisional balancing	Builds upon normalizing in order to solicit deeper response	What are some of the positive things about EHR you have experienced? What are some of the negative things about EHR you have experienced?
Deploy discrepancies	Identifies contradictions and helps people accept more positive attributes	Help me understand, you said this was … (negative), but then you also said this was … (positive).
Elicit self-confidence	Helps reinforce the positives and encourages additional positive changes	It seems you have been successful in doing X with the EHR. Could you use that approach to do Y?
Affirmations	Recognizes successes and efforts to change	It's clear you have been able to X successfully. That is really important.
Feedback	Enables comparisons with others to strength commitment to change	It has been reported by (name) that the EHR has been helpful in improving X. How do you compare with this? How can you get the same results?
Therapeutic paradox	Attempt to get person to argue for change	Have you thought about alternatives to practicing medicine/nursing in order to not have to use the EHR?

Source: Adapted from Sobell and Sobell 2008.

health and care and then select appropriate interventions to increase activation and promote positive patient behavior (Noteboom 2015). Research has shown that clinicians with strong patient-centered communication skills have patients who are more engaged, ask more questions, share more information, and are more adherent and generally healthier (Edgman-Levitan and Gandhi 2014). Similarly, empowering healthcare workers improves their ability to cope with change and more readily adopt change. Table 6.4 lists tips for empowering workers

Table 6.4.   Tips for empowering workers

Tip	Why	How
Foster open communication	Helps value input and further empowerment	Supply structured ways for workers to easily and regularly make known their thoughts, feelings, and observations. Acknowledge all input and reward valuable input. If input is not accepted, help workers understand why.
Talk straight	Honesty gains trust that supports empowerment	Communicate directly without sugar-coating messages or casting blame. Trust others so they will trust you.
Reward self-improvement	Supports continual learning, which help workers gain confidence in their empowerment	Budget and allocate time for training and development. Help each worker set a plan for growth and reward workers as they advance
Encourage safe failure	Recognizing that mistakes are a byproduct of innovative and changing organizations further provides confidence in empowerment	Give workers opportunity to try new things. Create checkpoints or set up a test environment to try out and learn from failures as well as successes. Use facilitation techniques to brainstorm about new ideas that will lead to reducing risk of failure.
Avoid dependency	Supports autonomy of knowledge workers in a safe environment	Provide vision, core values, purpose and direction. Have an open-door policy for workers who need assistance but avoid hovering and continually asking if workers need help.
Require and make accountability transparent	Encourages accountability for empowered actions	Tell workers when they are meeting expectations and when they are not. Hold all workers accountable for their actions.
Appreciate workers' efforts	Gives empowered people a greater level of satisfaction than simply financial stability	Find ways to say "thank you" and to openly and honestly appreciate workers' contributions and participation.

Source: Adapted from Daum 2013.

Check Your Understanding 6.1

Choose the best answer:

1. A characteristic of a knowledge work is:

    a. Ability to focus on only one project at a time

    b. Autonomy of decision making

    c. Extensive user of productivity software

    d. Systematic approach to learning

2. A change leader is always:

    a. A catalyst for change

    b. A designated leader in an organization

    c. Employed by the organization

    d. Upper management

3. An important skill of change leaders is:

   a. Aligning people

   b. Budgeting

   c. Controlling

   d. Problem solving

4. Which type of reaction to change is the easiest to recognize?

   a. Acceptance/modification

   b. Acquiescence

   c. Active resistance

   d. Opposition

5. When a person reacts to change with acceptance or modification, the organization should:

   a. Applaud the person's interest

   b. Ignore the person's interest

   c. Manage potential risk the modification may impose

   d. Work hard to adopt the modification proposed

6. Which new model of care can be modified to help strong resisters of an EHR?

   a. Motivational interviewing

   b. Patient engagement

   c. Personal motivation

   d. Shared decision making

7. Which of the following is helpful in empowering workers to accept change?

   a. Avoid dependency

   b. Provide incentives to initiate change

   c. Require attendance at all meetings

   d. Sanction those who do not change

Planning Communications for Change

Communication is one of the most difficult tasks in organizations seeking to make a change. To effectively plan for communications about a change, the following steps must be undertaken:

- Understand that communication is shared meaning.
- Understand the organization and what forms of communication are most effective in the organizational context.
- Develop a communication plan.
- Execute the five rights of communication.

Communication Defined

One of the best definitions of **communication** is "shared meaning." This definition gets at the crux of most communication problems—that the message is delivered but those who receive it do not understand it in the way that the deliverer intended. Even when the parties are not sharing information in real time, communication requires a conversation in order to verify that there is shared meaning.

To improve communication about change, recognize that communicating change is different than communicating other information. When communicating change, it is helpful to have a formal, documented communication plan that is checked frequently (such as every day). Finally, communication about change must reflect the systems development life cycle (SDLC), in which a need is identified, a communication is developed and delivered, feedback is obtained, success is celebrated, and course corrections are made where necessary. (See chapter 2 for more information on SDLC.)

Communicating Change

Communicating about a change is unique in several ways (Heathfield 2015a, b). Communicating about a change such as EHR and health IT must be done frequently, consistently, and via every possible channel, such as spoken presentations, written materials, videos, training sessions and materials, focus groups, bulletin boards, one-on-one conversations, intranets, e-mails, and text and instant messages.

Since change as massive as the EHR and some other types of health IT occurs over a fairly lengthy period of time and may involve changes even once a given plan is established, it is important to communicate as quickly as possible and ensure transparency. Sometimes, it may be necessary to acknowledge that a change is required but all details are not yet known; in these situations, offer reassurance that as soon as new information becomes available, there will be further communication. Then, be sure to follow through, so that such instant but incomplete communications will be trusted whenever they must be used.

Because communication is shared meaning, it is essential to help people share in the meaning. Some communication channels may seem less conducive to feedback than others, but all forms of communication must allow for opportunities for questions, clarifications, and input. Leaders should make a conscious effort to provide time after a presentation, a website for tracking information, a phone number to call, or any other effective means of obtaining feedback. When responding to comments and inquiries, leaders should provide answers only if the answer is known. It is better to acknowledge a lack of knowledge than to make something up that is incorrect. Leaders must also not be defensive or make excuses. Responses that are thoughtful are much more powerful than those that are off the cuff, flippant, and often wrong.

To strengthen the shared meaning, leaders should always set communication within the context of the organization's vision and mission and goals for the change. People need to understand why changes are being made, and they need help understanding how these changes will affect them. Stories can often be effectively used to illustrate relationships between what is about to happen and what the ultimate goal is, and how that goal fits within the stability of the environment.

If these communication strategies are put in place, communications should be proactive, which will diminish the likelihood of rumors. If rumors spread, that is a sign the organization has waited too long to communicate and must take corrective action. It is far better to admit mistakes and take corrective action than to ignore the rumors until they fester into resistance to change that may be impossible to repair.

Finally, leaders must seek feedback an ongoing, real-time basis—not just when a communication is delivered and questions are taken, or when a formal measurement system provides periodic information about performance improvements. Change leaders cannot sit in their offices and expect change to succeed. To the contrary, change leaders must be out and about, being accessible but also observing, sensing, feeling, and seeking out reactions to change. These interactions are also opportunities to express appreciation or give a pat on the back. Making a point of acknowledging the good work of one person or one group when speaking to another person or group is an excellent way of saying "thank you."

Developing and Using a Communication Plan

A formal, documented **communication plan** is a tool that helps ensure that the communications about change are carried out in the manner described above. Much like the "five rights of medication management," a communication plan ensures that the right message is delivered to the right people, by the right people, using the right media, and at the right time. A communication plan also supports the process of acquiring feedback.

This plan ideally should be available in an interactive software tool that can be accessed and updated by any given stakeholder in the plan. The project manager may be the person responsible for structuring the plan and performing routine maintenance on it, but he or she is not the sole communicator. In fact, many people are expected to deliver communications about change and must take responsibility for keeping their communication tasks updated.

Right Message

The **ADKAR model of communication** illustrated in figure 6.3 identifies generic types of messages used to communicate about an impending change. The ADKAR model recognizes a continuum of messages for projects that introduce a great amount of change, and it illustrates the relationship between types of messages and project phases:

- *Awareness* building needs to begin as soon as a new project or program need is identified

- *Desire* helps turn an uncertain concept into interest in specifics.

- *Knowledge* about any new project or program is essential for all stakeholders—although the knowledge needed is different at different levels. Throughout the planning process, stakeholders need to understand their role in making any new project or program successful.

Figure 6.3.   ADKAR model of communication

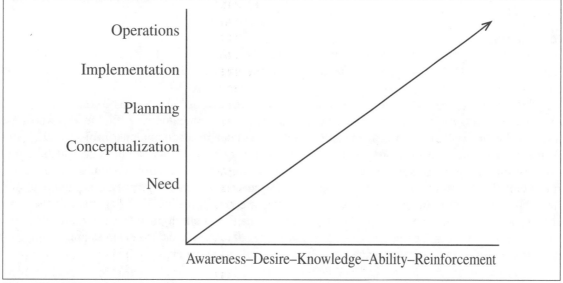

Source: Hiatt 2006

- *Abilities* to actually take part in a project or program implementation must be fine-tuned.

- *Reinforcement* of the benefits the new project or program helps ensure that ongoing operations are successful. Communication does not end with implementation. Continued success requires continual communications—about successes, challenges, course corrections, and more. (Hiatt 2006)

In addition to the content of the message, the context of the message is important. Context involves plain language, clarity, enough but not too much detail, and avoidance of "techno-speak." Depending on the message, an example, reference to additional information, checklists, or other tools can be helpful. When a message is delivered via media that support color, graphics, use of emoticons, and other visual aids, the aids selected should be suitable for the message and carry the same tone and demeanor as if the message were delivered in person. Excessive use of such aids should be avoided, as they often can convey unintended meaning and be easily misinterpreted. Similarly, in verbal communications, nonverbal forms of communication, such as gestures, body language, tone of voice, and so on, should fit the type of communication.

Right Sender
Selecting the right person to deliver any given message helps ensure that the message is successfully shared. Even when the sender delivers the message in person, the sender will be evaluated by the recipient and that assessment will influence the shared meaning. For example, the medical staff of a hospital will interpret a message from the chief of the medical staff differently than they would understand the same message from a deputy of the hospital administrator. If the message is very important, the ideal candidate to deliver it would be the chief of medical staff. The right sender should be designated for each type of message delivered (Hiatt and Creasey 2012).

Right Receiver
Any given message will have one or more right receivers and should be tailored based on who will receive it. For example, a message that announces that a new version of software will be installed may need to be sent to a wide range of staff. The message itself, however, may be more or less detailed based on whether it is sent to users, IT staff, or department managers.

Recipients must also be prepared to receive a message. They must take time to read or listen carefully, be able to ask questions for clarification, and trust that the information is correct. In a two-way communication, asking the recipient to paraphrase what the message says can help ensure that the communication is successful. Helping the recipient prepare to receive messages of different types should be a consideration of the sender.

Right Media
The method by which a message is delivered should be selected based on an assessment of what medium will most effectively convey the meaning of the message. Both the sender and the recipient must be accommodated.

The types of media with which to send messages are increasing, and all can be effective depending on the message and exchange participants. Smartphones with cameras, social media websites, and **groupware** (which is software used to facilitate exchange of documents, project plans, performance and outcomes measures, and other information) all have a very important place in communication. However in such an environment, in-person communication becomes increasingly important. In-person communication should not be considered only for special communications but also used on as frequent a basis as possible when communicating about change. In the long run, in-person communications take less time than managing the fallout from a poor, remote communication. Allowing for opportunities to obtain immediate feedback and express appreciation—even just for listening to the message—is a powerful way to effect change.

Holding huddles, conducting stand-up meetings, and picking up the phone are all good ways for senders to initiate communication. Huddles are short (10 to 15 minutes) stand-up meetings to bring a team together to review plans for the day and deliver project status checks (Vrabie 2014). Huddles are already used in healthcare in the form of rounds for physicians to learn about the status of their patients at the start of each day, or as shift-change reports for nurses when they hand off care of patients to the next shift. However, huddles to discuss an EHR or health IT project should usually be separated from these other meetings, unless the communication about health IT is absolutely vital and urgent and can be covered briefly (in less than five minutes).

Right Time

Delivering a message at the right time can help successfully convey its meaning. Obviously, delivering a message too late is bad. But messages that are delivered too early, too frequently, not frequently enough, and at poor times of the day, week, shift (and so on) also will not receive the desired attention from recipients. A communication plan that flags when it is appropriate to send a message and identifies the actual date and time the message is sent can be helpful.

Structure of Communication Plan

The structure of the communication plan should accommodate the five rights described here and provide a mechanism to track that each message was delivered and appropriate follow-up was performed. Figure 6.4 provides a sample structure. Figure 9.2 in chapter 9 provides an example of the types of communications that may be applicable in planning for an EHR or other health IT implementation. Software that supports such planning may also include other components that help manage exceptions and issues.

The communication plan should be prepared in chronological order. Ideally, any given sender should also be able to identify or extract just the messages he or she is responsible for delivering without altering the integrity of the overall plan. (It is also important for senders to understand what other messages have been sent by other senders.) There should be a protocol established for how messages can be added or removed from the plan.

Figure 6.4.   Sample communication plan structure

Message	Sender	Receiver	Medium	When	Date Done	Follow Up	Date Done

Check Your Understanding 6.2

Choose the best answer:

1. Which description best fits the definition of communication?

    a. Conversation

    b. Exchange of information

    c. Shared meaning

    d. Two-way communication

2. To strengthen a communication, it is helpful to:

    a. Add pictures, graphics, emoticons, and other visual elements to provide emphasis

    b. Encourage questions

    c. Establish context in light of the organization's vision

    d. Make sure all communications are two-way

3. In the ADKAR model of communication, *A* stands for:

    a. Acceptance of change

    b. Adoption of change

    c. Acquiescence about change

    d. Awareness of change

4. In planning communications about an EHR or other type of health IT change, it is best to:

    a. Designate one sender to send all messages

    b. Send all messages to all employees

    c. Deliver important messages in person

    d. Use technology to communicate all messages

Change Management Tools

The challenge of managing change has led to a wide variety of change philosophies and change management tools. Some of those most widely recognized are offered here as guidance for change leaders.

Making Change Management a Priority

Organization-wide change management—such as might be used in a major merger, initial push to adopt an EHR, or a campaign to embrace health reform in reimbursement (including significant risk to the organization and often also necessitating significant enhancements to health IT)—generally requires that a change management process be instituted and understood to be a priority. Often, organizations faced with a major change focus almost exclusively on implementing the business and technical features. The assumption is that people must accept the change because it was directed by executive management. But, over and over again, it is found that people do not accept such top-down change well, and, as a consequence, success with the major new initiative is less than desired (Jones and Recardo 2013).

Kotter (2012) describes an eight-stage process of creating major change. These eight changes are establishing a sense of urgency, creating a guiding coalition, developing a vision and strategy, communicating the change vision, empowering broad-based action, generating short-term wins, consolidating gains and producing more change, and anchoring new approaches in the culture of the organization. This process is reflective of the SDLC model, which may be why it so often is not used. (See chapter 2 for information about SDLC.) When the pace of change becomes ever more rapid, managers (who may not be change leaders) want to move from point A to point B virtually instantaneously, without intermediary steps, attention to people needs, or feedback loops. Change management needs to be **agile**—able to move quickly and easily, while still ensuring that an effective process is followed (Franklin 2014). At present, the expected lifespan of changes is continually growing shorter. As such, organizations need to become less hierarchical in order to avoid lengthy decision-making processes that cause changes to stall and take longer than necessary to put into effect. It must be recalled that knowledge workers, who often rise to formal leadership positions in healthcare organization, have no training in the SDLC. Indeed, the culture of many healthcare organizations today tends to get in the way of supporting a process for change.

Changing the Culture of the Organization to Support Change

Culture refers to norms of behavior and shared values among a group of people. Norms of behavior are "common or pervasive ways of acting that are found in a group and that persist because group members tend to behave in ways that teach these practices to new members, rewarding those who fit in and sanctioning those who do not." Shared values are "important concerns and goals shared by most of the people in a group that tend to shape group behavior and that often persist over time even when group membership changes" (Kotter 2012).

Linking the importance of an organization's culture to change management is reflective of the new models of care also being developed today, such as shared decision-making. In healthcare, shared decision-making moves away from the paternalistic model of medicine (do what the doctor says) to one in which patients are provided with evidence-based information on treatment choices and are encouraged to use the information in an informed dialogue with their providers to help the patients make healthcare decisions that best align with their values, preferences, and lifestyle (McClanahan 2013; Stratis Health 2014b). Shared decision-making is identified in health reform initiatives as a way to improve care and reduce costs because it is believed that when the treatment regimen is aligned with patient preferences, patients will be more willing to accept the regimen (Lee and Emanuel 2013). Similarly, a healthcare organization that embraces shared decision-making with regard to the adoption of new health IT is likely to be one whose culture supports holding everyone in the organization accountable for making the effort and embracing change (Connors and Smith 2012).

Recognizing Stages of Change

Three well-known works promote the notion that recognizing the stages of change that everyone goes through when faced with change will help appropriately target interventions that might help individuals move forward through the stages.

Grief Cycle

While controversial, the Kubler-Ross grief cycle (named after its original theorist, Elizabeth Kubler-Ross) is frequently cited as a way to understand the emotional stages people often experience when grieving a death. Since the grief cycle was first described in 1969, many have applied the model to any type of loss, including the loss experienced when change requires moving from doing things the old way to doing things a new way.

Although the model is called a "cycle," the stages of grief may occur in any sequence, and some people may skip stages. However, in general, the stages of denial, anger, bargaining, depression, and acceptance represent a roller-coaster of activity and passivity that a person experiences in an attempt to avoid change (Straker n.d.[a]). Getting through the cycle takes time. With regards to the death of a family member from natural causes, it is estimated that this process typically takes 6 months and may take up to 18 months (Maciejewski et al 2007).

Stages of Change

In the late 1970s, James O. Prochaska and Carlo DiClemente studied the experiences of smokers who quit smoking on their own and those who required treatment in order to understand why some people were capable of making the change on their own but others were not. They determined that a person quits smoking if he or she were ready to do so. The authors' **stages of change** model (also called the *transtheoretical model*) focuses on the decision-making of the individual experiencing intentional change. The model assumes that people do not change behaviors quickly and decisively. Rather, change occurs through a cyclical process, and each stage of change typically requires a particular amount of time. For each stage of change, there are appropriate intervention strategies, such as consciousness raising, self-evaluation, social liberation, self-liberation, helping relationships, counter-conditioning, and reinforcement management (Boston University 2013). Table 6.5 summarizes the stages and their timeline.

Three-Step Model of Change Theory

Kurt Lewin identified three stages of change that are the basis for many change management approaches today. The theory is based on a high-level approach to making a significant change, minimizing disruption during the change, and making sure the change is permanently adopted. The three steps are described as follows (Straker n.d.[b]; Morrison 2014):

- *Unfreezing*—preparing people to be "change ready." Unfreezing techniques include exposing a crisis that inspires people to change, providing evidence about the data for change that is difficult to ignore, educating about change, setting goals, visioning, and engaging everyone in planning.

- *Change* (also called *transition*)—providing time to complete the journey to a new state. Intervention strategies generally include breaking down the change into parts and providing support and facilitation to make incremental change.

- *Refreezing*—helping people establish a new stability. Current thinking about this step is to acknowledge that transitioning is a slow process that rarely stops cleanly, and that the next change is likely to be "just around the corner." Some commentators suggest a better term for refreezing is bringing people to a state of "slushiness." Interventions for this step include ensuring that there is no way back to old practices, introducing a new change to divert attention from existing change, demonstrating that the change is real, and devising appropriate rewards and rituals to confirm change.

Implications for Health IT Change Management

The various theories of change described here are similar to each other many respects, and, although not every aspect of the three models is applicable to change management related to health IT, the models do provide relevant insights into how to manage the emotional and psychological reactions of people facing change. First, these theories highlight that different intervention strategies work for different stages of change. Therefore, to achieve change, the intervention strategy must be selected according to where the person is in the process of change. Second, change of an emotional or psychological nature takes time. Notably, the timeframes given in the models for moving from

Table 6.5.   Stages of change model

Stage of Change	Timeline
Precontemplation (people may be told they need to change, but think only about the negative aspects of change)	6 months
Contemplation (people recognize the need to change and are weighing the positive and negative aspects)	6 months
Preparation (people are ready to make a change and start to take small steps toward change)	30 days
Action (people actually change their behavior and intend to continue to do so)	6 months
Maintenance (people sustain their new behavior and work to prevent a relapse)	Ongoing

Source: Boston University 2013.

introducing change to achieving a change that sticks are also roughly the same. More generally, change managers may find some comfort in knowing that change is slow and difficult, but effective and purposeful management of the phases of change can enable an organization to successfully weather the transition (Shaw and Elliott 2012).

Check Your Understanding 6.3

Choose the best answer:

1. Organizational culture refers to:

    a. Behavior norms and shared values in an organization

    b. Complexity of organizational structure

    c. Pace at which an organization adopts change

    d. Stages in which an organization manages change

2. In which stage of change theory is it recommended that introducing another change diverts attention away from an existing change?

    a. Kubler-Ross grief cycle

    b. Lewin's refreezing

    c. Lewin's unfreezing

    d. Prochaska's and DiClemente's stages of change

3. The average time for a change to result in acceptance is roughly:

    a. 6 months

    b. 18 months

    c. 5 years

    d. Unknown

4. To overcome the continually shorter lifespans of changes, an organization needs to be:

    a. Agile

    b. Futuristic

    c. More knowledge-oriented

    d. Paternalistic

Clinical Transformation with the EHR and Health IT

Many EHR and health IT projects have struggled to achieve full success because of the nature of the change the EHR brings about in the organization, which has been described as a clinical transformation, or the systematic modernization of the healthcare industry on the basis of new and evolving clinical information systems (King et al. 2003). The components of a clinical transformation as described by King et al. are listed in table 6.6 (2003)

Table 6.6.   Components of clinical transformation

- Integration of enabling technology throughout the redesign process to maximize technology's impact
- Untethering of information to make it available at the time and place it is needed
- Clinical process improvement and standardization across the health system and sharing knowledge across the system
- Evidence-based medicine and clinical care
- Sustained organizational and cultural change
- Transfer of knowledge and effective communication

Source: King et al. 2003, 40–41.

Because the EHR represents a clinical transformation, the organization must recognize the need for a culture that supports such a transformation. The clinical transformation often requires a cultural transformation. *Hospitals and Health Networks* (HHN) (2005) describes an organization with a culture that supports clinical transformation as one that is positive. Employees not only welcome change but actively look for ways to make improvements. The Baldrige Program (2015) identifies 11 core values and concepts for performance excellence. These are listed in table 6.7. The Baldrige Program's *2015–2016 Criteria for Performance Excellence* are shown in figure 6.5.

HHN also identifies barriers to cultural change, such as failure to set clear direction, lack of staff buy-in, fragmented communication, inadequate data collection and performance measurement process, failure to hold staff accountable for performance, lack of recognition and rewards program, satisfaction with the status quo, and insufficient leadership commitment and visibility (2005).

Project managers would do well to study the core values and barriers to change as they approach the EHR clinical transformation.

Change in Health Information Management

EHRs and other health IT have not only changed the way clinicians document and use health information but also significantly changed the nature of the information technology (IT) and health information management (HIM) departments. It is increasingly difficult to determine fixed departmental boundaries between HIM and IT.

Changes in the IT Department

Changes occurring in the IT department include significantly more outreach, user involvement, and focus on data and information. The implementation and maintenance of technology remain core IT functions, but these functions may be performed in a department-without-walls mode, often headed by a chief technology officer (CTO). IT staff physically and logically work much more closely with information system users. Rather than only focusing on the machinery used

Table 6.7.   Baldrige Excellence Framework core values and concepts

• Systems perspective	• Managing for innovation
• Visionary leadership	• Management by fact
• Customer-focused excellence	• Societal responsibility
• Valuing people	• Ethics and transparency
• Organizational learning and agility	• Delivering value and results
• Focus on success	

Figure 6.5. Baldrige Award criteria for healthcare

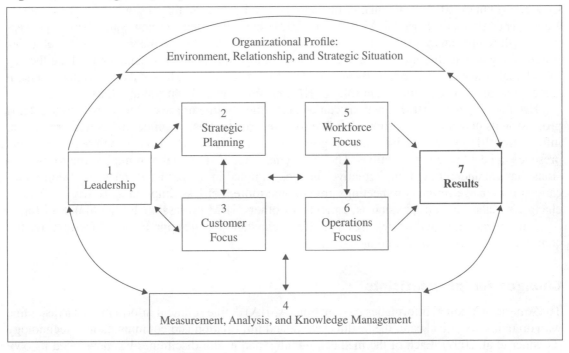

for data collection and storage, screen design, and report printing, technicians team with informaticists who are members of the medical, nursing, and allied health professions to gain a better understanding of the data and information being processed. The IT department has become an active, but not sole, participant in EHR selection.

Changes in the HIM Department

The HIM department has experienced considerable changes since the widespread adoption of EHRs. Kloss (2015) envisions information management as an enterprise-wide function. One HIM professional who has become the EHR project manager for her healthcare delivery system describes the shift in HIM as becoming ubiquitous and yet more centralized across settings—HIM professionals are everywhere, not just in one place. They are on the nursing unit, doing clinical documentation improvement and managing data quality; in the IT department, working as data analysts and data administrators; in compliance, providing HIPAA-related privacy support; in finance, supporting coding and other aspects of revenue cycle; in ancillary departments and clinics, providing EHR end-user support; and in registration or admission areas, working with patients and caregivers in new ombudsmen roles (AHIMA 2015), helping patients enter their own medical history into the EHR, and providing release of information services, among many others.

Some of the more traditional functions of HIM are increasingly outsourced, even as the workers who perform these jobs are tasked with new roles and new ways of performing functions. For example, medical coders are doing more auditing and validation. Transcriptionists have become auditors of voice-translated files. Master patient index specialists can merge records and ensure ongoing integrity of the index online from any location. Denial managers and data analysts can also perform their functions online. Some traditional HIM functions, such as document scanning, may become obsolete as organization operations become fully electronic and exceptions can be handled at the point of care. Release-of-information specialists will be needed less as patients increasingly obtain information online. In describing HIM 2025, however, Dimick (2012) notes that new roles will "blossom." For example, patient advocacy can be expected to gain greater prominence on the front end (Dimick 2012). Data quality management and data analytic roles will also grow considerably. The American Hospital Association (2014) envisions that the new value-based business model will require answers to many more questions,. and, according to the vice president of a data warehousing and quality improvement company, linking clinical and financial data will be the key to real quality and cost outcomes (Brown 2014). Much-needed workflow and process improvement leadership can also be an important role for HIM professionals (Amatayakul 2012).

Even though many HIM functions can be performed online or are no longer performed, HIM professionals play a role in information integrity, information use, confidentiality and protection, information life cycle, and information governance. Therefore, HIM must maintain a physical presence in healthcare organizations. The old saying, "out of sight, out of mind" is true for professions that are undergoing transformative change. As noted in the earlier discussion of communications for change, in-person meetings are become more, not less, important. To truly influence change, whether in staff, physicians, patients, or others, HIM professionals should use all forms of communication, including gestures that offer understanding and appreciation, to ensure that the communication results in shared meaning.

Changes for Informaticists

The American Medical Informatics Association (AMIA) defines clinical informatics as a discipline with domains in clinical care, the health system, and information and communications technology (Gardner et al. 2009). Each of the medical, nursing, and health disciplines has developed its own special areas of emphasis in informatics, and each discipline has particular approaches to the use of technology as an integral tool in helping organize, analyze, manage, and use information. A number of universities offer master's programs in one or more of the informatics disciplines.

References and Resources

Amatayakul, M. 2012. *Process Improvement with Electronic Health Records: A Stepwise Approach to Workflow and Process Improvement*. Boca Raton, FL: CRC Press.

American Health Information Management Association (AHIMA) 2015. HIM best practices for engaging consumers in their overall healthcare. *Journal of AHIMA*. 86(9):52–56.

American Hospital Association. 2014 (January). *Your Hospital's Path to the Second Curve: Integration and Transformation*. Chicago, IL: Health Research & Educational Trust. http://www .aha.org/content/14/your_hospitals_path_second_curve.pdf.

Baldrige Program. 2015. *2015–2016 Baldrige Excellence Framework: A Systems Approach to Improving Your Organization's Performance*. Gaithersburg, MD: U.S. Department of Commerce, National Institute of Standards and Technology. http://www.nist.gov/baldrige.

Boston University, School of Public Health. 2013 (January 22). The Transtheoretical Model (Stages of Change). http:// sphweb.bumc.bu.edu/otlt/MPH-Modules/SB/SB721-Models/SB721-Models6.html.

Bright, T.J., et al. 2012. Effect of clinical decision-support systems: A systematic review. *Annals of Internal Medicine*. 157(1):29–43.

Brown, B. 2014. Linking clinical and financial data: the key to real quality and cost outcomes. Health Catalyst. https:// www.healthcatalyst.com/linking-clinical-and-financial-data.

Brown, R. 2012. *The People Side of Lean Thinking: A Practical Guide to Change, Employee Engagement, and Continuous Improvement*. Mukilteo, WA: BP Books.

Connors, R., and T. Smith. 2012. *Change the Culture, Change the Game: The Breakthrough Strategy for Energizing Your Organization and Creating Accountability for Results*. New York, NY: Portfolio/Penguin.

Couros, G. 2013. 5 Characteristics of a change agent. The Principal of Change blog. http://georgecouros.ca/blog/archives/3615.

Daum, K. 2013 (September 30). 8 tips for empowering employees. *Inc.* http://www.inc.com/kevin-daum/8-tips-for-empowering-employees.html.

Dimick, C. 2012. Health information management 2025: Current "health IT revolution" drastically changes HIM in the near future. *Journal of AHIMA.* 83(8):24–31.

Edgman-Levitan, S., and T. Gandhi. 2014 (July 24). Empowering patients as partners in health care. *HealthAffairs* blog. http://healthaffairs.org/blog/2014/07/24/empowering-patients-as-partners-in-health-care.

Franklin, M. 2014. *Agile Change Management: A Practical Framework for Successful Change Planning and Implementation.* London, UK: Kogan Page.

Gardner, R.M., et al. 2009. Core content for the subspecialty of clinical informatics. *Journal of the American Medical Informatics Association.* 16(2):153–157.

Grenny, J., et al. 2013. *Influencer: The New Science of Leading Change.* New York, NY: McGraw-Hill Education.

Heathfield, S.M. 2015a (November 13). Why communication is important in change management. *About Money.* http://humanresources.about.com/od/changemanagement/a/change_lessons2.htm.

Heathfield, S.M. 2015b (November 30). Communication in the workplace. *About Money.* http://humanresources.about.com/od/glossaryc/qt/communication-in-the-workplace.htm.

Hiatt, J.M. 2006. *ADKAR: A Model for Change in Business, Government and Our Community.* Loveland, CO: Prosci Learning Center Publications.

Hiatt, J.M., and T.J. Creasey. 2012. *Change Management: The People Side of Change.* Loveland, CO: Prosci Research.

Holsapple, C. 2013. *Handbook on Knowledge Management 1: Knowledge Matters.* New York: Springer Science & Business Media

Hospitals and Health Networks (IIIIN). 2003. Cultural transformation. Special supplement sponsored by the Baptist Health Care Leadership Institute.

Jones, D.J., and R.J. Recardo. 2013 *Leading and Implementing Business Change Management: Making Change stick in the Contemporary Organization.* New York, NY: Routledge.

Kaplan, B. and K.D. Harris-Salamone. 2009. Health IT success and failure: Recommendations from literature and an AMIA workshop. *Journal of the American Medical Informatics Association,* 16(3):291–299.

Kloss, L. 2015 (September 25). Redefining the role of health information management in the new world of information governance. Iron Mountain. http://www.ironmountain.com/knowledge-center/reference-library/view-by-document-type/white-papers-briefs/r/redefining-the-role-of-health-information-management-in-the-new-world-of-information-governance.aspx.

Kotter, J.P. 2012. *Leading Change.* Boston, MA: Harvard Business Review Press.

Lee, E.O., and E.J. Emanuel. 2013 (January 3). Shared decision making to improve care and reduce costs. *New England Journal of Medicine* 368:6–8.

Maciejewski, P., et al. 2007. An empirical examination of the stage theory of grief. *Journal of the American Medical Association.* 297(7):716–723.

Malhotra, Y. 1997 (August 15–17). Knowledge management in inquiring organizations. *Proceedings of the 3rd Americas Conference on Information Systems.* Indianapolis, IN: Americas Conference on Information Systems, 293–295.

McClanahan, C. 2013 (February 19). Dinosaur doctors and the death of paternalistic medicine. Forbes Advisor Network. http://www.forbes.com/sites/carolynmcclanahan/2013/02/19/dinosaur-doctors-and-the-death-of-paternalistic-medicine.

Morrison, M. 2014 (July 7). Kurt Lewin change theory three step model—Unfreeze, change, freeze. RapidBi blog. https://rapidbi.com/kurt-lewin-three-step-change-theory/#.VohGU1Ijbwo.

National Learning Consortium. 2013 (April 30). Change management in EHR implementation. https://www.healthit .gov/providers-professionals/implementation-resources/change-management-ehr-implementation.

Noteboom, M.R. 2015 (May 1). What does "patient engagement" really mean? *Healthcare IT News.* http://www .healthcareitnews.com/news/what-does-patient-engagement-really-mean.

Robins, K., and F. Webster. 2005. *Times of the Technoculture: From the Information Society to the Virtual Life.* Taylor & Francis e-Library (first published by New York: Routledge, 1999).

Rollnick S., and W.R. Miller. 1995. What is MI? Motivational Interviewing. http://www .motivationalinterview.net/clinical/whatismi.html.

Shaw, P.L., and C. Elliott. 2012. *Quality and Performance Improvement in Healthcare: A Tool for Programmed Learning,* 5th ed. Chicago, IL: American Health Information Management Association.

Sobell, L.C., and M.B. Sobell. 2008. Motivational Interviewing Strategies and Techniques: Rationales and Examples. http://www.nova.edu/gsc/forms/mi_rationale_techniques.pdf.

Straker D. n.d.(a). The Kubler-Ross grief cycle. Changing Minds website. http://changingminds.org/disciplines/change_ management/kubler_ross/kubler_ross.htm.

Straker D. n.d.(b). Lewin's freeze phases. Changing Minds website. http://changingminds.org/disciplines/change_ management/lewin_change/lewin_change.htm.

Stratis Health. 2014a. Supportive communications. *Community-Based Care Coordination: A Comprehensive Development Toolkit.* https://www.stratishealth.org/documents/HITToolkitcoordination/4-Supportive-Communications .pdf.

Stratis Health. 2014b. Shared decision making. *Community-Based Care Coordination: A Comprehensive Development Toolkit.* https://www.stratishealth.org/documents/HITToolkit coordination/6-Shared-Decision-Making.pdf.

Vrabie, A. 2014 (May 15). How to run an effective team huddle: Why the morning huddle is the best meeting you'll ever have. Sandglaz blog. http://blog.sandglaz.com/how-to-run-a-morning-huddle-with-your-team.

Wartzman, R. 2014 (October 16). What Peter Drucker knew about 2020. *Harvard Business Review.* https://hbr .org/2014/10/what-peter-drucker-knew-about-2020.

Chapter 7
Health IT Vendor Selection and Contract Negotiation

Key Terms

Acquisition strategy

Ad hoc information requirements analysis

Applications inventory

Bidders' conference

Component producer

Due diligence

Functional capabilities inventory

Functional needs assessment

Key differentiator

Key selection criteria

Leasing

Objectives and measures for earning MU incentives

Outsourcing

Payment schedule

Reports inventory

Request for information (RFI)

Request for proposal (RFP)

Request for quotation (RFQ)

Retrospective analysis of decision-making

Rip and replace

Software as a Service (SaaS)

Standards and certification criteria requirements for certified EHR technology (CEHRT)

System integrator
Usability
User functional needs survey

Learning Objectives

- Summarize the critical role that advance planning plays in vendor selection for any EHR or other health IT system.

- Describe the scope and purpose of a functional needs assessment and explain how to conduct one prior to EHR vendor selection.

- Discuss financing and acquisition strategies for EHR and health IT.

- Describe the steps commonly taken in selecting a vendor.

- Differentiate between a request for information (RFI) and a request for proposal (RFP).

- Recommend how to manage the vendor selection process.

- Describe the critical tasks of due diligence and contract negotiation.

Many of the electronic health record (EHR) systems that are in place today in hospitals and physician practices are comprehensive, with one vendor supplying most of the core clinical components of the EHR and many of the source systems. In such situations, where an organization has already invested in an EHR and other health information technology (health IT) and uses one dominant vendor for the system's many components, some might conclude that the organization will have little need to select vendors going forward. However, vendor selection remains a highly relevant topic for health IT for the following reasons.

First, healthcare organizations will always need to select vendors for new types of health IT that the primary vendor cannot supply. In addition, some healthcare organizations want to replace systems, either to move to a single vendor for all applications to achieve better integration or to move away from a single vendor because they want to have the best of a certain component.

Second, organizations may become dissatisfied with a current vendor. For example, an organization may decide that functionality is missing in the vendor's productions, there is lack of support for the organization's strategic objectives, or there are service and reliability or uptime challenges.

Third, the current vendor could drop out of the marketplace. The EHR marketplace is highly dynamic, with vendors entering and leaving the market all the time. Over the past 20 years, there have been several thousand ambulatory EHR vendors, many of which have gone out of business or were acquired by other companies. In both the physician practice and hospital markets, only a very few vendors rise to the top with enough market share to sustain themselves. For example, in 2015, out of the top 10 ambulatory vendors, 5 had a market share of between 2.3 percent and 3.6 percent; in the hospital EHR marketplace, the top 3 vendors accounted for 60 percent of the market share combined, and only 10 vendors accounted for 90 percent of the market share combined (Green 2015).

Advanced Planning for the EHR and Health IT

This book emphasizes the importance of strategic and tactical planning for the EHR and other types of health IT. Although some organizations want to move into vendor selection quickly, thorough up-front planning without vendor influence pays tremendous dividends. Even for those undertaking a system replacement, careful planning before approaching vendors ensures that the organization is clear about its vision for the EHR or health IT, and that the EHR or health IT being acquired complements the organization's strategic initiatives. (See chapter 3 for information on strategic planning.) In describing "how to make the EHR replacement project a successful one," it is important to "take a little more time . . . to put forward an objective process" (Murphy 2015). Where the initial EHR selection was a daunting challenge, it pales in comparison to EHR replacement (Murphy 2015). "Second chances" to undertake such an expensive project have very little room for error.

Executive management commitment and support are critical success factors in any EHR or health IT project. By developing a migration path to achieve the vision of the EHR and health IT, the organization establishes a comprehensive plan that reduces the risk of reactive purchasing. Goal setting aids in establishing expectations for full utilization and benefits realization. Assessing the processes impacted by the EHR and other health IT and starting change management early helps clarify the functional requirements. These requirements are then available for use in assessing vendor products, and their consideration assures users that all due diligence has been performed in selecting a product that, then with training and workflow redesign—is most likely to help achieve specific, measurable return on investment (ROI). See chapter 3 for more information on the migration path.

Functional Needs Assessment

A **functional needs assessment** describes the key capabilities or application requirements for achieving the benefits of EHR or other type of health IT as the organization has envisioned it. It is a natural extension of the migration path and draws heavily from the workflow and process mapping activities discussed in chapter 5. Especially in replacement situations, the functional needs assessment becomes critical to differentiate among vendors whose products have the specific functionality desired and those whose offerings do not. A functional needs assessment also leads to better understanding of user preferences for **usability**, which is the extent to which a product can be used by specified users to achieve specified goals with effectiveness, efficiency, and satisfaction in a specified context of use. By specifying up front what those usability requirements are, the organization is more prepared to select a vendor that can address those issues.

Scope and Purpose of a Functional Needs Assessment

The federal government's incentive program for making meaningful use (MU) of EHR technology has focused primarily on the EHR. However, as the government and the healthcare delivery system look to the future and the Triple Aim goals (see chapter 4), the scope of health IT has broadened to encompass the sharing of data and information across all components both internal and external to a healthcare delivery organization/network (ONC 2015).

Even as healthcare moves forward with a broader view of health IT and looser coupling of health IT components among and across disparate organizations, the identification of key functionality that users need remains a key to successful use of health IT. A migration path that provides a "30,000-foot" view of the journey to health IT in general was described in chapter 3. This chapter helps drill down to define the specific functions as well as data requirements and technical capabilities that are needed to carry out any one component in the migration path. This set of requirements may be focused on the EHR in a replacement situation, or it may be focused on any other components, such as telehealth, population health, data warehousing, and much more. Functional requirements for any given project are used to screen vendors as product choices are made.

Models for Understanding Functional Requirements for EHR

A variety of models for understanding functional requirements for EHR have been developed over time. All have contributed in some way to the MU incentive program criteria, and each can also be used to contribute understanding of functionality for organizations setting out to conduct a functional needs assessment. The models of the Institute of Medicine (IOM; now the Health and Medicine Division of the National Academies of Science, Engineering, and Medicine), Health Level 7 (HL7), and MU program are highlighted here.

Institute of Medicine

The IOM, which was renamed in 2016 as the Health and Medicine Division of the National Academies of Science, Engineering, and Medicine (HMD), was the first entity to describe US requirements for an EHR. While others have subsequently built upon and refined these requirements, the original requirements may actually reflect the broadest vision for an EHR that many are currently striving to achieve.

In its first report on EHRs in 1991, the IOM identified a set of user requirements for patient records and record systems. The 1997 revised IOM report confirmed their validity, and the requirements continued to be reaffirmed through 11 years of work by Andrew and Bruegel (2005). The original IOM user requirements for patient records and record systems are reproduced in table 7.1. These user requirements remain valid today.

With renewed interest in EHRs occurring as a result of patient safety concerns, the federal government asked the IOM to provide further guidance on the key capabilities of an EHR system. In *Key Capabilities of an Electronic Health Record System* (2003), the IOM identified that an EHR system must address both primary and secondary uses of an EHR, as identified in table 7.2.

The IOM envisioned the critical building blocks of an EHR system to be the EHRs maintained by providers and by individuals; systems maintained by individuals are called *personal health records (PHRs)*. IOM updated the list of core functionalities, which are identified in table 7.3.

Health Level 7

In addition to publishing its guidance on EHR functionality, the IOM's 2003 work contributed to the work of HL7, which was the standards development organization targeted by the federal government to develop a standard for an EHR system functional model. The first HL7 EHR System Functional Model was on the ballot as a final American National Standards Institute (ANSI)–approved standard in spring 2007. Immediately thereafter, HL7 started work on a second version, which has is now on the ballot as both an ANSI standard (ANSI/HL7 EHR, R2-2014) and as an International Standards Organization (ISO) standard (ISO/HL7 10781). Figure 7.1 provides an elevated view of the framework of the HL7 EHR System Functional Model, including illustrating how various functional profiles for specific specialty applications, such as behavioral health, child health, clinical research, records management, meaningful use, public health, personal health record, and others, cut across all functional areas. The full HL7 EHR-System Functional Model, release 2, is available on the Internet under a free license (HL7 2014).

MU Incentive Program

In spring 2004, the federal government called for widespread deployment of health IT. Subsequently, the US Department of Health and Human Services (HHS) established the Office of the National Coordinator for Health Information Technology (ONC). In July 2004, ONC issued the Framework for Strategic Action, which included the "private sector certification of [health] IT products" in its broad goals (Thompson and Brailer 2004).

In response to this issuance, American Health Information Management Association (AHIMA), the Healthcare Information Management and Systems Society (HIMSS), and the National Alliance for Health Information Technology (the Alliance) funded and launched the Certification Commission on Health Information Technology (CCHIT). The commission's purpose was "to accelerate

Table 7.1.   Original IOM user requirements for patient records and record systems

Requirements Categories	Examples
Record content	Uniform core data elements
	Standardized coding systems and formats
	Common data dictionary
	Information on outcomes of care and functional status
Record format	"Front-page" problem list
	Ability to "flip through the record"
	Integrated among disciplines and sites of care
System performance	Rapid retrieval
	24-hour access
	Available at convenient places
	Easy data input
Intelligence	Decision support
	Clinician reminders
	"Alarm" systems capable of being customized
Linkages	Linkages with other information systems (e.g., radiology, laboratory)
	Transferability of information among specialities and sites
	Linkages with relevant scientific literature
	Linkages with other institutional databases and registries
	Linkages with records of family members
	Electronic transfer of billing information
Reporting capabilities	"Derived documents" (e.g., insurance forms)
	Easily customized output and other user interfaces
	Standard clinical reports (e.g., discharge summaries)
	Customized and ad hoc reports (e.g., specific evaluation queries)
	Trend reports and graphics
Control and access	Easy access for patients and their advocates
	Safeguards against violation of confidentiality
Training and implementation	Minimal training required for system use
	Graduated implementation possible

Source: IOM 1991. Reprinted with permission.

Table 7.2.   Primary and secondary uses of an EHR system

Primary Uses	Secondary Uses
Patient care delivery	Education
Patient care management	Regulation
Patient care support processes	Research
Financial and other administrative processes	Public health and homeland security
Patient self-management	Policy support

Source: IOM 2003. Reprinted with permission.

Table 7.3.   2003 IOM core functionalities for an EHR system

Core Functionalities	Examples
Health information and data	Key data using standardized code sets where available
	Narrative (clinical and patient) information
	Patient acuity/severity of illness/risk adjustment
	Capture of identifiers
Results management	Results reporting
	Results notification
	Multiple views of data/presentation
	Multimedia support
Order entry/management	Computerized provider order entry
Decision support	Access to knowledge sources
	Drug alerts
	Other rule-based alerts (e.g., significant lab trends, lab test because of drug)
	Reminders for preventive services
	Clinical guidelines and pathways
	Chronic disease management
	Clinician work list
	Incorporation of patient and/or family preferences
	Diagnostic decision support
	Use of epidemiologic data
	Automated real-time surveillance
Electronic communication and connectivity	Provider–provider
	Team cooordination
	Patient–provider
	Medical devices
	Trading partners (external)
	Integrated medical record within and across settings
Patient support	Patient education
	Family and informal caregiver education
	Data entered by patient, family, and/or informal caregiver
Administrative processes	Scheduling management
	Eligibility determination
Reporting and population health management	Patient safety and quality reporting
	Public health reporting
	De-identifying data
	Disease registries

Source: IOM 2003. Reprinted with permission.

the adoption of robust, interoperable [health] IT throughout the US healthcare system by creating an efficient, credible, sustainable mechanism for the certification of HIT products" (CCHIT 2005). Drawing from IOM and HL7 precedents, CCHIT created a robust set of functional criteria. Initially, CCHIT's certification process was voluntary for vendors. However, following the passage of the Health Information Technology for Economic and Clinical Health Act (HITECH) in 2009, the MU incentive program required product certification, and, at that point, several companies in

Figure 7.1.   HL7 EHR-system functional model, R2 overview

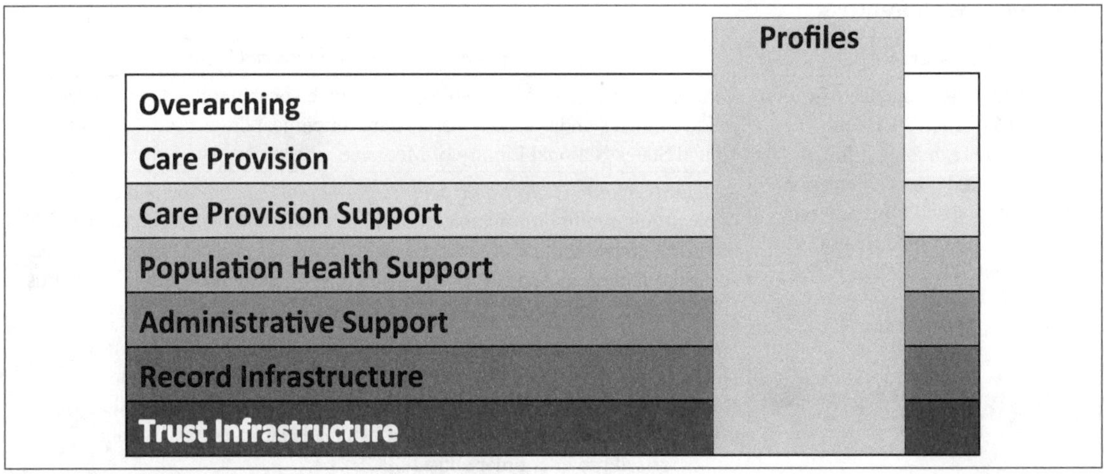

the business of certifying products across different industries joined the certification effort. Unfortunately, CCHIT, as a nonprofit organization, no longer had the business model to compete and dropped out of the EHR certification process. Its initial EHR functional requirements specification is now lost to the public.

According to current EHR functional requirements, products used for earning the MU incentives must include two types of specifications:

- **Standards and certification criteria for certified EHR technology (CEHRT):** CEHRT are developed by ONC and, ultimately, after soliciting public comment, codified in regulations. Vendors are required to have their EHR products tested in order to be certified. The ONC Health IT Certification Program website (ONC 2016) is the launchpad for information about product certification, the standards, the Certified Health IT Product List (CHPL), testing and test methods, and other resources.

- **Objectives and measures for earning MU EHR incentives:** The Centers for Medicare and Medicaid Services (CMS), which funds the MU incentive program, develops objectives and measures for eligible hospitals, critical access hospitals, and eligible professionals (CMS 2016). Just as ONC is required to solicit public comment and produce regulations specifying their standards for CEHRT, CMS must seek public comment on the MU criteria and publish the requirements in regulation. The healthit.gov site is the launchpad for information about the MU program requirements, Medicare and Medicaid incentives, Medicare adjustments in reimbursement for those not meeting the MU incentive program requirements, clinical quality measures and measurement, and information for those hospitals and professionals eligible to participate in the program.

In addition to identifying one's own functional requirements for EHR or other health IT (the process for which is described in the next section), anyone planning a vendor selection (or reselection) for EHR today should become thoroughly familiar with the MU incentive program, the standards and criteria for CEHRT, and the CMS objectives and measures for earning incentives. Table 7.4 provides a few of the standards and criteria from ONC and objectives and measures (including exclusions if applicable) from CMS. These examples are from stage 1 of the program (issued July 28, 2010). It should be noted that when subsequent stage final rules are published, the publication in the *Federal Register* provides only updates to the new stage, referencing back

Table 7.4.   Examples of standards and certification criteria for CEHRT and objectives and measures for earning MU incentives

Source	Examples (from Stage 1 for eligible professionals)
CEHRT Standards and Certification Criteria (45 CFR 170. Health Information Technology: Initial Set of Standards, Implementation Specifications, and Certification Criteria for Electronic Health Record Technology; Final Rule, July 28, 2010)	*Vocabulary standard:* Medications. Any source vocabulary that is included in RxNorm, a standardized nomenclature for clinical drugs produced by the United States National Library of Medicine
	Standards to protect electronic health information: Encryption and decryption of electronic health information. General. Any encryption algorithm identified by the National Institute of Standards and Technology (NIST) as an approved security function in Annex A of the Federal Information Processing Standards (FIPS) Publication 140-2.
	General certification criteria: Drug-drug, drug-allergy interaction checks—Notifications. Automatically and electronically generate and indicate in real-time notifications at the point of care for drug-drug and drug-allergy contraindications based on medication list, medication allergy list, and computerized provider order entry (CPOE).
Medicare and Medicaid Programs EHR Incentive Program (42 CFR 412, 413, 422, et al. Medicare and Medicaid Programs: Electronic Health Record Incentive Program; Final Rule, July 28, 2010)	*Objective:* Maintain active medication allergy list. *Measure:* More than 80 percent of all unique patients seen by the eligible professional have at least one entry (or an indication that the patient has no known medication allergies) recorded as structured data.
	Objective: Provide patients with an electronic copy of their health information (including diagnostics test results, problem list, medication lists, medication allergies) upon request. *Measure:* More than 50 percent of all patients who request an electronic copy of their health information are provided it within 3 business days. *Exclusion:* Any eligible professional that has no requests from patients or their agents for an electronic copy of patient health information during the EHR reporting period.

to stage 1 where applicable. Various organizations may publish summaries of the combinations of information for the stages, but it is always good to verify with the actual rule as published by the federal government.

Two important factors should be considered when reviewing the MU requirements. First, they are the *minimum* required for earning the incentives and focus only on core clinical components of an EHR, which do not even include charge capture for billing, which must be substantiated by a health record. As time goes on, it is important to appreciate that, with few exceptions (such a charge capture), these minimum requirements were the only requirements embedded in EHR products, even as additional requirements might have been desired. (This is one reason why many are looking to acquire enhancements to their existing EHR systems.) Second, it is uncertain whether or how the MU incentive program will extend beyond 2016. In 2016, changes were proposed that would keep the MU incentive program for hospitals but move the program under reimbursement models for physicians. Despite the proposed changes, it is always uncertain what view a new presidential administration will have on such programs.

Usability Requirements for EHRs

Although this chapter focuses on defining functional requirements and using them in vendor selection, many have called for greater usability in the functionality being sought. For example, a US Senate panel has been convened to look into EHR usability in light of the $28 billion taxpayer-funded dollars spent on subsidizing EHRs (through the MU incentive program) and complaints by physicians (Monegain 2015).

Figure 7.2.   Typical usability requirements of EHR

• Performance: response time, throughput	• Serviceability
• Scalability	• Security
• Capacity	• Regulatory
• Availability	• Manageability
• Reliability	• Environmental
• Recoverability	• Data Integrity
• Maintainability	• Interoperability

Figure 7.3.   HIMSS usability factors

• Simplicity	• Efficient interactions
• Naturalness	• Effective information presentation
• Consistency	• Preservation of context
• Forgiveness and feedback	• Minimize cognitive load
• Effective use of language	

Usability is often considered a functional requirement, although, technically, many experts separate functionality from usability. Functional requirements are "what a system or component must be able to perform," which is distinct from nonfunctional requirements that describe "how a system must behave" (Lessons from History 2011). As an example, "record/chart changes in vital signs" is one of the MU criteria for functionality, whereas "the display of the patient's vital signs must respond to a change in the patient's status within two seconds" is a complementary usability requirement. Figure 7.2 lists typical usability requirements for an EHR.

Evaluation of a product's usability is often subjective. As a result of the demand for better usability in EHRs, the federal government has begun addressing these important aspects associated with EHR functionality in attempt both to improve usability and remove the subjectivity from the assessment of usability.

In 2007, the ONC contributed to describing requirements for enhancing data quality in EHRs. The ONC work was extended, in conjunction with the Agency for Healthcare Research and Quality (AHRQ), to describe (human–computer) interface design considerations for EHR usability (Armijo et al. 2009a; Armijo et al. 2009b). In 2011, AHRQ published an EHR Usability Toolkit that describes usability issues in EHRs generally and by EHR functionality. This toolkit also provides methods and tools for measuring usability (Johnson et al. 2011). The National Institute of Standards and Technology (NIST), which ONC uses to conduct the product testing component of certification for EHR products, has taken these works and created a guide to the process approach for improving the usability of EHRs (Lowry et al. 2015).

HIMSS has also issued a white paper on usability in healthcare organizations (2011). This model recognizes the nine factors important for usability identified in figure 7.3.

Check Your Understanding 7.1

Choose the best answer:

1. The MU incentive program requirements do not address administrative processes.

2. When considering functional requirements for EHR and health IT, it is important to consider both primary and secondary uses of the technology.

3. As early as 1991, the IOM was addressing easy access for patients and their advocates to patient record systems.

4. Today, all EHR systems have the "laboratory test because of drug" core functionality identified by the IOM in 2003.

5. CMS specifies the standards that must be incorporated into certified EHR technology (CEHRT).

Functional Needs Assessment Process

From the issues described previously, it should be apparent that, despite the existence of functional requirements models, product certification, and usability tools, each organization needs to define its own functional requirements for its EHR or other health IT for a number of reasons, including the following:

- *Every organization starts from a different point,* with different levels of automation and a different mix of vendors.

- *Every organization has different needs.* What one organization may consider an essential requirement, another may consider only "desirable." Functionality will also evolve over time as a result of lessons learned from enhanced use.

- *Each vendor offers a somewhat different approach.* Although many vendors offer CEHRT, how they offer the MU functions and what additional functionality they may or may not offer varies considerably.

- *Other elements of product selection must be considered.* Factors that must be considered include the vendor's history and viability, staffing, and number and type of clients; the nature of implementation and training provided; the level and quality of support; and, of course, cost.

Any given organization's functional needs assessment, therefore, needs to use functional requirements models as resources, but those models must be adapted to reflect the organization's capabilities and needs.

Identifying Functional Requirements

A functional needs assessment often begins with a **user functional needs survey**. In such a survey, users are asked to identify the functionalities they need, and perhaps prioritize them. Although a user survey is important, users need to be sufficiently educated about EHR or other health IT functionality to provide meaningful responses. Consideration must also be given to variation in user needs, as not every user will have the same needs.

Surveying Users

Methods to survey users include small group facilitation, questionnaires, and rankings. Sufficient numbers of users must be surveyed to avoid bias. The process of surveying users should also be vendor neutral.

Use Cases

Another approach to defining functional requirements is the use-case technique (see chapter 5). Use cases are often relatively easy for clinicians to provide; they are essentially scenarios that describe a system's behavior as it responds to a request that originates from outside of that system. When engaging clinicians in use case development, one might simply ask them to identify and describe some patient care events that are typical, unusually complex, and unusually easy. Once the use cases are developed, each of the conditions, triggers, events, alternative paths, and business rules can be analyzed to determine what functions must be in the EHR or other type of health IT for their support.

Verifying User Requirements

In addition to interviewing users and engaging them in developing scenarios or use cases, other sources of information can contribute to functional specification. Some of these include the following:

- A formal **functional capabilities inventory** identifies the functional capabilities of systems already in place. This inventory not only helps potential users to see the scope of current capabilities but also establishes a foundation on which to understand what essential functional capabilities may be missing or desired. Existing and desired functional capabilities should be identified from workflow and process maps or use cases. These capabilities may be documented in the context of one of the functional requirements models or the organization's list of functional requirements. Another dimension of the inventory may be a survey of actual use of current functional capabilities, as many organizations have implemented systems that are not fully used. This assessment may help identify the degree of change management and education/training needed for an EHR. (See chapter 6 for information on change management.)

- An **Applications Inventory** identifies all the applications the organization currently has and how they may be related to one another (or not). Figure 7.4 shows a sample tool frequently maintained by information technology (IT) departments to describe information system (IS)

Figure 7.4.   Sample tool to describe IS interfaces

Information System Interfaces												
System	Interfaced with	User Dept.	Data	PHI	Support	Type	Frequency	Std	I/O	Medium	Transmission	Comments

interfaces. This tool is a good way to start an applications inventory. Any systems that are not interfaced and any applications that are an integral part of a larger system should be added to the list. Systems that are not interfaced but might exchange data with an EHR or other type of health IT may include, for example, operating room scheduling systems or emergency department systems.

- A **reports inventory** is a physical review of reports in which every report produced electronically or manually is reviewed first for whether the report is actually needed, and second for the information produced. "Report" should be carefully defined to include not only typical monthly summaries of performance distributed to managers but any information-generation process, including dashboards, notices, and others. For reports that are required or desired, the organization should assess whether all fields are complete and whether the information reported is current, accurate, and complete. Users should also be asked whether there are any desirable reporting activities in which they do not participate because they do not have sufficient or easily accessible data. If so, copies of these reports should be obtained and analysis of them included in the needs assessment. Finally, all requests for informational reports or access to specific data should be logged and evaluated to determine whether they also represent reporting needs for the EHR or other type of health IT.

- An **ad hoc information requirements analysis** aims to capture the most difficult of information needs, such as those that occur on a nonroutine or occasional basis. For instance, a physician treating a patient may decide that the symptoms are atypical and a differential diagnosis is elusive. Certain specialized knowledge helps the physician arrive at a more definitive diagnosis and determine a precise treatment plan. The organization may need health IT that supplies such support, such as special decision support utilities or literature searches, with data not routinely captured as part of the standard EHR templates. For instance, diagnostic decision support tools VisualDx (2015) and Isabel Healthcare (2015), now available as apps for mobile devices, enable comparisons of signs and symptoms, including photographs, with a reference library of rare and common diseases or conditions. Analysis of ad hoc information requirements may be done by making a series of observations or by developing use case scenarios with specialists.

- A **retrospective analysis of decision-making** is another approach to ad hoc information needs that are difficult to inventory. Whether executive management is making organizational decisions or providers are making clinical decisions, decision makers tend to rely more on instinct and past experience than on factual information. However, today's decision makers are realizing that solid data would be of immense help and may even be required for compliance with clinical credentialing. It is difficult for executives or clinicians to identify the types of data they need. Therefore, it can be helpful to have executives and clinicians identify the types of data they would have found helpful in making some recent decisions. This exercise can populate a set of data that should be captured routinely or provide a means of developing reports from existing data.

- A comparison of functions to benefits is a good way to conclude the functional needs assessment. This comparison involves making a list of the benefits cited by the organization in its EHR or health IT vision and migration path, identifying processes involved in achieving the benefits from process mapping, and mapping the processes to the list of functional requirements identified through the preceding processes. Figure 7.5 provides a sample structure for such a comparison. As the functional requirements are compiled into a usable document (such as a request for proposal or product analysis checklist), consideration needs to be given to using plain and simple words and illustrations or use-case diagrams so the requirements are clear to all potential users of the document (Cantoria 2011).

Figure 7.5.   Comparison of EHR functions to benefits

Benefits of EHR	Process	EHR Supporting Functions	Current State	
			Application	Needed
Patient safety	Order entry	Clinical and financial decision support	Order communication	CPOE
	Formulary	Managed care contract requirements	Automated formulary	Match to payer
	Pharmacy	Drug alerts	Drug–drug	Drug–other
	Medication administration	Drug identification	Point-of-care support	
		Person identity verification	Bar coding	

Copyright © 2016 Margret\A Consulting, LLC. Reprinted with permission.

Check Your Understanding 7.2

List five tools that are helpful in identifying and verifying user functional requirements for the EHR or another health IT system:

Financing Strategy

A financing strategy addresses how the organization is going to finance its EHR and health IT projects. Although the financing strategy is often included in strategic planning, it should be reviewed in advance of any preparations to approach vendors.

Financing options generally include a decision relating to whether an organization is going to self-develop a system ("build"), license clinical components from its incumbent vendor ("buy"), or acquire a product through an application service provider (ASP) or **software as a service (SaaS)** arrangement ("borrow").

Build Versus Buy

The question of whether to build or buy (acquire an EHR from a commercial vendor) is less commonly asked today than in the past. When there were few EHR and other health IT vendors and products were not comprehensive, some organizations considered building their own systems. Many of these systems were developed in academic medical centers or with a commercial partner that was interested in developing new products. Indeed, many of these projects were the forerunners to current EHR and other health IT systems. Now, most organizations recognize that commercial products can meet their needs and that most of these products will far surpass the functionality that could be self-developed. Still, some organizations want to at least consider the build option. Some physicians are intrigued with developing their own perfect system, and some hospitals have development teams they do not want to give up.

An organization's decision to build or buy should be based on a careful review of the marketplace—currently, it is more expensive to undertake self-development. Unless self-development is coupled with a vendor partnership that leads to commercialization, a self-developed system can be a drawback when attempting to integrate with commercial products as the organization grows, merges, or acquires affiliates.

Buy Versus Borrow

The choice to buy or borrow a system (using an ASP or SaaS arrangement) is often an economic decision. Licensing software and either buying or leasing hardware for an EHR or other type of health IT is a costly proposition. An EHR or health IT acquisition generally requires considerable initial access to capital as well as a considerable budget for ongoing maintenance, upgrades, and enhancements. Many organizations are therefore considering whether an ASP or SaaS model can be a less expensive way to obtain the functionality of an EHR or other type of health IT.

Essentially, an ASP or SaaS is an arrangement that involves a customer paying a subscription fee to access a software application and store their data on secure computers managed offsite by the vendor. In this model, the upfront capital outlay is less and fewer IT staff are required in-house. In fact, the ASP acquisition strategy may essentially be considered a financing model. The ASP or SaaS model of acquiring computing power is not new; many organizations shared computing services when computers were first being developed. Today, these models remain popular with customers, and many vendors find the steady stream of revenue from an ASP or SaaS arrangement is a good business strategy. New technologies have greatly enhanced the basic model of leasing access to sophisticated systems. (Note that these arrangements may go by other names, such as remote connectivity option [RCO] or service bureau.)

The difference between the ASP model and the SaaS model relates primarily to the underlying technology, not to the financing. Both models involve the hosting of various applications developed by a number of software vendors from a remote data center and the delivery of these applications to their customers over a secure Internet connection or a private network. However, the underlying technical architecture of the ASP model is client/server with a web front end. The SaaS model's technical underpinnings are based on pure web services architecture and often, although not necessarily, offered through cloud computing (Port 2009; Prasad 2011). See chapter 11 for a fuller description of these technologies. Some believe that the ASP offering lends itself to greater customization capability, whereas the SaaS model offers very little, if any, customization capability. In actual practice, however, neither model enables much customization—a limitation that can be desirable, especially for organizations that do not want to incur additional costs for customization and its ongoing maintenance.

The security and availability of data stored remotely or in the cloud is a concern when considering ASP or SaaS arrangements. Physician practices seem more willing to consider a cloud-based solution than hospitals; however, the reality is that any form of EHR or other health IT must use encryption and high-speed connectivity to ensure protection and access to the data (Nelson 2014).

Organizations that choose either the ASP or SaaS form of acquiring an EHR or other type of health IT should bear in mind they still have to acquire the hardware to be used by individual users. Hardware can be purchased or leased. Purchasing hardware allows the organization to take advantage of immediate ownership and the flexibility to do whatever it chooses with the equipment. However, purchasing also creates an immediate asset on the balance sheet, as well has implications for cash flow. **Leasing** hardware minimizes the burden of ownership, typically requires no down payment, and may remove the risk of obsolescence (depending on the length of the lease). Operating leases usually qualify for off-balance-sheet treatment for accounting purposes, will not affect financial ratios, and may conserve bank lines of credit for other acquisitions (Zadrozny 2005). It is a good idea to evaluate such options thoroughly from an accounting perspective, as paying over a period of time could ultimately be more expensive than buying. In addition to cost factors, the organization needs to be aware that confidentiality issues could arise if appropriate measures are not taken to destroy all data on the equipment prior to returning it to the leasing agent. Moreover, there may be monetary penalties for loss or damage to equipment or for returning it early.

Yet another option to acquiring an EHR or other health IT is outsourcing. **Outsourcing** is a contractual relationship with a specialized outside service provider for work traditionally done by the customer. In some respects, outsourcing is broader than ASP because ASP generally refers to the use of computer services, whereas outsourcing can include both computer services and various

Table 7.5.   ASP/SaaS advantages and disadvantages

Advantages	Disadvantages
Lower up-front costs for hardware and installation	Potential higher cost over long term
Software becomes an operating cost versus capital expenditure	Integration issues if ASP/outsourced functions must connect to in-house systems
Fewer data center headaches	Less ability to customize
Access to new and/or better technologies, especially for security	Loss of control/accountability issues

management services. Outsourcing is sometimes equated with the use of offshore services. However, outsourcing does not have to be offshore or even off-premises. Outsourced vendors can manage services directly at the customer's site.

The advantages and disadvantages to the ASP/SaaS model are summarized in table 7.5. As with any set of advantages and disadvantages, careful management of the process can offset disadvantages and capitalize on advantages. Perhaps the most critical element of ASP and SaaS models is a strong service-level agreement (SLA) that establishes the terms of service the ASP or SaaS vendor will provide (Karten 2009).

Other policies to be considered in the financing strategy include the purchasing requirements that stipulate the stability of the vendor business, the number of other installations it must have, the size and type of clients, and so forth. Some organizations are more willing to assume risk than others. The financing must reflect the degree of risk a healthcare organization is willing to accept.

Acquisition Strategy

Acquisition strategy refers to whether one primary vendor or a mix of vendors is preferred. Three popular types of acquisition strategies—best of fit, dual core, and best of breed—are described in chapter 3. Another acquisition strategy that is becoming more common is one in which an organization decides to switch to an entirely new (single) vendor, which has been termed **rip and replace**. This strategy may seem expensive and disruptive, and many experts recommend against it; however, a number of organizations are finding that it may be economically beneficial in an environment where the management of potentially hundreds of interfaces or where existing systems are out of date is costly. This strategy may be especially appealing to large hospitals or integrated delivery systems where there have been multiple mergers and acquisitions and it is desirable to get everyone on the same platform. Rip and replace is also being done in hospitals (and especially academic medical centers) where the original, home-grown EHR systems are becoming too costly to maintain and lack the standardization necessary for interoperability. Some physician offices and clinics are also ripping and replacing because they are dissatisfied with their existing products.

Check Your Understanding 7.3

Match the terms with the appropriate descriptions:

    A. Build

    B. Buy

    C. Borrow

    D. Lease

1. Using an ASP or SaaS arrangement

2. Developing one's own product

3. License applications from a vendor

4. "Borrowing" hardware from a vendor for a period of time

Selecting a Vendor

Whatever decisions are made about building, buying, borrowing, or replacing EHR and other health IT systems or components, a selection process must be undertaken. This process may be viewed as a funnel, where a series of steps are taken to narrow the potential field of vendors from many to one. The process involves using a set of filters to focus the candidate pool on the organization's specific requirements in order to negotiate a successful contract. Figure 7.6 illustrates these steps.

Planning

Vendor selection for the EHR and other health IT should begin with focused planning on how the selection process will be undertaken. There are two particularly important considerations: controlling the selection process and determining whether assistance is needed in the vendor selection process.

Controlling the Selection Process

As the organization begins to undertake vendor selection, it should control interactions with vendors to ensure a fair representation of products and keep marketing hype and accusations of unfair competitive advantage to a minimum. Most organizations require all vendor interactions to go

Figure 7.6.   Vendor selection process for EHR and other health IT

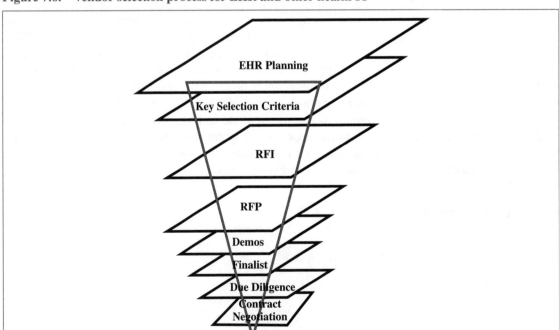

through one designated individual. The vendors who make the first cut should be treated equitably, with equal opportunity to demonstrate their products and interact with the selection team. In addition, the organization should select firm criteria for vendor selection.

The healthcare organization is buying a product or service, not salesmanship, and should not make decisions based whether the salesperson is poor or good. Potential customers can be highly swayed by friendliness, fancy dinners, and promises. Likewise, they can be turned off by surly salespersons who show little interest in the organization, even though their product may be outstanding. It is possible that the more marketing techniques a salesperson must apply to the product, the less likely the product meets the requirements to sell itself.

Controlling the selection process is as much about *looking past* the salesperson as it is about *looking at* the product. The vendor's salesperson will *not* be responsible for installation, training, or ongoing support. A good salesperson represents the company as a whole and should be a member of a collaborative team that learns the buyer's needs, understands its business requirements, and offers proactive suggestions. However, the bottom line is that the salesperson's responsibility is sales. He or she will generally not be around when there are implementation problems.

In the marketplace for EHRs and other types of health IT, it is important to recognize that the products are not commodities that have little to no qualitative differentiation. Although many good EHR products are on the market and many are certified as meeting the MU criteria, they still differ from each other significantly. A good product for one organization is not necessarily a good product for another. This fact emphasizes the need for thorough planning and a carefully controlled selection process.

Assistance with Vendor Selection

When an organization is relatively new to making large EHR or health IT investments, it can may want to seek the assistance of consultants. Consultants can typically provide everything from strategic planning, process redesign, and vendor selection to system integration, implementation, and ASP/SaaS services or outsourcing support. Any, all, or none of these types of consultants may be appropriate for an organization's project.

Many organizations find that a consultant facilitates definition of the vision for the EHR or other type of health IT, goal setting, and overseeing process assessment efforts. A consultant for this aspect of the project should be open-minded, an excellent communicator, and someone who values details but is not mired in minutiae. The organization's users should take ownership of process assessment but will likely need direction and support.

Many organizations also find it useful to have a consultant oversee the vendor selection process. In this case, the consultant should have a broad range of experience and be neutral regarding the pool of possible vendors. Many organizations take as much care in selecting their EHR or other health IT consultant as they do in selecting the system itself. However, many organizations also make the mistake of engaging a consultant who they perceive can carry them through all phases of the project—from visioning through implementation to ongoing support and benefits realization. This approach is often not the best strategy because a consultant who has sufficient experience in implementing a given product is likely to be highly biased toward that product. Therefore, this type of consultant is not recommended for the planning stages or the postimplementation benefits realization activities.

Most organizations need to supplement their own staff with people who can help implement the product. In many cases, the vendor supplies these individuals or outsources this function. In other situations, the organization may decide to obtain its own resources or use a mix of resources from the vendor and other companies. The involvement of too many different companies in the project can become a project management nightmare. However, with complex technology and interfaces or an accelerated timeline, organizations may need the services of multiple companies.

In addition to consultants who can lend expertise and/or human capital, **systems integrators** are companies, or parts of companies, that specialize in getting disparate vendor products to work together. They may write interface programs or supply an interface engine, which is a software tool that manages many interface connections among many disparate systems. An interface engine supports multiple communications protocols, including (but not exclusively) HL7, by mapping data formats among otherwise incompatible applications.

Organizations may also seek assistance from **component producers** that sell products that support the EHR and other types of health IT. Although the EHR relies on all source systems as well as the core clinical components to capture its data, there are a number of tools that manage the data in a variety of ways. Some of these may be data-capture tools, such as document imaging systems and voice recognition systems. Other tools serve to process the data. These might include a clinical decision support system, report writing tools, or data warehousing. The system integration tools mentioned earlier are component products.

Finally, niche or specialty products include EHRs or other forms of health IT that are primarily designed for one type of clinical specialty. For example, certain vendors support EHRs exclusively for behavioral health services, a field that is quite different from that of general medical and surgical services. Specialty-based EHR products and other specialized types of health IT have also been designed for physician office specialties, such as for cardiologists, nephrologists, and others. Many health IT products and services being considered for acquisition beyond the EHR are niche or specialty offerings. For example, the EHR vendor may be able to support a portal for patient access to their health information (and other functions), but this vendor may not offer a full-blown personal health record. Telehealth services, patient monitoring systems, care coordination systems, and many others are health IT products generally acquired separately from an EHR.

Narrowing the Universe of Vendors

No healthcare organization has the resources to evaluate hundreds of vendors to find one that will be the best fit. Some organizations narrow the universe of vendors by developing a short list of **key selection criteria** and issuing a **request for information (RFI)** to between 10 and 20 vendors (at most) in an effort to focus on perhaps 4 or 5 to evaluate seriously. Other organizations skip this step in favor of having users and other staff use the key selection criteria to review web demonstrations or attend trade shows in order to narrow the field. When the field is narrowed to a manageable number, the organization should issue a **request for proposal (RFP)** to obtain more detailed information concerning the full scope of the organization's functional requirements and/or a **request for quotation (RFQ)** (also called a *request for bid*) to obtain a price from which to negotiate.

Key Selection Criteria

Whether the organization uses an RFI and an RFP or RFQ or uses only an RFP or RFQ, it should draw from its planning activities to establish a set of initial vendor-screening criteria. Questions to ask include the following:

- Does the vendor share the organization's *vision* for the EHR?
- Does the vendor's product provide the *key functionality* needed to achieve the organization's vision?
- Does the vendor use the desired *technology*?
- Does the vendor qualify under the organization's *acquisition* policies, including MU certification and potentially other certifications or endorsements?
- Can the vendor support the organization's desired *implementation* strategy?
- What is the vendor's track record for *operations and maintenance* support?

- What is the vendor's understanding of the *implications* of implementing an EHR system?

- Is the vendor *viable* in the EHR market?

In the preceding list, key functionality refers not to a summary of the functional requirements specification, but to a list of functions that have been culled from the functional requirements specification that are considered absolute requirements critical to the successful achievement of the organization's goals for the system. A good way to determine this short list of key, or critical, functions is to rate each of the functional requirements previously identified as critical or noncritical. For example, every EHR that is certified has CPOE and must have drug-drug and drug-allergy checking. However, the CEHRT criteria do not require drug–laboratory value checking (for example, whether a specific drug is contraindicated for patients with poor liver function). The CEHRT criteria also do not specify that every person using the CPOE or EHR be alerted for every drug-drug contraindication. Users who encounter excessive alerts will experience alert fatigue and may come to totally disregard any alert. The ability to tier alerts based on risk may be a key functionality for community hospitals. Alternatively, a teaching hospital may not want or need such functionality.

Requests for Information

An RFI is basically a means to accumulate marketing literature. Because most vendors provide much of this information on their websites, RFIs are not used as often today as they were in the past.

When an RFI is used, the organization may wish to have an external adviser send it out on the organization's behalf (without identifying the organization). This approach allows the organization to understand the marketplace without being inundated with vendors attempting to make sales calls. A similar approach when soliciting information from websites is to use a generic email address for site registration. Generally, an RFI is limited to a two- or three-page set of questions on the following areas:

- *Company background:* Obtain information on the vendor's size, years in business, number of employees, and product lines. For instance, some EHR vendors also serve as clearinghouses for financial transactions or as analytics companies performing data mining. For certain medical specialties that must adhere to state-specific reporting requirements, it can be helpful to know the geographic area served.

- *Product information:* Obtain the product name, product history (how long has this vendor sold the product, versioning history, from whom may the product have been acquired), technical platform, and overview of product capabilities that will be matched with the functional needs assessment (discussed in chapter 8).

- *Market information:* Ask the vendor to identify its major competitors and explain how the vendor differs from them.

- *Installed base and clients:* Identify the number of EHR products the vendor has sold, is currently implementing, and has fully installed. Answers should indicate both the numbers of organizations and the numbers of users.

- *Special criteria:* Collect information on any unique features or functions the vendor has established as critical.

Figure 7.7 is an example of a vendor comparison map that can be used to plot the responses to the RFI. The letters in the figures represent specific vendors. The vendor comparison map can accommodate any limited number of key criteria that an organization wishes to evaluate. The example suggests that the organization considers new technology and a full product suite with an ambulatory

Figure 7.7. Vendor comparison map

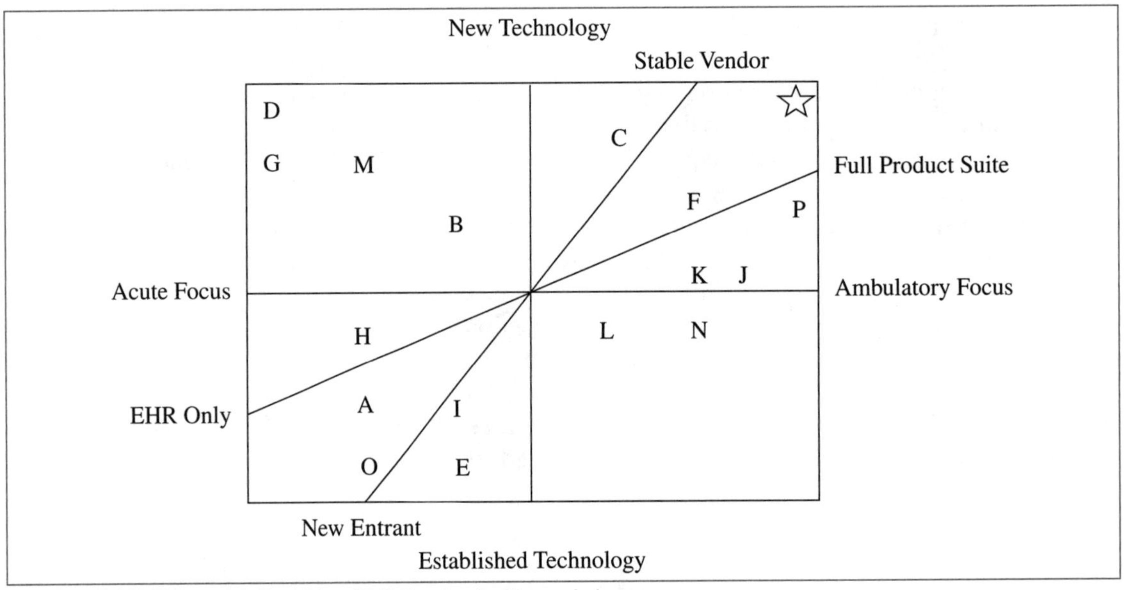

Copyright © 2016 Margret\A Consulting, LLC. Reprinted with permission.

focus to be the most important factors to the organization. This tool helps narrow down a large list of vendors.

Requests for Proposals

An RFP is a formal document sent to vendors inviting them to submit bids for the organization's EHR or another health IT project. RFPs should be sent to at least four or five vendors that seem to best fit the organization's overall criteria after it has studied the marketplace. The number of RFPs sent may depend on whether the healthcare organization is public or private. Public organizations may be required to send RFPs to every eligible vendor.

A well-constructed RFP serves two important purposes. First, it solidifies the planning information and organizational requirements into a single document. In a way, it is the culmination of the organization's strategic EHR and health IT planning—including workflow and process improvement and functional needs assessment. The EHR or health IT steering committee and the organization as a whole benefit from the RFP bringing all this information together. Second, when developed and managed correctly, the RFP will garner responses that provide valuable insights into each vendor's operations and products and it tends to level the playing field by asking all the vendors the same questions. It serves as a source document for the contract that provides the license to use the vendor's software.

RFPs do not serve their intended purpose if they lack substance and vendors supply canned responses. The intent of the RFP should be to elicit a description of *how* the vendor believes its product will solve the healthcare organization's specific problems and meet its requirements. Writing an RFP that will result in more than a set of checkmarks in a "yes" column on a form takes skill.

The RFP usually has some fairly standard components, including the following:

- *Organizational profile:* The first section describes the healthcare organization, including its basic demographics, mission and goals, vision for the EHR or other type of health IT, current information infrastructure, and specific constraints (such as the project's particular timeline). This section also contains the organization's instructions for responding (for example, to whom the bid should be sent, how many copies will be sent, and how vendor questions will be handled).

- *Vendor information:* This section, which may be placed immediately after the organizational profile or at the end of the proposal, asks the vendor for a description of its demographics. The description should include the vendor's size and longevity (years in business, revenues, profitability, number of employees), product research and development history and plans, types of installations (number, size, status), corporate composition (organizational makeup, employee qualifications and tenure, state or country in which most work is performed), references, user group information (leader, size, frequency of meetings), and contract history (any defaults, pending lawsuits, Internal Revenue Service status).

- *Functional specifications:* In this section, the organization requests a description of functional capability, such as the processes and workflows the product supports, and compares these against its redesigned workflows and processes. Alternatively, the organization may develop a script describing a scenario, or use case, based on its redesigned workflows and processes and ask the vendor how its product would perform the inherent functions. This approach can be useful for avoiding "yes and no" responses.

- *Operational requirements:* This section should elicit information on the EHR or other health IT product's data architecture, analytical processes supported, necessary interfaces, reliability and security features, system capacity, expansion capabilities, response time, downtime, and other issues associated with system maintenance. Questions in this section should be drawn from the organization's data infrastructure assessment.

- *Technical requirements:* In this section, the vendor should propose the appropriate technical architecture to meet the organization's functional specifications and operational require ments for the EHR or other type of health IT, delineating the specific hardware, networking, and software requirements. Many organizations now ask vendors to describe both minimum and optimum requirements, as some vendors have only supplied minimum requirements that have not worked well after implementation. Questions in this section should be drawn from the organization's data and information infrastructure assessment and information technology infrastructure assessment (discussed in chapters 10 and 11, respectively).

- *Application support:* The vendor uses this section to propose an implementation schedule and describe data conversion, acceptance testing, training, and documentation, as well as the ongoing support, maintenance, and upgrades it will supply.

- *Licensing and contractual details:* In this section, the vendor is asked to supply its specific bid for one-time and recurring costs based on the organization's requirements. This section should also include a request for the vendor's standard contract, financing arrangements, proposed relationships with hardware vendors, and warranty information. This section should include clauses that protect the healthcare organization in the event the vendor goes out of business. Many organizations request the pricing information be provided in a separate section of the response. This approach removes the influence of cost from other critical evaluation factors. Because pricing models and proclivity to discount vary so much among vendors, it is often easier for a financial specialist to attempt to normalize these aspects of vendor responses for comparison purposes before the EHR or health IT steering or selection committee reviews them. This individual would also construct a spreadsheet to compare products on their ability to generate a desired ROI and benefits realization.

- *Evaluation criteria:* Some organizations add their evaluation criteria to the RFP so the vendor knows up front the most important elements of the evaluation. This section would indicate how the organization weighs various factors. For instance, evaluation criteria may identify that cost is weighed at 50 percent of the organization's decision-making criteria or that the organization will permit the vendor to outsource interface development but not maintenance.

Requests for Quotations

An RFQ is used as the basis for selection on price among very similar products. It may be more suitable than an RFP if the organization has thoroughly studied products and concluded that a small number are very similar. It is important to bear in mind, however, that virtually all EHR and many other health IT vendors include confidentiality clauses in their proposals. As a result, revealing one vendor's price to another in the hopes of getting that vendor to lower its price will put the customer in the potential position of being sued for breach of contract.

Managing the Vendor Selection Process

If an organization uses an RFP, managing the RFP issuance, receipt, and evaluation is as important as preparing its content. RFPs should be sent to all vendors on the organization's short list at the same time, and all vendors should be given the same amount of time to respond. If a vendor requests an extension, it should be granted only for extenuating circumstances and only before any other vendor has submitted a response. At that point, all vendors then should be notified immediately that they have an equal extension period. A request for an extension may be viewed as a red flag for potential problems, although with the current surge in momentum for acquiring an EHR or other form of health IT, such requests are becoming more common and should not necessarily deter consideration of the vendor. Alternatively, if a vendor does not respond to an RFP, it may be that the vendor recognizes that its product is not a right fit for the organization or simply has to make choices based on its own capacity. If an organization is interested in such a vendor, it may contact the vendor to find out why a proposal was not received and decide whether to accept one late if the vendor becomes interested in responding.

Issuing an RFP may instantly launch a competitive feeding frenzy. Vendors seem to be able to sniff out the fact that the organization is looking for an EHR or some other health IT, and it can often feel like salespeople are descending on the organization in droves. The steering committee should discuss the potential (inevitability) of a deluge of solicitations and plan for it directly. Some organizations try to keep potential vendors' identities confidential; others include the potential vendors' names in the RFP. A middle ground is perhaps more common: The shortlist is not revealed, but respondents are not kept secret (which is often impossible anyway). Most organizations do not accept proposals from vendors other than the ones to whom RFPs have been directed. If an exception is made, the steering committee should vote on it and should not give the vendor extra time, unless the committee deems the omission to be an oversight on the part of the organization. This scenario should not occur when sufficient planning and careful construction of the selection criteria have taken place.

Some organizations hold a **bidders' conference** to respond to questions about the RFP. In this situation, the RFPs include the specific date, time, and location (sometimes virtual) for the conference. Any vendor may attend and ask questions. Thus, all vendors hear all questions and obtain the same answers, keeping the playing field even. However, most vendors either do not attend or attend only to learn who other vendors are who are bidding and what other vendors are asking.

When no bidders' conference is scheduled, the organization should decide whether it will respond to questions, who will respond, and how. Responding to questions and sharing the responses with all vendors receiving the RFP can serve the same purpose as a bidders' conference. How tightly the bidding process is controlled is up to the organization.

Many organizations use codes of conduct for vendor selection to advise and remind the members of their steering committee and others of the practices to which they want to adhere. This type of code helps achieve an objective and fair vendor selection process.

Evaluating the RFP Response

A first step in RFP evaluation may be to assess the vendor's overall response: Was it received early or on time? Did the vendor ask appropriate questions or were its questions simply intended to gain competitive advantage? Did the vendor follow the organization's instructions on how to respond? The answers to these and other such questions can be revealing. The organization also may want to learn why certain vendors did not respond.

After obtaining some initial impressions, the organization should do an in-depth analysis of the responses and how they compare to the overall selection criteria. Because a comprehensive EHR and some other health IT projects are large and complex, some organizations find it useful to allocate sections of the responses to the RFP to different subject teams for thorough evaluation. Organizations may also consider developing a **key differentiator** tool. This tool identifies the key selection criteria relative to the functional requirements and potentially some additional factors relative to the nature of the vendor. For example, if the organization wants to be able to use a mix of operating systems, that may be a key differentiator because not all products have such capability. The teams then report back to the steering committee as a whole, perhaps only that they have verified all of the requirements but are scoring exclusively on key differentiators. Many organizations use some form of scoring methodology to evaluate the proposal against the key differentiators and a formal group process technique to ensure everyone's input.

A Likert scale may be used to do a quantitative analysis on the results of the RFP. Figure 7.8 provides an example of a Likert scale, which compares six vendors (A through F) against 10 weighted selection criteria. The figure illustrates the following example:

> A hospital has prioritized 10 criteria. It has assigned a simple numeric weight to each criterion, ranging from 1 (least important) to 10 (most important). (It is possible to use a different scale and assign different weights to each criterion. For example, a scale of 1 to 5 may be used. The first two criteria may be considered most important and both weighted as 5, the next three may be weighted as 3, and the remaining 5 weighted as 2.)

Figure 7.8. Vendor comparison on Likert scale

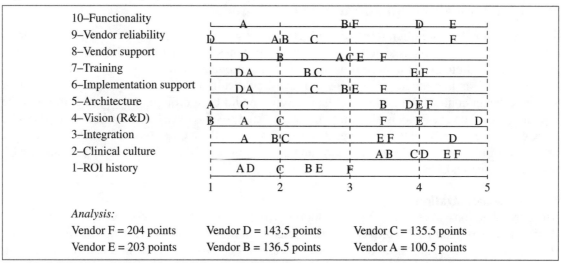

To calculate each vendor's score, the sum of each criterion's weight is multiplied by the vendor's rating on that criterion. (In figure 12.3, vendor A earned 1.5 on the first criterion weighted 10, thus the 10×1.5 equals 15; the remaining criteria are calculated and then totaled. In this case, vendor A earned a total of 100.5 points.)

In the final analysis, vendors F and E have the most potential for this organization because they are 60 points ahead of the next group of vendors, which consists of D, B, and C.

Some organizations evaluate EHR products on what they call an "MU checklist." Although this process may seem unnecessary if the product is certified for MU, the checklist can serve two important purposes for the organization. First, where there are "menu set" criteria, exclusions, and optional clinical quality measures (CQM), an organization may have preferences for which criteria and measures to use and report. In addition, while each certified product includes the required functions, how the products deliver those functions may vary. So, because these are the most important functions, differentiating among the associated processes and workflows can be important. A second reason to use such a checklist is to focus on the MU criteria as an aid in setting expectations for users. The checklist simply helps the organization confirm that the product provides for these functions and establish that users will be expected to use the functions in the intended manner.

At the conclusion of the evaluation of RFP responses, one vendor may rise to the top or several vendors may warrant further, in-depth review. At this stage, it is important to rule out any vendors who are subpar.

One thing few organizations discuss but might consider at this stage is the concept of good customership. Customers often chide vendors for their sales tactics and vaporware (software that is described by way of a slideshow or other marketing presentation but does not yet exist), but vendors often expend considerable resources in responding to RFPs, conducting demonstrations, and performing other legitimate sales activities. Although expenses associated with sales are factored into the price of the product, organizations should avoid making frivolous demands of vendors. When the organization is not serious about a particular vendor after reviewing its response to the RFP, the organization should notify the vendor as simply and politely as possible that it is not getting the project and extend appreciation for the vendor's response. Prompt elimination of noncontenders also makes management of the rest of the due diligence needed to make a final selection easier and less expensive. Other factors associated with good customership include removing internal bias from the selection process by requiring individuals in the selection process to acknowledge any conflicts of interest, not accepting gifts from the vendors, respecting the vendor's intellectual property rights, and maintaining confidentiality about the process.

Due Diligence to Determine the Vendor Finalist(s)

The next set of steps are often referred to as **due diligence**, or a formal process of investigation to ensure that the product is as stated in the vendor's response to the RFP or RFQ and is truly right for the organization. Due diligence is an analysis of the product via demonstrations, site visits, reference checks, and corporate visits. This process should culminate in identifying the vendor with whom to begin contract negotiation. Organizations should be thorough and not rush through the due diligence; however, this is also the time when "analysis paralysis" can set in and needs to be managed. It can be helpful to remember that acquiring an EHR or other type of health IT is not just about the product, but that people, policy, and process play a tremendous role in how successful one can be with an EHR.

Product Demonstrations

Most organizations invite the finalist vendors (typically, two or three companies) to conduct a demonstration of their EHR products on site. Demonstrations are valuable for several reasons, even in cases where the organization has previously viewed demonstrations from these vendors. First, the demonstration acquaints as many of the potential users as possible with the product, which makes everyone feel that they are a part of the process and gives the organization an opportunity to obtain feedback. Potentially hundreds of people may view a demonstration or series of short demonstrations, and so a feedback mechanism should be devised to focus on the highlights. A second reason to conduct a demonstration is to evaluate products side by side. Finally, the demonstration illustrates the vendor's understanding of the organization's specific requirements. The post-RFP demonstration should be tailored to the organization's specific needs and requirements; earlier demonstrations probably would have been generic.

As with the RFP, one option at this stage is to prepare a script the vendor must follow during demonstrations to highlight the key processes the organization wants to observe. This type of demonstration is an excellent test of whether the vendor fully understands the organization's situation. If the vendor cannot meet a specific requirement and indicates this fact during the demonstration, its honesty is a point in its favor as long as the requirement was not a major factor.

It is important to be sure that the EHR or other health IT product being demonstrated in response to the RFP is based on the current, real release of the product, not vaporware or a version still under development. A demonstration may be conducted in several segments. One segment is for many users who will spend just 5 or 10 minutes at the demonstration to get a sense of the look and feel of the product. A small but important use of the product should be scripted for such a purpose. Another segment is a longer (one- or two-hour) demonstration of a more comprehensive scenario for members of the steering committee. In this segment, committee members should challenge the vendor and encourage the vendor to ask questions. The steering committee should include users of all types, including physicians, other clinicians, and administrative professionals. This range of participants ensures that all aspects of the EHR or other health IT product are evaluated thoroughly. A separate demonstration also may be planned for the organization's technical team to evaluate the interfaces, understand modification procedures, and so on.

Vendors should be given adequate time to set up their equipment and test their software and network connections. Some organizations try to have all the vendors demonstrate at the same time, but in separate locations. When this approach is not feasible, it is important for comparison purposes to conduct the demonstrations as close together in time as possible. As soon after the demonstrations as possible, evaluations should be collected and the selection committee debriefed.

Site Visits

Once the organization has reviewed the formal demonstrations, it should be possible to further narrow the field. Ideally, after the demonstrations, there should be just two vendors left in the mix. Organizations may then visit client sites of those vendors. These sites should be as similar as possible to their own. The purpose of the visits is to assess the vendor's product in action and learn about the installation process and obtain feedback from direct users. Site visits also can be valuable for learning other information from clients, even apart from their relationship to the product. Even though most vendors arrange site visits at their "best" sites (and often compensate the client in some way for the time it spent hosting the site visit), organizations can still learn worthwhile lessons from these excursions. (The purchasing organization should pay for the trip and not accept the vendor's offer to do so.)

The site visit team should include a representative group composed of clinician users, information management representatives, and others. Typically, this team is a core group of the larger steering committee. It is preferable to have the same group go on all visits. Generally, one or two visits per vendor are made.

It is advisable to establish an agenda for the site visit. The vendor may be present during introductions, but the rest of the site visit must be done without the vendor present to prevent vendor bias. If the vendor wishes to stay, the team should be large enough and prepared to release one of their members to stay with the vendor while the remaining team members conduct the rest of the visit. Team members should not hesitate to speak to people other than those scheduled (who may potentially be primed by the vendor). It is useful to observe as many people as possible who are not on the formal agenda. (Insofar as possible, these individuals should be typical users.) Even so, because the client at the site needs its vendor to survive, people working at the site rarely give the vendor bad marks. In addition, the visitors will need carefully crafted questions so that the responses reveal important insights about the vendor's level of service and support without offending the vendor's representatives, even if they are not present. Another reason to proceed cautiously is that vendors may have outsourced staff to the site; thus, it is possible some of the IS staff, trainers, and others at the site may actually be employees of the vendor.

At the conclusion of each site visit, participants should be debriefed immediately before their impressions and reactions are forgotten or confused with other site visits.

Checking References

At the same time that site visits are being conducted, the organization should make reference calls to as many of the vendor's other clients as possible. The organization has the right to ask for a complete list of the vendor's clients, and any vendor that does not provide a list at this point should be suspected of having something to hide. Some vendors may ask the organization to sign a contract not to contact clients other than those the vendor identifies. Obviously, such an agreement is not something desirable for the organization, and the steering committee should think twice about this vendor.

The people calling references need an agenda to ensure that they do not forget no key questions. A conference call or a series of calls to talk with equivalent users, technical staff, and administrators might be a useful tactic. Moreover, conversations with the leaders of the vendor's user group and reviews of meeting agendas and attendance lists can be helpful in supplementing reference checks.

Corporate Visits and Vendor Walk-Throughs

After site visits and reference checks are completed, an organization still may not be ready to narrow the field to one vendor. At this point, representatives from the healthcare organization, such as the chief executive officer, chief financial officer, and medical director, may want to make a corporate visit to meet with their counterparts at the vendor's company. The chief information officer may meet with the vendor's chief technology officer.

Corporate visits are particularly helpful as vendors start to merge and acquire other companies. The culture of the vendor can make a difference in how well the healthcare organization may interact with the vendor in the future, the trust the organization places in the vendor's promises, and so on.

When making the finalist selection, another useful activity is to request that the vendor's technical staff conduct a walkthrough of the healthcare organization. This activity helps ensure that the vendors fully understand the technical infrastructure that exists and any customization that may be required. The walk-through should result in a detailed implementation plan and firm up any potential change in the initial cost estimates provided in the RFP.

Creating the Implementation Plan

Most organizations phase in EHR projects and some other types of health IT because these projects are so large and impose significant change. Developing an implementation plan with the vendor to learn of their recommendations on how to construct the phasing can be very insightful as part of the selection process.

When an organization phases in an EHR or other health IT project that either replaces paper-based processes or systems that cannot be converted, the organization should consider whether a direct cutover or parallel conversion will be used. The direct cutover has the advantage of not having to maintain two processes, but it requires considerable up-front preparation, including uploading data for active patients either before the cutover or as each patient is scheduled. Parallel conversion is more comfortable because the organization knows that everything is backed up, but it sometimes extends reliance on paper systems into perpetuity.

Often the nature of the organization (inpatient or outpatient, size, number of locations) and the extent of data already automated determine the form of conversion. Straight cutovers and parallel conversions are rarely done for an entire EHR implementation except in a small facility or office. However, parallel conversions are often performed for revenue cycle management, inventory, and other systems that require some form of reconciliation over time.

Making the Final Decision

Ultimately, the organization must narrow the field to a single vendor of choice. Usually, the steering committee is responsible for recommending the finalist, although the decision is best made with input from all participants.

No product will exactly meet every one of the organization's requirements. Customization is possible, but adapting the organization's requirements to adjust to a close match keeps costs down. Moreover, customization can have a long-term impact on the organization's ability to implement system upgrades successfully.

Even at this point in the project, members of the organization may tend to hold on to old, familiar ways. Vendors may even encourage an organization to buy a product that most closely matches its current processes. (Is there any wonder that ROI opportunity is low for such products?) New users of such systems tend to look for products that seem easy to use—even though those products may not be sophisticated enough and could end up frustrating users later on. It is important for an organization to facilitate a true understanding of its EHR or health IT vision and goals in those individuals who will make the selection decision or recommendation.

Price should be the last factor considered in finalist selection. Many factors influence the pricing of the EHR and other health IT products. Hard-line negotiation over costs seldom proves beneficial over the long run. At this point, prices should not be significantly different across the vendor finalists unless the products are significantly different. If the products are significantly different, the decision is often one of price versus functionality. When balancing concerns about functionality and price, the organization must consider its migration strategy carefully. It may be appropriate to phase in functionality, and good vendors should be able to show how this can be done. Alternatively, being "penny wise and pound foolish" can result in problems down the road, as the following scenario illustrates:

> A large group practice bought a comprehensive EHR system and expected to achieve significant cost savings through clinical decision support. Unable to fund workstations for every examining room, the practice decided to provide interim functionality through printouts and have physicians use the workstations centralized at the nurses' stations. Even though queues rarely formed at the workstations, physicians found the practice inconvenient and got their nurses to enter their data. This not only defeated the opportunity to benefit from clinical decision support at the point of care, it also reduced the expected benefit to nursing personnel. The bottom line was that the physicians were essentially unhappy with the system. Although an investment in more workstations would have paid for itself, the physicians would not agree to the additional expenditure, seeing the entire system as being less than successful and beneficial only from an operational, not a clinical, view.

The following example illustrates a successful implementation:

> An integrated delivery system (IDS) with many small and medium-sized physician practice affiliates scattered across nearly an entire state needed a way to improve communications. Physician practices in the IDS varied greatly, from not having an EHR to having fairly sophisticated systems. The IDS considered investing in the purchase of a single system for all affiliates. At the time, the cost was prohibitive, but the IDS believed that supporting a web-enabled system to exchange data and to begin feeding a repository was a significant advantage to all practices. Such a system would also accomplish a common look and feel among the hospitals and the

practices. As practices decided that they wanted more functionality or upgrades for their current systems, they migrated to a common vendor.

Performing Final Due Diligence and Negotiating the Contract

The final steps before signing on the dotted line are the final due diligence to investigate the vendor of choice and contract negotiation.

Final Due Diligence

Demonstrations, site visits, and reference checks are all parts of due diligence. However, these activities focus primarily on the product. For a major investment such as an EHR, the healthcare organization also needs to assess the vendor's viability and how well the organization believes the vendor and organization can work together. This assessment may be conducted in a corporate site visit or a vendor investigation.

The healthcare organization should ask the vendor how many implementations are currently under way, what the average tenure of employees is, what plans exist for mergers or acquisitions, and what their projected growth is (Williams and Samarth 2011). The organization may choose to obtain credit checks on the vendor and its officers, especially if the vendor is not well established. Depending on whether the vendor is public, some information about its operations may be easier to obtain than other information. Still, considering the size of the investment the healthcare organization is making, even a nonpublic company should disclose reasonable financial information at this point. The market status of other products in the vendor's product line is also a good indicator of its financial status and ability to meet contractual obligations. In fact, with the rapid market evolution of EHR vendors in response to the MU incentive program, the number of vendors in the EHR marketplace today is not sustainable. Even in other forms of health IT, considerable consolidation of vendors is happening.

Contract Negotiation

The following discussion is not a substitute for legal advice but provides some tried-and-true suggestions for effective contract negotiation.

Before beginning the actual contract negotiation, the organization must decide whether to negotiate with one or two vendors. Some consultants suggest that the wisest approach is to narrow the field to two vendors and negotiate with the primary candidate first, leaving the second choice available in the event contract negotiations with the first one break down. Again, good customership is advised. If the process of contract negotiation is expected to be fairly rapid, an organization can keep a second vendor waiting for word of its decision. However, there are many variables in contract negotiation, and a second vendor kept waiting for a long time may become frustrated and not provide the best second choice. This vendor will surely figure out that it is not the primary choice by the fact that the organization has turned off communications. If the negotiation fails with the first vendor, the organization may opt to restart the process instead of returning to the second vendor.

Contract negotiation with a vendor begins by folding in a copy of the original RFP and the vendor's response into the vendor's standard contract. The beginning of contract negotiation should also include a thorough review of exactly what is being acquired. This step may seem unnecessary after the comprehensive selection process just performed, but it is needed to ensure that the organization is getting what the vendor promised. Determining what the vendor is actually providing in terms of software licenses, hardware, and services may involve clearing up many nebulous details. For example, will the vendor provide and install the hardware (or will the organization do one or both of these tasks)? How many hours of training are included? Does the license agreement include only the EHR or other health IT provided by the company, or does it also include licenses to third-party software necessary to support coding (for example, the license to use Current Procedural Terminology [CPT] from the American Medical Association), the drug knowledge database, and even the database design? (Sterling 2005) The final implementation plan also should be included in the contract. By themselves, the vendor's response to the RFP and the implementation plan are not legally binding documents.

Contracts for certified technology should also address MU from the perspective of the vendor maintaining certification throughout the stages as products are expected to change and measures require additional utilization by users (Jackson et al. 2011). If the health IT being acquired is not an EHR or includes other non-EHR components, such as a new practice management system for a physician practice, the contract should include the requirement for keeping current with applicable other regulatory requirements. A lesson learned in planning for the change to ICD-10-CM was that some contracts had no provision for this transition or had no timeline for initiating planning.

Contracts should include a milestone-based **payment schedule** based on actual accomplishments, not dates. Milestone payments may be linked, for example, to installation of software, completion of system configuration and testing, training, and go-live, with a large sum held back for acceptance after some period of use (Ames et al. 2011). Such a payment schedule relates primarily to the straight license approach to acquiring an EHR, but similar considerations can and should be included for whatever up-front fees an ASP or SaaS vendor requires. Compensation adjustments for product delivery delays and nonperformance should be specified. Maintenance contracts should include a clause that correlates problems with appropriate response times.

The Healthcare Financial Management Association (HFMA) has compiled a guide to IT contract negotiation that identifies 10 critical components (HFMA 2004). These are included in table 7.6.

In addition to these critical components, some organizations look to protect themselves in the event the vendor goes out of business or is acquired by another vendor. Terms of the contract should stipulate that the vendor will keep the product up to date for a specified number of years as long as the client pays maintenance agreement fees. The contract also should obligate any company acquiring the vendor to uphold these terms. To protect against the vendor going out of business, some organizations require the vendor to put the source code and data schema for the product into an escrow account, making it available to a programmer the organization may acquire to assist in keeping the product current, at least until a new selection process can be undertaken. Some vendors require a separate fee for this process (O'Connor 2005; Uretz 2005).

The organization may also want to ask the vendor to supply evidence that the data retained in the EHR system can be converted to another platform if necessary. Some companies have been developed to perform just such services. If the organization uses an ASP, the contract should also stipulate that data will be returned to the organization. If the organization is using a SaaS model and the data are also held by the vendor, the contract should also address return of the data. (In some SaaS models, the organization holds the data and only uses the SaaS to process them, returning the data and results of the processing after each processing activity.) The process of negotiating an ASP or SaaS agreement has a number of elements that are different from negotiation of a straight licensure contract. These include ensuring disposition of data should the vendor go out of business as well as protection of data, so they are not comingled with any other organization's data and are not de-identified and sold without the organization's knowledge. With ASP and SaaS models, it is critical to put even more attention on service level, especially with regard to connectivity. The extent to which the organization wants to incorporate such protections in the contract will depend on the risk profile of the organization and the perceived stability of the vendor in the marketplace (Amatayakul 2010, 169–171).

Table 7.6.   Critical contract negotiation components

Component	Description
1. Product definition and contract structure	• Define the system components covered by the contract; include response to the RFP to ensure comprehensive functionality description • Determine whether software license agreement maintenance provisions (including service-level agreement), and installation are included in one contract or separate contracts
2. Scope of license	• Recommends a fully paid, perpetual, royalty-free, nonexclusive, nontransferable license for use by, or on behalf of, affiliates, as specified • Reviews a vendor's standard set of restrictions on licenses and negotiates incremental pricing, if necessary
3. Pricing structure	• One-time costs • Ongoing maintenance, including response to federal regulations • Operational changes
4. Implementation	• Includes specific work plan for implementation • Includes provisions for breach of agreement
5. Key personnel	• Qualifications • Replacement provisions • Third parties • Selection rights for key staff
6. Acceptance testing and payment terms	• Define testing stages (unit testing, integration testing, interface/network testing, stress testing, and live testing) • Define acceptance at each stage • Provide for correction of errors • Provide for testing and remedies
7. Performance warranties	• Response time • Uptime • Batch processing throughput assurance
8. Limitations on liability	• Ensure mutuality of liability • Insurances
9. Change in vendor control and product obsolescence	• Defines triggering events • Identifies remedies if a triggering event occurs • Identifies exclusions for limitation of liability
10. Dispute resolution and exit strategies	• Process • Mediation or binding arbitration • Exit clauses that outline right to deliverables and interim payment

Source: Adapted from HFMA 2004.

Check Your Understanding 7.4

Choose the best answer:

1. In selecting a vendor for EHR or health IT, the primary criterion for an organization should be the vendor who:

    a. Currently supplies most applications for the organization

    b. Is number 1 in the marketplace

   c. Passes all stages of due diligence conducted by the organization

   d. Sells for the lowest price

2. The *least* important tool to be used in selecting a vendor for most organizations is:

   a. Request for bid

   b. Request for information

   c. Request for proposal

   d. Request for quotation

3. Which of the following tools is most helpful for narrowing the field of vendors from all to a manageable number to study in depth?

   a. Functional needs assessment

   b. Key selection criteria

   c. Recommendations from other organizations

   d. Request for proposal

4. Which of the following questions is *not* appropriate to ask a vendor during vendor selection?

   a. How frequently do you supply updates to the software?

   b. How many times and for what reasons have your clients filed lawsuits against you?

   c. How much do you spend on research and development?

   d. How successful have your clients been in achieving ROI with your product?

5. When is it recommended that the organization's steering committee evaluate the price of a product under consideration?

   a. After the initial phase of narrowing the field of vendors

   b. As part of planning for vendor selection

   c. At the conclusion of all due diligence

   d. Before reviewing the response to the RFP

6. In order to understand the culture of the vendor organization, it is appropriate to:

   a. Ask clients if the vendor is easy to get along with

   b. Check Better Business Bureau vendor reviews

   c. Conduct corporate site visits

   d. Poll the vendor's current clients

References and Resources

Amatayakul, M. 2010. *Electronic Health Records: Transforming Your Medical Practice*, 2nd ed. Denver, CO: Medical Group Management Association.

Ames, E., V. Ciotti, and B. Mathis. 2011. Meaningful abuse: The rush toward EHR implementation. *Healthcare Financial Management.* 65(2):70–73.

Andrew, W.F., and R.B. Bruegel. 2005 (May). An exclusive look at the EHR system marketplace: 2005 EHR systems review. *ADVANCE for Health Information Executives.* http://www.health-care-it.advanceweb.com.

Armijo D., et al. 2009a (October). *Electronic Health Record Usability: Evaluation and Use Case Framework.* Agency for Healthcare Research and Quality (AHRQ) publication no. 09(10)-0091-1-EF. https://healthit.ahrq.gov/ahrq-funded-projects/use-dense-display-data-and-information-design-principles-primary-care-health-2.

Armijo D., et al. 2009b (October). *Electronic Health Record Usability: Interface Design Considerations.* Agency for Healthcare Research and Quality (AHRQ) publication no. 09(10)-0091-2-EF. https://healthit.ahrq.gov/sites/default/files/docs/citation/09-10-0091-2-EF.pdf.

Cantoria, C.S. 2011 (January 26). Tips for writing functional requirements. Bright Hub Project Management. http://www.brighthub.com/office/project-management/articles/11954.aspx.

Certification Commission on Health Information Technology (CCHIT). 2005. https://www.cchit.org/

Centers for Medicare and Medicaid Services (CMS). 2016 (July 14) Electronic health records (EHR) incentive programs. https://www.cms.gov/Regulations-and-Guidance/Legislation/EHRIncentivePrograms/index.html?redirect=/ehrincentiveprograms.

Green, M. 2015 (July 6). 50 things to know about the EHR market's top vendors. *Becker's Health IT and CIO Review.* http://www.beckershospitalreview.com/healthcare-information-technology/50-things-to-know-about-the-ehr-market-s-top-vendors.html.

Healthcare Financial Management Association (HFMA). 2004. *Dotting the I's and Crossing the T's: Ensuring the Best IT Contract* (promotional material). Westchester, IL: HFMA.

Healthcare Information Management and Systems Society (HIMSS) Usability Task Force. 2011. Promoting usability in healthcare organizations: Initial steps and progress toward a healthcare usability maturity model. http://www.himss.org/ResourceLibrary/ResourceDetail.aspx?ItemNumber=10910.

Health Level Seven (HL7). 2014. (April). HL7 EHR-System Functional Model, release 2 (ANSI/HL7 EHR, R2-2014). http://www.hl7.org/implement/standards/product_brief.cfm?product_id=269.

Institute of Medicine (IOM). 1991. *The Computer-Based Patient Record: An Essential Technology for Health Care,* edited by Dick, R.S., and E.B. Steen. Washington, DC: National Academies Press.

Institute of Medicine (IOM). 2003. *Key Capabilities of an Electronic Health Record System: Letter Report.* Washington, DC: National Academies Press. http://www.nap.edu/books.

Isabel Healthcare. 2015. Differential diagnosis: Use Isabel diagnosis tool to broaden your ddx, http://www.isabelhealthcare.com.

Jackson, J., S.J. Fox, and V. Schick. 2011 (March). Negotiating the EHR vendor contract. *Bulletin of the American College of Surgeons.* 96(3):12–17.

Johnson, C.M., et al. 2011 (August). EHR usability toolkit: a background report on usability and electronic health records. Agency for Healthcare Research and Quality (AHRQ) publication no. 11-0084-EF. https://healthit.ahrq.gov/ahrq-funded-projects/electronic-health-record-usability-toolkit/citation/ehr-toolkit-background.

Karten, N. 2009. Establishing service level agreements. In *How to Establish Service Level Agreements.* Randolph, MA: Karten Associates. www.nkarten.com.

Lessons from History. 2011 (February 23). Functional versus non-functional requirements and testing. http://www.lessons-from-history.com/node/83.

Leventhal, R. 2014 (August 26). KLAS: One quarter of ambulatory EHRs could be replaced. *Healthcare Informatics.* http://www.healthcare-informatics.com/news-item/klas-25-percent-ambulatory-ehrs-could-be-replaced.

Lowry SZ, et al. 2015. Technical evaluation, testing, and validation of the usability of electronic health records: Empirically based use cases for validating safety—enhanced usability and guidelines for standardization. National Institute of Standards and Technology (NIST). http://nvlpubs.nist.gov/nistpubs/ir/2015/NIST.IR.7804-1.pdf.

Miliard, M. 2015 (August 18). Community hospitals replacing EHRs: More than half unhappy with usability. *Healthcare IT News.* http://www.healthcareitnews.com/news/community-hospitals-look-replace-ehrs

Monegain, B. 2015 (April 30). Senate panel to look into EHR usability. *Healthcare IT News.* http://www.healthcareitnews.com/news/senate-panel-look-ehr-usability.

Murphy, K. 2015 (December 23). How to make the EHR replacement project a successful one. *EHR Intelligence.* https://ehrintelligence.com/news/how-to-make-the-ehr-replacement-project-a-successful-one.

Nelson, R. 2014 (September 11). Is a cloud-based EHR solution for you? *MedPageToday.* http://www.medpagetoday .com/Columns/PracticePointers/47606.

O'Connor, K.J. 2005. Everything you always wanted to know about software escrow agreements—and then some! *Journal of Healthcare Information Management.* 19(1):10–12.

Office of the National Coordinator for Health Information Technology (ONC). 2007 (May). *Recommended Requirements for Enhancing Data Quality in Electronic Health Records.* Washington, DC: ONC.

Office of the National Coordinator for Health Information Technology (ONC). 2015. Connecting health and care for the nation: A shared nationwide interoperability roadmap, final version 1.0. https://www.healthit.gov/sites/default/files/ hie-interoperability/nationwide-interoperability-roadmap-final-version-1.0.pdf.

Office of the National Coordinator for Health Information Technology (ONC). 2016 (August 5). ONC health IT certification program. https://www.healthit.gov/policy-researchers-implementers/onc-health-it-certification-program.

Port, L. 2009 (June). ASP vs. SaaS. Doing more with less. *Peer to Peer.*

Prasad, A. 2011. Web based EMR—ASP vs. SaaS? Should you really care? RevenueXL blog. http://www.revenuexl .com/blog/bid/22325/Web-based-EMR-ASP-vs-SaaS-Should-you-really-care.

Sterling, R. 2005 (July 8). 6 EMR contract terms that avoid big headaches later. Presentation at the Electronic Medical Records for Physician Practices Conference, Washington, DC.

Thompson, T.G., and D.J. Brailer. 2004 (July 21). *The Decade of Health Information Technology: Delivering Consumer-centric and Information-Rich Health Care—Framework for Strategic Action.* Washington, DC: Office of the National Coordinator for Health Information Technology.

Uretz, M. 2005. How to survive your EHR contract. The EHR Group. http://www.ehrgroup.com.

VisualDx. 2015. VisualDx—visual clinical decision support system (CDSS). http://www.visualdx.com.

Williams, T., and A. Samarth. 2011. *Electronic Health Records for Dummies.* New York: Wiley Publishing.

Zadrozny, B. 2005. Joining the HIT revolution: Should you buy or lease the tools you need? *Healthcare Informatics.* 22(2):97.

Chapter 8
Health IT Project Management: Roles in Design and Implementation

Key Terms

Balanced scorecards
Benefits portfolio
Change control
Change management
Coaching
Conflict management
Critical path
Dashboard
Domain team
Gantt chart
Information silo
Issues log
Key performance indicator (KPIs)
Managing
Negotiation
Planning
Program
Project
Project champion
Project charter
Project management
Project management office (PMO)
Project manager
Project plan

Project risk
Project scope
Project sponsor
SCODF typing model
Steering committee
Team building
Trust
Work breakdown structure

Learning Objectives

- Identify the prerequisites for a successful EHR or other health IT project.

- Describe the scope and characteristics of an EHR or other health IT project.

- Identify human resources requirements, organizational structure, and team-building characteristics for a successful project.

- Assess potential interest in and skill at being a project manager and gaining EHR project involvement.

- Recognize project planning and management techniques and tools useful to an EHR project.

Project management is a well-planned and organized effort to accomplish a specific mission, such as implementing an electronic health record (EHR) or other type of health information technology (health IT). A **project manager** aids an organization in planning the tasks required to achieve the project goals and objectives, determining what resources are needed, associating budgets and timelines for completion, and then managing the project; however, it also takes many other people, in a variety of roles, to implement an effective EHR or other health IT system. All stakeholder groups must be directly involved.

Prerequisites for EHR and Health IT Success

Virtually every healthcare organization is in some stage of implementing or optimizing use of an EHR and planning for new health IT. Wherever the organization is on its migration path toward an EHR or other type of health IT, it needs to develop and manage a **project plan**, which documents and describes the status of accomplishing the project's goals, tasks, milestones, and resource utilization.

An important part of project management is to recognize the scope of the project and distinguish *project* from *program* (see table 8.1). According to the Project Management Institute (PMI) *Guide to the Project Management Body of Knowledge* (PMBOK Guide), a **project** is "a temporary endeavor undertaken to create a unique product, service, or result" and a **program** is "a group of related projects managed in a coordinated way to obtain benefits not available from managing them individually" (PMI 2013). Thus, programs often extend beyond the life of a project, and programs have a greater mission and scope than any single project would. With regard to the EHR and health IT, it can be difficult to draw a definite distinction between projects and programs, because EHR and health IT projects often seem like long-term, not temporary endeavors, and because there can be so many of them that they blend together into something that looks like a program. However

Table 8.1.   Project vs. program

	Project	Program
Activities	Many short, performed once	Variable, performed repetitively
Sequence	Defined pathway	Repetitive
Connectivity	Dependencies among activities	Independent or possible pass-off
Purpose	Single, well-defined goal	General objectives
Time	Defined start/end, intense pressure	Ongoing, pressure ebbs and flows
Money	Fixed costs avoid overruns	Budget, focus on profit and loss
Specification	Vision	Mission
Scope	Boundaries of project	Limitations of authority/responsibility
Quality	Continual assurance tests	Quality improvement projects
Resources	Variable, multidisciplinary	Dedicated
Organization	Matrix	Line and staff

a given organization chooses to use these terms, the important element to bear in mind relative to project management is that a project has a defined beginning and end. This point aids the organization in determining the value of a given project and if, when, and how the organization will proceed forward with other, related, projects.

Another distinction that can be helpful to bear in mind for successful project management is that between **planning**, which is about preparation, and **managing**, which is carrying out the plan. Although this distinction may seem to be a subtle nuance, many organizations lament that their project manager spends so much time managing the project plan that there is no time for managing the project itself. Project management requires following the project plan and keeping it up-to-date, but the bulk of a project manager's time should be spent on project management, not planning.

Prerequisites for a successful project, then, include planning that reviews the SMART goals established for the EHR and health IT during the organization's strategic planning process and incorporating these into a project charter (see below). This approach helps focus the project on gaining the desired results. Executive management support, including clinician leadership, is another important prerequisite. For the project to succeed, there must be clear evidence of that organization executives and leaders understand and are committed to the EHR or other type of health IT. They must actively carry that message to all users and other stakeholders and must allocate appropriate resources to achieve success. Executive management should also require adherence to applicable standards of practice for project management. See chapter 3 for a discussion of strategic planning, chapter 4 for information on SMART goals, and chapter 6 for guidance on communicating messages to users and stakeholders.

Planning

Virtually every organization will start project planning with review of a budget or budgets for EHR and other health IT projects. While a separate budget for each project is important for managing the project, EHR and health IT projects should not be viewed as exclusively information technology (IT) projects or be totally isolated as separate initiatives. They support infrastructure for the broader goals of the organization's strategic plan. In fact, project managers should begin their planning with a review of the organization's strategic plan, its goals, and how the EHR or other health IT projects, once implemented, support achievement of the goals (see chapter 3). It must also be recognized that these projects can transform into ongoing programs. For this reason, some organizations refer to their EHR or other health IT projects as implementation projects, thereby distinguishing them from the ongoing activities associated with maintenance and optimization. Marx (2010) notes, "Each element of EHR implementation requires continual care and feeding—indefinitely. Implementation is just the forerunner of optimization." A process that tightly aligns the EHR and other forms of health IT to the organization's corporate strategic initiatives and incorporates these into an ongoing information management program in no way diminishes the importance of the EHR or other health IT. Rather, such a process treats these projects as integral features of virtually every other organizational initiative.

One way to emphasize the project nature of the EHR or other health IT implementations is to use a project charter. A **project charter** includes a statement of work that defines the specific scope of a given project, the business case for the project, agreements relative to who does what and the size of the budget, environmental factors that must be monitored to control project risk, and organizational process assets that can be put to the project. Executive management signs off on this charter, providing the project manager the authority to apply organizational resources to project activities. By signing off on the project charter, both executive management and project manager formalize the project's scope of importance.

Executive Management Support

Support from executive management is crucial to the success of a health IT project, and absence of support can doom the project. EHR projects are long-term, expensive undertakings. Their payback period often extends well beyond the three-year timeline that most chief executive officers (CEOs) use when looking for a return on investment (ROI). Unfortunately, some executives simply look upon the EHR or other health IT project as a necessary cost of doing business and a project for which the chief information officer (CIO) is responsible. Several factors can influence the level of management support, including the following:

- If members of the executive suite, including CEOs, chief financial officers (CFOs), and even CIOs, as well as many members of the board of directors, do not fully understand the concept and purpose of an EHR and some other types of health IT initiatives, they may not fully support these projects. One chief medical officer (CMO) observed that although many of his colleagues understood an EHR at the *intellectual* level, it was not until they would actually use the EHR that they would understand it at the *intestinal* level. At that point they could fully appreciate the level of change it brought about, not just in documentation or accessing information but in the way they practiced medicine. Education is a key element in gaining leadership support. Educating executive management entails building trust and benchmarking. It may be necessary to find multiple venues and multiple supporters over time to persuade leaders that an EHR or other health IT initiative is an appropriate undertaking that will support the organization's corporate strategic initiatives.

- CEOs may legitimately question whether the medical staff will use an EHR or other types of health IT to the fullest extent possible. CEOs want to know whether there be an ROI or continuous ongoing costs. Benchmark data, to the extent that they are available, can help make the case for the project to executives. An increasing number of research findings demonstrate the value of health IT. Demonstrating that the project shows a sufficient level of attention to workflow and process improvement (see chapter 5) and change management activities (see chapter 6) is also necessary. Outlining these efforts can reassure executive management that the EHR or other form of health IT will be supported beyond the initial implementation of the product. Furthermore, a project that has the direct support of the organization's medical staff and involves them in planning and implementing activities may be more likely to get executive approval and support.

- CEOs want to see a business case for the project and expect the business case to be realistic. There is no need to attempt to determine the monetary value of every benefit. A **benefits portfolio** is a mix of monetary and qualitative benefits. While qualitative benefits should be quantified in the business case, they do not need to be quantified in monetary terms. For example, patient satisfaction is very important to executive management and is associated with the Triple Aim goal of improving the quality of the care experience. (See chapter 4 for information on the Triple Aim.)

Medical Staff Buy-in

Although executive management must support the EHR or health IT project to provide the appropriate resources and demonstrate the project's importance to the organization, the medical staff is going to be one of the primary users, and therefore their buy-in is essential. To get the buy-in of medical staff, the physicians must be convinced that the EHR or other type of health IT is necessary, time-saving, and trustworthy. Historically, physicians have not valued documentation in the same way that people in other industries do. For example, pilots will not fly planes without documentary evidence about weather, load, and other key factors, but physicians are trained to at least initiate emergency treatment for a patient without any information other than what is available from rapid observation. Even in nonemergency situations and with a complete health record, physicians tend to rely on their powers of questioning and observation to reach diagnostic and therapeutic decisions. It is a rare physician who does not ask a new patient (or one not seen for some time) questions already answered in the health record. Unfortunately, such an approach takes time, relies on the probability of the physician matching responses to recalled knowledge, and can frustrate patients. Physicians may have concerns about others' data collection abilities or the age of existing information in the record, or worry that the patient may have been confused or less than completely truthful in reporting previous data. These are certainly legitimate reasons for reviewing data with the patient. However, validating the older data rather than reentering the data may be less time consuming for the provider and may ease patients' frustration with repeating data. Unfortunately, most EHRs are not designed to support such validation activity in a way that is meaningful for physicians (or auditors).

Today's healthcare environment is truly information based, and members of the medical staff are coming to that realization and recognizing better ways to use information. Education and communication with the medical staff are critical for helping physicians identify the benefit of such changes and gaining their support.

Physician and Other Clinician Champions

Another important ingredient in a successful EHR and some other health IT projects is a **project champion** or champions who support colleagues in their adoption of a new technology or program. Project champions may hold formal positions, such as chief medical informatics officer (CMIO) or medical director of information systems (MDIS), or they may simply be engaged physicians who volunteer to support colleagues who struggle with or resist outright the concept of the EHR or other health IT. Physician champions do not have to be the highest-ranked physicians, but they must be respected by their peers.

In their zeal to promote EHR systems, some physician champions have been viewed by their peers more as mavericks out of touch with reality than as true leaders seeking to improve the lot of their colleagues. In such a case, it is best to cultivate several physician champions. Recruiting effective champions may require heart-to-heart talks with potential candidates or with someone who can influence potential candidates to persuade them of the value of volunteering. The more physicians behind an EHR or other health IT initiative, the more likely others will become involved. Figure 8.1 provides a sample job description for a CMIO/MDIS. If the organization is not large enough or

Figure 8.1.   Sample job description for CMIO/MDIS

Purpose

This physician will be responsible for supporting the design and development of the electronic health record (EHR) and other health information technology (HIT) that will assist clinicians in the delivery of effective and efficient patient care. The CMIO participates as a member of both the EHR Steering Committee, representing the needs and requirements of the physician community, and serves as an advocate of management in promoting the use of HIT in the clinical setting.

Tasks

1. Participates in clinical advisory groups to provide broad-based input into the design of the EHR in order to support excellence in patient care, quality measurement, and economic value to the organization
2. Engages patient care providers with varying roles including physicians, physician extenders, nursing staff, ancillary department personnel, and health information management professionals to contribute to the development and use of the EHR
3. Develops empathy and understanding of physician needs and builds trusting relationships with physicians to gain support of EHR initiatives. Is responsive to users' needs, including training and support requirements, to assure widespread acceptance and provider use of the clinical systems
4. Reviews medical informatics trends, experiences, and approaches; develops technical and application implementation strategies; and assists in the development of strategic plans for the EHR
5. Works in concert with the EHR Project Manager and Information Systems (IS) staff to design and implement systems supporting the organization's goals
6. Works in concert with the physician quality team in the design of evidence-based guidance, clinical decision support, and other health care models utilizing the EHR to gain maximum efficacy and support for patient care protocols
7. Champions the use of clinical decision support and other EHR features supporting protocol management to leverage clinicians' time and optimize clinical quality outcomes
8. Supports development and adoption of health information exchange strategies to enhance communications among affiliates and referring physicians and with patients and their authorized caregivers
9. Participates in the development and deployment of solutions for clinical quality measurement, reporting, and improvement. Designs and evaluates collection of data for clinical purposes, including tracking and interpretation of outcomes
10. Leads development of clinical documentation user interfaces and their interrelationship with other clinical information relative to clinical documentation improvement in support of correct coding/billing
11. Participates in clinical activities, providing patient care in appropriate clinical settings as applicable. Reviews patient assessments and management plans. Participates in applicable clinical research

Special Skills

- Possesses excellent interpersonal skills and is able to work effectively with a diversity of personalities. Must be approachable and be able to present data with effective communication and presentation skills. Must be an effective consensus builder
- Has a good grasp of clinical workflow and has an interest in EHRs, clinical quality measurement and outcomes improvement, and patient-centric care
- Strong leader with a mature sense of priorities and solid practical experience who can design and implement EHR within the framework of technical boundaries
- Politically savvy, has a high tolerance for ambiguity, and can work successfully in a matrix management model
- Systems thinker with strong organizational skills
- Adaptable and has a strong collaborative management style—a creative thinker with high energy and enthusiasm, and a team player who promotes the concepts of people working together versus individual performance
- Is a contemporary clinician who understands major trends in healthcare and is familiar with point-of-care products and medical informatics trends and tools, while being actively engaged in the practice of medicine

does not have the resources to hire such an individual, the job description can still supply insights into some of the functions and characteristics that volunteer physician champions may find useful to consider.

Project planning may also need to identify project champions among other types of clinicians. Nurses, especially, have not historically been accustomed to using computers as part of their work. During the implementation of the EHR and other types of health IT, Nurses' needs for support are often somewhat different than those for physicians. Nurse champions also can speak up about issues associated with the EHR or other health IT during implementation that other nurses may feel uncomfortable raising. Nurse champions may be found among those who simply have a keen interest in information technology, have experience elsewhere, or have special training, perhaps as nurse informaticists.

Involvement of Users and Other Stakeholders

User involvement from the start is another prerequisite of successful EHR and other health IT projects. Users include the full spectrum of clinicians as well as administrative and financial staff and other persons who rely on the health record to carry out their responsibilities. Examples of such functions include assessing quality of care, managing healthcare risk issues, providing patients access to services (scheduling, registration), wayfinding (directions to patients to find their way around a facility), obtaining reimbursement (eligibility verification, coding, billing), identifying potential product lines for the organization, and many other functions.

User involvement in EHR and health IT planning does not simply mean the organization convenes a committee composed of selected potential users; there should also be a groundswell of users who are seriously interested in the project. As with executive management commitment, a groundswell of user interest does not happen suddenly. Change management must be undertaken to develop a climate of interest in the user community. (See chapter 6 for information on change management.) For example, nurses adopting a bar code medication administration record (BC-MAR) system may need coaching with respect to process improvement and communication with patients. Without such coaching, nurses have to find all sorts of ways to work around perceived problems with bar code medication administration, which only creates new work for themselves and does not really ensure the "five rights" for safe medication administration (right patient, right drug, right time, right dose, right route). It may seem surprising how limited many users are in their knowledge of computers in general, let alone EHR systems and other health IT. While a great many users may have experience with smartphones and home computers, that experience involves very different types of activities than those performed in an EHR or other form of health IT. The following example illustrates this point:

> A physician in a clinic had heard that EHR systems often generated significant revenue by making it more efficient to conduct clinical trials. It was explained that patient candidates for clinical trials could be selected at the time the physician entered visit notes. This process would supposedly decrease the nursing time required to review records for potential candidates, improve candidate participation because the physician could answer questions directly and immediately, and, ultimately, increase the number of participants in clinical trials. When asked how physicians would keep track of the criteria and then match them to the visit notes, it became apparent that the physician had spent little time understanding the nature of the EHR even as it was used for routine documentation. Interestingly, after an explanation was provided, the physician identified an entire set of desired activities and became hooked on this use for the EHR.

Users need to understand how an EHR or other form of health IT can make their job easier and more gratifying. For example, nurses need to believe that technology that saves an hour per day of nursing time is not going to result in the loss of a job or lower pay but instead will free nurses to spend their time providing better patient care, patient instruction, and followup. One way to help educate users is to make SMART goals come alive for them. SMART goals should be top of mind as workflow and process improvements are identified and change management is instituted. (See chapter 4 for more about SMART goals.)

One-on-one communications, such as those described in chapter 6, may be necessary to identify and address each person's fears and anxiety points. Physicians in particular do not like to appear uninformed within their peer group. Multiple, short meetings with key naysayers may clarify issues that can turn them around in support of an EHR. The result of an educational process will be a better informed set of users who are interested in achieving success with EHR.

Resource Allocation

A final major prerequisite for EHR and other health IT success is the provision of appropriate and sustained resources for which there is accountability. Clearly, one major resource is funding. However, resources also include people, policies, and processes.

Project managers, physician and other champions, informaticists, health information management (HIM) professionals, IT support personnel, other clinician users, and other stakeholders are all necessary to achieve success. In addition to the time commitment, people with the appropriate skills for the various jobs must be available. Resource leveling is the project management task of taking available resources and comparing them to project or projects demands (Faucheux 2013). When multiple IT projects are underway, allocation of existing resources may be difficult. A form of resource leveling is also necessary when EHR and other health IT projects involve users who are needed full time at the bedside of patients. When users with the right skills are not on staff or are unavailable to participate in the project when needed, the organization may have to bring special expertise in house by either hiring people with certain skills (many of whom will be needed long term) or contracting with consultants for temporary, specialized assignments. When consultants are used, someone in the organization should learn about the tasks they are performing, both for oversight purposes and to ensure ongoing continuity of processes.

Alternatively, an organization may decide to train certain staff members who demonstrate interest and related skills to participate in the project. Organizations should recognize that their staff members might already have expertise in areas outside of their usual job responsibilities. For example, an engineer may be studying IT unrelated to his or her job. HIM professionals may be tapped as data analysts and workflow analysts. Protective services personnel are greatly enhancing their information security knowledge and expertise. Staff may welcome the opportunity to stretch by using such knowledge and skills, although care must be taken not to overburden them with new responsibilities if they are required to continue performing at least some of their former responsibilities. Many organizations find that such responsibilities evolve into new full-time jobs. Some staff members may also have very strong interest and inclination suitable to acquire new skills. Tapping these individuals for a vendor's certification can be good for the employee and the organization. However, it is also important to recognize that now that an organization has trained staff in new responsibilities, the staff may be recruited by other care delivery organizations or vendors. Many vendors include in their contracts that organizations may not hire their employees; similar contractual language should also be in place to protect the organization from the vendor hiring its staff. If an organization invests in special training for an employee who does not already have an employment contract that requires new trainees to stay on the job or repay the cost of training, this agreement should be instituted prior to the training.

Standards of Practice

Organizations also should establish and enforce clear policies, business rules, and applicable standards of practice for a project. Creativity and innovation are usually desirable, but it is clearly inappropriate to jeopardize a project or the organization itself by stepping out of applicable standards of practice.

Policies may include anything from requiring use of standards recognized by the federal government where they exist for EHR or health IT applications to using standardized medical vocabulary, formulary, or practice guidelines.

Business rules dictate how an organization will carry out its functions. For example, one organization implementing the Health Insurance Portability and Accountability Act (HIPAA) transactions and code set standards had a business rule that it would not seek copayments in advance of providing services. Although many organizations see the HIPAA eligibility verification process as one way to enhance their collection process, this particular hospital viewed it as a way to plan financial counseling for patients after care services had been delivered. Business rules also encompass determining who can access patient-specific information, what level of signature is required on an order, the content to include in a patient history and physical examination, the required components for a medication order, and many other issues that must be addressed in an EHR and other types of health IT.

A formal standard also exists for project management. The PMBOK Guide (PMI 2013) is a standard approved by the American National Standards Institute (ANSI). This standard is extremely comprehensive, and, for any given project, it may be used more as a guide than an absolute standard that must be followed to the letter. Still, an organization with many large and complex projects would be well served by having a project manager certified by the Project Management Institute (PMI n.d.).

Finally, well-defined systems development life cycle (SDLC) processes should be used. (See chapter 2.) A disciplined approach to managing the project and steps needed to see systems through their life cycle from conception, through planning, selection, acquisition, installation, testing, training, and implementation, to ongoing maintenance, upgrading, and enhancements will help ensure that the EHR or other health IT project is implemented on time, within budget, and in the most effective manner.

In addition to finding the people to provide project management, the processes themselves must be agreed upon and adhered to (as noted earlier). Some people are uncomfortable following a formal process or are uneasy requiring others to follow formal structures. Time and again, however, projects waste time and cause frustration because formal processes are not in place. When everyone recognizes that formal project management processes are valuable, there will be no turning back.

Scope and Characteristics of the EHR and Other Health IT Projects

The general characteristics of most projects are that they:

- Have a defined beginning and end, usually follow a standard SDLC, and have a defined budget

- Are a line function (in which staff report to the project manager), although may also use special staffing, often through volunteerism from many parts of an organization

- Concern something new and therefore involve uncertainty and change

- Require great attention to detail as well as the ability to see the big picture

Most EHR projects and many other health IT projects have these characteristics, except for the first one. The lack of a clear beginning and end does not to suggest that an EHR or other type of health IT project should not be completed on time, standardized, or held accountable to a budget; however, most EHR projects follow a spiral life cycle that in reality includes a series of many new projects that implement new components or modules over potentially many years. In addition, the EHR and other forms of health IT require ongoing maintenance, because they change as the practice of medicine and health services change. Because of the complexity of an EHR and many other health IT projects, each new upgrade or maintenance requirement may be considered a mini-project in its own right.

Regarding the EHR or other health IT initiative as an ongoing program instead of a project can help ensure that it is properly maintained. (Refer to table 8.1, earlier in this chapter, for the key distinctions between projects and programs.) However, the programmatic nature of health IT can also be problematic. Sometimes, the result is lack of project-type accountability for a budget, with overexpenditures and an uncertain ROI.

Project Management Resources for the EHR and Health IT

Most projects follow a fairly standard pattern of human resource allocation. A project manager typically reports to a **project sponsor**, who is the person who provides resources and support for the project and is accountable for enabling success (PMI 2013). For a very large, complex project such as the EHR and some other health IT projects, project sponsor could be the chief operations officer (COO) or another person from executive management. Some large organizations may have a **project management office (PMO)**. In this case, there are multiple project managers with direct responsibility to the director of the PMO and also responsibility to the project sponsor as each different project is worked on. Some organizations have decentralized PMOs, with one located in the IT department, another in finance, and others elsewhere. In this case, each focuses on a domain of expertise. In a centralized PMO structure, the PMO has a portfolio of projects, supporting construction, mergers and acquisitions, procurement and implementation of medical devices, and many others, including EHR and health IT (Schwalbe 2013).

In addition to the project manager, many other individuals are involved in carrying out the work of the project, with the project manager providing oversight, facilitation, and coordination. Some of these individuals work for the organization in other capacities and also work on the project because they either have been assigned to do so or have volunteered to help. These individuals often become members of the EHR or other health IT **steering committee** (a committee composed of representative stakeholders that advises the project manager and others on matters relating to the project implementation overall) or other subcommittees, commonly called **domain teams**, which are groups of people that work on aspects of the project that relate to their specialized areas of expertise. Other individuals may be hired as new employees to help implement and maintain the project, or they may be temporary employees or consultants primarily available to help during implementation and the go-live phase.

Project Organizational Structure

Most hospitals will construct a fairly structured organization to undertake their EHR project or other large-scale health IT project. Health IT projects that are smaller in scope may not require as structured an organization. In many organizations, an initial steering committee for an EHR or health IT project is chosen to be responsible for guiding the process of visioning and product selection, and then it is dissolved when that process ends. Another steering committee then forms to be involved in high-level implementation activities. This later steering committee may be aided by subcommittees and/or domain teams that focus on specific aspects of the project and report back to the steering committee. Some organizations not only create such a committee structure but also assign specific decision-making authority to it. This practice can be helpful because clarity about who can make what decisions improves the chances for the project to stay on task, on time, and on budget.

Even when projects have steering committees, a project manager is necessary for ongoing coordination and support. This is because steering committees are essentially composed of a volunteer group of individuals who carve out time from their normal days to participate or who may be assigned a small number of hours from their routine tasks.

Composition and Role of the Steering Committee

Steering committees for the EHR or other health IT may vary in their composition depending on organization preference. Sometimes, the committee is composed of senior managers or executives. In this case, there will be a number of specific domain teams. Although it is advantageous to have executive management engaged in the EHR or health IT project, their myriad commitments may make it difficult for them to attend meetings, and their representatives may not be given the same level of authority to make decisions, which can delay progress. In addition, the domain teams that form to do the nuts-and-bolts work are then often homogeneous and continue the **information silo** effect (where information is not shared across organizational units or their information systems [Shaywitz 2015]) that an EHR or other health IT is intended to overcome.

Another, often better way to lend executive support to the project is for an executive sponsor to be committed to a steering committee that is composed of individuals more representative of the end users. The composition of such a steering committee for an EHR is described in table 8.2, with some variation based on the size and type of organization. Subcommittees or domain teams may still be needed in this structure because of the volume of work. Some of these subcommittees may focus on nursing, physician, or other specific clinician interests; however, where feasible, they should focus on interrelated sets of functions that involve different types of clinicians, such as medication management, care planning, or quality improvement. During the vendor selection process, there may be a small group that reviews technology and another that studies the cost-effectiveness of the products; there may be a large group that reviews demonstrations and a small group that goes on a site visit. All such groups, however, need to either come together as the steering committee or provide representatives to the steering committee on a regular basis. By doing so, this limits the effects of information silos that previously dominated the workplace.

Table 8.2. Composition of the EHR steering committee

Members	Purpose
EHR project manager	Provides EHR project direction and support
User representatives (from major functional and business units, including their informaticists, as well as medical staff, research, quality improvement, and other major clinical data users or suppliers)	Understands current data requirements and workflows, evaluates functionality of new systems and ability to implement new workflows and processes, gains buy-in for EHR adoption
IT professionals (e.g., applications, operations, network, telecommunications)	Understands and evaluates technical capability of current and proposed systems and level of "fit"
HIM professionals	Perform data analysis, ensure data quality, support operations and data flow, oversee data sets, act as data brokers
Internal consultants (as needed, e.g., financial analyst, contracts manager, human resources, labor relations, legal, etc.)	Provide probability and criticality estimation, offer ways to implement controls, represent customer interests
Trainers	Gain insight into creating training and programs
Corporate compliance official Information privacy official Information security official	Coordinates with compliance activities
Executive sponsor	Represents executive management, can help interpret message for executive management

Check Your Understanding 8.1

Match the terms with their appropriate descriptions:

A. Domain team

B. Program

C. Project

D. Project charter

E. Project champion

F. Project plan

G. Project sponsor

H. Resource allocation

I. Resource leveling

J. Steering committee

1. Document that defines the scope, business case, and agreements for a given project

2. Comparison of available resources to needed resources

3. Coordinated activities designed to continuously carry out a specific mission

4. Group that provides overall advice to the project manager relative to a project

5. Person who provides resources and support for a project and is accountable for enabling success

6. Person who supports colleagues in their adoption of a new technology or program

7. Group that works on aspects of the project that relate to a specialized area of expertise

8. A temporary activity undertaken to create a unique product, service, or result

9. Document that identifies and describes the status of accomplishing the project's goals

10. Person who assigns resources to a project

Role of the Project Manager

As noted previously, the project manager supports the steering committee and is responsible for overseeing that all aspects of the EHR or health IT project are completed. A project manager requires skills much like a general contractor for a building project. A general contractor hires the mason, plumber, electrician, painter, and so on. He or she may not be technically skilled in any one of these roles but can read a blueprint and understands the skills needed to perform each role. Thus, the general contractor knows when to bring an individual on board to perform a particular job and how to evaluate the end product.

Like a general contractor, the project manager for an EHR or other health IT project should have a good understanding of what health IT is, have some healthcare background, and understand project management tools and techniques. Above all, however, the project manager should have strong leadership skills to work with many different people, provide compelling direction, build trust, manage conflict, and use influence to get things done (Doll 2005).

Bennatan suggests that a project manager needs to possess a "magic suit of clothes" to accomplish the project goals (2009). EHRs and other large-scale health IT projects are not typical IT projects, and IT skills or even strong technical project management skills are less important to the EHR project manager role than vision and leadership. The projects are sufficiently large in scope that IT skills, ability to use project management software, and even clinical knowledge can all be achieved by team members led by the project manager.

Table 8.3 provides a checklist to identify the characteristics of successful project managers for EHRs and other health IT. (A person who answers yes to all or almost all of the questions has the potential to succeed.) A sample EHR/health IT project manager job description is provided in figure 8.2.

Table 8.3.   EHR project manager checklist

❏ **Are you entrepreneurial? Do you care what's next?**
(If a project should have a defined end, that may also mean an end to the job, or at least a shift to a different project. Some people thrive on such constant change; others prefer a more stable environment.)

❏ **Do you generally get tasks done on time?**
(Some individuals always are procrastinators, have "hope creep" where they believe they can get the work done even though they cannot, or have "effort creep" where they are working very hard but not producing the desired work. A proven track record of getting a project done early or on time—and correct—is essential.)

❏ **Do people respond well to your requests?**
(An internal candidate for EHR project manager sometimes carries "baggage" that is difficult for others to see past. If you are viewed as a nag, servant, geek, or having other negative characteristics, these may be difficult to overcome, even with the best of skills. In addition, because the project manager does not have line authority over the members of the project team, influence must be used to get team members to complete tasks they agree to undertake.)

❏ **Do you like to share the spotlight?**
(An EHR project requires a team effort. While the project manager should get credit for a job well done, others must also be recognized. The chair of the EHR steering committee, for example, may have the spotlight while the project manager is the force behind the scenes.)

❏ **Are you comfortable communicating with all?**
(Individuals with limited experience in communicating to large groups, persons with authority, or highly technical individuals may find it difficult to be as assertive in communications as necessary. A project manager must be able to build trust and interpersonal relationships to achieve project goals.)

❏ **Do you see "all sides"? Value opposing viewpoints?**
(A project manager needs to be able to present alternatives clearly and without bias, but also to steer a group to make unbiased and objective decisions. If you carry personal biases or always play devil's advocate, it may be more difficult for you to be neutral.)

❏ **Are you a diplomatic "straight-shooter"?**
(In some cases, a project manager must convey bad news or take tough stands in order to move the project along. This must be done, but done with diplomacy or respect can be quickly lost.)

❏ **Do you see the big picture, while attending to detail?**
(EHR projects can include hundreds if not thousands of tasks, many of which have dependencies and all of which must be managed. However, the project manager must also motivate the team to keep it moving forward and be mindful of the overall project purpose and goals.)

❏ **Are you comfortable with change?**
(A project manager not only faces the end of the project as a change, but must be able to help others with process improvement and a truly clinical transformation that brings enormous change to users.)

❏ **Do you delegate appropriately?**
(A project manager must delegate the work of the project to individuals who have the knowledge and skills to perform the work. Taking on tasks others can and should perform leaves the project manager with no time to manage the project.)

Figure 8.2.   EHR/health IT project manager job description

JOB TITLE: EHR/Health IT Project Manager

SUPERVISORY RELATIONSHIPS:
Reports to: Director, Project Management Office
Supervises: Administrative support staff as applicable for project

BASIC FUNCTIONS:
The EHR/Health IT Project Manager works closely with stakeholders to understand project requirements and business needs, and to identify, evaluate and select solutions to business problems; assists in the design and maintenance of project definitions and deliverables; plans and manages the delivery of business system solutions in support of the organization's business objectives including developing project plans, estimates, specifications, flowcharts, presentations; communicates the status of projects in both formal and informal settings; proactively identifies and resolves project risks/opportunities that may impact a project or its deliverables; is responsible for execution and control of the project from inception to project close; and interfaces with all functional business groups to ensure the efficiency and effectiveness of system solutions deployed support business goals and objectives. The position is also responsible for technology vendor relationship management and negotiation of contract business terms and contract administration.

1. Demonstrates an understanding of the organization's mission, vision, and values as described in the Associate Handbook by:
   a. Displaying a positive attitude and providing solutions
   b. Assuming a sense of ownership by staying informed and taking initiative to provide excellence with every encounter.
   c. Demonstrating excellent communication abilities by asking questions, providing suggestions, thanking others, and solving disagreements in a face-to-face, polite, and respectful manner
   d. Promoting exceptional teamwork by working across departmental lines, with the medical staff, and internal and external organizational customers
   e. Performing all position duties and responsibilities in accordance with standards of The Joint Commission and the organization's performance evaluation and competency assessment policies
2. Manages multiple, concurrent projects, which may involve large numbers of users, multiple departments, and other organizations, using defined project management methodologies.
3. Provides direction in identifying project requirements and in identifying, evaluating, and selecting solutions.
4. Assists in writing business cases and calculation of project costs and ROI to support project requests.
5. Determines the project approach, staffing, and schedule and defines team member roles and responsibilities.
6. Creates and manages project plans, risk mitigation plans, communication plans, resource requirements, project costs, and all other project management–related documentation.
7. Manages relationships among vendors, subcontractors, and internal teams. Travel may be required.
8. Performs day-to-day management of all phases of the projects, including record maintenance, report preparation, and correspondence to coordinate all project activities with all stakeholders.
9. Measures and monitors progress to ensure that projects are delivered on timeand within budget and meet expectations.
10. Communicates effectively with leadership and stakeholders to provide project risk analysis, status, and analysis of requirements that might impact strategic direction.

OTHER DUTIES:
Performs additional duties as assigned.
Keeps informed about current technologies in the health care information systems field.
Maintains an understanding of organizational operations.

POSITION QUALIFICATIONS:
Education: Baccalaureate level college degree. Experience with Microsoft Office Suite and Microsoft Project software as well as technical writing. Advanced degree preferred.
                         Training in project management and systems analysis preferred.

(continued)

Figure 8.2.   EHR/health IT project manager job description (Continued)

Experience:	4 years' experience as a project manager with formal project management methodologies. Project management experience in healthcare preferred.
License/Certifications:	Project Management Professional (PMP) preferred.
Special Skills:	Demonstrates excellent interpersonal skills, building trust and confidence with all stakeholders.
	Employs excellent communication and listening skills to ensure effective relationships and clear exchange of information. Communicates technical terminology at level appropriate to audience.
	Actively participates in, or leads, meetings.
	Ability to take strategic direction from management and participate in strategic planning activities throughout the lifetime of the project. Has a broad view of organizational goals and objectives and is cost-conscious, pragmatic, and resourceful.
	Ability to see tasks through to completion with minimal guidance.

Source: Adapted from job descriptions for IS Project Manager and Process Implementation Nurse, Watertown Regional Medical Center, J. Mueller, MBA, RHIA.

Project Manager Skills

The PMBOK Guide (PMI 2013) identifies 11 critical skills for a project manager to possess: leadership, motivation, communication, influencing, decision making, political and cultural awareness, trust building, negotiation, conflict management, coaching, and team building. A special consideration in team building is meetings facilitation.

Leadership

Leadership skills involve focusing the efforts of a group of people toward a common goal and enabling them to work as a team. An effective project leader inspires a shared vision. These skills are distinguished from management knowledge and skills (Barry 2010). Management of an EHR or other type of health IT project may require general management knowledge of finance and accounting principles; research and development; strategic, tactical, and operational planning; organizational structures, organizational behavior, and personnel administration; work relationships, including motivation, delegation, supervision, team building, and conflict management; and self-direction through time management and stress management. Management of an EHR or other health IT project also entails knowledge of EHR/health IT concepts, although detailed technical skills are not required.

Although the EHR or health IT project manager is expected to manage and lead, he or she generally—and ideally—shares the leadership tasks with others. It is hoped that a physician champion, other clinician leaders, executive management leadership (including the CIO), and others who are needed will head up teams and assume responsibility for project tasks.

Motivation

To motivate project teams, the project manager fosters an environment that is conducive to performing project tasks while providing value to the individuals on the team. Motivation starts with making sure everyone understands the big picture. The general purpose and functionality of an EHR or other type of health IT may be fairly well understood, but the scope of the project implementation may not be as clear. The project manager needs to be upfront about all that is entailed and reassure team members that they will have the right tools to do their part. Even for a team composed primarily of volunteers, establishing performance goals and tracking results for the team demonstrates the importance of the tasks at hand. Finally, motivation includes working side-by-side with team members and celebrating successes with them.

Communication

Communication involves the ability to convey information in a clear, unambiguous, and complete manner. (See chapter 6.) The schematic in figure 8.3 illustrates the scope of communication requirements for the project manager of an EHR or other health IT project. The scope is very broad. There are internal and external communications, from communicating specific tasks to and receiving reports from team members to potentially preparing media releases with the organization's public relations staff and creating informational materials for patients. The project manager must be equally at ease communicating with peers, with those individuals engaged in specific tasks who may be anywhere within the organization's hierarchy, and with executive management and the board of directors. Written and oral communication skills are a given, but the art of listening and the ability to quickly gain knowledge are possibly even more important.

The project manager must have not only general communication skills but also the ability to manage project communications. Project communication skills are listed in table 8.4. Effective communications for an EHR project should begin with not only an effective communicator at the helm of the project but also a communication plan (see chapter 6).

Influencing

The PMBOK Guide (PMI 2013) describes influencing as a strategy of sharing power and relying on interpersonal skills to get others to cooperate toward common goals. To influence team members, the PMBOK Guide suggests leading by example and following through with commitments, clarifying how a decision will be made, using a flexible interpersonal style and adjusting the style to the audience, and applying power skillfully and cautiously.

Adjusting interpersonal style to fit the audience is especially important when working with multiple generations of people who bring different expectations and behaviors to their work in healthcare, and vastly different skill sets with respect to technology. Hospitals and Health Networks (HHN 2013) ran a series of articles about generations in the workplace, defining characteristics of

Figure 8.3.   Management communication skills

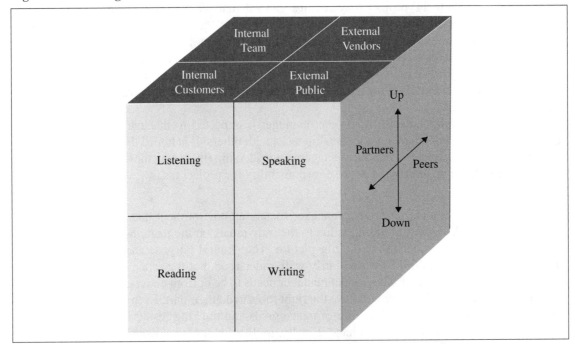

Table 8.4.   Project communication skills

Project Needs	Communication Skills
Instruction	• Select appropriate medium: oral, e-mail message, informal memo, demonstration, formal procedure. • Use appropriate communication style: active versus passive voice, sentence structure, word choice, body language.
Feedback	• Understand sender–receiver models of communication. • Construct feedback mechanisms. • Recognize barriers to communication.
Meeting management	• Prepare agenda. • Facilitate discussion: ice-breaking, energizing the group, gaining input from all, managing the verbose. • Manage conflict. • Prepare minutes.
Building consensus	• Be logical, not emotional. • Avoid "win–lose." • Avoid changing minds only to achieve harmony. • Avoid majority voting or bargaining. • Value different views. • View initial agreement as suspect. • When individuals understand and accept the logic of a different point of view, you have reached consensus.
Follow-up	• Select appropriate aids to manage schedules, calendars, and communication among team members. • Select appropriate time frame: regular, intermittent, key milestones only, based on exception reporting. • Select appropriate medium: oral, e-mail message, informal memo, formal request. • Document follow-up.
Data collection	• Determine scope of required data: high-level, detailed; identified, deidentified; quantitative, qualitative; anecdotal, trend, or benchmark. • Select appropriate collection tools: interview, observation, questionnaire, survey.
Reporting	• Understand the audience and scope of required report: executive-level, general, specific, exception reporting, status reporting. • Select appropriate medium: oral, written; informal, formal. • Use appropriate presentation techniques: body language, visual aids, written report binder.

those in the silent generation, baby boomers, generation X, and millennials. Project managers and team leaders would be well advised to learn about and consider these differences in their work.

Decision Making

Individuals can have different types of decision-making styles, including command, consultation, consensus, and random. The PMBOK Guide (PMI 2013) suggests that there are four factors that affect the decision style: time constraints, trust, quality, and acceptance. To some extent, these decision styles can also reflect the culture of the organization or one's personal style preferences.

Following a consistent decision-making process can help overcome the negative aspects of any of the separate styles. Such a process might include the following:

- *Problem definition* to fully explore, clarify, and define the problem about which a decision must be made

- *Problem solution generation* to explore fully the potential solutions to a problem to ensure the best possible course of action

- *Ideas-to-action* to select evaluation criteria, rate the pros and cons for each potential alternative solution, and ultimately identify the best solution

- *Solution-to-action planning* to engage stakeholders and ensure successful implementation of the solution

- *Solution evaluation planning* to ensure postimplementation evaluation

- *Evaluation of the outcome and process* once a decision has been implemented

Political and Cultural Awareness

The people involved in an EHR or other type of health IT project are likely to be a culturally diverse group, and their cultural differences can either lend strength to the project or be a source of political conflict. As noted above, understanding differences in the various generations of people working in healthcare can help with communication and consensus-building. Age, however, is not the only factor to consider. Many organizations conduct cultural awareness training to help employees understand often subtle but powerful cultural nuances that can affect the working environment and the ability of people to collaborate successfully. A project manager may find it useful to request that such training be provided across the entire organization (Chebium 2015).

Trust Building

Trust, or feeling confident that one can rely on others to act as they should and achieve what is expected of them, is empowering. It helps people stay engaged and increases the quality of collaboration necessary in carrying out a project such as an EHR or other health IT implementation (Young 2015). Dearborn (2014) identifies the core principles of trust to be giving trust first, communicating effectively, and being genuine. Of course, there is nothing wrong with President Ronald Reagan's philosophy of "trust, but verify" in situations where verification can support the transparency necessary to accomplish trust.

Negotiation

In the context of project management, **negotiation** is a discussion that resolves an issue in a way that all parties find acceptable. Project managers often find that there is more than one approach to most activities associated with EHR and health IT implementation. Examples include whether clinical decision support will be tailored to user type or not, or whether ICD-10 or SNOMED will be used to encode the problem list.

Often the best way to gain alignment on options is to invoke the primary principle of negotiation, which is to achieve a win-win resolution. To do so, the project manager should anticipate points of negotiation and be prepared to illustrate the pros and cons of each option. Each member of the group should be asked to contemplate and raise any conflict of interest they have with the options and to recuse themselves from the discussion if necessary. This process helps remove bias and aids in creating trust. Each group member should also be asked to contribute any additional information known about each option. It is at this point that most people start bargaining. The project manager should help the group focus on common interests. Reminding the group that the ultimate goal is what is best for the patient can help trigger unbiased thinking. The conclusion of a negotiation process is finding the option that all can agree to accept. The project manager should restate this option and by show of hands or other formal process observe that agreement has been reached. Documenting the negotiation is also important for future reference.

Conflict Management

Conflict is inevitable in project environments. It can result in poor outcomes, or it can be healthy for a project team when managed properly. **Conflict management** is the practice of being able to identify and handle conflicts efficiently and fairly (McKinney 2015). It is very important for project managers to be able to manage conflict. Minor disagreements can easily turn into major problems when conflict is ignored or not dealt with immediately. Like negotiation, the best conflict management results in a win-win situation.

There are generally five ways people deal with conflict:

- Avoiding or ignoring conflict is a lose-lose situation. Either the conflict festers forever without resolution, or one side effectively takes what it wants. Unfortunately, the side that gets what it wants in this way is usually the side that has the least desirable resolution.

- Accommodating is a lose-win situation. Accommodating is often done to appease others by downplaying conflict. When an undesirable resolution wins out, the only benefit to the accommodation strategy is that the resolution is usually not as onerous as in the avoiding strategy.

- Competing is a win-lose situation. Competition can be healthy, but where there must be a resolution, there cannot be a loser. Dealing with conflict through competition could be effective in a crisis situation, but in general it is more desirable to get to resolution.

- Compromising is sometimes described as a bend-bend situation. Both parties have to give up something. If the something is very minor, compromise may ultimately be viewed as win-win. But if the something is fairly significant, the best approach is collaborating.

- Collaborating is a win-win situation where ideas are integrated into finding a creative solution that is acceptable to all. The process of collaboration can require considerable time, in which case the compromise often ends up being the resolution (Dontigney n.d.; SNU 2015).

Coaching

Coaching in a team environment is a way to develop the team to a higher level of competency and performance. It utilizes empowerment, actual skill development, and formal or informal training. For example, a project team working to optimize EHR use by nurses might want to have some formal training on workflow and process improvement. At the same time, change management interventions may help a few of the members of the team overcome resistance to EHR use, or all of the team may wish to have some skills building on how to roll out the improved workflows.

The PMBOK Guide notes that coaching is also used to address poor performance. Coaching is different than counseling; the latter focuses on addressing situations where team members willfully do not do something, whereas coaching helps members who cannot do something (PMI 2013). Coaching is viewed as a motivator because those who are coached often come away from the experience not only satisfied with a job well done but also recognizing they have a new skill that can be applied in other contexts.

Team Building

Team building is essentially an important subset of all other interpersonal skills required of a project manager. It can be viewed as having two parts. First is the recognition of what help a project needs and then dividing up the work into various components that individual teams can address. The second part relates to helping each person in a team work together as a team.

As noted previously, every EHR and most other health IT projects will have a steering committee, and large projects will likely involve several additional teams. Teams also may form and disband as the need arises. Some common teams used in EHR and health IT projects are described in table 8.5. For whatever teams may be required in these types of projects, including the steering committee, the ultimate goal is problem solving and decision making to achieve the success of the project. However, good results from teams do not happen automatically. Team building encompasses selecting the right team members and understanding and managing group dynamics:

Selecting the Right Team Members

Organizational culture often determines how individuals come to be part of a team. Some organizations simply appoint people based on their knowledge, skills, and perceived or expressed interest. Others call for volunteers to form teams and generally accept anyone who volunteers. For an EHR or health IT project, it may be necessary to have some control over team composition, although volunteers can help achieve buy-in that is critical for adoption. During team formation, it is important to consider the personalities of the team members. One well-recognized measure of personality is the Myers-Briggs Type Indicator. The questions in figure 8.4 are used to characterize an individual on four scales (for example, ESTJ), with the result being 16 different personality types.

Sometimes, the Myers-Briggs personality typing is too much to introduce into a steering committee or other type of team. A smaller, more manageable number of characteristics that may help distinguish roles in a group is the **SCODF typing model** (created by the author). This model identifies traits that individuals may have relative to their project contributions. Each SCODF

Table 8.5.   Types of EHR and health IT teams

Type of Team	Purpose
Steering committee	Provides oversight and represents broadest number of stakeholders in the EHR or other health IT initiative.
Vendor selection team	Responsible for developing functional specifications and the request for proposal to narrow field of vendor candidates with which to perform due diligence and make recommendations. May be a subset of the steering committee or a separate team.
Negotiation team	A special team that negotiates the contract. May be composed of a mix of selected members of the steering committee, vendor selection team, other individuals with experience in large or specialized procurements, consultants, and legal counsel.
Implementation team(s)	Responsible for the implementation of the EHR or other type of health IT. Large projects may require domain teams (see below).
Domain teams	Provide special expertise and represent direct users in various aspects of implementation. For example, there may be separate nursing and medical domains to build clinical decision support rules for an EHR. For connecting with a health information exchange organization, domain teams may include those who specialize in workflow and process improvement, privacy and security controls, and data/information governance. For a data warehouse integrating clinical and financial information to support data analytics for health reform, domain teams may include those from information systems, patient accounting, revenue cycle management, and care coordination.
Training team and/or super users	Responsible for learning the system well and supports users throughout rollout. May exist prior to or separate from domain teams.
Ongoing maintenance team and/or clinical advisory team	Ensures clinical, financial, and/or new business aspects of the EHR or other health IT are kept current and ongoing users' concerns are addressed.

Figure 8.4.   Myers-Briggs Type Indicator questions

Guiding Question	Types	
Where do you direct your energy?	Outer world (Extroversion)	Inner world (Introversion)
How do you process information?	Through known facts (Sensing)	Through possibilities (iNtuition)
How do you make decisions?	On the basis of logic (Thinking)	On the basis of personal values (Feeling)
How do you organize your life?	In a way that is structured (Judgment)	In a way that is flexible (Perception)

type has both positive and negative characteristics, and each person usually displays one predominant trait:

- **S**tarters are individuals who are anxious to get started, even when planning may not yet have been finalized. Their strength, however, is to push and not let projects languish.

- **C**reators are those who are constantly generating ideas throughout the project, but they may never succeed at carrying them out. Their strength is to ensure that new ideas do not get lost and to instill innovation in a project.

- **O**verseers are those who promote decision making and delegate well, but they may be seen as manipulative. Overseers can be natural leaders if they learn to be discerning and diplomatic.

- **D**oers are those who can turn good ideas into reality. They are not innovators, but they are cooperative and get their assigned jobs done.

- **F**inishers are conscientious and deliver on time, but they may be too painstaking and anxious to complete the project, potentially putting it at risk for not ensuring that all control points have been tested or new ideas considered.

Teams may also occasionally need and want advisers, who are knowledgeable about a specialty area but do not know or care about the big picture. Regardless of the professional backgrounds of the team members, it is a good idea to have as broad a mix of personality types as possible on a team.

Understanding Group Norms, Managing Group Dynamics, and Valuing Diversity

Understanding personalities may not only ensure that a balanced group is involved but also can help individual members relate to each other, manage conflict, and negotiate to achieve consensus. Another important aspect of team building is valuing diversity and making it work for the team instead of dividing it.

Understanding how formal teams work and facilitating this work is an important task for the project manager. In a classic work, Tuckman (1965) describes five stages of group development (table 8.6) that the project manager may find useful to understand and address as the steering committee forms and starts its work. A common challenge in an EHR or health IT steering committee is that, although healthcare delivery requires teamwork, the healthcare team is quite different from a project team. The healthcare team has a specific leader (the physician) who directs other specialists (nurses, therapists, technicians, and so on). Everyone understands the structure of the healthcare team and his or her position in it. The healthcare team does not undergo the stages of team building. In some respects, the fact that healthcare is so dependent on a specific type of teamwork may make creating effective EHR or health IT project teams more difficult. Physicians, who are always in the position to direct, may find themselves in other roles on project teams, and those who typically take direction may be called on to direct. Any tools the project manager can use to convey the nature of

Table 8.6.   Five stages of group development

Stage	Description	Aids to Move to Next Stage
Forming	Stage where personal relations are characterized by dependence on other group members for guidance and direction. Group members desire acceptance by the group and so attempt to keep things simple and avoid controversy.	Formal orientation processes, potentially including "fun" break-the-ice exercises or formal member characterization activities, such as Myers-Briggs personality assessments. Each team member must relinquish the comfort of nonthreatening topics and risk the possibility of conflict.
Storming	Stage characterized by competition and conflict in personal relations. Because of fear of exposure or failure, team members seek structural clarification and commitment. Typically some members will become completely silent and others will attempt to dominate.	Group members need to move from a "testing and proving" mentality to a problem-solving mentality. Listening and conflict management techniques are essential. To manage the natural conflict, the project manager needs to be firm about setting goals, communicate frequently, encourage team members to be open and honest about concerns and differences, let team members create something, and emphasize the importance of following project management techniques.
Norming	Stage where group members demonstrate cohesion and are engaged in active acknowledgment of all members' contributions. This is when team members experience trust and the sense of group belonging and even relief as a result of resolving interpersonal conflicts. Data will flow freely and creativity is high.	The major drawback of the norming stage is that members may begin to fear the inevitable future breakup of the group and may resist change as a result. No one will own up to this concern, but the project manager should suspect this is occurring when the group cannot settle down and make decisions. Change management techniques must be employed to get the group to the next stage.
Performing	Stage where the team genuinely solves problems leading toward optimal solutions. In this stage, members can work independently, in subgroups, or as a total group with equal facility. Individual members are self-assured and no longer need group approval but respect other members' contributions.	This is the ultimate goal of team building. Unfortunately, experts report that many groups do not achieve this stage. The project manager must be skilled in advancing the group through the earlier stages as quickly as possible, while recognizing that each stage is unavoidable and must be managed to get to the next stage. Once in the performing stage, however, the project manager must also prepare the team to adjourn.
Adjourning	Stage that terminates the task and members disengage from the group's relationships. Sometimes this creates apprehension and may be regressive.	The most effective interventions in this stage are celebration and recognition. Individual members can also be recruited for ongoing monitoring activities, trainers for new staff, and subsequent projects. However, promises for such activities should only be used when they advance the disengagement process and are real.

Source: Adapted from Tuckman 1965 (384–399) and Tuckman and Jensen 1977 (419–427).

a project team, how individuals can be valuable and equal members of project teams, and what to expect on a project team can help work the team through the team-building stages.

Some organizations or members of teams find it uncomfortable or believe it unnecessary to participate in team-building activities, especially where participants may be required to adhere to a special methodology or engage in game playing or another unfamiliar activity. Instead of avoiding the activities and missing their value, however, team leaders should find ways to overcome participants' concerns. Team members who are uncomfortable with such activities may find it even more difficult to change processes and adopt new technology.

Figure 8.5.   The seven sins of deadly meetings and their salvation

Sins	Salvation
1. People don't take meetings seriously. They arrive late, leave early, and spend most of their time doodling.	1. Adopt the mindset that meetings are real work; have an agenda, know your role, and follow the rules for minutes.
2. Meetings are too long. They should accomplish twice as much in half the time.	2. Track the cost of your meetings; use technology for providing feedback.
3. People wander off the topic. Participants spend more time digressing than discussing.	3. Get serious about agendas and store distractions in a "parking lot."
4. Nothing happens once the meeting ends. People don't convert decisions into actions.	4. Convert from "meeting" to "doing" and focus on creating a document.
5. People don't tell the truth. There's plenty of conversation, but not much candor.	5. Consider anonymity through technology—but avoid gamesmanship through facilitation.
6. Meetings are always missing important information, so critical decisions are put off.	6. Get data, not just furniture, into meeting rooms (maybe remove the furniture).
7. Meetings never get better. People make the same mistakes.	7. Monitor meetings and apply quality improvement techniques.

Source: Matson 1996.

Meeting Facilitation

With teams generally comes the requirement for meetings. In many organizations, meetings are both the most universal part of work life and the most despised part of work life. So many meetings are unproductive that the mere thought of another one may deter a valuable member from participating in the EHR or health IT project. Despite new collaboration software that allows teams to communicate without meetings or hold virtual meetings, face-to-face meetings continue to be the primary form of achieving project work. In 1996, Eric Matson wrote a treatise on meetings he called "The seven sins of deadly meetings." Figure 8.5 provides a summary of these and some salvations that project managers may want to deploy.

Check Your Understanding 8.2

Chose the best answer:

1.   Most EHR and health IT project managers are:

   a. Clinicians

   b. Entrepreneurial

   c. Procrastinators

   d. Resistant to change

2.   A project manager's communications extend to:

   a. End users

   b. Executive management

   c. External public

   d. Local vendors

3. In conflict management, the best way to achieve a winning result for everyone is to:

   a. Accommodate

   b. Avoid

   c. Compromise

   d. Collaborate

4. When a project manager needs to address willful inaction by a project worker, what is needed?

   a. Coaching

   b. Counseling

   c. Facilitating

   d. Negotiating

5. When a group gets together to perform work on a project, a competitive situation is often experienced during which of the stages of group development?

   a. Forming

   b. Storming

   c. Norming

   d. Performing

6. A good way to facilitate a meeting when the participants wander off topic is to:

   a. Ask the sergeant at arms to remove the offending participants

   b. Call the worst offender to task by making him or her facilitate the meeting

   c. Put the topic of discussion in a parking lot

   d. Stop holding in-person meetings

EHR Project Management Techniques and Tools

Whether a professional project manager is used or an individual who is well organized and well respected in the organization assumes this role, formal project management techniques are essential for ensuring that EHR and other health IT projects engage all relevant parties and stay on time and on budget.

Project Management Standards

By now it should be clear that project management is the application of knowledge, skills, tools, and techniques to project activities to meet project requirements. This work can be done informally, but formal project management is often required when a project competes with other projects or day-to-day activities for scope, time, cost, risk, and quality. Formal project management also helps bring convergence among stakeholders with different needs and expectations. As previously alluded to, the field of project management has a formal body of knowledge, the PMBOK Guide, developed by the PMI that is approved as an ANSI standard (ANSI/PMI 96-001-2013). PMI has a worldwide membership of more than 100,000. It oversees development and maintenance of the standard, develops the PMBOK Guide, and offers certifications in project management. Table 8.7 lists the project management knowledge areas and excerpts of key tasks from the PMBOK Guide (PMI 2013).

Project Phases and Life Cycle

By their nature, projects are differentiated from day-to-day work activities because the former are unique undertakings, generally with a specific start and finish. The start-and-finish aspects of a project are qualified by the word *generally* because, as has been discussed, some projects do not have firm finish dates. As has also been previously covered, projects with no clear end point are risky because it is hard to determine whether goals have been met, if users are satisfied, or even if the system is being used. It may be necessary to break up the EHR or other health IT project into phases with key milestones that signify the end of each phase. Not only is it difficult to sustain a project for too long a period of time, but, at some point, the project must be folded into the day-to-day activities and enter a maintenance mode—a phase that includes the ongoing monitoring and evaluation of results with course correction as necessary. The course correction itself may entail an entirely new project.

In addition to defining the project's boundaries and potential phases that can be treated as separate projects, each project has process groups within it that need to be recognized. The PMBOK Guide (PMI 2013) describes a project as having five major process groups: initiating, planning, executing, monitoring and controlling, and closing. Figure 8.6 illustrates that these process groups often overlap, with monitoring and controlling processes crossing the entire project.

Table 8.7. Project management knowledge areas

Knowledge Areas	Summary of Key Tasks
Project integration management	Project planning Change control
Project scope management	Project authorizaton Scope planning
Project time management	Activity definition, sequencing, and duration estimating Schedule development and control
Project cost management	Resource planning Project cost estimating, budgeting, and control
Project quality management	Evaluating overall project performance and monitoring specific project results
Project human resource management	Organizational planning Staff acquisition and team development
Project communication management	Communications planning and distribution channels Project performance reporting Administrative closure on key phases or project completion
Project risk management	Managing adverse events that may stall or derail project
Project procurement management	Planning solicitations Source selection Contract management
Project stakehodler management	Identifying stakeholders Planning stakeholder management Managing stakeholder engagement Controlling stakeholder engagement

Source: Adapted from PMI 2013.

Figure 8.6.　Phases of a project's life cycle

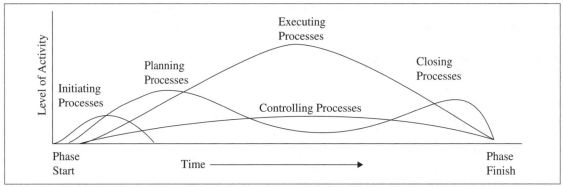

Initiating Processes

As described in the PMBOK Guide (PMI 2013), the initiating process involves project formulation, feasibility studies, strategic design, and approval to proceed to planning and acquisition. Many healthcare organizations consider this initiating process to be part of their overall strategic planning. If so, individuals participating in the initiating processes for the specific EHR or other health IT project should review the strategic plan, the EHR and health IT migration path, and any feasibility studies that provide background on organizational readiness, ROI expectations, and technical assessments of various parts of the health IT infrastructure.

For most EHR and health IT projects, the primary purpose of this phase should be to ensure an understanding of the **project scope**, which is the embodiment of the work that needs to be accomplished so that the specified features and functions are in place. Defining the scope of an EHR or health IT project may not be easy because of the many components that often comprise such systems. Because, ultimately, the full scope of the EHR and other health IT will likely be implemented, defining the scope for any one subproject may seem artificial. However, defining scope for each milestone within the full scope of the project, or formally limiting the scope of each project in a series of projects can be beneficial psychologically.

Scope creep is a term often used to describe the situation where a project's features and functions have expanded beyond the originally defined scope. The result is almost always delays and cost overruns, which will make executive management, who must approve additional expenditures, unhappy. Scope creep can result in dissatisfaction with the way the project is being managed, which in turn can translate into dissatisfaction with the project as a whole. An initiating project scope definition and the realization that project add-ons must be considered separate projects help project managers manage scope creep (Stachowiak 2014).

Planning Processes

The project planning process focuses on specifics. In fact, because many healthcare organizations jump right into specifics and do not conduct a formal initiation phase, they often are less prepared for the ultimate cost and level of change required for an EHR and some other health IT initiatives.

Upon approval for a project to proceed, a specific, highly detailed project plan is developed. This includes identification of phases, milestones, human resources, and expenditures (see section later in this chapter on project management tools).

Executing Processes

The executing (or conducting) phase of a project includes the carrying out of the project plan. For an EHR or other health IT *selection* project, the typical steps include assessment and definition of functional requirements, obtaining information about the universe of vendors that offer products to meet these requirements and narrowing the field, distribution of a request for proposal, vendor selection, due diligence, and contract negotiation (see chapter 7). For an EHR or health IT *implementation* project, the typical steps include taking delivery of and installing the hardware and software, system configuration, revising workflows, testing, training, and supporting end users during go-live (see chapter 9). In projects relating to *optimization* of EHR or other health IT, the steps often start with establishing a formal outcomes monitoring program if that was not performed as part of the implementation project. A benefits realization study should result in identification of areas for improvement. Once these are identified, the root cause(s) of issues are identified and solutions found. Solutions may be workflow and process improvements; systems reconfiguration, enhancements, or addition components (which would require a new vendor selection and/or implementation process); retraining, reinforcement, coaching, or counseling; or even adjustment of goals that were too aggressive or not aggressive enough. Chapters 3, 4, and 5 are focused on why and how to understand the need for optimization, and chapters 14 through 20 address specifics in different healthcare settings.

Closing Processes

The closing phase of any project should include implementation of benefits realization studies using the metrics defined earlier. This phase supplies the feedback mechanism to correct course, fine tune, or prepare for the next major phase in the migration path for the EHR or other type of health IT. Closing processes also should ensure that team members are given appropriate recognition and return to their day-to-day activities. Finally, this phase ensures operational and production support for ongoing use of the EHR or other type of health IT.

Monitoring and Controlling Processes

Monitoring and controlling processes run through the entire scope of a project. They are often considered to be the project management functions of communication, team management, procurement, time management, risk management, integration, and configuration management. These functions are very similar to the functions performed by any operations manager: The project manager must communicate project assignments, project status, and issues. Team members must be managed with respect to completing tasks, by applauding their efforts or correcting course where necessary. Project managers may be involved in procurement of technology. They will certainly be involved in keeping the project on track for timely completion. Project managers must also recognize potential risk areas and address these before they occur. For example, if interface development is consistently delayed by a vendor, the risk that the entire system go-live timeline will be delayed must be recognized. It may be necessary to escalate the delay issue to higher levels in the vendor's organization or even find another vendor to perform the work. Breaking down the information silos so that people work together to ensure that data can be well integrated is a critical function of the project manager. Finally, as the EHR or other type of health IT is configured to meet the organization's unique requirements during an implementation or optimization project, the changes made must be thoroughly documented. This step is called *configuration management* (or *change control*).

Project Management Tools

In addition to the knowledge and skills that give a project manager unique techniques for managing complex projects, several tools are available to aid the project manager in project planning. The project plan is the project's manager's roadmap. A good outline of the elements of a project plan adapted from Hughes (2000) and Egeland (2011) is listed in table 8.8.

Project Charter, Scope, Deliverables, and Approach

The EHR or health IT migration path provides a good way to appreciate the scope of a project, although a project charter provides further detail about the exact boundaries and agreements that surround any given EHR or other health IT project. *Deliverables* are specific milestones in

Table 8.8.   Components of a Project Plan

- Project charter, scope, and deliverables
- Description of project approach
- Work breakdown structure
- Budget management
- Capacity plan
- Start dates
- Major milestones and target end dates
- Dependencies
- Risks, constraints, assumptions, and contingencies
- Controls
- Performance measurement baselines
- Supporting detail

implementation, adoption by users, or achievement of goals. A project manager should understand what the deliverables are because they define the scope of the project.

An organization's culture and the vendor's culture both determine the project approach. Evaluating the vendor's standard implementation plan should have been a part of the vendor selection process to ensure that the two organizations' cultures do not clash over the implementation. (See chapter 7.) It is not unusual for a vendor to want to come into an organization, take over the project management, implement the project, and quickly move on to the next project. If the healthcare organization prefers a more staged approach or more active involvement by its own project manager and project team or has other ideas, these differences need to be reconciled before a contract is signed and may be one element that prevents the acquisition of a specific product.

Another element of project approach relates to how a project is actually initiated. Initiation may include conducting a project kickoff meeting or series of meetings with key stakeholders in the project (executive management, steering committee, domain team leaders, champions, others). Such an activity sets the tone for project communications (VanBruaene 2011).

Work Breakdown Structure

The **work breakdown structure** refers to the specific tasks within the project and how they are divided into various phases of the project, as illustrated in figure 8.7. A *task* is work to be performed.

Figure 8.7.   Portion of a project work breakdown structure

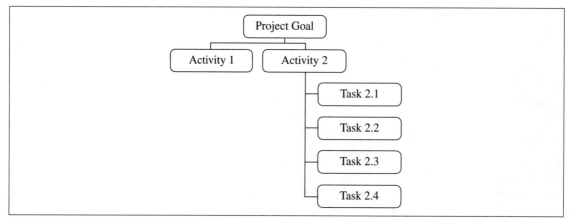

An *activity* is a collection of related tasks. Highly complex projects, such as EHR implementations, may have several major project goals, often called *milestones* in project planning. Where a task consumes time, or has duration, a milestone is an event or goal that a task has achieved. Frequently, project planning software is used to document the work breakdown structure. Figure 8.8 illustrates the use of Microsoft Project for this purpose. Project management software not only helps illustrates tasks but can help manage a budget, keep projects on time, identify dependencies between tasks, measure performance, manage risk, and track open issues (Rouse 2015).

Budget Management

Some healthcare organizations want to assign cost to each task or activity to manage the project's budget. Although this approach certainly provides information about the total cost of ownership, many of the human resources used to accomplish the tasks involved in the project have already had their time allocated to their primary work functions. The value of the human resource time spent on a project may be of interest to a healthcare organization, but it is not commonly tracked. However, vendors will track the time vendor resources are spent on each task because implementation time may be billed on an hourly basis. Additionally, there may be contractual limits to the amount of overall time a vendor spends to accomplish the project or specific activities and tasks for which the vendor will charge. Healthcare organizations should understand their contracts and track their usage of the vendor's human resources accordingly.

In general, a healthcare organization is more concerned about an overall budget and managing to the budget instead of managing cost estimates on a project plan.

Capacity Plan, Start Dates, Major Milestones and Target End Dates

Keeping a project on time requires a capacity plan in which staff resources are identified and assigned. Establishing start and target end dates for each task helps level resources so they will

Figure 8.8.   Project plan Gantt chart

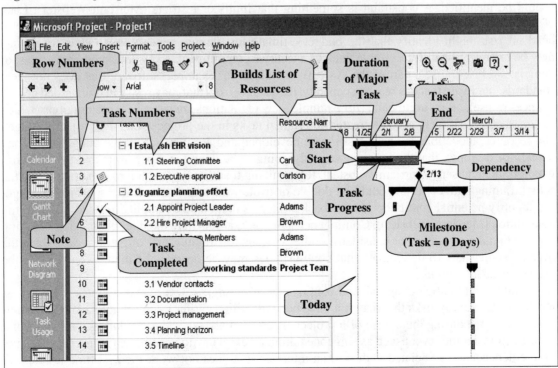

be available when needed. Start and target end dates are important not only because each initial task should be scheduled but also because the start dates of subsequent tasks may be dependent on completion of previous ones. Most healthcare organizations do not fully realize the enormity of the EHR and other health IT implementation tasks, but delays carry the risk of substantial consequences for patient care or the bottom line, such as not earning meaningful use incentives along the stages defined by the federal government, or becoming subject to downward reimbursement adjustments. Delays also generally add cost because consultants or contractors have to be retained for a longer period of time, and cost savings are delayed.

Identify Dependencies

As previously defined, a dependency exists where one task relies on another in order to be completed on time, on budget, or both. It is critical to identify dependencies between tasks for several reasons. First, identifying dependencies helps keep a project on time. When plotting tasks and their start dates on a project plan, the tasks that have dependencies are often the most critical to accomplish to keep the project on time. A project's **critical path** is the sequence of the tasks in which there is no slack. In other words, if one task in the critical path cannot start on time because another has not been completed, there is no slack and the project will be delayed. If a task can be performed at any time, or if there is some range of time within which it can be completed, there is some slack in the schedule. A second reason to identify dependencies is to establish controls. Several types of controls should be built into a project plan. These include work authorizations, change controls, and testing.

Risks, Constraints, Assumptions, and Contingencies

Project risk is an uncertain event or condition that, if it occurs, has an effect on at least one project goal (PMI 2013). All projects have risk, and, as Mar has suggested, a risk-free project achieves nothing; it is not possible to build great businesses "by hiding under a rock" (2015). Risk management, then, is about identifying risks early on and planning how to manage them.

In managing a project plan, the project manager should identify as many potential risks as possible up front. To the extent possible, the constraints, assumptions, and contingencies of each risk should be identified. A constraint is something that limits or restricts (Merriam-Webster). Lack of funding is a common constraint. During the initiating phase, a project manager who looks to head off risk might identify that the budget estimate for training appears low. Other constraints may be organizational (for example, lack of executive commitment, a key staff member resigns, or clinicians refuse to use a part of the system), technical (for example, software that does not meet standards, hardware that has reached capacity, or system errors that may result in unintended consequences of use), or environmental (for example, new regulations are issued). If assumptions (which are the factors that were used to create the original tasks in the project plan, the project's budget, and resource allocations for each task) were developed and are included in the budget, they may reveal, for example, that the training was only going to be done for super users and they, in turn, would train end users (Merriam-Webster). Recognizing that this assumption may be faulty and the actual training budget needed could be double or triple what was is planned, the project manager can identify potential contingencies (fallback strategies that could be applied instead of the initial assumption [Merriam-Webster]). Contingencies in this example may include seeking authorization for additional expenditure or considering other options for training that might at least reduce the overrun somewhat. To determine what contingencies may be needed, "if-then" scenarios can be used to evaluate options.

In addition to anticipating risk and contingency planning, project managers must track issues, which are essentially risks that may not have been identified earlier or could not have been anticipated, that arise during the course of a project. There will always be issues during the course of a project, from a minor event such as someone taking an extra day to accomplish a task that does not have a dependency associated with it to an interface that does not work the first time it is tested. Issues may be related to many different factors. Most project managers keep an **issues log** for this purpose. When the project manager is satisfied the issue has been resolved, it can be recorded into the log. Open issues, however, need to be tracked and their completion managed.

Controls

One important reason for managing project risk is to institute controls so that the risks can be mitigated. Controls may be alternatives that are equivalent or better to the original, or they may be contingency plans. To the extent possible, controls should be proactive. If a project milestone is at risk for being late, the project manager should identify this issue as early as possible and take specific steps to avoid delays. All of the project manager's skills surrounding communications, team building, and other aspects of project management come into play to help avoid risks from materializing.

Beyond control of the project plan, **change control** refers to the requirement for determining what changes can be made and by whom, when, and for what reason. It is a formal process of tracking every request for change in a system, determining the impact of the potential change on other elements of the project or the system itself, obtaining the necessary authorization for the change to be made, keeping track of the change in the event that a future action is dependent on understanding what has been changed, and then carrying out the change with the necessary resources. During project implementation, changes can result in scope creep, where suddenly the project has taken on new directions, added features or functions, or expanded to areas of the organization not included in the original plan. Although not all changes in an EHR or other health IT project result in scope creep, any change to the system can have a profound effect on another part of the system and must be documented and maintained. A change to a single data element may impact a clinical decision support process; in this scenario, it will be necessary to remember that a change occurred and its impact on any future system release can be determined.

Change generally involves additional resources. A change request can come about during a project or after the project has been completed—sometimes, there are so many requests for change that they all cannot be accomplished at once. To address change requests, most organizations implement a formal change control process for all IT and often for other projects and programs as well. Using this process, the project management team evaluates each request, determines whether the request is feasible and appropriate, and then assigns priority to potential change. Because change in general is such an enormous part of implementing or optimizing an EHR or other type of health IT, change management is addressed as a separate topic in chapter 6.

Performance Measurement Baselines

In many cases, implementation of controls depends on understanding a baseline and desired performance measures. For example, if an organization plans to have all its end users trained on computer navigation prior to training them on the EHR system, it can be helpful to have a baseline measurement of how many people have such skills, what skills others need, and when training has been accomplished. It can also be helpful to identify various milestones for the training, such as 50 percent of staff will be trained by a certain date; by another date, 75 percent will be trained; and so on.

Most project planning software includes tools to document actual end dates and actual expenditures for each task that rolls up to a milestone, or project goal. Performance measurement baselines, such as the target end date or budget, should be described with specific metrics that can be measured (see chapter 4).

Supporting Detail

In some projects, a spreadsheet can be used for simple tracking purposes. However, as previously mentioned, a project manager frequently uses more sophisticated project planning software to manage the myriad tasks and other project elements. The basic component of any such software is a Gantt chart (illustrated in figure 8.8). A **Gantt chart** is a type of graphic used to illustrate project tasks, phases, and milestones and their start, targeted end, and actual completion dates. It helps illustrate where more than one task must be performed simultaneously.

Figure 8.9.   Dashboard example

Department of Veterans Affairs OIT PMAS Dashboard
Active Projects Report

Project Name	Sponsor	Overall	Rqmts	Sched CURR	Sched PREV	Cost CURR	Cost PREV	Total Cost	Acq Plan	Prime Contractor
National Teleradiology Program	VHA	G	G	G	G	G	G	G	G	dNovus
National Utilization Management Integration (NUM)	VHA	G	G	G	NA	NA	NA	NA	G	ProSol
Nationwide Health Information Network Adapter Gateway	VHA	G	G	G	G	G	G	G	G	SPAWAR
Nationwide Health Information Network Direct	VHA	Y	G	G	NA	G	NA	G	Y	CACI
Network Based Call Routing	VBA	G	G	G	G	NA	G	NA	G	Verizon
North Chicago VA and USN Navy Great Lakes Hospital Merger	VHA	G	G	G	G	NA	NA	NA	NA	–In House–
Oncology Tumor Registry (ONC)	VHA	G	G	G	G	G	G	G	G	Patriot Tech—Harris Corp
Personal Identity Verification	OSP	G	O	G	G	G	G	G	G	HP
Pharmacy Legacy Enhancements—DME	VHA	G	G	G	G	NA	G	R	G	HP
Pharmacy Re-Engineering (PRE) 0–5	VHA	G	G	G	G	G	G	G	G	HP

Project planning software such as Microsoft Project can also show dependencies among tasks (where completion of one task depends on the start, specific progress, or finish of another) as well as actual completion dates for each task, which can help the project manager estimate whether the entire project will be completed on time. Project planning software can be coupled with document sharing and collaboration software, such as Microsoft's SharePoint, which permits the exchange of project information with team members and others so various task alerts and files can be shared.

Some project managers may find it helpful to use balanced scorecards, key performance indicators, and dashboards in addition to project management software. A **balanced scorecard** is a system that measures and manages defined metrics derived from institutional sources and aligns the metrics with the strategic goals of the organization (Balanced Scorecard Institute 2010). **Key performance indicators (KPIs)** are quantifiable measurements, previously agreed on, that reflect the organization's critical success factors (Parmenter 2010). A **dashboard** is a tool that collects data from multiple sources to unify a variety of metrics into a single view (Borden et al. 2008). An example of part of the stoplight, color-coded dashboard that the US Department of Veterans Affairs Office of Information Technology (VA OIT 2011) uses to track the status of their many projects is illustrated in figure 8.9.

As the project manager works through issues, supporting detail should be documented. This documentation might be in the form of an email or a formal report saved in a file associated with the plan. Communication with the vendor also should be maintained. If the vendor indicates it can start later with no impact on cost or overall project completion but later claims the loss of time was to blame for additional costs, the project manager will need to have supporting documentation to challenge the billing. Most documentation deals with issues, meeting agendas and minutes, invoices, testing results, training scores, progress reports to executives, and so on. It may be appropriate, however, to keep track of other communications, such as newsletter announcements and even celebrations.

Check Your Understanding 8.3

1. Match the project life cycle phase with the task:

   Initiating

   Planning

   Executing

   Closing

   Monitoring and controlling

   1. Carrying out a project plan
   2. Benefits realization
   3. Project management
   4. Understanding project scope
   5. Development of project plan

2. Match the terms used in a work breakdown structure to their description:

   Activity

   Dependency

Goal

Milestone

Task

1. Status of achievement, with zero days' duration.

2. Step to be performed in a project

3. Same as a milestone

4. A group of tasks

5. A constraint upon when a task may start

3. Provide a brief description of each of the following project risk management terms:

Risk

Constraint

Assumptions

Contingencies

References and Resources

American Health Information Management Association (AHIMA). 2010 (August). eHIM practice transformation (updated). *Journal of AHIMA.* 81(8):52–55.

Balanced Scorecard Institute. 2010. Balanced scorecard basics. http://www.balancedscorecard.org.

Barry, T.R. 2010. Top 10 qualities of a project manager. Project Smart. http://ProjectSmart.co.uk.

Bennatan, E.M. 2009 (June). *Software Project Management: The Magic Suit of Clothes.* Advanced Project Solutions.

Borden, M.P., M. Murray, and A. Yorkos. 2008. Developing a dashboard to aid in effective project management. SAS Global Forum, paper 052-2008. http://www2.sas.com/proceedings/forum2008/052-2008.pdf.

Chebium, R. 2015 (January 7). How to create an effective cross-cultural training program. *HR Magazine: Society for Human Resource Management.* (6)1. https://www.shrm.org/hr-today/news/hr-magazine/pages/010215-cross-cultural-training.aspx.

Dearborn, J. 2014 (July 9). Does trust in the workplace matter? *Forbes Brand Voice.* http://www.forbes.com/sites/sap/2014/07/09/does-trust-in-the-workplace-matter.

Doll, B.A. 2005. Project management 101. *Journal of AHIMA.* 76(1):50.

Dontigney, E. n.d. 5 conflict management strategies. *Houston Chronicle.* http://smallbusiness.chron.com/5-conflict-management-strategies-16131.html.

Egeland, B. 2011 (February 28). Components of the project plan. Project Management Tips. http://pmtips.net/Blog/components-project-plan.

Faucheux, M. 2013 (June 27). What is resource leveling? Juggling your resources. Bright Hub Project Management. http://www.brighthubpm.com/resource-management/14644-what-is-resource-leveling.

Hospitals and Health Networks (HHN). 2013. Generations in the workplace. http://www.hhnmag.com/articles/5919-generations-in-the-workplace.

Hughes, G. 2000. The value of project management expertise. *Journal of AHIMA.* 71(10):72–73.

Mar, A. 2015 (November 29). 130 project risks (list). Simplicable. http://management.simplicable.com/management/new/130-project-risks.

Marx, E. 2010 (June 23). The secret to successful CPOE adoption—revealed. HisTalk CIO Unplugged blog. http://histalk2.com/2010/06/23/cio-unplugged-62310.

Matson, E. 1996. The seven sins of deadly meetings. *Fast Company*. http://www.fastcompany.com/26726/seven-sins-deadly-meetings.

McKinney, P. 2015 (January 14). What is conflict management? Definition, styles, and strategies. Study.com: Introduction to Management. http://study.com/academy/lesson/what-is-conflict-management-definition-styles-strategies.html.

Merriam-Webster. N.d. Assumptions. http://www.merriam-webster.com/dictionary/assumptions.

Merriam-Webster. N.d. Constraint. http://www.merriam-webster.com/dictionary/constraint.

Merriam-Webster. N.d. Contingencies. http://www.merriam-webster.com/dictionary/contingencies.

Parmenter, D. 2010. *Key Performance Indicators*, 2nd ed. Hoboken, NJ: John Wiley & Sons.

Project Management Institute (PMI). 2013. *A Guide to the Project Management Body of Knowledge (PMBOK Guide)*. Newton Square, PA: PMI.

Project Management Institute (PMI). n.d. Certifications. www.pmi.org/Certification.aspx.

Rouse, M. 2015 (April). Microsoft Office Project. TechTarget Software Applications Glossary. http://whatis.techtarget.com/definition/Microsoft-Project-Microsoft-Office-Project.

Schwalbe, K. 2013. *An Introduction to Healthcare Project Management*. Minneapolis, MN: Schwalbe Publishing.

Shaywitz, D. 2015 (March 24). Data silos: Healthcare's silent shame. *Forbes*. http://www.forbes.com/sites/davidshaywitz/2015/03/24/data-silos-healthcares-silent-tragedy.

Southern Nazarene University (SNU). 2015 (January 21). Conflict management strategies and styles. https://home.snu.edu/~hculbert/conflict.htm.

Stachowiak, S. 2014 (March 19). Scope creep—the two dirtiest words in project management. Team Gantt. https://www.teamgantt.com/blog/scope-creep-the-two-dirtiest-words-in-project-management.

Stack, L. 2013 (November 5). 7 tips for motivating your team (even when the going gets tough). *Talent Management and HR*. http://www.eremedia.com/tlnt/7-tips-for-motivating-your-team-even-when-the-going-gets-tough.

Tuckman, B. 1965. Developmental sequence in small groups. *Psychological Bulletin*. 63:384–399.

US Department of Veterans Affairs Office of Information Technology (VA OIT). 2011. Department of Veterans Affairs OIT PMAS dashboard: Active project report. http://www.oit.va.gov/docs/dashboard/201101_OIT_PMAS_Dashboard_Active_Jan_2011.pdf.

VanBruaene, M. 2011 (September 21). Key elements for successful project planning and implementation (blog post). http://www.advancingyourorganization.com/?p=915.

Young, V. 2015 (October 6). 3 ways a culture of trust drives productivity. Reinventing HR: A Blog by Reflecktive. http://blog.reflektive.com/3-ways-a-culture-of-trust-drives-productivity.

Chapter 9
Health IT System Implementation and Ongoing Maintenance

Key Terms

Abstracting

Acceptance testing

Adoption

Auditing

Big-bang approach

Celebration

Change control

Chart conversion

Configuration management

Conversion strategy

Critical path

Customer service

Data conversion

Dependencies

Favorites list

Go-live

Go-live rehearsal

Issues management

Milestone completion

Optimization

Patient satisfaction survey

Phasing strategy

Pilot testing

Preload

Resource leveling

Risk management

Roll-out strategy

System build

System configuration

System documentation

Turnover strategy

User satisfaction survey

Walk-through

Learning Objectives

- Identify and reinforce the need for implementation planning and management, including risk management.

- Describe infrastructure preparedness for hardware installation, workflow and process improvement, and stakeholder readiness.

- Describe the need for system build or configuration and the importance of system configuration management, including its ongoing documentation.

- Describe the need for testing and a test environment, and define testing stages.

- Plan training and support strategies.

- Explain data conversion, chart conversion, and other activities prior to go-live.

- Describe ongoing strategies for successful adoption and optimization of health IT.

The implementation process for an electronic health record (EHR) or other type of health information technology (health IT) begins after the contract with the vendor is signed. While implementing some types of health IT is not as enormous a task as implementing an EHR, all implementations require careful planning and execution. However, if the steps outlined in the previous chapters have been carried out as part of planning for the EHR or other health IT, much of the implementation process should be to carry out the plans—while still expecting the unexpected. In the migration path model and the systems development life cycle (SDLC), neither planning nor implementation is ever finished. However, implementation of one or more of the components of the migration path can be a defined project and should be treated as a milestone to reach and celebrate.

Implementation Planning and Management

As described in chapters 3 and 4, strategic planning for an EHR and other health IT includes alignment of organizational goals with when and how the EHR and other health IT initiatives are carried out. Strategic planning establishes the framework for ensuring that workflow and process improvement (chapter 5) and change management (chapter 6) are precursors to any health IT implementation. Finally, specific implementation planning and management (chapter 8)—whether a vendor is hired to provide a significant level of implementation support or not—is essential to successful implementation.

The importance of thorough planning for the EHR implementation cannot be emphasized enough. The College of Healthcare Information Management Executives (CHIME) describes the need for not only executive support but also executive champions to lead the charge to EHR "or it becomes 'just an IT project'" (CHIME 2010). Experts today urge hospitals to take their time and plan a project as thoroughly and carefully as if a loved one were a patient on the go-live date." They also suggest that no amount of disruption that risks lives offsets the cash flow of any incentive program or return on investment goals (Ames et al. 2011). "EHR implementation [has been described as] a journey, not a destination" (Vaughan 2009). Yet, while the journey is one reflecting the SDLC, that does not mean milestones and their goals along the journey should not be met. (For more information on SDLC, see chapter 2.)

Stakeholder Engagement

To effectively implement EHR and other health IT, the organization must establish an appropriate organizational structure for the implementation, and key stakeholders must participate in workflow and process improvement, change management, and system configuration. Some organizations dissolve their EHR or other health IT vendor selection committee after vendor selection has occurred and create a new implementation committee and/or domain teams to assist dedicated staff and/or vendor/consultant staff with the implementation functions (see chapter 8). The scope of the EHR or other type of health IT project and the nature of the organization determine the approach, although most organizations find that input from stakeholders/users is essential for implementation. Stakeholders include physicians, nurses, and other clinicians whose patient care work will involve the technology, as well as health information management (HIM) professionals who are involved in clinical documentation improvement and quality measurement, reporting, and improvement (Computer Science Corp. 2009). Virtually every list of "best practices for EHR implementation" identifies the need to create a strong project governance structure, establish a program office for the EHR that focuses on clinical workflow, and engage physicians early and often (DerGurahian 2011).

Engaging physicians in the implementation process is not easy, but it is important. Physicians are vital to the process because they are the drivers of clinical care delivery. Physicians' diagnoses, orders, notes, and conclusions direct what others do, and clinical quality measurement and improvement depend on physician documentation and engagement.

Implementation Approach

Early in the implementation planning, if not in the strategic planning for health IT in general, it is necessary to determine the roll-out and turnover strategies for how the new technology will be used throughout the entire organization, as well as strategies for (paper) chart conversion and data conversion.

Roll-Out Strategy

Roll-out strategy describes whether an organization will phase in the components of the EHR or other health technology or follow a "big bang" approach where the whole system is implemented at once or in a short period of time. Because an EHR implementation typically is a huge undertaking, most organizations implement an EHR using a phased roll-out strategy. (See table 9.1.) However, the phasing may vary, and may be constructed in a multilevel, matrix-like approach.

Due to the complex nature of an EHR with its many clinical components, its connections to source systems, and the staged requirements of the federal government's meaningful use (MU) incentive program, hospitals almost always need to phase in an EHR via components, such as those described in chapter 1. However, when implementing each component, many organizations also adopt a phasing strategy, such as roll-out by nursing stations, departments, physician specialties, sites, and so on. Sometimes the phasing strategy depends on the module being implemented

Table 9.1.   Summary of roll-out and turnover strategies

Type of Roll-out Strategy	Consider Using if Healthcare Organization Is:
Phased • Implementation of an EHR component, or functions of a component, in one or a few organizational units at a time • Plan exists to follow on with full roll-out in same manner	• Multispecialty clinic • Medium- to large-sized clinic or hospital • Multisite facility • Implementing a complex EHR
Big Bang • Implementation of all aspects of an EHR component (or entire EHR in an ambulatory setting) in all organizational units virtually simultaneously	• Single-specialty clinic • Small clinic or very small hospital • Other size/type clinic or hospital with considerable staff resources and vendor support
Pilot • Application of straight turnover or parallel processing in one or a few organizational units • Determination whether to proceed to full roll-out is made after some period of use • (Often not acceptable to vendors because level of effort needed to represent product fairly is too great)	• Implementing a product new to market • New to computerization • Medium to large size • One with previous bad experience with EHR

Type of Turnover Strategy	Consider Using if Healthcare Organization Is:
Straight Turnover • Paper processes cease shortly after go-live • Close monitoring and cycle checking ensure system works as planned	• Most EHR environments
Parallel Processing • Paper processes continue until system works as planned • Requires diligence in keeping both paper and electronic systems complete, accurate, and timely	• Select processes, such as patient accounting • Some BC-MAR applications (with poor results) • Organizations new to computerization in general • Implementing a product new to market

and the interest of the users. For example, a computerized provider order entry (CPOE) might be implemented first on a medical-surgical inpatient unit because that is where it might have the greatest impact. Alternatively, some hospitals chose to initiate MU participation by first implementing CPOE in the emergency department (ED). The ED was a good choice for first implementation of CPOE because the MU regulations dictated that only 30 percent of a hospital's orders had to be placed via CPOE for the organization to earn the stage 1 incentives, and because the ED is a relatively small, controlled environment with a limited number of physicians who are affected at one time. When planning the roll-out strategy, careful consideration should be given to the size of the organizational unit (not too big or too small), balancing the level of interest of the users (are they curmudgeons or "techno-docs"?), the complexity of the unit (complexity influences the degree of customization needed), and so on.

Another element of the phasing might relate to the functions performed by the component being implemented. For example, some organizations get everyone up to speed on rudimentary processes and then phase in more specific processes. This strategy has advantages and disadvantages, and its advisability often depends on what module is being implemented. For example, bar code medication administration record (BC-MAR) could be implemented first through electronically generated medication administration record (MAR) forms and then through a full bar coding process. This phasing may help acquaint nurses with computer systems and achieve patient safety benefits while the organization works on upgrading its pharmacy system, acquiring medication supply systems, adding bar code processing, and so on. Alternatively, some hospitals initially implemented CPOE only for medication orders or for orders with limited need for clinical decision support. Neither of these approaches may be acceptable to physicians, who often find it time consuming to have to enter orders in both electronic and manual modes and who consider order entry without clinical decision support to be merely a clerical duty. In clinics, physicians may decide to first use the EHR only to retrieve laboratory test results and documents from the hospital, then to perform eprescribing, and finally move to documenting via templates.

As part of the roll-out strategy, the organization must decide whether it will require all users (within the organizational units targeted for implementation) to use the system or allow those who are not interested to opt out. In general, the opt-out option only applies to physicians. Currently, fewer hospitals are adopting an opt-out strategy than in the past—primarily because it is a burden on staff to run parallel processes and because it is a patient safety concern. Although these issues are also concerns in physician offices and clinics, some clinics opted to permit some physicians not to adopt the EHR because the MU incentives are per physician, not per organization. Organizations save money in license fees if a physician will not use the system; however, there may be other costs associated with this strategy. In one large clinic, for example, the physicians decided to acquire licenses only for those interested in using the EHR and allow others to continue to use paper records, but the latter group would be charged paper-processing fees. In this case, only a few physicians opted for paper records initially, and even they quickly realized that they would have to learn the system anyway to manage their partners' patients. The need to process paper records in parallel with electronic records was phased out at this clinic within a year. In another example, a hospital initially decided to exclude its behavioral health unit from EHR implementation because the general EHR was not suitable for such documentation and there were concerns about confidentiality.

Most healthcare organizations prefer to allow for some phasing of health IT but desire ultimate adoption by all. As noted, maintaining a hybrid environment is costly and may affect patient safety. In any hybrid record situation, it may never be completely clear where the latest information is available. Unfortunately, because of the need to implement an EHR in components and phases in most hospitals, the hybrid record situation has all too often been the norm. Still to this day, hospitals have areas that rely on paper because a component not required by the MU program was not implemented or was unavailable from the vendor. Most hospitals are managing this small amount of paper by scanning the documents and making them available through an add-on application in the EHR (see chapter 18). Hybrid record-keeping is less common in physician offices, where the phasing can be accomplished more quickly.

Because of concerns about hybrid records, or even simply gaining full adoption, some organizations have tried and successfully accomplished implementing at least the major components of an EHR in a **big-bang approach** (also called *rapid implementation*). This strategy requires extremely careful planning up front, commitment by all users (or almost all), and an enormous amount of support during the go-live (Badger et al. 2005). Some small hospitals chose this approach because they wanted to acquire and implement an EHR in time to get MU incentives (Quammen 2011). Some physician offices also consider the big-bang approach, both to reduce the overhead of maintaining a hybrid system and to ensure that every physician is on board. Big bang roll-outs tend to be more successful in smaller practices.

Phasing is sometimes called pilot testing. **Pilot testing** usually means that an information system is tested with one group of users, and, if they do not like it, use of the system is discontinued. However, when the term is used to describe a roll-out strategy, it more commonly means that one group of users will go live first and how they use the system will be evaluated before the it is rolled out to other groups of users. Although the intent of such a pilot group is to work out bugs in the software and workflows, fewer organizations are adopting this strategy than in the past. Vendors today have greater deployment of their software so it is less buggy, and organizations often are not willing to take the time that pilot testing entails. Nevertheless, such a pilot roll-out strategy can be a good idea—organizations that choose not to take the time to attend to workflows typically have poor results.

Turnover Strategy

Turnover strategy is the plan for how users will first transition to the new EHR or other type of health IT—will the they have to stop using the previous system on go-live, or will it be run parallel to the new system for some period of time after go-live?

- *Straight turnover* refers to having everyone in the designated group go live at one time, with previous processes (such as paper records or legacy systems) ceasing virtually immediately. This form of turnover has been the most typical one for organizations transitioning from paper to EHRs or from legacy systems to newer systems, because most organizations find that any reliance on former processing activities ends up being too time-consuming and sends a message that the new system is not to be trusted. Although this strategy may seem risky, it is frequently found that staff cannot perform both two processes accurately, completely, or on a timely basis. Furthermore, a straight turnover does not imply that quality checks are forsaken. Part of the go-live support should be to ensure that new processes are performed correctly and completely, verifying accuracy against actual activity rather than previous forms of documentation. This enables staff to quickly move to the new environment, for the sake of patient safety and to begin realizing the organization's expected return on investment (ROI).

- *Parallel processing* is a turnover strategy where the organization continues using the old system while introducing the new (for example, processing records in manual form as well as electronic form). The intent is to validate the outcomes of the new system (for example, comparing electronic processing to the manual processing periodically, such as at the end of a day, week, or month). Most organizations find this validation process to be too time-consuming and prone to errors. For instance, in one hospital, nurses wanted to run parallel processing when implementing the BC-MAR system. The result was that some nurses primarily used BC-MARs, often forgetting to document on paper as well, whereas other nurses did the opposite. The staff checking the accuracy of the system thought there were major problems, until it was recognized that this was an implementation problem, not a system problem. Some form of double-processing may be necessary during the initial stages of go-live (for example, a clinical department might use paper worksheets until it is certain that the EHR documentation is reliable), but that is not what is typically meant by parallel processing, where *every* action is duplicated. Some organizations find parallel processing to be helpful when implementing new patient accounting systems or practice management systems. However, even in these cases, the labor effort may not justify the end result. In addition, many newer such systems have many forms of quality control and processes that older systems did not have; therefore, even if the process is deemed highly accurate, the results may not be the same.

Conversion Strategy

Closely related to roll-out and turnover strategies is the **conversion strategy**, which refers to the proportion of the existing paper records (chart conversion) or data in other electronic systems (data conversion) will be moved to the EHR or other type of health IT prior to or during go-live. This section focuses on chart conversion. Data conversion is discussed later in this chapter.

Chart conversion may be somewhat less of an issue for acute care areas of a hospital than for clinics or the ambulatory areas of a hospital. Most hospitals apply a straight turnover approach to chart conversion, where the new system is used on go-live but users must rely on paper records (which may or may not be scanned) for past admission information. This approach is generally acceptable in the acute care setting because the typical admission is a unique episode of care. Past records can be useful, but an updated, comprehensive history and physical examination are needed for every hospitalization. However, if the hospital has a high readmission rate, it may need to consider some of the chart conversion strategies identified for the ambulatory environment (see discussion later in this chapter).

More often, the issue for a hospital is the hybrid record, where only parts of the health record are available electronically and some parts remain on paper. For example, a hospital may have had a digital dictation system (for the history and physical exam, radiology, and some other diagnostic studies results) and a laboratory results reporting system for some time. It then may add a CPOE system and a BC-MAR system, but progress notes and nursing graphics may continue to be hand-written. Unless the hospital prints everything out and scans everything back into a single system or is able to integrate the electronic content with scanned images, a hybrid record is the result. Where a hospital declares its electronic components of the chart to be the official legal health record, it usu-ally finds the need to include reminders in the paper chart that certain documents or data are only accessible electronically. Such a system can lead to confusion, especially if not all users are willing to use both the electronic and paper chart components. For example, those physicians not interested in EHRs may request that the electronic content be printed. If the physician writes notes on printed charts, their notes then may become "original health record" content that needs to be filed into the paper chart, potentially resulting in more than one version of information. If other physicians or clinicians rely on the fact that the electronic source is the "official source," the annotation may be missed, presenting a potential patient safety issue. Still other physicians may prefer to access the electronic system and ignore paper content.

In a clinic or other ambulatory environment an episode of care can last for several visits, and reliance on previous visit information is therefore often more essential than in a hospital. For chronic disease patients, information from several years ago may remain pertinent. Furthermore, the time spent with a patient during any given clinic visit is usually not long enough to re-create an entire medical history for the new EHR. As such, the chart conversion strategy requires careful consideration of what data from the charts need to be converted, how, and when. Some organiza-tions choose a chart conversion strategy in which they use document imaging, abstraction, or a combination of both, to back-file six months or a year of content of active charts.

Although all forms of chart conversion have their pros and cons, document imaging is often touted to be an easy and cost-effective solution. In reality, it may be neither easy nor inexpensive. One physician office found that scanning an average primary care provider record took a clerical staff person 45 minutes or longer. The number of staff hours plus the cost of heavy-duty scanning equipment for bulk scanning, even if leased temporarily, was cost-prohibitive. In addition, most physicians find that it is time-consuming to locate scanned images unless they are carefully indexed (which costs more up front), and they dislike having to look at scanned images. A good alternative to scanned records is to COLD feed digital dictation of a comprehensive note into the EHR. (COLD refers to "computer-output to laser disk"; the acronym is still used, even as laser disks have been replaced with other technology.) Digital dictation places key information into the EHR in one loca-tion, although is not structured data that serves to prepopulate the record in advance of its first use by the provider. Scanning all charts could provide an ROI if it frees up storage space. However, if that is not the case, it might make more sense to perform scanning in combination with abstracting or consider abstracting only.

Abstracting, also called **preload**, is the process of extracting information from a document or record, often to create a brief summary of a patient's illness, treatment, and outcome, or enter them into an automated system for subsequent processing. Like scanning, abstracting can also be time-consuming and costly, but it potentially can be more controlled, thereby reducing cost. During

Table 9.2.   Chart conversion strategies

Technique	Advantages	Disadvantages
Continue pulling paper chart	• Makes entire chart available • Often acceptable for hospitals, especially those with a relatively low readmission rate	• Requires paper charts to be available for many years after EHR go-live • May result in a hybrid record if some clinicians will not use EHR for current care
Scan paper charts of active patients	• Makes entire content of paper chart available electronically • Acceptable process for both acute and ambulatory care • Allows destruction of paper chart, unless only parts of paper chart are scanned	• Does not provide discrete data for processing in clinical decision support, so for some period of time, an electronically hybrid record results • Cost/benefit issues of degree of indexing must be addressed
Abstract data from paper charts of active patients	• Makes data available for electronic processing of reminders and alerts • Some vendors are supporting templates that capture key data and distribute them to appropriate place in EHR	• Error prone if performed by nonphysician • Time-consuming if performed by physician • Rarely used by hospitals; increasingly used by clinics
Use a combination of above	• Achieves all benefits relating to access • Most often used for a short period of time in which chart is pulled for any additional scanning or abstracting	• May be confusing if not consistently applied • Probably most costly to implement due to variations in instructions

chart conversion for EHR implementation, a limited amount of data (for example, problem list, immunizations, most recent laboratory test results, and potentially medications and allergies, if this information is not available for interfacing through an existing eprescribing system or from a pharmacy benefits consolidator) can be abstracted by skilled staff (transcriptionists, coders, pharmacy technicians, and nurses are suitable). Data abstracted will need to be validated by the provider during the first visit after go-live. A timing issue may also arise—if a chart is converted too early and another visit occurs prior to the EHR go-live, the chart must be abstracted again later. However, the result of abstracting key data is a significant improvement in productivity for the physicians (Jankowski 2010). In some cases, clinics find that the physicians can abstract a small amount of data more efficiently and accurately than staff. One clinic required each of its physicians to abstract their own charts or lose their bonus for the year. Some physicians performed this task the night before or in the early morning prior to seeing patients, or they opted to take longer with each patient during the initial visit after go-live. Either way, they found the experience was an important contribution to patient care and helped them become more acclimated to the EHR so they were able to return to their standard productivity rates faster than anticipated. Table 9.2 compares paper chart conversion strategies.

Time Frame for Implementation

Another part of the overall planning approach is the time frame for implementing each phase. The vendor should be able to offer estimates of the time it will take for any given organizational unit to go live on the system or each of its components. The organization should track how much time the roll-out takes in the first organizational unit that is phased; this information can be used to obtain a solid estimate of the time it takes to install, train, and obtain adoption. Subsequent units should take less time, but the organization may decide to give every unit the same amount of time or step up the process where some units are implemented in parallel. The level of staff availability and experience and the scope of the project are the determining factors.

Installation Versus Implementation

When overall phasing and time frames are established, detailed tasks should be plotted on an implementation plan. An implementation plan usually begins with the first steps of implementation. This is perhaps where the distinction between installation and implementation is most apparent. As noted in chapter 4, *installation* refers to merely setting up and plugging in hardware, and loading software onto the computer, whereas *implementation* includes all of the tasks associated with preparing for and readying the software and users for actual use. Key differences between installation and implementation are illustrated in table 9.3. Note that, in an application service provider (ASP) or software as a service (SaaS) environment, many of the installation steps are performed at the vendor location, although the site acquiring the system will still have some hardware and networking installation requirements for user devices.

Because the tasks, people involved, budget, and myriad other details need to be tracked, each implementation plan for an EHR or another large-scale health IT system could well include thousands of tasks. Many vendors use detailed implementation plan templates when working with healthcare organizations. Such plans should be a part of the contractual agreement when acquiring the system. However, it should be the task of the organization's project manager to manage the organization's own implementation plan. This plan should carry forward the key milestones of the vendor's plan as well as include the tasks for which the organization itself is responsible. The project manager should be directly involved in harmonizing the plans as well as the following objectives:

- Reviewing and signing off on completion of tasks (a set of actions for completion)

- Monitoring project for risks associated with the following:

  - Procurement issues (delivery of software, hardware, or task completion performed by consultants or otherwise outsourced)

  - Communication issues

  - Time management

  - Task **dependencies** (where one task cannot proceed without an earlier task being completed)

  - **Milestone completion** (reference points in the implementation plan that indicate progress)

Table 9.3.   Installation versus implementation

Installation	Implementation
Assemble hardware components	Review contract and develop detailed implementation plan
Connect devices	Establish issues/risk management system and documentation requirements
Run hardware setups	Prepare infrastructure, such as data center enhancements, user area shelving, and so on
Lay network cable	Procure hardware, accept delivery, inventory, and tag components
Install network devices, including wireless access points	Design process improvement changes
Test network connectivity	Configure applications
Load application software	Test applications
	Train users on applications
	Go-live
	Monitor results

    ◦ **Resource leveling** (where the right staff and funding are available at the time needed)

    ◦ Budget overruns

Issues and Risk Management

Because of the number of tasks and their complexity and dependencies, it is important to have an issues management program. An **issues management** program (also called **risk management**) serves to receive and document issues and track them to their resolution (Arredondo 2012). Figure 9.1 shows a sample issues log.

    The project manager is tasked with receiving reports of issues (or personally identifying issues, where applicable), logging them, identifying the resources needed to take corrective action, and documenting resolution. He or she must understand the scope of issues that need to be tracked as well as the nature of issues that need to be escalated to a higher authority (Santamarina 2015). The project manager should acknowledge issues that may take the implementation off the **critical path** (that is, the series of tasks where there is no slack and which if not performed in sequence and on time will delay the project). For example, a week's delay in obtaining extra printers is not as critical as a report from the system integrator that an interface will require several hundred hours of additional work. The project manager probably can find a work-around for the shortage of printers but will need to report the issue of the interface to the chief information officer (CIO), board, or other authority. Any issue that would have a material bearing on the project's timeliness, budget, or desired outcome is a risk that needs to be escalated.

System Documentation

Often left to the end of an information technology (IT) project is documentation of the system configuration, policies and procedures for performing improved processes, and many other necessary records relating to the system. **System documentation** is documentation about the system itself—the user manuals, practice guidelines that support templates, decision support rules, and other system documentation—and it must be performed virtually for every step of the implementation process. There are so many steps in an implementation of an EHR or other health IT system that not documenting issues with current status and completion makes the implementation project very difficult to manage.

    System documentation is also critical for ongoing maintenance, and, in some cases, it may be needed in a legal dispute. Two actual examples illustrate this fact:

Example 1:

A hospital was sued over a clinical incident in its ED. In addition to the clinical aspect, there was lack of documentation corroborating a system crash alleged to have occurred at the time of original dictation of the visit note, necessitating redictation. This suggested a cover-up to the plaintiff's attorney. Upon further questioning, the hospital reported it did not know it was required to keep such records. The hospital had to pay a higher

Figure 9.1.   Issues log and sample entry

#	Issue	Source	Date ID	Reference	Escalation	Resolution	Date Tested	Sign Off
33	Screen does not display error correction	Mary	3/2	M3.S4.D2	No	Source code correction (vendor)	3/10	J.P.

settlement than it might otherwise have needed to pay for the clinical incident alone, and it was reported to the US Department of Health and Human Services (HHS) Office for Civil Rights (OCR) for violating the Health Information Portability and Accountability Act (HIPAA) Security Rule requiring information system review activity to be documented.

Example 2:

IT staff adjusted a clinical decision support rule in an EHR after numerous complaints by physicians that they did not like the constant alerts the system provided and wanted it changed. Sometime later, a clinical incident occurred and a malpractice suit was initiated against a physician. The physician claimed that there had been no alert from the EHR to the fact that the patient was at risk; as a result, the physician believed he should not be held accountable. However, the plaintiff's attorney found that a clause in the contract for licensing the EHR that stated the EHR was not a substitute for professional judgment and that the vendor was not liable for any consequences relative to use of the EHR. The case was settled for a substantial amount of money. After the settlement, the physician attempted to get IT staff fired for changing the alert, but the staff had documented when the alert was changed and that the physicians who had requested such change included the physician who had been sued. The practice manager did not fire the IT staff.

Policies and procedures that reflect the directives relative to use of the EHR or other health IT in various processes are also important to document. Many organizations do not have policies with respect to EHR and health IT system use, relying instead on general policies for professional credentialing, compliance, privacy and security, human resources, and other issues. However, EHRs and other types of health IT provide enhanced opportunities to improve upon all forms of policy-related matters. Policy and procedure changes related to these technologies should be codified as revisions to existing policies and procedures or added to the existing set of policies. For example, under HIPAA, individuals have the right to request restrictions on use and disclosure of protected health information (PHI). In a paper-based operation, many healthcare organizations must turn down such requests because they are impossible to manage. With an EHR, some restrictions may be more feasible to implement (and some may become required). Policies on PHI should therefore be reviewed and revised, if applicable. Moreover, the EHR brings about new ethical dilemmas. For example, should documentation of a rationale be required when a clinician overrides an alert from a decision support rule? There is considerable difference of opinion on this question (Rollins 2005), but each organization should state its preferences in policy. Other policies may center on tighter access controls, disaster recovery planning, release of information, and acceptance of content from a personal health record.

Check Your Understanding 9.1

Indicate whether the following statements are true or false (T or F):

1. Implementation planning and management are not necessary when a vendor is hired to supply implementation services.

2. A roll-out strategy in which all EHR or other health IT components are implemented at once is referred to as *straight turnover*.

3. Parallel processing, in which paper processes are continued during initial use of health IT, is not recommended for most clinical applications.

4. In most physician practices, it is helpful to pre-load data abstracted from paper charts into the new EHR for active patients.

5. A milestone is a step in an implementation plan that must be performed prior to another step.

6. An example of an issue to log onto an issues/risk management log is when a domain team leader is habitually late in performing tasks.

7. Documentation of changes made to the application during system configuration can be done at the conclusion of the implementation when things are less hectic.

Infrastructure Preparedness

When the implementation plan has been established, there are a number of tasks associated with preparing hardware and telecommunications equipment and physical plant of the organization as well as preparing stakeholders and especially new users for using new equipment and working with improved processes.

Hardware, Telecommunications, and Physical Plant Infrastructure

Preparing the organization's hardware, telecommunications, and physical plant for the EHR or other health IT is among the first implementation tasks. This step may entail purchasing and installing hardware, upgrading telecommunications network, and even making changes in the physical plant. For example, some organizations must do extensive cabling, add wireless capability, or expand or rebuild their data center. These organizations may need additional space, hardware, cabling, and air conditioning for servers as well as space to use as a "war room" where system configuration can occur, meeting rooms, and a separate training room. If the organization acquires a product through an ASP or SaaS arrangement, it may not need a fully functional data center, but it will probably need space to set up, test, and fix hardware and any onsite servers, as well as for meetings and training.

There often are physical plant issues associated with workstation location, ability to use workstations on wheels (WOWs; also called *wireless on wheels*), mobile devices, patient kiosks, printers, and so on in non-IT parts of the facility. For example, a hospital built a brand-new facility but found that WOWs could not be moved into the patients' rooms due to their configuration. All of the patient care devices were suspended from the back of the patients' beds, but no accommodation was made to even place a mobile device on a small table or shelf. If an organization decides to launch a large-scale scanning program or chart abstraction process for chart conversion, it may need considerable extra space for staging charts, high-speed scanners, and so on. This type of project may entail a completely separate area apart from the file area, and often involves a courier process to move charts from the file area to the scanning operation and then to a temporary archive location. Additional storage devices and sometimes off-site disaster recovery sites must be added.

Hardware purchasing and delivery are also two important early tasks in implementation. For example, the organization must decide how many devices to acquire, their type, and whether they will be purchased in advance of other tasks or just-in-time for actual use. Most hospitals have a procurement office to help manage purchasing and delivery, but small physician practices do not. If organizations acquire devices before they are actually needed, then storage space must be found for them.

Healthcare organizations also must decide a bring your own device (BYOD) policy. Allowing users to do work on their personal computers, smartphones, and tablets may seem like an effective way to manage costs, but the time required for IT staff to configure each user's unique device exceeds the cost of setting up only one or a limited number of standard devices. (See also chapter 12 on the security issues relating to BYOD.) The increasing use of multiple devices simultaneously (such as, phones, tablets, pagers, and workstations) also affects workflow. Voltz (2015) describes the workflow issues of managing multiple devices as the "dizzying pace of context switching."

Workflow and Process Infrastructure

Other infrastructure preparation issues include workflow and process assessment and redesign (if not performed earlier). Tackling these issues early in the planning is advisable. Many workflows and processes can be improved even before the EHR or other health IT is implemented. However, it is also important to recognize that the organization may not be able to redesign all of the workflows in advance of working through the EHR or other health IT implementation. Although organizations want to tailor their EHR or health IT to fit within desired staff workflows to the extent possible, they cannot force a system to function a specific way just because staff are accustomed to a workflow, nor can they create one generic workflow that everyone must be forced to use (Thompson 2010).

Moving to more standardization in workflows and processes can contribute to better patient care and easier use of the EHR or other health IT (Vang 2014). For example, the EHR can facilitate the use of clinical pathways, standard order sets, and evidence-based guidelines (Carter 2014). Although these tools are not new, not every clinician has used them or documented against them. In a paper environment, such tools were often treated as general guidance rather than required processes. Clinicians frequently did not give much consideration to the standardization of terminology such use would require, and they were not held accountable for their use as there was virtually no means to document whether standards were followed. In the EHR, however, the pathways, order sets, and evidence-based guidelines support improvement—so long as clinicians have reviewed and approved them in advance and continue to apply professional judgment in their use. Clinicians could begin preparing for the transition from a paper environment to full EHR implementation by reviewing what clinical tools exist, understanding and agreeing to use of the standard terminology they include, developing new tools or modifying existing ones as needed, and starting to use them more fully. Such efforts in advance of implementation could help clinicians understand the EHR better and establish expectations for use of the EHR.

New workflows often drive policy changes. Individuals who work on creating the workflows and processes for use with the EHR or other type of health IT are in the best position to recognize these policy changes and advocate for them.

Identifying and obtaining agreement on all forms of standards is something to prepare for in advance of software installation. For example, some vendors offer a proprietary vocabulary or the option to adopt a standardized vocabulary. Although this organization's preferences may be partially decided prior to contract negotiation, reviewing the vocabulary and deciding specifically how it will be used may be necessary before the contract is finalized. Perhaps only a limited portion of standardized vocabulary will be adopted. For example, an organization could select to use the Clinical Observations Recordings and Encoding (CORE) Problem List Subset of SNOMED CT, which is the set of terms most useful for documenting and encoding clinical information at a summary level, such as for a problem list (NLM 2016). Some mapping from the vendor's vocabulary, or even a standardized vocabulary, to standard data sets used prior to software installation may be required. Performing as many of these types of tasks prior to system build, the next major task, helps the build go smoothly (and keeps costs in line with budget).

Certainly, policies, procedures, training materials, and user manuals can be developed, or at least initiated, in advance of the roll-out. Clinicians responsible for using clinical guidelines, templates, macros or smart text, structured data-entry screens, and decision support rules need to be involved in reviewing, developing, and acquiring these components. Physicians should be creating their **favorites list** of medications, problems, or other frequently generated data. In some cases, the EHR can "learn" what a clinician's favorites are by frequency of use. However, many organizations take proactive steps to ensure that each clinician's favorites are already built into the system prior to go-live.

Stakeholder Preparation

As part of infrastructure preparedness, the process of preparing new users and other stakeholders for the level of change that the EHR and health IT may bring about should begin in earnest as soon as the implementation is initiated. People skills are vital—not only for the project manager but for all supervisors and managers who must "carry the word" and be supportive of the EHR for their staff. In fact, in one discussion of a successful CPOE implementation, the primary attributes identified were motivation, vision, leadership, personnel, value, workflow, project management, training, support, and evaluation—with technology listed only once (Fenton et al. 2006).

However, a realistic picture must be painted of what life will be like during and after go-live. Giving staff false expectations may be worse than not communicating with them at all. For example, telling staff that an EHR will save time and money while improving patient care could be setting the project up for failure. Staff may conclude from this message that their jobs are at risk, and they may therefore potentially sabotage the project, even if unintentionally. Although saving time and reducing costs might be goals for the EHR that may be recognized in the future, they should be discussed in a way that acknowledges the journey to achieve those goals and that those goals include better use of existing staff (Fields 2010). See chapter 6 for more information on change management.

The project manager should have a defined communication strategy and plan. (See chapter 6.) Figure 9.2 shows a sample communication plan. The organization may create a newsletter that provides updates on implementation of the EHR or other health IT system, post a general status report on the organization's intranet, or start an online discussion of frequently asked questions. Some one-on-one communication with key individuals who need to be convinced may also be in order. Anything that will help the clinical transformation and ease the minds of staff is essential.

As discussed in chapter 6, staff reticence and uncertainty can make implementation difficult, affect productivity, cause an increase in errors, and have other negative effects on the organization. Sometimes it is difficult to see that these issues are arising. The smart project manager must anticipate them and offer appropriate reassurance to members of the organization.

An EHR or other form of health IT does not typically result in significant staff cutbacks in most departments of a healthcare organization. However, it is also important to be honest with staff. For instance, some staff may find that their jobs become quite different. Some jobs might be eliminated, but there may well be other opportunities for staff. For example, some clerical staff members have been redeployed from paper chart filing to helping patients access the computer to fill out forms. As one clinic converted to an EHR, it anticipated that it would no longer need transcribers. Rather than cutting staff, it decided to sell transcription services to other providers until transcription could be phased out through attrition. In reality, the clinic itself continued to need transcription, so transcriptionist staff actually had to be increased.

Preparing stakeholders to use computers continues to be an issue—but in new and unforeseen ways. Even today, some physicians and nurses have never used a computer. They require basic training, such as on Windows functions or how to use a mouse or other navigational device. Familiarity with computer systems as a whole can help these individuals become comfortable once the specific training for the new technology takes place. To this end, organizations may want to institute policies that encourage or require the use of computers for many functions. For example, a facility may require that everyone obtain his or her schedule from the computer, all meeting announcements only be posted electronically, and all quality improvement reports be provided online. However, organizations should recognize that some resistance to the use of technology may not be related to an overall lack of computer skills. Clinicians may easily be able to perform tasks such as keeping a calendar on the computer or entering data but feel that such tasks are clerical work and come to resent these requirements.

Figure 9.2.   Sample communication plan

Key Messages	To (All Staff, BOD, EHR Team, MDs, Patients)	From (Med Dir, Admin, EHR Team, MDIS, Proj. Mgr)	Medium (E-mail Blast, Hotline, Intranet, Media Kit, Meeting, Newsletter, Personal Comm., Pol. & Proc., Poster, Report, Script, Website)	Date(s) or Milestones
EHR planning				
EHR education				
Computer skills				
EHR migration path				
Stakeholder engagement				
Benefits/Value				
Selection process				
Code of conduct				
Process improvement				
Expectations				
ROI				
Contract signing				
Implementation plan				
Chart conversion strategy				
EHR testing				
EHR training				
Suggestions				
Celebration				
Adoption rate				
Patient satisfaction				
Physician satisfaction				
Staff satisfaction				
Quality measures				

Another potential issue is that the EHR and other types of health IT are often created on a client/server platform rather than using web services architecture. Staff members who are facile with new technology may find it difficult to use the older platform (Dunbrack 2015).

The organization must also prepare to communicate with patients about the new EHR and other significant health IT innovations. For example, many vendors provide big signs that describe the organization as undergoing "EHR construction" and a short pamphlet explaining what an EHR is, how it changes their provider's access to information, and how it will benefit patients. One organization undergoing EHR implementation perhaps said it best: "You cannot overcommunicate!"

System Build and Configuration

System build, also called **system configuration**, is the process in which the software is configured with all the various data dictionaries, table development, rules logic, data and code set mapping, file designs, screen layouts, data quality edits, report designs, repository structures, and technical controls, including security access controls and error correction routines.

Need for System Build and Configuration

EHRs and other types of health IT vary in their degree of customizability, but all, including ASP and SaaS models, have some system build requirements. Some vendor products have a low degree of flexibility; others can be almost totally customizable. Part of the vendor selection process is to determine the degree to which the organization needs and wants to customize its system. Some organizations make a conscious effort to reduce the level of customization simply because they think standards are a good thing. Other organizations want to accommodate every conceivable nuance and may have the resources to do so. Most are somewhere in the middle, recognizing the system needs to accommodate many of their unique aspects while still improving processes through standardization. (See chapter 7 for more information on vendor selection.)

System build includes the most detailed of tasks and is often the most labor-intensive step in the overall implementation process. It is the most fundamental step to making the EHR and other health IT systems work. However, it should be noted that, although a basic system platform should be established initially, some aspects of system build can, will, and should go on for many years. A prime example is clinical decision support. Most organizations decide to have just the right amount of decision support on go-live, and then build it up as users become accustomed to the system (Campbell 2013). It can be difficult to determine the right amount for an organization; however, choices are becoming easier due to the MU incentive program, heightened attention to all forms of clinical quality measurement and improvement, and increasing evidence of the effectiveness of clinical decision support.

As part of its commitment to help support EHR implementers, Office of the National Coordinator for Health Information Technology (ONC) has nine developed SAFER (safety assurance factors for EHR resilience) self-assessment guides (see figure 9.3). Each SAFER guide begins with a checklist of recommended practices. A practice worksheet gives a rationale for and examples of how to implement each recommended practice as well as likely sources of input into assessment of each practice. The worksheet also includes team members and follow-up action (ONC 2014).

With respect to system configuration of clinical content, the SAFER self-assessment guide best practice states that "Clinical content used, for example, to create order sets and clinical charting templates and to generate reminders within the EHR, is up-to-date, complete, available, and tested." Suggested sources of input are clinicians, support staff, or clinical administration. Several practice scenarios are included, such as fixing broken links to Internet-based clinical information resources. Another is that the organization has a naming convention and unambiguous synonyms for common orders, results, procedures, order sets, charting templates, and macros (for example, dot phrases or canned text). Yet another is that the organization has a clinical informatics committee to review content (ONC 2014).

Figure 9.3.   SAFER self-assessment guides

- High Priority Practices
- Organizational Responsibilities
- Contingency Planning
- System Configuration
- System Interfaces
- Patient Identification
- Computerized Provider Order Entry with Decision Support
- Test Results Reporting and Follow-Up
- Clinician Communication

Source: ONC 2014.

Configuration Management

An important part of system build is configuration management. Sometimes referred to as *change control* (see chapter 8), **configuration management** is generally somewhat narrower in scope than change control and is the process of identifying, recording, evaluating, tracking, coordinating, reporting, and controlling changes to a system (HHS n.d.). Configuration management is not the same as change management. Change management (see chapter 6) is the process of changing human behavior as part of an overall business solution (Wallace 2007). The purpose of configuration management, where a record is kept of every change made to customize the EHR or other health IT system to the organization's specifications, is to ensure that the change is well planned, appropriately documented, approved, and audited (Chamberland 2014). This goal is especially important in a clinical environment, where a single change—such as in the valid values of a data element or whether a data element is required or optional—can directly affect clinical decision support. Configuration management should be linked to metadata (which refers to data that describes the properties of data to be collected in an information system; see chapter 10) in the system's data dictionary in a data dictionary control log, such as the one shown in figure 9.4.

After go-live, changes will continue to be made to the configuration of the screens, reports, decision support rules, and other processes. Because a change to any one part of the system potentially affects many other parts, it is essential to thoroughly understand the information flow and data model that the change request impacts. Such changes are generally made at the request of an individual or group. The organization should have a policy concerning who may make a change, how it should be documented and authorized, and what priority it will be given. Many organizations require that all changes be made using a formal change request process, which would include a master change control log and request forms (Carman 2013).

Figure 9.4.   Data dictionary change control log

Data Element Characteristic	Original	Change	Change Requested by:	Change Approved by:	Change Performed by:	Change Tested by:	Final Change Date:
Name of entry							
Table							
Physical name							
Synonym(s)							
Definition							
Reference							
Source of data							
Derivations							
Valid values							
Conditionality							
Default							
Lexicon							
Relationship							
Access restrictions							
Process rules							

Testing

Testing is critical, but it is sometimes overlooked or shortchanged, especially in smaller organizations. In fact, some vendors (especially those selling to physician offices) assume that, because they have run their software through developmental testing processing and have previously implemented their product in numerous other client organizations, further testing is not necessary, or that testing will take place during end-user training. However, it should be clear from the previous discussion on system build that every implementation is different and needs to be tested. Furthermore, new users should not be put into the position of "testing" the system. That scenario will only frustrate new users to the point that they will not trust the new system.

Establishing a Test Environment

The first step in testing is to establish a test environment (sometimes called a *development environment*) or ensure that the ASP or SaaS vendor has a test environment. A *test environment* refers to an instantiation of the software on a separate, or virtually separate, server (Ashraf 2015). Because testing will continue throughout the implementation process, it is important that the tests do not disrupt the production environment. In addition, fixes, upgrades, and modifications will be needed routinely in the future and should be tested in a manner that does not slow down or cause errors to occur in the actual system used on a day-to-day basis. At a minimum, the test environment should include separate hardware and installation of software. Ideally, it would include test data. Many vendors provide test data, but some organizations prefer to develop their own test data to ensure that all conceivable issues are tested.

Some vendors and organizations recommend using actual data (though not "live" data) for testing. This strategy can be advisable because it is sometimes difficult to create test data from scratch that cover every type of data to be encountered, but the approach raises the issue of whether the data should be de-identified. In response to a frequently asked question, the website maintained by the OCR, which oversees HIPAA privacy and Security Rule compliance, offers that such test data do not have to be de-identified because their use is part of the organization's operations. Still, many organizations prefer not to take the chance that the actual data will include records for a current employee, a relative or friend of an employee, or a person with a public profile, and will at least change the names of the actual patients.

Developing a Test Plan and Schedule

Once a test environment is established, a test plan and schedule should be developed to include the necessary tests. Table 9.4 describes tests that typically should be performed. The names of the testing types in the table are not standardized, but their descriptions should be sufficient to guide the project manager to ensure that all appropriate testing is performed.

Test Scenarios and Testing

Test data are required to conduct the various levels of testing. However, without a scenario or story that sets the data in context and describes expected inputs, processes, and outputs, testing is not as thorough as it could be. Many organizations utilize use cases that describe the sequence of actions a system should take with respect to a specific task or function. Chapter 7 describes use case development with respect to defining EHR functional requirements.

Users or domain experts must develop the clinical use cases and also should be the ones to conduct their testing. Only clinicians can explain the nature of a thought process that the EHR should support, and therefore they are the only ones to ensure that a system has been built properly.

Table 9.4.   Types of system testing

Test	Description
Unit and function testing	Testing of individual modules or applications. This is the most basic test to ensure that each separate component works as expected. This test would look at screen design to ensure that all the tables load properly, reports are generated correctly, and so on.
System testing	Tests how well modules or applications work together. It also looks at work flow within a department or other organization unit and across units. If data are to flow from one department to another and do not, this is a problem.
Integrated system testing, or interface testing	Testing of systems that had to be interfaced to ensure the proper exchange of data.
Performance and stress, or load, testing	Testing of system performance, including response time, with volumes of data as anticipated in a live setting; and testing of performance that simulates peak volumes.

Engaging users to not only write but also conduct the tests helps their peer group develop trust in the system. In many situations, anyone responsible for conducting an EHR system test is required to sign off that the system performed the test to specifications. An issue log, or separate testing log, should be maintained to ensure that all test failures are corrected. Figure 9.5 uses a variation of use case modeling (Larmon 2002, 53) to describe part of a scenario that might be used for testing a CPOE system. Not every conceivable drug ordered via a CPOE system needs to be tested; however, a small number of typical, complex, and unusual scenarios from each clinical specialty should be constructed and tested. Obviously, if any of the tests reveal problems, the problems need to be fixed by the vendor. Contract language should cover the vendor's obligation to do so.

Acceptance testing is a term used in EHR implementation to describe the point at which the organization signs off that the implementation is working as expected. This usage is somewhat different than the way acceptance testing is understood in typical software development, where it is the completion of use case testing that triggers acceptance. The vendor and organization should agree on the criteria with which an implementation is accepted. For an EHR, acceptance typically occurs at least 30 to 60 days (or longer) after go-live. Acceptance occurs after go-live because not every conceivable scenario can be anticipated in advance. Some issues go unidentified until the system is working in the production environment for some time. Some vendors plan to retain their staff in an organization until the formal sign-off on acceptance occurs; others have staff return later to review the system's performance with organizational representatives. At a minimum, before an organization signs off on acceptance, it should ensure that all issues have been satisfactorily resolved, that users are adopting the system as expected and their satisfaction is acceptable, and users have completed one "cycle" of processing on their own without issues. Such a cycle should ensure that all charges have been captured, regular reports can be run, and information needed for subsequent care is available.

Performance warranties also may be considered part of acceptance testing. In many cases, vendors make claims about productivity or performance capabilities and will go "at risk" for these performance criteria. In other words, they will accept a late payment or provide other forms of compensation should the vendor's product fail to perform as warranted. However, vendors will require that the organization provide appropriate metrics, baseline data, and documentary evidence of improvement (or lack thereof). If the vendor is unwilling to go "at risk," the organization may still wish to conduct its own benefits realization studies to take corrective action internally where needed (and to celebrate success).

Figure 9.5.   Portion of sample use case model for CPOE system test

Provider	System
Primary Success Scenario: Receive appropriate D-D, D-L, D-A, D-W, and D-Dose	CPOE with interface from ADT, Problem List, Medication List, Allergy Documentation, Laboratory, Pharmacy, and Referral systems
Secondary Success Scenario: Retrieve list of patients who may be pregnant, become pregnant, or nursing to advise them of birth defect warning	Data mining capability
Basic flow: 1. Provider enters order for Paxil 2. D-D contraindication alert if patient taking MAOIs or thioridazine 3. D-L alert if patient has severe renal or hepatic impairment 4. D-A alert if patient has a hypersensitivity to paroxetine (active ingredient in Paxil) or any inactive ingredients 5. D-W (obtain psych consult reminder) if patient is at risk for suicide 6. D-dose recalculation for starting dose in pediatric patients	1. System finds structured product label (SPL) information from drug knowledge base 2. System compares D-D contraindications from SPL to active medication list 3. System compares most recent creatinine clearance with SPL warning of <30 mL/min 4. System compares ingredients in Paxil to drug allergy information on SPL 5. System checks patient problem list for suicide risk 6. System recalculates starting dose for patients under specified age, height, and weight
Extensions (or alternative flows): 2-a: Alert with respect to MAOIs or thioridazine fires 1. Cancels order 2. Requests to see detailed SPL 3. Selects alternative antidepressant 4. Overrides alert and retains for Paxil 2-b: Override presents list of potential rationales required for order to be accepted 1. Selects rationale 2. Cancels order	1. System deletes order for Paxil 2. System supplies content of SPL 3. System performs checks as above on alternative order 4. System accept override request and supplies rationale requirement per organizational policy
Secondary flow: 1. Request system to search for all patients for whom Paxil was ordered AND who are women between 12 and 50 years old . . . 2. Produce mailing labels of all patients on report	

Training

Training is an aspect of implementation that occurs at various points in the process, targeted at different individuals, and for different purposes. Training of varying intensity, methodology, and purpose occur periodically and strategically throughout the implementation process. Table 9.5 lists the various types of training that should be incorporated throughout the entire SDLC for the EHR or other health IT system.

Fields (2010) observes that "staff will always need more training than you expect," but, on the other hand, Guerrero (2013) recommends training people only on areas they are going to use. Both of these statements are especially true for physicians. They may not find the EHR or other health IT to be intuitive to use and could form bad habits if they are not trained in appropriate use

Table 9.5.   EHR and health IT training throughout the SDLC

Type of Training	Target Audience/Modality	Key Message(s)
Introduction	• Everyone in the organization • Short sound bytes at meetings, in newsletters, and so on	• An EHR and health IT is an essential technology for patient safety, quality of care, and user satisfaction • An EHR and health IT is a complex system with which the organization will migrate to and with all users involved
Education	• Initially steering committee, executive management, and other decision makers • Ultimately all developers and super users • Seminars and briefings that introduce theoretical and practical knowledge targeted to specific audience	• An EHR and health IT introduces a clinical transformation • An EHR and health IT is a system of systems designed for knowledge management • An EHR and health IT requires thorough planning and highly detailed and specific implementation, testing, and training
Briefings	Project sponsors • Project managers (organization and vendor) • Dashboards, regular meetings to keep key individuals up to date	• Current progress, issues, and successes with EHR and health IT implementation
Skills building	• Super users in person classroom/online training to build process mapping competencies, screen layout design competencies, and so on • End users on computer navigation using classroom or personal training tools, then on EHR and health IT functionality in various forms of communications, including demos	• An EHR and health IT is a tool that aids clinician decision making • Data entry should be performed by the individual closest to the source of the data, including the patient where possible • An EHR and health IT requires competency in navigating a computer
Instruction	• Super users on vendor-specific requirements, usually at vendor training seminar or on-site hands-on • End users to perform specific functions using train-the-trainer, training workstations, instruction manuals, "cheat sheets," and automated help function	• How this EHR and health IT works, may be customized, should be trained on • How this EHR and health IT works and tasks performed
Support	• End users provided standby assistance for navigating screens or any other assistance during go-live	• Achieve comfort using the EHR and health IT to gain full adoption
Retraining/ Refresher training/ coaching	• Super users to relearn or refresh for later upgrades often via online or seminar • End users who have created work-arounds to use of system in meeting • End users who are not fully adopted by one-on-one training	• Ongoing monitoring of system use and continue to support system as it evolves • Achieve comfort using the EHR and health IT to achieve benefits

and even sanctioned shortcuts. However, physicians may not do well in a group learning experience. Fields observes that "physicians are used to practicing by themselves and relying on their own knowledge to treat patients." When put in a group learning situation, they may therefore feel reluctant to ask questions because they do not want to reveal to others what they may consider to be a failure in themselves, even though it may seem absurd to expect anyone to know how to use a sophisticated tool with no training. Therefore, conducting one-on-one training with physicians is recommended.

Unfortunately, it is common for organizations to not budget appropriately for skills building, instruction, or support for end users. Skimping in these areas results in users who are not properly trained and either do not make maximal use of the system or are reluctant to use it. The overall result is that the system's anticipated benefits are not realized. Executive management is then (rightly so) in the position of wondering where its ROI is.

Some vendors are at fault for portraying their systems as easy to use and intuitive to learn. However, busy professionals need hands-on training and reinforcement to ensure that what may appear intuitive to an information systems technician or EHR developer is discernible to the end users. As much training as possible should be done early on, although further training will have to occur after testing and just prior to go-live, and continue after go-live.

Training Approach and Modalities

Many organizations follow a train-the-trainer approach for user training. When trained staff members have completed the initial training, they become trainers for other staff members. Of course, use of this approach varies with the size of the organization and who is being trained. Some physician practices find that train-the-trainer is not as effective as it could be because the method puts pressure on trainer-physician relationships and may only focus on how to operate the technology rather than how it will actually affect the workflow (Hyden 2013).

Using a mixture of training modalities should be considered. In general, some classroom training is required, with on-the-job support also provided. However, the classroom training could be web-based or help screen–based, where users are not only guided by trainers but learn to use such training modalities for greater independence. Different types of users have been found to have different preferences. For example, nurses generally prefer classroom training of at least one to two hours. Physicians prefer one-on-one training. Many hospitals and large clinics find that a required short introduction to a new system in a classroom setting but not necessarily hands-on training is helpful for physicians and can be followed with a reduction in patient load for a period of a few weeks after go-live. Additionally, organizations should make trainers available to provide almost instantaneous assistance, and many have their trainers wear distinctive clothing, such as red jackets, for this purpose.

The first group of users to go live often ends up serving as both partial system designers and testers because glitches almost inevitably occur. The more the system can be tested in advance, the better the live process will be and the more likely users will be to adapt to the new system. Another issue with the first group of users is that they sometimes become trainers. New users often turn to the first group of users for help, especially when the number of trainers available is insufficient for subsequent implementations. There is some risk in this approach. First, it is time-consuming for the initial group of users, who by now should be in full production mode. Second, the initial users may have developed bad habits because they had to learn intuitively or did not learn correctly the first time. (This potential for spreading bad habits also points to the need for adequate initial training and also monitoring to ensure that ongoing use is appropriate.)

Theoretically, by the time the later groups of users go live, system problems will have been worked out and only operational problems will need to be addressed. In actual practice, as more data flow through the system, odds increase that unforeseen system problems will occur, although they should be less frequent than in the beginning.

Finally, it is very important to train users not only on the screens, templates, and other parts of the EHR or health IT but also, as noted above, on the new workflows. In one clinic, physicians were observed walking their patients to the laboratory, to the front desk for check out, to the nurses' station, and so forth. When asked why, physicians stated they were unsure whether the task they had placed in the EHR was getting to the intended destination and wanted to check on that directly. Had workflow been a part of their training and dress rehearsal, they would have been able to see the flow of information through the office. Of course, workflows need to have been evaluated and altered appropriately by this stage of the project. One physician described the EHR implementation in his office as one in which it felt like the office staff was "redesigning an airplane in flight" (Gerson Lehrman Group 2009).

As part of their workflow training, physicians need training on how to use EHRs or other health IT systems during the actual patient encounter. Terry (2013) notes that use of the EHR in the exam room need not harm the doctor-patient relationship if the EHR is used properly. A family physician and his coauthors note that a major reason why many physicians become too absorbed in their computers to pay adequate attention to their patients during office visits is because their training—which must include learning to type, typing without neglecting patient needs, telling the patient in real-time what they are doing, encouraging patients' participation in building their charts, and looking at the patient instead of the screen—is insufficient (Ventres et al. 2006).

Human Resources and Labor Relations Issues

Various human resources and labor relations issues are associated with training and should be planned for in advance. One issue in a union shop is the extent to which unionized jobs change. Early collaboration with union representatives can forestall many problems with union staff. Another issue for all types of organizations is how and when training will occur—during the workday, in overtime, or on personal time. Will users be required to achieve a certain level of competency that is tested and certified? Users are often given new access and authentication mechanisms that may be accompanied by signing a confidentiality agreement. For physicians, incentives or compensation for training may need to be considered.

Another issue is the subsequent role of staff members who worked on the EHR or other health IT project. On an individual level, physician champions of health IT may move into an informatics role, supporting ongoing knowledge development. Nurse trainers may assume technical support roles or provide informatics support for nursing care. Nurse educators continually monitor and update materials made available to the healthcare organization's consumers. HIM professionals can serve as excellent monitors of ongoing use of the EHR or other health IT, evaluate emerging technology, conduct benefits realization studies, and contribute to ongoing process improvement, operations analysis and redesign, and workflow changes. Other roles for that may suit some staff include database maintenance, data quality monitoring, outcomes management, consumer informatics (merging consumer education with individual health data), information security, knowledge management, and user relations.

Check Your Understanding 9.2

Choose the best answer:

1. Workflow and process improvement during EHR implementation is focused on:

   a. Determining functional requirements

   b. Documenting changes the EHR requires in workflows

   c. Modifying the EHR to fit current workflows

   d. Redesign of workflows for more standardization

2. Stakeholder preparation during EHR implementation includes:

    a. Assessing which potential users need more training than others

    b. Creating a plan to retire or terminate staff who will no longer have jobs

    c. Developing a communication strategy about the implementation

    d. Orienting users to the purpose for an EHR

3. Configuration management refers to:

    a. Arranging for software to be tested

    b. Changing the physical plant to accommodate new technology

    c. Configuring data dictionaries and clinical decision support rules

    d. Controlling what changes are made to a system

4. Testing interfaced applications to ensure that they exchange data properly is:

    a. Function testing

    b. Integrated system testing

    c. Performance testing

    d. Unit testing

5. Which of the following types of training ensures that end users can navigate the EHR for specific functions?

    a. Briefing

    b. Education

    c. Skills building

    d. Support

Data Conversion and Other Activities Prior to Go-Live

The final phases of testing, conversion, and training are often performed in overlapping time frames. Obviously, training must occur early for those users who will help configure the system and perform tests, but end-user training can and should wait until closer to the go-live.

Data Conversion

Pre-live conversion may include data conversion. **Data conversion** in the strictest sense refers to changing data in one file type (for example, a word-processing document) to another file type (for example, a spreadsheet). There are many data conversion programs—some freely available on the Internet—that support such conversion, and most do a very good job. However, if a text document, database, or spreadsheet format is not supported in a packaged conversion program, the data must either be converted to an intermediary format (ASCII text) and then converted to the new format. Page format settings as well as macros and other attributes are often lost during the conversion process. If the application or the "export to ASCII" option is not available, the only recourse is to have a custom conversion program written from scratch.

If the organization is lucky, data in one system are compatible with the system being implemented. Then, data conversion just involves transferring data from the old application to the new one. Such data conversion may not require any special program. However, since the purpose of getting a new application is to acquire additional functionality, it is very likely that the existing data set does not include all the data needed to support the new functionality. As a result, the new functionality may not work as effectively as desired with the old data. Depending on the application being changed, it may be that data conversion can be avoided by simply retaining the old software for a period of time until data processes performed on it are no longer needed. For example, an old billing system can be retained until all current bills have been produced and a large percentage have been paid (Zielinski 2012). An older inventory system, similarly, could be retained until all inventory documented in that system is used.

Movement of data to a new application is more difficult where the existing data, such as patient demographics, are needed for a long period of time. In this case, extensive mapping of the old applications to the new ones is needed to reconcile the location, format, and characteristics of data between the old and the new systems (Frech 2015). It may be determined that some data that are unavailable in the older application are not needed in the future; some data may be available from other sources; and, in some cases, data may need to be manually abstracted. As a simple example, an old system may not include the ZIP+4 postal code. Some organizations may decide not to worry about that, or they could obtain a program from the post office that fills this field.

The existence of error in the old system and its potential impact on the new system must also be considered. For example, master person indexes (MPIs) are known to have an error rate of between 9 percent and 10 percent (Banton and Filer 2014). It may be necessary to do a MPI cleanup project before converting an old MPI to a new system. Some organizations, especially large hospitals with antiquated and often self-developed systems, have found the differences between the old system(s) and new system to be so significant that they only convert a portion of their data for only certain applications. Much as with chart conversion (described earlier in this chapter), manual abstraction of some key data may be required (Gettinger and Csatari 2012). Decisions about how and when data conversion will take place are essential in planning any implementation, but they become critical when replacing one system with another. Generally, such decisions will have been made earlier in the planning process, but actual data conversion would occur at this point.

Go-live Rehearsal

A **go-live rehearsal** is a relatively new but highly effective phenomenon. In this process, staff members take turns role-playing themselves and patients as they run through a typical workflow and process with the EHR or other health IT system in the test environment. For physicians in their offices, this rehearsal has proven to help them to be more comfortable using the EHR in the examining room with the patient. The fear of patient disruption prevents many physicians from fully adopting an EHR, even though most patients have favorable reactions to most EHR operations (Gerson Lehrman Group 2009).

Support

Finally, the day of go-live is the day on which users actually use the system in a production mode. Vendors often measure **go-live** as the first instance that a user logs onto the production system. This should be the time when "all hands are on board." Many organizations will attempt to go live during a "light" period, such as a weekend day, night shift, or other time when fewer patients are expected and the minimum number of users are required. If a light period cannot be identified, the organization might create one by not scheduling as many patients or by closing part of a unit and shifting patients to another unit. Whatever strategy is adopted, a full complement of support personnel should be available to provide assistance. For a major EHR implementation, a full complement of vendor support staff also should be made available. If the EHR or another health IT system is being implemented in a small physician office and vendor support staff will not be on site, there should be assurances that vendor support will be available via telephone.

Organizations should anticipate that Murphy's law, which suggests that if anything can go wrong, it will, may play out during go-live. To avoid mishaps, preparedness is crucial.

EHR Adoption and Optimization

Although go-live signifies the time when the end user starts to use the system, go-live should not be considered the end of the EHR implementation activities but the start of the adoption phase of implementation. The RAND Corporation makes a distinction between a system being installed versus a system being adopted. It notes that "an organization may invest in [installing] a system and expose clinicians to it, but **adoption** requires acceptance and use of the system on a regular basis" (Fonkych and Taylor 2005, 18).

In keeping with getting more value from an EHR or other health IT, however, even adoption is insufficient. **Optimization** of systems significantly improves productivity and contributes to the clinical transformation intended from an EHR and other types of health IT. The National Learning Consortium (2013) has developed a checklist on strategies for optimizing an EHR system that focuses on special opportunities in point of care charting, CPOE, clinical decision support, and BCMAR applications.

Monitoring System Usage

A first step in ensuring adoption and then optimization is to determine the extent to which the system is being used and used appropriately. During go-live and immediately thereafter, support staff must be readily accessible to troubleshoot any problems. These staff should also keep their eyes and ears open for any signs of potential nonuse or misuse. For example, if one staff member who is anticipated to have difficulty has no questions or apparent problems during go-live, that may be because the individual is actually not using the system. A special point needs to be made to touch bases with every user, not just those communicating problems directly. Observation alone may not be enough to detect issues. A person clearly at the computer workstation entering data may be struggling to locate information or not using templates appropriately. Actual use should be monitored to be sure that every user is using the system as intended.

Auditing data entry by running simple reports can be an effective way to check that systems are used properly. For instance, at the end of the first week after go-live, generating a list of all patients and their smoking status would not only check that such data had been entered (hence, every expected user entered one data element) but also verifies that this data element (which is required for the MU incentives) is being captured. If there are fewer entries than anticipated, a list of patients without such entries can identify potential user issues. However, before assuming that users were not entering the data, the system configuration should be checked. It may be possible that there is a comment field associated with this data element that is capturing information that should have been put into a structured format. There may also have been a training issue, where expectations were not set or were not clear.

It is appropriate to begin collecting productivity and performance data soon after go-live, especially if the information can be generated directly from the system itself or an indirect measure can be used as a surrogate. For a physician office, for example, a way to infer that the system is being used is to monitor that the amount of dictation has gone down or number of lines of transcription is reduced.

Conducting Satisfaction Surveys

Conducting a **user satisfaction survey** is a visible way for the organization to recognize the importance of adoption and obtain some consistent feedback. Two or three short satisfaction surveys might be used to gauge adoption, especially because intervention efforts may be taken after each one, if needed.

Especially for ambulatory care environments, a **patient satisfaction survey** also can be a powerful tool. Many providers find that patients value having online access to their medical records and that physicians are significantly more likely than patients to have concerns about the EHR (Ross et al. 2005). Evidence that patients are satisfied (assuming they are) may help physicians overcome concerns that their patients do not like them using the EHR.

While patient satisfaction surveys can help alleviate physician concerns about patient acceptance of EHR use, they can also be used to evaluate how the use of EHRs and other types of health IT affects the physician–patient relationship in terms of quality of care. Although performed on psychiatric outpatients, which may not be the norm for medical practice, a study by Stewart and colleagues (2010) used patient satisfaction surveys of psychiatric outpatients (adults with chronic mental illnesses) before and after the implementation of an EHR and found no significant difference in psychiatrist-patient relationships when the psychiatrist used an EHR. Providers participating in the study observed that attention to communication style, interpersonal manner, and computer proficiency helps maintain the quality of the relationship following EHR implementation. In another study also related to behavioral health, Klein and colleagues surveyed patients of a family practice group about depression screening using an automated questionnaire and concluded that the screening was feasible and resource-efficient; additionally, the physicians anecdotally noted instances in which previously resistant patients felt more comfortable with this screening method (Klein et al. 2006). As a last example, a public health professional practicing in a low socioeconomic status community found that teenagers were more likely to admit to risky behavior when answering questions on the computer than when face to face with the professional (Medical Net Systems n.d.).

Emphasizing Celebration

Celebration involves the recognition of achievements and the expression of appreciation to users for their extra effort. It is also an opportunity to obtain informal feedback.

The value of celebration in the implementation of the EHR or another health IT system cannot be overemphasized. Ideally, celebration should occur at strategic milestones throughout the project's implementation phases. Timing celebrations with achievement of milestones also allows recognition that progress is being made and that implementation is not an endless journey but a series of steps. Individuals, departments, and others should be recognized for their contributions.

Celebration does not have to be loud and raucous. It can be tasteful and in keeping with the culture of the organization.

Conducting a Benefits Realization Study

Formal benefits realization studies are not easy to do and require baseline data to be valid. However, they can reassure users (and executive management) that the system is having an impact and is worth bearing with any interim issues. See chapter 11 for details on conducting a benefits realization study.

Creating a Customer Service Attitude

Another important strategy to help gain adoption is to create a **customer service** attitude within the organization—where the customers are the end users of the system (as well as the patients). Achieving this perspective may be easier said than done, but there are many ways to take small steps toward this goal. For example, holding a pizza lunch or donut breakfast once a week after go-live is an opportunity to obtain feedback in a nonthreatening way. Remember, individuals struggling to use the system may think their jobs are at risk, may be embarrassed in front of their peers, or may have other misperceptions that need to be debunked. Furthermore, if they are struggling or not using the system at all for some reason, that absolutely must be addressed. All support staff, help desk personnel, supervisors, and others need to understand the importance of a customer service attitude when a system such as the EHR is being implemented. The level of change and potential risk in the system is one that many find stressful.

Conducting Walk-throughs/Rounding

A final way to promote better adoption is to conduct **walk-throughs**, much like physicians perform rounds (Nelson 2013). Walk-throughs should first be done shortly after go-live to thank everyone, and then again several weeks or months after go-live and periodically after that. These walk-throughs may provide surprising insights into what is really happening—despite the best of intentions, good customer service, and other efforts, it is conceivable that individuals who should be fully using the system are still using workarounds, putting up with slow response time, or simply are not sure what an icon on the screen means. Additionally, walk-throughs are a terrific way for staff to realize that leaders are genuinely interested in the EHR or other type of health IT and its continued success.

Walk-throughs should be conducted by a variety of staff and should become a routine means of gaining feedback. Done en masse and only once or twice, walk-throughs can imply an investigation with the potential for blame. Citizens Memorial Hospital is a Healthcare Information and Management Systems Society (HIMSS) Davies Award winner and has achieved stage 7 (the highest level) on the HIMSS EHR Adoption scale (HIMSS Analytics 2011). During an interview with the CIO (Fluckinger 2010), it was learned that "seven years after going live, Citizens Memorial still staffs a physician resource room near the medical-surgical unit with an information systems specialist or a super user to help docs or other EHR users who have questions about or problems with the system." Whereas the CIO at Citizens Memorial talks about taking questions and fielding problems, others who perform outreach to users on a continuing basis find they also get many new ideas and thoughts for future enhancements to their EHR or other health IT systems.

Ongoing Strategies

Most healthcare organizations claim that no EHR system is ever fully implemented. If, as Vaughan (2009) suggests, the EHR is "a journey, not a destination," this journey really never ends. Initial installation may be done, but modifications, enhancements, and upgrades are virtually ongoing. Some of the decision making related to the level of customization and benefits realization, for instance, requires as much facilitation and finesse as the initial selection process.

Many lessons will be learned throughout the implementation process. Whether formally tracked and documented or simply recognized and dealt with, the lessons learned should be anticipated and accepted. It may be the culture of some organizations that lessons learned are seen as failures and blame is quickly placed. This approach is not healthy and should be avoided. In fact, it would be wise to discuss this issue in one of the early steering committee meetings and reinforce the value of open and constructive communication, without fear of retribution, in training sessions. Although EHRs are not completely immature products, they are relatively new and the changes they bring are often more comprehensive than any other change the organization has dealt with in the past. Undoubtedly, lessons will need to be learned; ideally, organizations will be willing to write articles and contribute case studies so that others can benefit from the lessons they have learned.

Finally, the EHR is not only implemented in phases but also in a migration path that will continue to be enhanced with new technology, new knowledge sources, and new ideas. Generally, it is understood and accepted that vendor upgrades need to be applied, new regulatory initiatives must be incorporated, and routine system maintenance must occur. In addition, it can be expected that when the EHR is on its migration path, users will see the path enhanced continuously.

Check Your Understanding 9.3

Write a brief description in your own words of the differences between the following states of EHR or health IT systems:

1. Installation

2. Implementation

3. Adoption

4. Optimization

References and Resources

Ames, E., V. Ciotti, and B. Mathis. 2011. Meaningful abuse: The rush toward EHR implementation. *Healthcare Financial Management.* 65(2):70–73.

Arredondo, R. 2012 (December 4). A working healthcare project risk management approach. Sierra-Cedar blog. http://www.sierra-cedar.com/2012/12/04/a-working-healthcare-project-risk-management-approach.

Ashraf, U. 2015 (June 11). The five essentials for software testing. LinkedIn Pulse. https://www.linkedin.com/pulse/five-essentials-software-testing-umar-ashraf.

Badger, S., et al. 2005. Rapid implementation of an electronic health record in an academic setting. *Journal of Health Information Management.* 19(2):34–40.

Banton, C.L., and D.L. Filer. 2014 (October). The impact of multiple master patient index records on the business performance of healthcare organizations. *Journal of Technology Research.* http://www.aabri.com/manuscripts/141877.pdf.

Campbell, R. 2013. The five rights of clinical decision support: CDS tools helpful for meeting meaningful use. *Journal of AHIMA.* 84(10): 42–47.

Carman, C. 2013 (May 8). 4 steps to effective change control. *Insights.* http://insights.dice.com/2013/05/08/why-change-control-isnt-for-sissies.

Carter, J. 2014 (January 20). Modeling clinical workflows and processes. EHR Science. http://ehrscience.com/2014/01/20/modeling-clinical-workflows-and-processes.

Chamberland, B. 2014 (September 18). EHR Success: 4 change management process tips. *InformationWeek.* http://www.informationweek.com/healthcare/electronic-health-records/ehr-success-4-change-management-process-tips/a/d-id/1315823

College of Healthcare Information Management Executives (CHIME). 2010 (September 13). Hospital executives' leadership critical to EHR implementation. In *The CIO's Guide to Implementing EHRs in the HITECH Era.*

Computer Sciences Corp. 2009 (April 27). *Report: Hospitals Must Change Priorities During EHR Implementation.* Falls Church, VA: Computer Sciences Corp.

DerGurahian, J. 2011 (March 3). Concord Hospital's 10 steps for EHR implementation. *Health IT and Electronic Health News.* http://searchhealthit.techtarget.com/news/2240033057/Concord-Hospitals-10-steps-for-EHR-implementation.

Dunbrack, L.A. 2015 (December 14). New EHR technology to spur EHR replacement, other predictions. EHR Intelligence. https://ehrintelligence.com/news/new-ehr-technology-to-spur-ehr-replacement-other-predictions.

Fenton, S.H., K. Giannangelo, and M. Stanfill. 2006 (June). Essential people skills for EHR implementation success. *Journal of AHIMA.* 77(6):60-A–D.

Fields, R. 2010 (August 13). 5 Mistakes that derail an EMR implementation. *Becker's Hospital Review.* http://www .beckershospitalreview.com/healthcare-information-technology/5-mistakes-that-derail-an-emr-implementation.html.

Fluckinger, D. 2010 (October 21). Ten tips for a hospital EHR implementation process. Tech Target Search HealthIT. http://searchhealthit.techtarget.com/tip/Ten-tips-for-a-hospital-EHR-implementation-process.

Fonkych, K., and R. Taylor. 2005. *The State and Pattern of Health Information Technology Adoption.* Santa Monica, CA: RAND Corporation. http://www.rand.org/pubs/monographs/MG409.html.

Frech, T. 2015 (June). Switching EHRs? Get the data conversion correct. *For the Record.* 27(6):30. http://www .fortherecordmag.com/archives/0615p30.shtml.

Gerson Lehrman Group. 2009 (April 28). Obstacles to EHR adoption lie in small group practices. http://www.glgroup .com/NewsWatchPrefs/Print.aspx?pid=38092.

Gettinger, A. and A. Csatari. 2012. Transitioning from a legacy EHR to a commercial, vendor-supplied, EHR: One academic health system's experience. *Applied Clinical Informatics.* 3(4): 367–376.

Guerrero A. 2013 (May 17). Five best practices for training staff on using a new EHR. Software Advice. The Profitable Practice blog. http://profitable-practice.softwareadvice.com/five-best-practices-for-training-staff-on-ehr-0513.

Healthcare Information and Management Systems Society (HIMSS) Analytics. 2011. EMR adoption model. http:// www.himssanalytics.org/hc_providers/emr_adoption.asp.

Hyden, M. 2013 (February 19). 4 common technology mistakes. Medical Group Management Association (MGMA) Connection Plus. http://www.mgma.com/practice-resources/mgma-connection-plus/online-only/2013/february/ 4-common-technology-mistakes.

Jankowski, K. 2010 (August 13). Key decisions to increase productivity in preparation for an EHR implementation. Santa Rosa Consulting. https://www.santarosaconsulting.com/SantaRosaTeamBlog/post/2010/08/13/Decisions-to-Increase-Productivity-in-Preparation-for-an-EHR-Implementation-NextGen.aspx.

Klein, E.W., et al. 2006. Depression screening interfaced with an electronic health record: A feasibility study in a primary care clinic using optical mark reader technology. *Primary Care Companion Journal of Clinical Psychiatry.* 8(6):324–326.

Larmon, C. 2002. *Applying UML and Patterns: An Introduction to Objected-Oriented Analysis and Design and the Unified Process,* 2nd ed. Upper Saddle River, NJ: Pearson Prentice Hall.

Medical Net Systems. n.d. Improving her patient encounters: Changing patients' lives with the EncounterSuite's patient generated medical history. http://www.medicalnetsystems.com/index.php/patient-encounters.

National Learning Consortium. 2013 (September 30). Strategies for optimizing an EHR system. https://www.healthit. gov/providers-professionals/implementation-resources/strategies-optimizing-ehr-system.

National Library of Medicine (NLM). 2016 (May). UMLS®: The Clinical Observations Recordings and Encoding (CORE) Problem List Subset of SNOMED CT. https://www.nlm.nih.gov/research/umls/Snomed/core_subset.html.

Nelson, R. 2013 (July 10). 7 golden rules for EHR optimization. *MedPageToday.* http://www.medpagetoday.com/ Columns/PracticePointers/40363

NLM. 2011. UMLS®: The CORE Problem List Subset of SNOMED CT. National Library of Medicine.

ONC (Office of the National Coordinator for Health Information Technology). 2014 (January). SAFER self-assessment guides: System configuration. https://www.healthit.gov/safer/safer-guides.

Quammen, B. 2011 (March 2). Big-bang EHR: The right choice. *Health Data Management.* http://www .healthdatamanagement.com/opinion/big-bang-ehr-the-right-choice.

Rollins, G. 2005. The prompt, the alert, and the legal record: Documenting clinical decision support systems. *Journal of AHIMA.* 76(2):24–28.

Ross, S.E., et al. 2005. Expectations of patients and physicians regarding patient-accessible medical records. *Journal of Medical Internet Research.* 7(2):e13.

Santamarina, R. 2015 (July 22). The implementation of risk management. Project Management.com. http://www.projectmanagement.com/articles/299628/The-Implementation-of-Risk-Management.

Stewart, R.F., et al. 2010. Do electronic health records affect the patient-psychiatrist relationship? A before and after study of psychiatric outpatients. *BMC Psychiatry*. 10:3.

Terry, K. 2013 (July 1). Doctors need more training on how to use EHRs during patient encounters. InternetMedicine.com (originally published on iHealthBeat). http://internetmedicine.com/2013/07/07/doctors-need-more-training-on-how-to-use-ehrs-during-patient-encounters./

Thompson, J. 2010 (October 25). Six best practices for EHR implementation. *Healthcare IT News*. http://www.healthcareitnews.com/news/six-best-practices-ehr-implementation.

US Department of Health and Human Services (HHS). Practices guide: Configuration management. HHS Enterprise Performance Life Cycle Framework. http://www.hhs.gov/ocio/eplc/EPLC%20Archive%20Documents/08%20-%20Configuration%20Management%20Plan/eplc_configuration_management_practices_guide.pdf.

Vang, S. 2014 (October 8). The underappreciated workflow: Why standardization offers path to efficiency. Hayes Management Consulting blog. http://meetings.hayesmanagement.com/blog/the-underappreciated-workflow-why-standardization-offers-path-to-efficiency.

Vaughan, C. 2009 (September 29). EHR implementation is a journey, not a destination. *HealthLeaders Media*. http://www.healthleadersmedia.com/technology/ehr-implementation-journey-not-destination.

Ventres, W., S. Kooienga, and R. Marlin. 2006. EHRs in the exam room: Tips on patient-centered care. *Family Practice Management*. 13(3): 45–47. http://www.aafp.org/fpm/2006/0300/p45.html.

Voltz, D. 2014 (June 20). EHR proliferation hurts physician workflow. *InformationWeek*. http://www.informationweek.com/healthcare/electronic-health-records/ehr-proliferation-hurts-physician-workflow/a/d-id/1278721.

Wallace, S. 2007. Scope and change control. In *The ePMbook*. http://www.epmbook.com.

Zielinski, L. 2012. How to avoid conflicts between your new EHR and your old billing company. *Family Practice Management*, 19(1): 14–17 http://www.aafp.org/fpm/2012/0100/p14.html.

Chapter 10
Data Infrastructure

Key Terms

ABC Coding Solutions
Algorithms
Analytical database
Big data
Business intelligence
Checklist
Classification
Code
Code set
Coding
Comment fields
Continuity of Care Record (CCR)
Controlled vocabulary
Core measures
Customer relationship management (CRM)
Data
Data architecture
Database management system (DBMS)
Data denormalization
Data dictionary
Data Elements for Emergency Department Systems (DEEDS)
Data entry aid
Data infrastructure

Data mapping

Data mart

Data modeling

Data normalization

Data provenance

Data Quality Management Model

Data repository

Data set

Data warehouse

Discrete reportable transcription (DRT)

Executive decision support

General Equivalence Mappings (GEMS)

Granular

Healthcare Effectiveness Data and Information Set (HEDIS)

Health Intelligence

Heuristic thought

Information

International Classification of Functioning, Disability, and Health (ICF)

International Health Terminology Standards Development Organization (IHTSDO)

Institute for Safe Medication Practices (ISMP)

Knowledge management

Lexicon

Logical Observations Identifiers Names and Codes (LOINC)

Macro

MEDCIN

Medical Dictionary for Regulatory Activities (MedDRA)

Metadata

National Drug Code (NDC)

National Quality Forum (NQF)

Natural language processing (NLP)

Nomenclature

Online analytical processing (OLAP)

Online transaction processing (OLTP)

Ontology

Optical character recognition (OCR)

ORYX

Protocol

Registry

Registry functionality

RxNorm

Semantics

SNOMED CT

Standard order set

Syntax

Taxonomy

Terminology

Transaction

Transactional database

Unified Medical Language System (UMLS)

Uniform Hospital Discharge Data Set (UHDDS)

Unique Device Identification (UDI)

Universal Medical Device Nomenclature System (UMDNS)

Value

Variable

Vocabulary

Vocabulary server

Wisdom

Learning Objectives

- Define the role of data infrastructure in the creation of the data-information-knowledge-wisdom continuum.

- Describe types of data, their formats, and their processing requirements.

- Connect vocabulary standards, code sets, and their mapping that support data sharing across the continuum of care.

- Distinguish between types of data architectures, including data sets, databases, data repositories, and data warehouses, and how each supports the EHR and other types of heath IT.

- Define data management and describe the purpose and techniques for data modeling.

- Describe the purpose and construction of a data dictionary and the importance of metadata in an electronic environment.

- Discuss the importance of data, information, and knowledge governance and data quality and data integrity.

Data are the lifeblood of any organization. However, the difference between data in healthcare organizations and data in most other industries is that healthcare data are a greater challenge to capture, store, and process because of their textual and contextual nature. Moreover, the data documented in healthcare often are not raw facts and figures, which are typically considered data in the "data processing" sense, but the results of analyzing these data into information (Amatayakul and Cohen 2008). Where a computer typically relies on data to process into information, clinicians want to mentally process data and prefer to document information. This results in a true paradigm shift in how clinicians document—whether or not they use a computer. This means that the value of an EHR and other health IT is highly dependent on the design of its data infrastructure, including its architecture, vocabulary, and quality. Although most commercial electronic health records (EHRs) and other health information technology (health IT) products are based on a proprietary data infrastructure, it is important for those individuals implementing such systems to have an overall understanding of how the data infrastructure works to ensure the quality of the data, optimize system performance, and aid clinicians in adoption. In addition, the federal government is mandating an increasing number of standardized vocabularies that provide broader adaptability to national reporting structures, data sharing, and other uses of health information.

Data Infrastructure

Data infrastructure refers to the data needed to operate an enterprise and how they are defined (vocabulary), structured and processed (architecture), and quality assured.

Chapter 2 reviews the data-information-knowledge-wisdom (DIKW) continuum. As a refresher, **data** are the raw elements that make up our communications. Humans have the innate ability to combine data they collect and, through all their senses, produce **information** (which is data that have been combined to produce value), enhance that information with experience to produce knowledge, and with insight produce **wisdom** that can be used as best practice This processing of data (also known as **heuristic thought**) is what affords humans their intelligence. Computers, on the other hand, are machines that, although they can process data very rapidly and tirelessly, cannot create knowledge without humans programming them with complex structures that attempt to simulate human brain power and heuristic thought. However, computerized sources of data, information, and knowledge can be immensely helpful when we have to rapidly collect and process numerous facts and quickly make decisions based on recalling a tremendous volume of information. Computers are now capable of applying pattern analysis and other highly sophisticated techniques to help healthcare providers do their jobs. For example, a computer can generate a list of the medications that a given physician tends to order most often or recognize a person's handwriting and convert it into typed form.

Today, information technology is a key element of knowledge management and the learning organization. Knowledge workers have come to be better understood, and their relationship to organization performance is being emphasized, such as by Mostashari (2011), a former deputy national coordinator in Office of the National Coordinator for Health Information Technology (ONC), in describing the importance of the EHR in a learning health system. The concept of knowledge management is receiving renewed interest because it is recognized that "quality care of patients requires evaluating large amounts of data at the right time and place and in the correct context" (Wickramsinghe et al. 2009). The concept of the DIKW continuum has also matured. When it was first described, it was considered a logical progression, where each step forward in the continuum would enhance the value of data. Some critics (Weinberger 2010) have suggested that "the depiction is too clean. That knowledge is more creative, messier, harder won, and far more discontinuous." Other researchers (Booker et al. 2008) and even proponents of the DIKW model (Bellinger 2004) observe that data, information, knowledge, and wisdom are more than simply collections; the whole represents more than the sum of its parts and has a synergy of its own. Such observations certainly are suggestive of the challenges EHR developers face in incorporating best practices and evidence-based guidance into clinical decision support (CDS) systems. The progression of how data are used to support knowledge, the insights into knowledge workers discussed in chapter 6, and the importance of learning to healthcare in general, and EHR in particular are very relevant concepts today as the industry considers how transformative it is for clinicians to be recording data rather than information in the EHR, how they learn to use the EHR and other health IT, how well they trust the knowledge provided through these systems, and ultimately how they can be optimized for maximum value.

Data architecture for an EHR and other health IT, then, is the structure that must support the ability of the information technology (IT) to create the knowledge continuum—as messy as it may be! (Bali and Dwivedi 2007; Alavi et al. 2010). Data architecture for an EHR or other type of health IT is built on an information infrastructure that includes various types and formats of data, creation of various structures in which to store and process data, and various measures that ensure data quality and integrity.

Formats of EHR Data

Clinical data come in many different forms. Figure 10.1 illustrates seven different formats of data and gives examples of their various sources. Essentially, these seven different formats of data are stored in an information system in one of two ways: as an electronic reflection of the original or as a structured data model.

- *Reflections of original data,* often referred to generally as *image data,* include document images, unstructured text data, video, audio, vectors, and diagnostic images. Image data without any further processing are stored in an indexed manner and may be recalled from storage using the index. The *index* is a database that contains the patient's name, health record number, and potentially other identifying information. Information to identify and describe the image and the information it contains may be entered into a database in a variety of ways, depending on the nature of the image. For paper documents that are scanned and stored, such information may be entered by the person who is operating the document imaging scanner or by a bar code that is printed on the document or affixed as a label to the document. If the document is a word-processed document, it can be converted into XML (extensible mark-up language), which tags various elements within the document according

Figure 10.1. Clinical data types and their sources

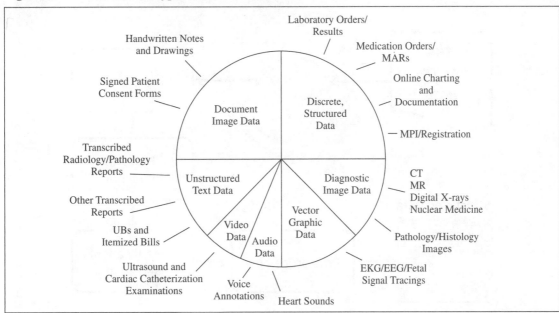

Source: Kohn 2002.

to predefined parameters; these tags enable the computer to find data by searching for specific element types. Alternatively, much more **granular** (that is, at a more detailed level of specificity) indexing may be accomplished by **optical character recognition (OCR)** Current "tried and true" forms of OCR include optical mark recognition, intelligent character recognition, voice recognition, and discrete reportable transcription (see below). Additionally, new OCR applications are being investigated by EHR vendors as an alternative means of data entry (Fea 2016). Research is currently being performed on combining various OCR technologies with neural networking for even more sophisticated outputs. For example, applications may extract textual words from photographs or scanned images of a handwritten document and stored them as structured data (see figure 10.2) (Spillman 2013).

- *Structured data* (sometimes also referred to as *discrete data*) are stored in databases without further processing being necessary and can have significant operations performed on them. Structured data are the values associated with variables that are the important information to be captured about a patient. As in mathematics, a **variable** is a function that may assume any given value or set of values. A **value** is any point or attribute in the range of a function. Values for variables in EHRs and other health IT are generally captured via checklists, pull-down (or drop-down) menus, or templates that guide a user in entering the values for each of the required variables. (Refer to figure 1.8 for an example of such data capture techniques.) The ability to enter structured data is one of the key elements that distinguishes an EHR from its paper counterpart. For example, temperature is a variable; 99.8°F is one value that may be entered, perhaps at the time of the patient admission. If the patient spikes a fever later in the admission, the value entered at that time may be 101.0°F. Appropriate medication may cause the temperature to decrease over time, and these data points may also be captured—in fact, they could be captured through human entry or via a connection to a monitoring device. Because these values are entered as structured data,

Figure 10.2.   Example of intelligent OCR

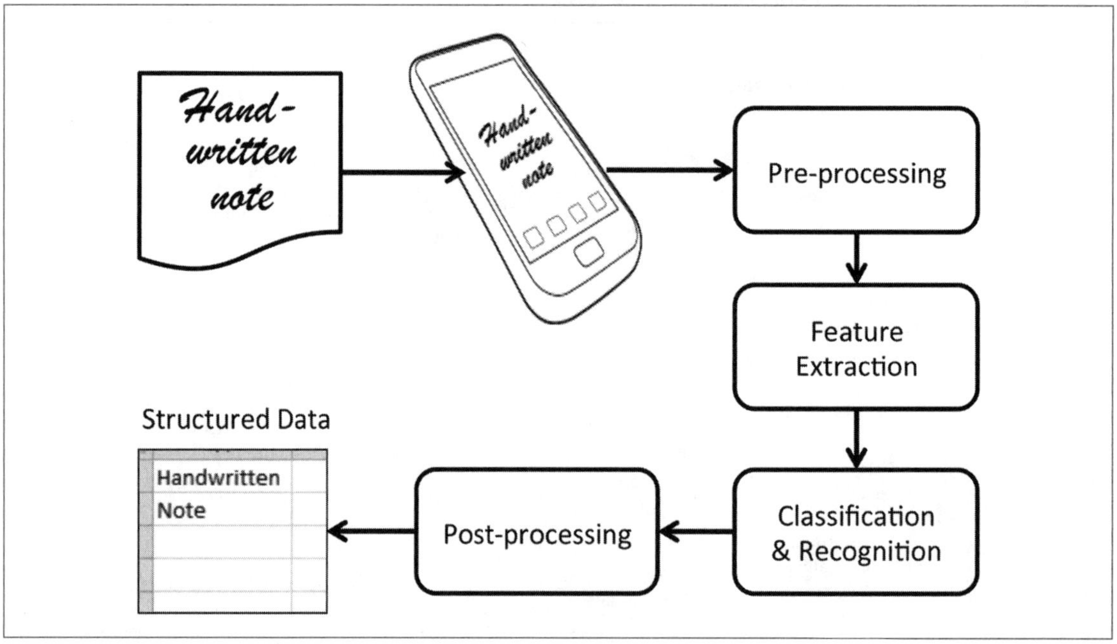

Adapted from Spillman, A (2013) Captricity.

they can be graphed automatically by the computer, illustrating the patient's variations in temperature. The range of valid values may also be specified in the database programming, and the computer can check that only values within that range are entered. In the example of temperature, a valid range can be specified numerically. For values that are narrative, such as drug names, descriptions of pain, and so forth, the values may be limited to a set of predefined terms that are displayed in a checklist or drop-down menu. The basis of all CDS in EHRs is structured data.

Some debate the relative value of unstructured versus structured data. However, two important points essentially make the debate moot.

First, both forms of data have an important place in an EHR and other types of health IT. For example, it may be equally important to retrieve a streaming video of a cardiac catheterization as it is to retrieve the discrete values of the last set of vital signs. It is, however, somewhat less possible to retrieve individual data elements from unstructured data, such as document images or narrative text, although sophisticated indexing and search strategies are making it easier to do so.

Second, the debate usually compares narrative text keyed in as a stream of human thought as compared to data entered into a computer as structured data elements (such as from pick lists or pull-down menus). Again, there is value to both narrative text and structured data, although their value are different, and there are trade-offs in using either format. For example:

- Narrative text allows an individual to record context and conveys subtle differences that structured data often does not. The trade-off is that such data may take longer to enter and be more difficult to process. The time it takes to enter narrative data depends on the volume of data, any available dictation or transcription support, and the keyboarding ability of the user. Narrative data are more difficult to combine with other data (for example, on a graph) to form new information.

- Structured data can be easily captured and are very accurate. Experienced users of an EHR can move rapidly through a series of structured data collection processes. However, these processes must be well designed and tailored to each user or the process could take longer than keyboarding or dictating. Structured data are generally based on a standardized data dictionary, if not a controlled vocabulary, that makes use of the data very precise. The ability of the user to select the exact elements needed for the communication makes the process accurate as well. Structured data also allow data to be processed into graphics for trending and other analyses.

A significant part of system build during EHR implementation is to construct tables of structured data for use in data capture, and to review how those may be used for various presentation purposes, decision support processing, reporting, and generation of narrative notes. For example, specific values may be entered for vital signs. Often, a range of values is specified as valid values, with anything outside the range generating a flag as part of the system's CDS system. In addition to use in CDS, the clinician may want to see these vital signs trended against the level of medication administered. A variety of **data entry aids** are available to help users in selecting the desired data to be input. A *pick list* is one form of data entry aid that may be used for medications. In this case, everyone who will use the system, including the ordering physician, dispensing pharmacist, and nurse who administers the medication, must agree on the data options that affect the computerized physician order entry (CPOE) system, pharmacy information system, and medication administration record system. Often, one or more clinical vocabularies are referenced to ensure use of standardized terms.

Those who are implementing the system must also decide when the entering of narrative data will be accommodated. For example, narrative data may be very appropriate at the conclusion of a report of history and physical examination findings to describe a unique situation not accommodated by the structured data selections. Narrative data can be added to templates via **comment fields** that enable a small amount of text to be input. In some applications, however, such as CPOE, narrative in comment fields has been found to lead to inconsistencies that could cause harms to patients (Singh et al. 2009). For example, Singh and colleagues found that a structured data selection was "Warfarin 10 mg orally every day," but an entry in a comment field was recorded as "Take 7.5 mg a day on Monday–Friday only."

In addition to being able to add a narrative note to a structured data entry template, another form of data entry aid that combines the concept of structured and unstructured data is the use of **macros**, which are commands that a user can create and retrieve later that produce a specific set of terms, phrases, or sentences. In EHRs, macros are sometimes called *smart text* or *dot phrases*. In documenting a progress note, a physician could key in a series of codes representing the desired text. The text may include the place where variable data must be inserted. For example, a procedure performed on an ear would require a place for "right" or "left" to be entered. Each macro must be created by either the system implementer or user. In sophisticated EHRs, the system may "learn" a user's common phraseology and, after a few times of entering narrative, offer to create a macro for the user. In using such a system, however, it must be recognized that only a specific set of smart text and the variables within the text are able to be processed. Any element within the narrative that is not a variable is not structured data.

There are also data entry aids that permit narrative context to be applied to structured data and to parse unstructured data. Computers can be programmed to wrap narrative text around structured data elements to form complete sentences. For example, many EHRs contain programs that can produce a narrative report about the history and physical examination for which structured data were selected. For example, a user enters history of present illness (HPI) for a patient presenting with chest pain, the user selects "mild" for severity of symptoms, "stable" for changes in severity, and "dyspnea" in column Yes and "palpitations" and "dizziness" in column No; from these selections, the EHR can create the following sentences: "The symptoms are described as mild. The symptoms have been stable. Associated symptoms include dyspnea accompanying the chest pain, but not palpitations or dizziness." In comparison to the example of the smart text, this narrative reflects fully standardized and structured data. Figure 10.3 illustrates this example. ("Chest pain" was recorded on a previous screen). A number of EHRs offer this feature, although many clinicians find that the result is a much longer, less user-friendly note than what would have been produced if handwritten on paper or dictated. In addition, there are concerns that all records start to read the same, putting into question the quality of the data collection process.

Computer programs called *natural language processors* also can break apart (or parse) narrative text by words or phrases and encode the words and phrases for later processing. This is essentially the reverse of the preceding process. **Natural language processing (NLP)** enables narrative data to be converted into structured data elements and stored in a database. NLP is still somewhat immature with respect to being a common function in an EHR system; however, there are a growing number of successful experiments in using NLP for extracting data from narrative notes in EHRs. A survey of five major provider settings (HealthPartners, Park Nicollet Health Services, Billings Clinic, Kaiser Permanente, and Geisinger Health System) found that using EHRs with a typology for categorizing electronic measures of quality and safety (dubbed *e-indicators*) through an NLP process gave much more clinical relevancy to the measures (Fowles et al. 2008).

NLP has been combined with speech dictation to result in **discrete reportable transcription (DRT)**, which enables tagging elements in a document transcribed into an XML format so they can be placed into structured data collection templates. DRT still requires human intervention; however, the best of both worlds (a narrative document and structured data) can be achieved when DRT is associated with speech dictation, a dictionary of narradata (discrete data derived from narrative reports), and NLP tools that automatically move the dictated and tagged speech to the template (Catuogno 2010; Schwartz 2015).

Figure 10.3.   Narrative notes from structured data

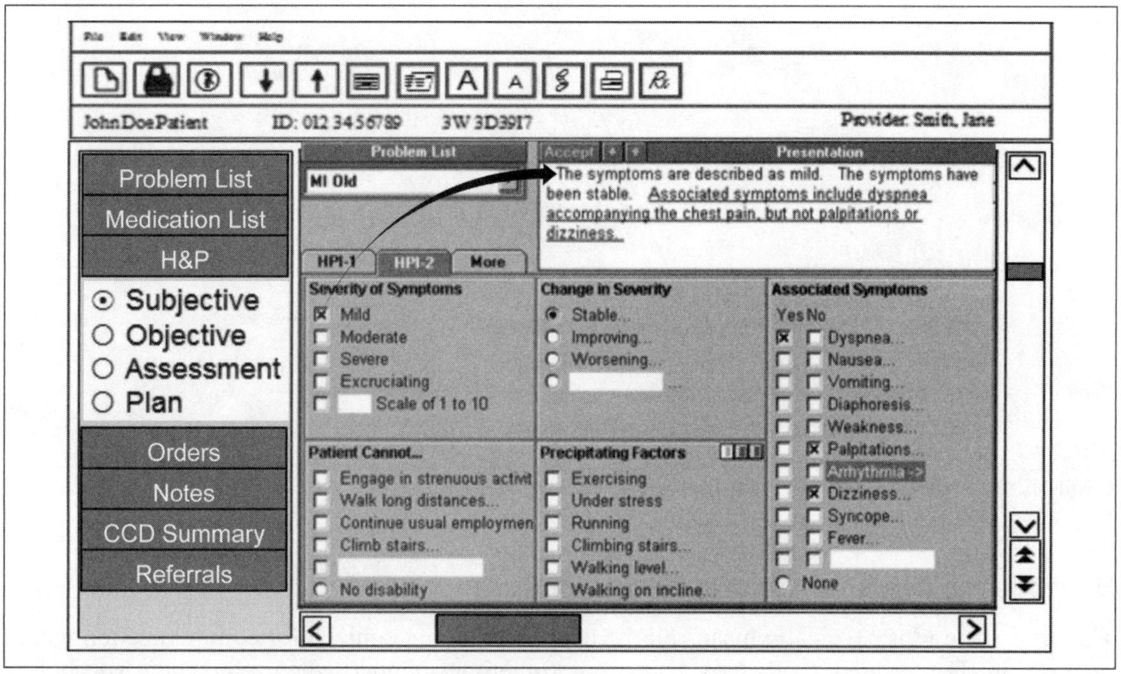

In summary, both structured data and narrative text in an EHR afford much greater access to data than when recorded in a paper record. Structured data may provide a more automated approach to achieving the knowledge continuum, whereas unstructured data rely more on human intervention to achieve knowledge from the data.

Vocabulary Standards

As should be clear from the preceding discussion, it is important to adopt standards to define and structure the language used to supply the values for structured data—however those data may be generated. The primary purposes of using such standards are to reduce inconsistency and ensure understanding.

Unfortunately, in healthcare there are many ways to define, classify, and represent how a language can be structured and used. One way to view the interrelationships among language components is illustrated in figure 10.4.

Language

Language generally refers to a system of communication using an arbitrary set of vocal sounds, written symbols, signs, or gestures in conventional ways with conventional meanings. In the schema proposed in figure 10.3, language is the broadest possible set of words available for communication among a group of people.

People often refer to "the language of medicine," meaning a subset of words used primarily in medicine. This subset sometimes is referred to as *vocabulary* and other times as *terminology*. Dictionaries identify vocabulary and terminology as synonyms. Figure 10.3 suggests that vocabulary is a somewhat broader set of terms than terminology. In addition to the number of terms, a subtle but important difference relates to usage of the terms.

Figure 10.4.   Taxonomy of healthcare language components

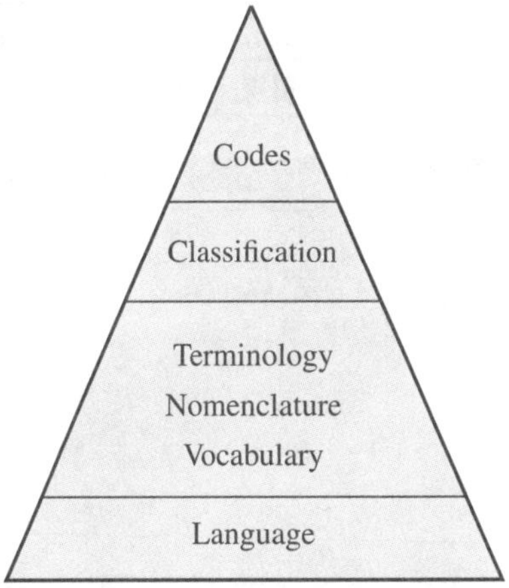

Copyright © 2016 Margret\A Consulting, LLC. Reprinted with permission.

Vocabulary, Terminology, and Nomenclature

The term **vocabulary** typically means all the terms that are recognized for communication within the domain. The term **controlled vocabulary** is sometimes applied when referencing vocabulary standards, suggesting that the terms within the vocabulary are carefully selected for their inclusion and terms outside the boundaries of the vocabulary are not acceptable—or in an EHR might not be able to be processed in various applications. Each term has a unique meaning, and there may be explicitly identified synonyms.

In contrast, the term **terminology** often includes a prescribed set of terms authorized for a specific use. For example, the Common Procedural Terminology (CPT) published by the American Medical Association (AMA) is a set of terms used for professional billing.

The term **nomenclature** refers to a defined system for naming. The Systematized Nomenclature of Medicine (SNOMED) is the most widely recognized nomenclature in healthcare. It is developed and maintained by the College of American Pathologists. Its current version, SNOMED Clinical Terms (**SNOMED CT**), is intended to provide a set of concepts and relationships that offers a common reference point for comparison and aggregation of data about the healthcare process. SNOMED is discussed in more depth later in this chapter. For the purposes of this book, *vocabulary, nomenclature,* and *terminology* are used as synonyms to mean a body of terms and their definitions.

Classification

A **classification** is a grouping of terms of similar meaning, often for defined purposes. The most widely recognized medical classification is the International Classification of Diseases (ICD); its primary purpose is to categorize diseases for morbidity and mortality reporting. For many years, the United States used a clinical modification of ICD (ICD-9-CM) for the additional purpose of reimbursement. The World Health Assembly of the World Health Organization (WHO) endorsed ICD-10 in 1990, and WHO member states began using the classification system in 1994 for both morbidity and mortality reporting. In 1999, the United States began using ICD-10 for reporting mortality and began using a clinical modification of ICD-10 in 2015. The clinical modifications for diagnoses (ICD-10-CM) and procedures (ICD-10-PCS) contain substantial increases in content over ICD-9-CM.

Although the concept of a classification would appear to be straightforward and different from a system of naming, some specialists in medical language use the terms *classification, vocabulary, terminology*, and *nomenclature* synonymously. For example, CPT is essentially a classification of procedures and professional services, maintained by the AMA and used for professional service billing. Similarly, the *Current Dental Terminology* is maintained for the same purpose by the American Dental Association.

This synonymous use of terms can be confusing, especially with respect to developing a data infrastructure for an EHR. For an information system whose primary function is charge capture, a classification system is sufficient and actually more desirable (Bowman 2005). For an EHR where CDS rests on very specific data, a classification system may not be granular enough to generate alerts based on multiple data parameters. However, classification systems and vocabularies can—and should—be coordinated. If a highly granular nomenclature such as SNOMED is used to standardize data capture, it should be able to be mapped into a broader classification system for statistical, reimbursement, and other purposes. **Data mapping** is the process of identifying relationships between two distinct data models. It may be used both to coordinate data among different classification systems and when transitioning from one version of a classification system to another. The National Library of Medicine (NLM) maps versions of ICD and other classification systems to SNOMED (NLM 2015). The Centers for Medicare and Medicaid Services (CMS) and Centers for Disease Control and Prevention (CDC) created the General Equivalence Mappings (GEMs) for temporary use to ensure consistent national data during the time the United States moved from ICD-9-CM to ICD-10-CM/PCS. It is important to be aware when considering use of mapping that one size does not fit all; also, there can be a loss of fidelity when mapping among classification systems that have different levels of granularity is performed (AHIMA 2013).

In addition to mapping various classifications for coordination and version transitioning, mapping serves other purposes within a health IT environment. Mapping may be performed to mediate between a data source and a destination, to consolidate multiple databases, in de-identifying data, and for other purposes. However, mapping alone is not sufficient to share unambiguous data across different components of an EHR or other health IT system. The ability to use multiple vocabularies across different applications in an EHR system is the function of a **vocabulary server** (Browsers 2006; 3M 2014). The Health Level 7 (HL7) Common Terminology Services (HL7 CTS) is the functional specification standard that provides the interfaces across such applications in support of a vocabulary server.

Taxonomy

A term often associated with classification is **taxonomy**, which is the science or technique of classification. Specialized classifications in use in healthcare may be called taxonomies instead of classifications, especially where the intent is to show "parent-child" relationships between terms in a controlled vocabulary that may form a natural hierarchy (Garshol 2004). For example, figure 10.3 represents a taxonomy of healthcare language. Another important taxonomy is the Taxonomy of Medication Errors, which was developed by the National Coordinating Council for Medication Error Reporting and Prevention (NCC MERP) and has been widely adopted by CMS, the Food and Drug Administration (FDA), the US Pharmacopeia, and other organizations (NCC MERP 2005; FDA 2016). Another common taxonomy in healthcare is the Healthcare Provider Taxonomy code set developed by the AMA, maintained by the National Uniform Claim Committee (NUCC), and freely available on the Washington Publishing Company website (AMA 2008). This taxonomy is used to digitally encode physician specialties on electronic claims (CMS 2010).

Codes, Code Sets, and Coding

In discussing concepts associated with vocabularies and classification systems, the term **code** refers to a representation of words to enable machine processing. Codes may be applied to vocabularies or classification systems. Code systems may have a structure associated with them or be random representations. For example, ICD has a hierarchical structure. In this context, **coding** is the term applied when representations are assigned to the words they represent. Coding diagnoses and procedures is the assignment of codes from a code set that follows the rules of the underlying classification or other coding guidelines.

Encoders are computer software programs that assist human coders in assigning appropriate codes by making the classification systems available electronically. EHR systems may include an encoder. In addition to encoders, many EHRs developed for use by physicians in offices or clinics incorporate documentation support to help physicians assign the correct evaluation and management (E/M) codes from CPT based on their documentation to support optimal reimbursement. CMS also uses codes from the Healthcare Common Procedure Coding System (HCPCS) for certain procedures or services performed by physicians, physical therapists, and others (CMS 2015). Totally automated code assignment, which is called computer-assisted coding (CAC), also is possible. NLP technology can read the data contained in the EHR and apply various **algorithms** (rules-based approaches) or statistical approaches to assign codes (Sagence 2014). If the codes to be applied are highly **granular** (that is, related very specifically to individual words or short phrases) and include codes for relationships between words (for example, causes), CAC can improve accuracy and productivity of coders (Crawford 2013; Dougherty et al. 2013). Where codes are more reflective of broad classifications (such as ICD or CPT), the quality of the underlying documentation drives the success with which NLP can succeed (Schnitzer 2000; Fenton 2002).

The term **code set** is frequently used to refer to a group of associated codes. The codes may represent individual terms in an inventory or dictionary of terms. When associated with an entire language or terminology, an inventory or dictionary of terms often is referred to as a **lexicon**. The codes also may represent classes of terms in a classification, such as ICD. In its Transactions and Code Sets regulation (for standard billing transactions), the Health Insurance Portability and Accountability Act (HIPAA) includes medical code sets (such as ICD and HCPCS, including CPT) as well as nonmedical code sets, such as revenue codes and claims adjustment reason codes. The phrase "HIPAA code sets" is frequently used to describe the medical code sets permitted to be used in the HIPAA transactions.

Another usage of the terms *code* and *coding* should also be observed. In information technology (IT), *code* refers to the representation of instructions used to direct the processing of a computer. *Coding* then refers to writing the instructions. This is the software that makes our computers work. Obviously, precision in language matters.

Finally, there is also a distinction between *code set* and **data set**. The latter refers to a predefined list of data, often to be collected for contribution to a registry or special database for analytical purposes. Data sets are described later in this chapter.

Check Your Understanding 10.1

1. The data architecture of IT:

    a. Affords standards for use of code systems and classifications of data in health IT

    b. Describes how the structure of the technology supports the knowledge continuum

    c. Offers a means to identify functional requirements for health IT

    d. Provides for the governance of information as processed by technology

2. The benefit of narrative text in an EHR or other type of health IT is to:

   a. Convey subtle differences not easily captured with structured data

   b. Ease human use of information technology in health care

   c. Ensure accuracy of data entry and use

   d. Reduce data entry time for end users of EHR or other health IT

3. The process of converting narrative data to structured data for storage in a database is:

   a. Classification

   b. Coding

   c. Discrete reportable transcription

   d. Natural language processing

4. The purpose of SNOMED-CT is to:

   a. Ensure unique meaning for all medical terms, hence standardizing the language of medicine

   b. Group terms with similar meaning for different purposes

   c. Provide a common reference point for comparison and aggregation of data

   d. Replace all other medical terminologies and classification systems with a single system

5. In which case is computer-assisted coding MOST successful?

   a. Codes are highly granular

   b. Codes reflect broad classifications

   c. Underlying documentation reflects high-level, summary information

   d. Coding is performed for reimbursement only

Classifications and Vocabularies in Certified EHR Technology

The National Committee on Vital and Health Statistics (NCVHS) was tasked under HIPAA to make recommendations for uniform data standards for patient medical record information. After several years of analyzing the many candidate terminologies (there are reportedly more than 100 different terminologies, of which NCVHS reviewed 46) and hearing public testimony, NCVHS recommended that the federal government recognize a "core set of terminologies" (NCVHS 2003) and that Department of Health and Human Services (HHS) direct government agencies to become early adopters to accelerate the process for incorporation of standardized terminologies in private sector information systems.

As a result, the Final Rule on the Initial Set of Standards, Implementation Specifications, and Certification Criteria for Electronic Health Record Technology (CEHRT) (45 CFR 170[b] 2010) for the meaningful use (MU) incentive program included the following classifications and terminologies.

ICD-10-CM and ICD-10-PCS

ICD-10-CM is a standardized classification of diseases, injuries, and causes of death. ICD-10-PCS provides a standardized classification of procedures. The National Center for Health Statistics (NCHS) maintains the diagnosis part of the classification and CMS maintains the procedure part of the classification. Codes are updated each year, effective with start of the federal fiscal year (October 1). Guidelines for coding and reporting are approved by four organizations that make up the Cooperating Parties: American Hospital Association (AHA), American Health Information Management Association (AHIMA), CMS, and NCHS. In addition to their use in mortality reporting, morbidity reporting, and reimbursement, ICD-10-CM/ or SNOMED CT is required for compiling the problem list in certified EHR technology (CEHRT) used to earn MU incentives.

ICD-10-CM greatly expands the number of diagnosis codes (from 13,600 in ICD-9-CM to 69,000). Because the international version of ICD does not include a procedure code system, the United States has created an extensive procedure classification system (PCS). In ICD-10-PCS, the United States greatly expanded the number of codes, from 4,000 procedures to 71,000 procedures. ICD-10-PCS includes much more precise definitions for operations than ICD-9-CM. In addition to there being many more codes (and more extensibility due to use of alphabetical characters in the codes) in ICD-10-CM compared to ICD-9-CM, the ICD-10-CM codes are designed for capturing much greater detail. They include explicit laterality, greater specificity, extensions, and combination codes to support greater diagnostic accuracy, improved quality measurements and outcomes analysis, better statistical precision for public health reporting, and improved payment accuracy, value-based purchasing analysis, and trending (Hazelwood 2003).

SNOMED CT

SNOMED CT is a comprehensive clinical reference terminology that allows for consistent capture of detailed clinical information. It was originally developed in 1965 as the Standardized Nomenclature of Pathology (SNOP) before being converted to the Systematized Nomenclature of Medicine (SNOMED) and undergoing several versions by the College of American Pathologists (CAP). Starting in January 2004, the NLM made SNOMED CT core content and all version updates available free of charge. In 2007, CAP transferred the intellectual property rights of SNOMED CT to the Denmark-based International Health Terminology Standards Development Organisation (IHTSDO 2009). As a member of IHTSDO, SNOMED CT is subject to the IHTSDO Affiliate license provisions (incorporated in the License Agreement for Use of the UMLS Metathesaurus), and is free to users in the United States (NLM 2015). SNOMED CT is an official standard, an attribute necessary for the United States to adopt the code system for use in the EHR. Supporting tools that aid software developers in using SNOMED CT continue to be available directly from SNOMED Terminology Solutions, a division of CAP.

As a core terminology for the EHR, SNOMED CT provides a common language that enables a consistent way of capturing, sharing, and aggregating health data across specialties and sites of care. SNOMED CT has several components, including the following:

- A concepts table containing 344,000 concepts with unique meanings and formal logic-based definitions organized into hierarchies (see figure 10.5)

- A descriptions table containing more than 913,000 English-language and 660,000 Spanish-language descriptions or synonyms for flexibility in expressing clinical concepts

- A relationships table containing approximately 1.3 million semantic relationships to enable robust reliability and consistency of data retrieval

As part of its goal for a nationwide, interoperable health information technology infrastructure to improve the quality and efficiency of healthcare, HHS supports the NLM to fund, coordinate,

Figure 10.5. SNOMED CT concepts

SNOMED CT concepts are organized into the following top-level hierarchies, subject to change as requirements, scientific, and ontological developments occur:

- Clinical finding
- Procedure
- Situation with explicit context
- Observable entity
- Body structure
- Organism
- Substance
- Pharmaceutical/biologic product
- Specimen

- Special concept
- Physical object
- Physical force
- Event
- Environments and geographical locations
- Social context
- Staging and scales
- Qualifier value
- Record artefact

Source: SNOMED CT Starter Guide, version 2016-08-17, IHTSDO.

and/or perform official mappings between standardized clinical terminologies and HIPAA code sets (that is, ICD and CPT). NLM uses its Unified Medical Language System (explained later in this chapter) to support such mapping. Integrated terminology management depends on the ability to capture key clinical data in detailed, standardized form (using standardized vocabularies, codes, and formats as applicable) as close to their original sources (patients, healthcare providers, laboratories, diagnostic devices, and so on) as possible (Campbell and Imel 2005). As such the NLM is undertaking a number of mapping projects and supporting investigations into their effectiveness.

The UMLS CORE project is an example of one such investigation into the use of problem list terminologies. Studying use of the SNOMED Problem List Subset in six large healthcare institutions, Fung et al. (2010) found that most institutions use their own local terminologies; however, when evaluated together, most of the frequently used problem list terms (PLTs) could be found in standardized terminologies. Furthermore, with developing mappings and crosswalks, the SNOMED Problem List Subset could be effectively used to reduce variability in PLTs and enhance interoperability of problem list data.

LOINC

Logical Observation Identifiers Names and Codes (LOINC) terminology is widely used for representing laboratory data in ordering laboratory tests and reporting laboratory test results. It has been further enhanced to include other observational data, such as vital signs, and is widely used for implementing standardized assessments and care management in nursing home and noncritical access hospital swing beds (MDS 3.0) and home health (OASIS-C). It is maintained by the Regenstrief Institute and supported in part by grants and contracts from NLM, the Hartford Foundation, and other HHS funding sources (LOINC from Regenstrief 2010). It is required for use in the MU incentive program for documenting laboratory data.

LOINC also provides codes that can be used to describe the nature of documents being exchanged using the HL7 Clinical Document Architecture (CDA) standard. This aspect of LOINC is particularly important because the HIPAA Administrative Simplification provision mandates the adoption of standards for electronic claims attachments. A claims attachment includes the clinical and administrative information sometimes necessary to adjudicate claims. This information may include a discharge summary, diagnostic imaging report, invoice for special pharmaceuticals, and others (LOINC from Regenstrief 2015).

RxNorm

RxNorm is a standard notation for clinical drugs developed by NLM, the Veterans Administration (VA), and the FDA in consultation with the message standards development organization,

HL7. It represents a drug's ingredients, strength, and dose form and includes various relationships to other drugs, such as equivalencies, trade names, and so on. The RxNorm provides normalized names for clinical drugs and links its names to many of the drug vocabularies from commercial drug-knowledge bases that are commonly used in pharmacy management and which are often used in EHR systems as knowledge sources for drug decision support (such as Multum, Micromedex, First Databank, Gold Standard Drug Database, and MediSpan). RxNorm also includes the National Drug File–Reference Terminology (NDF-RT) from the Veterans Health Administration, which is a terminology used to code clinical drug properties, including mechanism of action, physiological effect, and therapeutic category (NLM 2014). RxNorm is also the standard code set for clinical drug names required under the MU incentive program.

Other Important Classifications and Terminologies in EHRs

In addition to the previously discussed terminologies that are included in the requirements for the MU incentive program, the following additional vocabularies (listed in alphabetical order) are important for specialized data capture:

ABC Coding Solutions (formerly Alternative Link) is a joint venture of the Foundation for Integrative Healthcare and Alternative Link. It provides more than 4,500 codes to describe complementary and alternative medicine and nursing services (integrative healthcare) (ABC Coding Solutions 2016). In 2003, CMS approved a pilot test of the codes as a means to fill gaps left by HCPCS codes. The intent was to facilitate comparisons of the economic and health outcomes of convention, complementary, and alternative health practices (Dunkleberger 2003). In 2006 the pilot was discontinued. CMS (2010) issued a statement that ABC (Advanced Billing Concept) codes would not be permitted in HIPAA transactions (that is, claims). Commercial insurers, however, continue to find these codes helpful in evaluating nonphysician and alternative medicine health services.

Diagnostic and Statistical Manual of Mental Disorders, Fifth Edition (DSM-5) from the American Psychiatric Association (APA) is widely used in behavioral health both to encode data as well as to supply standard criteria in naming conditions. DSM-5 links with the U.S. implementation of ICD-10-CM (APA 2015).

International Classification of Functioning, Disability, and Health (ICF) is a health and health-related classification system maintained by the World Health Organization (WHO) that reports body functions and structures, activities and participation, and environmental factors. Implementation of ICF started in 2001, and the classification is used in clinical settings for functional status assessment, goal setting and treatment planning and monitoring, as well as outcome measurement (WHO 2015).

MEDCIN is a proprietary medical vocabulary developed by Medicomp Systems. It includes more than 250,000 terms for symptoms, history, physical examination, tests, diagnoses, and therapies. A number of EHR products incorporate the MEDCIN Engine directly. The company also offers a web-enabled tool that works with all major browsers. Its purpose is to enable rapid entry, retrieval, and correlation of relevant clinical information, including with CPT, ICD, LOINC, RxNorm, SNOMED CT, and other vocabularies, at the point of care and to produce narrative reports from the same data (NLM 2015). Although the content coverage of SNOMED CT as a reference terminology outperformed MEDCIN in a direct comparison conducted in 2007 (Brown et al.), MEDCIN remains a well-liked way for physicians to enter structured data into an EHR for aggregation, analysis, and data mining while also generating narrative notes.

MedDRA is the **Medical Dictionary for Regulatory Activities** and was developed by the International Conference on Harmonisation. It is owned by the International Federation of Pharmaceutical Manufacturers and Associations. Now in its 18th version (September 2015), its purpose is to enable entry, retrieval, and analysis of data relating to all phases of drug development and to the health effects and malfunction of devices (MedDRA 2015). It is used internationally by drug regulatory agencies and the pharmaceutical industry to more readily exchange and analyze data related to the safe use of medical products (NLM 2015).

Nursing terminologies are becoming increasingly integrated into EHRs. Nine terminology sets unique to nursing are recognized by the American Nurses Association (ANA). These nursing sets contain terms to represent nursing diagnoses, outcomes, and intervention (Thede and Schwirian 2014). Figure 10.6 lists terminology sets unique to nursing that have been approved by the ANA (2012). In addition, ANA recognizes nursing diagnosis terms in SNOMED CT and additional nursing terms in ABC Codes and LOINC. Many of the ANA terminology sets are also mapped to SNOMED CT (Kim et al. 2011). A license from SNOMED Terminology Solutions must be acquired to map organizational nursing data elements to SNOMED CT.

National Drug Code (NDC) is a universal product identifier for human drugs. For each product trade name, a unique 10-digit, 3-segment number is applied. The segments identify the labeler (the firm that manufactures or distributes the drug), the product (the strength, dosage form, and formulation), and the trade package size. The labeler segment is assigned by the FDA, and the other segments are assigned by the manufacturer or distributor. The FDA maintains a directory of these names, codes, and approved application number, which is updated twice a month. In addition to its regulatory use, NDC codes are widely used for managing drug inventories in clinical and retail pharmacies (FDA 2016).

Unique Device Identification (UDI) is being established by the FDA to improve the quality of information in medical device adverse events reports. The UDI is a unique identifier that identifies the device model, current production information (such as the lot or batch number), and the device's serial number or expiration date. The FDA is also creating the Global Unique Device Identification Database (GUDID), which will include a standard set of identifying elements for each UDI and will be available to the public so that users of a medical device can easily look up current information. The database will not contain any information about who uses a device (that is, protected health information is not included). The UDI and this database will help the FDA identify product problems more quickly, better target recalls, and improve patient safety (FDA 2015).

Universal Medical Device Nomenclature System (UMDNS) of the ECRI Institute (formerly the Emergency Care Research Institute) is an international standardized nomenclature and coding system for more than 8,842 unique medical device concepts and definitions, with an additional 15,702 entry terms to facilitate classifying biomedical information. It is used to facilitate identifying, processing, and communicating data about medical devices, and is being used in applications ranging from hospital inventory and work order controls to national agency medical device regulatory systems, and from e-commerce and procurement to medical device databases (ECRI Institute n.d.; NLM 2015).

Unified Medical Language System (UMLS)

NLM provides the nation's principal biomedical bibliographic citation database, MEDLINE/PubMed. There are more than 5,600 titles of reference works and more than 23 million citations

Figure 10.6.   Nursing terminologies

• NANDA-Nursing Diagnoses, Definitions, and Classifications	• Nursing Management Minimum Data Set (NMMDS)
• Nursing Interventions Classification System (NIC)	• PeriOperative Nursing Data Set (PNDS)
• Clinical Care Classification System (CCC)	• Nursing Minimum Data Set (NMDS)
• Omaha System	• International Classification for Nursing Practice (ICNP)
• Nursing Outcomes Classification (NOC)	

in this database (NLM 2016). To index its journals for the databases, NLM developed the Medical Subject Headings (MeSH) controlled-vocabulary thesaurus. It consists of sets of terms naming descriptors in a hierarchical structure that permits searching at various levels of specificity (NLM 2015).

From its extensive experience in controlled-vocabulary thesaurus development and usage for biomedical literature, NLM designed the **Unified Medical Language System (UMLS)** in 1986 to help health professionals and researchers retrieve and integrate electronic biomedical information from a number of sources, not just bibliographic databases. With respect to EHRs, the purpose of the UMLS is to "facilitate the development of computer systems that behave as if they 'understand' the meaning of the language of biomedicine and health" (NLM 2015).

Semantics and Syntax

To help in understanding why NLM with the UMLS should play a coordinating role in terminologies for the EHR, two terms related to the study and use of language should be thoroughly understood: semantics and syntax.

- **Semantics** is the branch of linguistics dealing with the study of meaning, including the ways meaning is structured in language and how changes in meaning and form occur over time. Semantic, then, refers to the meaning of a word or other symbol. For example, the term *attending* may have a general meaning, such as when describing any physician attending to (taking care of) a patient, or the term can be used specifically to mean the particular physician designated to be responsible for the care of a specific patient.

- **Syntax** is the study of the patterns of formation of sentences and phrases from words and the rules for the formation of grammatical sentences in a language. In the example used to describe semantics, it is clear that the pattern (or syntax) in which the terms *attending physician* or *physician attending [to]* are sequenced results in different meanings of *attending* (the first being an adjective that describes a type of physician and the second being a verb that describes what the physician is doing).

For vocabularies to support the language of medicine, both the meaning of terms (semantics) and their format (syntax) must work together to form communications.

Knowledge Sources

To further its goals of serving as the means to retrieve biomedical data from multiple sources, the UMLS develops knowledge sources that can be used by a wide variety of application programs to help retrieve data caused by differences in terminology and the scattering of relevant information across many databases. There are three UMLS knowledge sources:

- *UMLS Metathesaurus* provides a uniform, integrated distribution format from more than 100 biomedical vocabularies and classifications and links many different names for the same concepts. It supplies information that computer programs can use to interpret user inquiries, interact with users to refine their queries, identify which databases contain information relevant to particular inquiries, and convert users' terms into the vocabulary used by relevant information sources. The Metathesaurus is intended for use primarily by system developers but also can be a useful reference tool for database builders, librarians, and other information professionals.

- *SPECIALIST Lexicon* contains syntactic information for many terms, component words, and English words that do not appear in the Metathesaurus.

- *UMLS Semantic Network* contains information about the types or categories to which all Metathesaurus concepts have been assigned and the permissible relationships among these types (for example, virus "causes" disease).

As can be seen from these knowledge sources, the UMLS has a vested interest in controlled vocabularies and ensuring the many different vocabularies of the different domains of clinical care are not only kept up to date but also freely available.

Even as NLM, through its UMLS project, maps vocabularies, mapping at a local level is also an important element of keeping EHRs up to date. The EHR in any given healthcare organization frequently uses both proprietary and standardized vocabularies and data sets and must be mapped to the local environment. Organizations should adopt a strategy to ensure that each EHR upgrade also addresses clinical vocabulary mapping (Bronnert et al. 2011; Assar 2013; 3M 2013).

Check Your Understanding 10.2

1. A predefined list of data to be collected for a specific purpose is a:

    a. Code set

    b. Data set

    c. Taxonomy

    d. Vocabulary

2. Which classification/vocabulary is required to be used in an EHR per the MU incentive program?

    a. ABC Codes

    b. NANDA

    c. RxNorm

    d. UMDNS

3. Nursing terminologies are used to represent which of the following?

    a. Disabilities

    b. Drugs

    c. Interventions

    d. Procedures

4. Semantics is:

    a. Data integration

    b. Study of meaning

    c. Study of patterns

    d. Thesaurus

5. SNOMED CT provides a consistent way to describe:

    a. Concepts

    b. Diagnoses

    c. Document types

    d. Patient identity

Data Architecture

Data architecture refers to the specific way each individual data element is used in the information system. On a practical level for providers seeking to implement an EHR system, a set of data (often predefined or anticipated) that have standardized meanings defined by a controlled vocabulary would be placed in a database for processing. The nature of the processing (for operational use or analytical purposes) determines the type of database. The quality of the outcomes of the processing is first determined by the quality of the data entered and then the quality of the software used for processing.

Data Sets

Data sets were one of the first ways data were structured for use in healthcare, and they continue to be a critical way consistency is achieved in sharing data (Davoudi et al. 2015). A data set is a predefined group of data elements to be collected. Data sets are often defined for the collection of data for various quality reporting programs, such as those used by the federal government, the Joint Commission, and other accreditation programs. Each individual data set encourages healthcare providers to collect and report data in a standardized manner. Although they do not necessarily require use of a controlled vocabulary, most data sets make reference to at least some of the standardized vocabularies or common code sets in healthcare, or may provide a data dictionary that defines data elements for purposes of use within the data set. (See the next section in this chapter for a discussion of these data management functions.)

One of the issues with healthcare data sets is that there are so many, and there is no single standardized data set for all of the EHR—and it is probably not feasible for there to be such. Standardized definitions and ways to collect, populate, and access, display and store common data elements are probably the best actions that can be taken (Fridsma 2013). One of the initiatives that aims to achieve such common data elements is the Structured Data Capture Initiative in the Standards and Interoperability (S&I) Framework. The S&I Framework was adopted by the ONC to enable harmonized interoperability specifications to support national health outcomes and healthcare priorities. It creates a forum where healthcare stakeholders can focus on solving real-world interoperability challenges (S&I Framework n.d.). (See also chapter 13.)

An early initiative to align data sets is the core measures project undertaken by CMS and the Joint Commission, which attempted to align a number of their data requirements into what is referred to as *core measures*. Healthcare organizations continue to find themselves compiling very similar (but not precisely the same) data for different purposes. This proliferation of data sets is a burden on the healthcare delivery system; also, with potentially differing data definitions in each data set, the data may not be comparable (AHIMA Workgroup 2003). The lack of standardized expression and definition of data makes aggregating and using the data for quality assessment or any other purpose difficult. This situation is especially troublesome because there is an increasing demand for care coordination across the continuum of care, and for aggregating data to study populations. If data coming from a hospital are defined differently than data coming from a physician's office, the resultant analysis of the data will be flawed.

In addition to a lack of standardized data definitions, data to be collected as defined by any given required data set may have to be manually abstracted from paper records and even in some cases from EHRs. Such manual abstraction is time-consuming and error-prone, but it has been necessitated in part by the lack of common data definitions and also because many EHRs have been designed primarily for direct patient care functions, not data collection or analysis. (See the next sections in this chapter for discussion of data management functions and potential solutions.)

The following standardized data sets are actively in use today:

- The **Uniform Hospital Discharge Data Set (UHDDS)** is the core set of data elements that form the basis of hospital discharge data systems. Claim forms are the major vehicle for collecting the UHDDS, and definitions, such as for principal diagnosis and other diagnoses, are consistent with the requirements of HIPAA's Transactions and Code Sets requirements. NCHS coordinates the state data collection for national survey data (unpublished interview with M. Greenberg, January 7, 2004).

- CMS quality measure reporting is a requirement for all providers who participate in the Medicare program. Each quality measure reporting program includes its own set of quality measures that include specific data sets. CMS implements quality initiatives to ensure quality health care for Medicare beneficiaries through accountability and public disclosure. The goals for CMS quality measurement are to provide effective, safe, efficient, patient-centered, equitable, and timely care. CMS uses tools that help measure or quantify healthcare processes, outcomes, patient perceptions, and organizational structure and/or systems that are associated with the ability to provide high-quality healthcare (CMS 2015a). CMS has a Measure Management System for developing and maintaining the quality measures used in its various accountability initiatives and programs, including the Hospital Inpatient Quality Reporting (IQR) program, Hospital Outpatient Quality Reporting (OQR) program, Physician Quality Reporting System (PQRS), Value-based Payment Modifier, and others, such as for long-term care settings and ambulatory care settings (CMS 2016). These quality programs are linked to various incentives and/or adjustments to reimbursement, and are subject to change. Medicare is rapidly moving from paying for volume to paying for value and has developed a Quality Measure Development Plan that is significantly revamping its quality measure reporting program to focus on clinical care, safety, care coordination, patient and caregiver experience, population health and prevention, and efficiency and cost reduction. This plan also requires CMS to work collaboratively with federal and state partners, private payers, and organizations such as the **National Quality Forum (NQF)** to create an aligned set of measures that reduces provider burden. Under recent legislative action, the Medicare Access and CHIP Reauthorization Act (MACRA) of 2015, some of the payment adjustments for the PQRS, value-based payment modifier (VM), and MU programs are being sunsetted. Details of the changes in measures and their impact on reimbursement are anticipated to be made public in 2016 (CMS 2016c).

- **ORYX** was established by the Joint Commission to provide rigorous comparison of the actual results of care across hospitals. Performance measurement using ORYX data helps healthcare organizations support performance improvement and demonstrate accountability to the public and other interested stakeholders through the Joint Commission accreditation process (Joint Commission 2015). As previously stated, in 2003, the Joint Commission and CMS began to align measures that were common between them to reduce data collection efforts. These are often referred to as **core measures**.

- The **Healthcare Effectiveness Data and Information Set (HEDIS)** is a tool developed by the National Committee for Quality Assurance (NCQA) and used by more than 90 percent of US health plans to measure performance on important dimensions of care and service. The results are contributed to the NCQA accreditation programs (for health plans), certification programs for service organizations (for example, utilization manager credentialing), and physician recognition programs. NCQA has been very active in the establishment of Physician Practice Connection—Patient-Centered Medical Home (PPC-PCMH), which is designed to improve coordination of care. The PCMH has also been adopted by CMS as a means to demonstrate the highest level of care coordination in its value-based payment initiatives (CMS 2016). Many health plans report these data to employers as they evaluate health plans in offering insurance benefits to employees. Consumers have access to HEDIS results in the NCQA Quality Compass web-based comparison tool (NCQA 2016).

- **Continuity of Care Record (CCR)** is a data set maintained by ASTM International, an international standards development organization, as ASTM E2369-12 Standard Specification for Continuity of Care Record (CCR) (ASTM International 2012). It identifies the most relevant administrative, demographic, and clinical information facts about a patient's healthcare, covering one or more healthcare encounters. The standard specifies not only the data elements to be included but also the XML coding required when the CCR is created in a structured electronic format. ASTM International notes that this is not a core data set for the EHR but a means for one provider to aggregate pertinent information about a patient to forward it to another provider in support of continuity of care. HL7 has developed an implementation guide for sharing the CCR, known as the Continuity of Care Document (CCD), which uses the Hl7 Version 3 Clinical Document Architecture (CDA), Release 2 (HL7 n.d.[a]).

There are many data sets that have been developed for specialized purposes. Some of them continue to stand alone (for example, Surveillance, Epidemiology, and End Results [SEER] Program from the National Cancer Institute, National Institutes of Health), some have been subsumed into various standards (for example, the Data Elements for Emergency Department Systems [DEEDS] in HL7 Version 3), some remain for a limited audience (for example, AHIMA [2003] Core Data Sets for the Physician Practice EHR), and some have been retired (for example, the Patient Care Data Set for nursing terms [ANA 2012]).

Data Registries and Data Registry Functionality

A data **registry** is the collection of the data that have been predefined by a data set. For example:

Data Set	Data Registry	
What data are needed for the registry	*Collection of actual data in accordance with data set specifications*	
Patient Name	Smith	Johnson
Age	12 years	15 years
Dx Code	250.01	250.11
Date of Dx	Sept. 18, 2016	Oct. 21, 2015

Two of the most common registries in healthcare are cancer registries, which are used primarily to track and follow-up on the progress of cancer patients as well as to support cancer research, and immunization registries, which serve to verify that an immunization has been performed and track immunization rates within populations. The California HealthCare Foundation has observed that "studies show that people with chronic conditions get recommended care only about half the time" (quoted in Reese 2008). The foundation points out that a disease registry is a convenient tool to compile key data about specific populations of patients for the purpose of monitoring progress and ensuring follow up. Such registries are deemed so important, in fact, that the Stage 2 MU incentive program offers eligible professionals the option of reporting data from the EHR to a cancer registry, other registry, or both (42 CFR 412, 413, and 495 2012).

Registries are also important to support providers in managing health reform with new payment methodologies under the Affordable Care Act (ACA) of 2010. Federal regulations stemming from ACA have initiated the development of accountable care organizations (ACOs) to improve continuity of care that is believed will ultimately improve the healthcare value proposition (42 CFR 425 2011). ACOs need access to data across the continuum of care to provide continuity of care. ACOs also need better data about quality and cost of care because they are also a payment mechanism wherein providers share the financial risk for patients who are unnecessarily readmitted or have other excessive costs. Registries can support care management across the continuum of care—especially for patients with chronic illnesses such as diabetes, hypertension, asthma, and depression—by reducing potentially duplicative services, better managing drug therapy, and alerting providers of when a patient appears to be at risk for complications. Registries are capable of rapidly providing data that can be aggregated to identify quality of care and cost improvement opportunities. For example, a registry in Sweden helped reduce the revision burden of hip arthroplasty to a small percentage of patients, reducing cost and improving patient quality of life (Larsson et al. 2011).

Registries are generally separate databases that exist apart from a provider's EHR system, and often outside of a given provider's organization. Registries are frequently maintained by a state's public health department, the CDC, or other federal agency. For instance, the CDC provides the National Program of Cancer Registries (NPCR) (CDC n.d.) Narrowly focused registries may be developed and maintained by a hospital, academic medical center, or other affinity group, often in association with a specialty society. For example, the MODY (Monogenic) Diabetes Registry was developed by the University of Chicago and is sponsored by the Juvenile Diabetes Research Foundation and the American Diabetes Association (University of Chicago School of Medicine n.d.). Medical societies and vendors may maintain registries for their members, especially supporting data collection for the Physician Quality Reporting System (such as the American Academy of Dermatology [AAD n.d.]) and the CMS and the Joint Commission core measures. Increasingly, vendors are supporting near-real time data aggregation services to provide quality improvement feedback from these registries.

Because the primary purpose of a registry is population health management, registry functionality in an EHR is not always present, although it can be highly desirable. **Registry functionality** refers to functions that can be performed on a panel of patients simultaneously, rather than functions typically performed in an EHR, which relate to only one patient at a time. For example, a registry function would be to generate a list of telephone numbers of patients who need to be called for follow-up or a mailing list of patients who need to be notified that a drug has been recalled, to evaluate how many patients with certain attributes a provider has treated, to help determine whether joining an ACO is financially viable, and to make any number of other queries. Registry functionality may also be the means by which a provider submits data to an external registry, giving the provider the best of both worlds: registry functionality integrated within the EHR and the ability to contribute to a larger registry that can be tapped for population health data comparisons.

Big data refers to the massive amount of data available to study, which is often in unstructured formats. With big data, traditional databases and methods of analysis are difficult to use. In 2012, IBM observed that 90 percent of the data in at that time had been created between 2010 and 2011 (Zikopoulos et al. 2012). McKinsey Global Institute describes big data as "the next frontier for innovation, competition, and productivity" (Manyika et al. 2011). While big data are often thought of in reference to the retail or manufacturing industries, McKinsey Global Institute describes the US healthcare system as one of five major domains with the biggest potential for transformation through the use of big data. A frequently cited example of how analysis of big data can rapidly provide important discoveries is the case in which big data analytics performed by the California-based integrated managed-care consortium Kaiser Permanente identified that thousands of patients had major cardiac events after taking the drug Vioxx for arthritis. This problem was so quickly identified with such a large population of patients that the drug was withdrawn from the market within only five years of its entry (MSNBC 2004). Applications of big data analytics can be used to identify waste, address known operational inefficiencies, and improve productivity in health care. Such results, however, do not come without challenges. Again, citing the McKinsey Global Institute, investment in technology will be needed to take full advantage of big data, and challenges associated with data access, talent acquisition, and changing mindsets and behaviors will need to be addressed (Manyika et al. 2011). See also chapter 20.

Databases

Electronic data are typically retained in databases. However, not all databases are designed in the same way. Different types of databases perform different functions.

Whether a standard data set has been established by an external entity or a set of data has been captured for internal documentation purposes, the most common data structure for information processing is a file, which contains related records and is housed in a database. In paper-based systems, a file room houses numerous records. Each record is related to a given patient, and an indexing system helps with record location. Within each record, there are a number of forms that guide what data are to be captured. Some forms are simply lined sheets of paper on which certain categories of unstructured data are to be recorded, such as progress notes and orders. Where information is dictated and transcribed, there may be an outline of content, or **protocol**, prescribed in a policy as to what content should be included, such as for discharge summaries and operative reports. Other forms may include **checklists** for recording somewhat more standardized data, such as the checklists for a patient's medical history and physical examinations and many nursing forms to record medication administration, vital signs, and other information. Some healthcare organizations promote use of structured paper forms as they make the transition to an EHR. For instance, paper-based **standard order sets** can be an effective precursor to CPOE. During system build, these paper forms can be used to correctly program the standard order sets that will be embedded in the EHR. The **Institute for Safe Medication Practices (ISMP)** has published guidelines for standard order sets. They note, however, that "if standard order sets are not carefully designed, reviewed, and maintained to reflect best practices and ensure clear communication, they may actually contribute to errors" (ISMP 2010).

Paper file systems are easy and less costly to create than computer systems, but the former are not flexible enough to support relationships needed to describe data in clinical practice. There are limitations to the extent to which their data content can be indexed, extracted, analyzed, and, of course, they are accessible to only one person at a time.

Files of records where the content has been scanned into a computer system basically have many of the same limitations as a paper file system of records. However, electronic documents are stored in a database where indexing capabilities exist, so that it is somewhat easier to identify a particular form or page. In simple document scanning systems, indexing may be applied only to the entire record, group of forms, or individual document; however, document content systems provide more ability to structure some of the content of the documents. Beyond that, documents rendered in XML include metadata tags that further add structure to data within documents (Viola and Mookencherry 2012). Any of these forms of electronic documents make the records accessible to many persons at one time.

To overcome the limitations of scanned and somewhat static documents, most industries have sought to capture more structured data. Over time, a variety of types of databases and **database management systems (DBMSs)**, the software and data structures used to support a database, have been developed to store and process structured data. There are a variety of ways to describe types of databases, and new structures for databases are rapidly being developed. The most traditional database categorization is by their structure, such as the following (Stephens and Plew 2001) and as illustrated in figure 10.7.

- A *flat file database* is the oldest form of database structure. It stores data in a plain text file, where each line of the text file holds one record, with fields separated by delimiters, such as commas or tabs. Although this structure is a simple way to store files, there are no folders or paths to organize the data. Despite the fact that there are many newer, much more functional forms of databases, and most newer forms of databases can import and use the data from flat files, there are many flat file databases still used in health plans and healthcare provider organizations—especially in older patient accounting systems.

Figure 10.7. Database formats

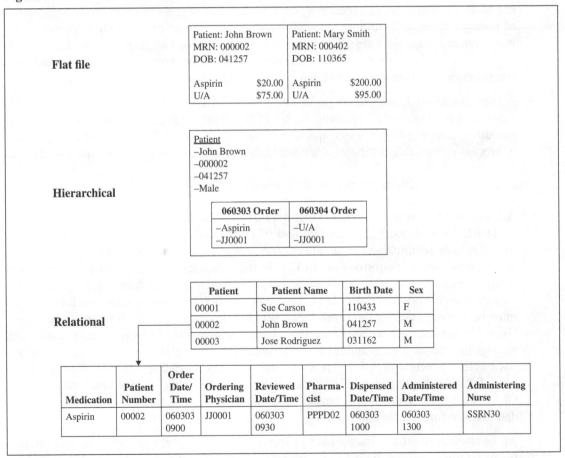

- A *hierarchical database* is the next oldest structure. Although it is no longer used in the development of new EHR systems, it may be found in existing, legacy systems within healthcare organizations. It is modeled from a treelike structure, with a root, multiple branches, and multiple leaves. Records at a branch level are sometimes referred to as *parents*, with records at the leaf level referred to as *children*. Unfortunately, a major constraint of the hierarchical structure is that each child can have only one parent, meaning that multiple copies of the same record may have to be retained to show multiple relationships. Furthermore, programs that retrieve data from hierarchical databases must navigate through the branches from top to bottom to get to the desired record, requiring predefined access paths and slower response time.

- A *relational database* departs significantly from the first two types and currently is the most common form of database. Relational databases are constructed using tables instead of tree structures. The tables do not specify how to retrieve the required data or navigate through predefined paths. Users write queries that reference the data of interest. Software supporting these queries then identifies the tables and specific columns in the tables to retrieve the requested data. Maintenance of the tables is easy. Because rows in a table have no inherent order, they are simply added to as they grow (Mon 2003).

- An *object-oriented database* is one of the more recent approaches to database management. This type of database is derived from object-oriented programming and has no single inherent structure. The structure for any given class or type of object can be anything a programmer finds useful—a linked list, a set, an array, and so on (hence not illustrated in figure 10.7). Furthermore, an object may contain different degrees of complexity, making use of multiple types and multiple structures. As a result, object-oriented DBMSs emphasize programming language integration rather than programming language independence. Interfacing with the database may mean using object-oriented programming language functions (such as C++) rather than embedding a separate database access language (such as SQL).

- A *multidimensional database* might best be considered a hybrid between a hierarchical database and a relational one, capturing the benefits of both database structures so that a large amount of data can be processed quickly. A multidimensional database enables the ability to process various data attributes at a time, including within various hierarchies and levels.

Another way to classify databases is by their function (Rodriguez 2011):

- A **transactional database**, also called *operational database,* enables data to be entered, retrieved, updated, modified, trended, and (if authorized) deleted by the user (rather than by a database administrator or another database specialist). Each operation (that is, entry, retrieval, and so on) performed on the data in this relational type of database is commonly referred to as a **transaction**. Any transaction performed on the database logically represents a single unit of work. For example, in retrieving a laboratory result, the request for the result must be accompanied by the result being supplied to a workstation. A request cannot just "hang" in the database without reaching a logical conclusion. The tools used to create and manage the transactions to and from an online database are referred to collectively as **online transaction processing (OLTP)** tools. (Databases may receive and provide data in offline, batch form, but for use in an EHR, transactions must be online, in real time.) In summary, OLTP deals with many small transactions, in real-time operations, where queries on the database are foreseeable and recurring.

- An **analytical database** is designed to maintain data on which complex analysis is performed. Often, such analytical tools are referred to collectively as **online analytical processing (OLAP)** or *fast analysis of shared multidimensional information* (FASMI). The most common form of database used for OLAP is the multidimensional database. Examples of such analytics are budgeting, forecasting, predictive modeling, and data mining. OLAP is very commonly used to develop **customer relationship management (CRM)** software and game building. CRM can help healthcare providers manage physician credentialing and recruitment, referrals, clinical trials, and other information management tasks that require building and manipulating large contact databases (Microsoft Dynamics 2012). CRM tools will play an increasingly important role in care coordination where health coaches must track patients, their caregivers, providers, and community services. OLAP has most often been used in **executive decision support**, where it may also be called **business intelligence**. Dashboards and other aids are also being used by healthcare executives to gather **health intelligence**, such as to monitor quality, cost, and experience of care measures (Burke 2013). OLAP is also used extensively in CDS system development, and it is used to create computer games that are playing an increasing role in care delivery and management of health and wellness (Cella 2015). OLAP performs complex queries on an occasional, ad hoc basis for research, strategic planning, and knowledge generation.

Data Repository

Each automated application in healthcare uses a database to manage the data collected, processed, and stored by the application. For example, the laboratory information system will maintain data about all the laboratory tests the particular laboratory performs, the nature of the specimen to be collected, data about normal values for the test results, a record of the quality controls applied to the test results, and many other data, including, of course, the results of each test for each patient. These databases are typically created by a vendor or data supplier, making them proprietary to the given application. As a result, an organization that has many applications will likely have many databases, and there will most likely be much duplication of data within those databases. Furthermore, the databases may not be interoperable. In other words, retrieving data from two different databases may require two different queries. Interfaces may be developed to exchange data between databases, but their programming is time-consuming, and the data to be shared must be determined in advance.

A **data repository** is a transactional database designed with an open structure that is not dedicated to the software of any particular vendor or data supplier. It contains data from multiple, disparate application systems so that an integrated, multidisciplinary view of the data can be achieved. A data repository requires the following data integration functions:

- *Data transformation:* This integration function is the process of reconciling and standardizing data content being acquired from numerous data sources. It may be achieved through the application of message standards, SGML/XML languages that define data in documents, off-the-shelf products that make it easier to link and share data between databases, or custom-written interfaces between o products from one vendor and those from another. Clearly, this function would be made easier if there were a standardized data model, a data dictionary, controlled vocabularies and coding schemes, and knowledge representation. (See the next section for a discussion of these data management functions.)

- *Data cleansing:* This refers to detecting and restructuring bad data to ensure quality and usefulness.

- *Linkage:* This integration function is achieved through an enterprise-wide master person index (EMPI).

Not all healthcare providers with EHR systems have a data repository. Either their vendor does not sell one or they have been able to manage without one due to limited need. However, new requirements, such as those in stage 2 of the MU incentive program, demand much more integration of data from multiple sources for clinical decision support and other uses. As providers start to acquire a repository, they often look first for products from their primary incumbent vendor. In some cases, this vendor has developed a viable option. However, these products still may be limited in functionality, and they may be created in a proprietary manner that makes it difficult to move data from other vendors' products into the repository. As a result, organizations may acquire a data repository from a third-party vendor (that is, a vendor other than the one that sells the core clinical components of an EHR or other type of health IT system).

Data Warehouse

In addition to a data repository that is updated in real time and used for transaction processing, healthcare organizations may want to collect and reorganize data into a format more suitable for ad hoc querying and analytical processing. These secondary, or derived, databases are optimized to perform sophisticated analysis on data, and are generally called a **data warehouse**. They are not used directly in patient care—they may not even include patient-identifying information. Figure 10.8 illustrates the relationship between a clinical data repository (CDR) that supports the EHR and a warehouse.

Figure 10.8.   Data warehousing

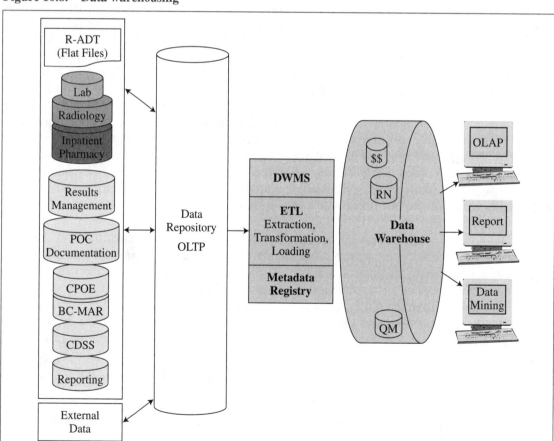

Just as for any database, there is software that manages the data warehouse structure. It is called a *data warehouse management system (DWMS),* and it extracts data from the data repository (or directly from individual application databases), transforms the data so they are suitable for the type of processing to be performed in the warehouse, and then loads the data into the warehouse. This set of functions is often referred to as *extraction, transformation, and loading* (ETL). The transformation process is one of understanding the exact nature of the data based on the metadata in the data dictionary, tagging and indexing the data, and providing supporting data integrity routines.

The data integrity routines may normalize or denormalize the data. **Data normalization** is a process that eliminates redundancy. It is critical for databases intended for OLTP, but it may not be desirable for a data warehouse because storing subsets of redundant data may improve analytical efficiency. The **data denormalization** process is one where intentional redundancies are created. It is important, however, that the redundancy be a true redundancy. Synonyms are not redundant data. When such subsets of data are created, the subset is often referred to as a data mart. Of course, not all data in the data marts may be redundant. For instance, a data mart may be created for executive decision support, another for nursing research, and a third for clinical quality outcomes analysis. Each may have some data that are the same and other data that are unique to the particular data mart (Sharma 2011). In a multidimensional database, which is increasingly used for OLAP, data marts may be used to populate a cube (which is structure that holds data in a more compressed format) for reporting purposes (Cuthbert 2011).

Data warehousing is the most effective way to achieve a consolidated view of the healthcare enterprise and the trends affecting it. However, considerable skills are required to build and maintain a data warehouse and to use it to perform sophisticated analysis. In addition, the data warehouse must have sufficient data to produce statistically valid, meaningful results. Most clinical data warehousing is performed by companies on behalf of providers, large insurance companies, registry services, and government agencies. Clinical data warehouses may be found in academic medical centers or corporate headquarters of integrated delivery networks. Data warehouse applications have been primarily used as follows:

- In *revenue management,* no single transaction system can address all the different contractual and regulatory reimbursement formulas to which a typical integrated delivery system is subject. With revenue based on a mix of fee-for-service, capitation, and risk pooling, a data warehouse is often necessary to obtain a picture of the organization's revenue stream and the factors controlling it.

- *Clinical management* provides one of the greatest returns on investment for warehouses, where day-to-day patient data can be fed into highly sophisticated analytical applications to contribute to best practices and identify areas of excessive variation from best practices.

- *Outcomes management* goes a step beyond clinical management by studying factors such as treatment regimens and response to treatment to develop best practices and contribute to improved clinical outcomes.

- *Operations management* refers to the management of administrative functions. For example, cost accounting, case-based budgeting, and variance analysis help improve the healthcare organization's operational efficiency.

- *Population management* contributes to proactively managing the health of a group of individuals, such as the members of a health plan, by predicting healthcare utilization and identifying at-risk members requiring case management.

Check Your Understanding 10.3

Choose the best answer:

1. How a data element is used in an information system is referred to as:
   a. Data architecture
   b. Data set
   c. Data management
   d. Vocabulary

2. Which statement is *true*?
   a. CMS defines the data set for EHR.
   b. ONC defines the data set for EHR.
   c. There is no one single data set for EHR.
   d. Standards development organizations define minimum data sets for EHR.

3. The Continuity of Care Record is used for:
   a. Aggregating data to forward to another provider
   b. Classifying data for continuity of care
   c. Compiling a registry
   d. Exchanging documents across the web

4. Registry functionality is:
   a. Collection of data for claims processing
   b. Functions that an EHR performs to alert a provider about a potential adverse event
   c. Processes that can be performed on a panel of patients simultaneously
   d. Separate databases for specialized data

5. The database structure in most EHRs is:
   a. Flat file
   b. Hierarchical
   c. Multidimensional
   d. Relational

6. Online transaction processing (OLTP) is performed in what type of database?
   a. Flat file
   b. Hierarchical
   c. Multidimensional
   d. Relational

7. A transactional database for housing data from multiple disparate application is:

   a. Analytics database

   b. Data repository

   c. Data warehouse

   d. Registry

8. Development of games for health is an example of:

   a. Customer relationship management software

   b. Data warehousing

   d. Online analytical processing software

   e. Online transaction processing software

9. In which type of database does data normalization ensure one source of truth?

   a. Analytics database

   b. Data warehouse

   c. Transactional database

   d. Registry

10. Which of the following is *false*?

   a. A data repository contributes data to a data warehouse.

   b. Data repositories are important for integrating data.

   c. Most EHR systems come with a data repository.

   d. Most hospitals do not have their own data warehouse.

Data Management

Data management involves managing the technology of the database; configuring systems to ensure that all required data elements are accommodated and processes produce accurate information; ensuring the quality, confidentiality, and integrity of the data being collected (data governance); and verifying both that processes correctly produce information (information governance) and that knowledge can be derived from the information (knowledge governance). Database administrators, data administrators, HIM professionals, and others participate in data management.

Data Management Components

The basic components of data management include data modeling, data dictionary maintenance, controlled vocabulary and coding system usage (described earlier in this chapter), and knowledge representation. While not every user of an EHR or other health IT needs to be able to manage the data as discussed here, an appreciation for data management helps end users understand the importance and complexity of the systems they are using. It also must be noted that EHR vendors vary significantly as to whether end users (or more likely their staff) have access to and can make changes in any or all of the elements of data management. In general, vendors of lower-priced products give end users minimal or no ability to make changes or reconfigure their systems, whereas higher-priced products may provide sophisticated toolkits that support reconfiguration. In situations where such access is not given, appreciation for what is entailed in data management and the sophistication of the processes associated with it helps end users understand the cost that may be associated with any reconfiguration requested of such vendors.

Data Modeling

Data modeling is a representation of the data structures for a specific database to ensure that the information requirements of an organization are met (Gao 2010). It is often performed during application software design and development (Rouse 2010), but it is also required whenever any changes are made to data elements to be collected in the database (ER/Studio Data Architect 2015). The entity relationship diagram (ERD) illustrates the relationships among a system's different elements (entities). An example is provided in figure 10.9. Although ERDs were first created in the development of relational databases, they are useful in object-oriented databases as well. Figures 10.10 and 10.11 illustrate how the basic ERD has been enhanced with object-oriented notation and used in modeling (Ambler 2006).

Data Dictionary

A **data dictionary**, also called a *metadata repository* or *registry,* is used to capture the results of data modeling, which are **metadata** (data about the data in the data model for a given database or set of databases). The data dictionary is usually stored in a database. It must be very carefully managed, as any change made in it impacts the way software that collects, processes, and shares data is able to use the instructions that derive from the data dictionary.

Because many source systems supply data for use by the core clinical applications that comprise an EHR and also receive data from these applications, healthcare organizations must be aware that a change to one application may have a ripple effect throughout other applications. In addition, external parties conducting quality measurement or using data for other purposes must understand

Figure 10.9.   Entity relationship diagram

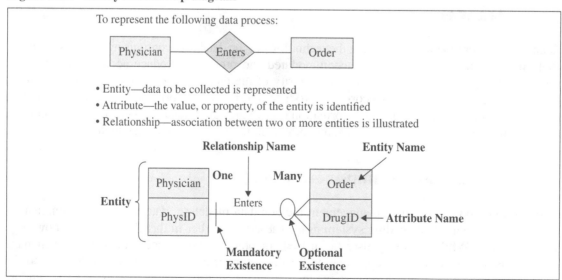

Figure 10.10.   Object-oriented notation

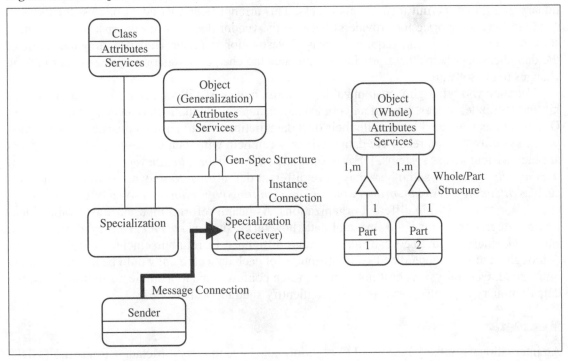

Figure 10.11.   Example of object model

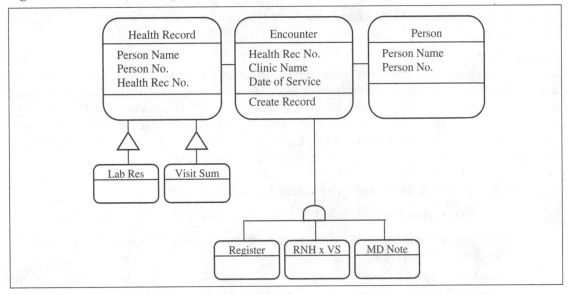

that any changes they make to metadata can have consequences for a provider organization (and its vendor). For example, reconciling differences in metadata may entail countless hours of detailed examination of each required data element. Zafar (2008) describes an incident in which a commercial laboratory suddenly, and without notice, changed a data field originally containing only units to contain both units and the unit of measure. The result was the generation within minutes of thousands of error messages, which took three months to repair.

Because of the complexity and risk of data management, some vendors maintain the data dictionary and do not permit their clients access. This arrangement cuts down on cost for the vendor (and lowers the price for providers) because the vendor does not run the risk of the provider staff making errors that may require extensive investigation to repair. Understanding the nature of the data dictionary helps these providers appreciate the charges a vendor may require for making changes in the software.

Vendors who sell highly customizable software, however, will supply a wizard or other toolkit that facilitates at least limited and controlled changes to the data dictionary by the customer. Organizations may need to compile their own data dictionaries to ensure consistency across disparate systems. A comprehensive data dictionary can help with data processing when terms that are inconsistent across systems. Phrases such as *patient number*, *health record number*, *account number*, *visit number*, and others may have different definitions. Moreover, definitions of terms such as *attending physician*, *primary physician*, *admitting physician*, and so on often have different interpretations within different organizations. As health reform imposes considerable attention to integrating clinical and financial data, how terms such as *episode, encounter, admission, stay*, and others are defined can make a huge difference in reimbursement (Delbanco 2014). Although a unique, standardized set of attributes for each data element would be ideal, it is likely impossible. Generally, it is best not to try to force conformance to a single definition. Thus, the data dictionary must also serve as a map to identify such inconsistencies.

Metadata

An international standard, ISO/IEC 11179, Information Technology—Metadata Registries (MDR) (ISO/IEC 2010) describes how a data dictionary should be maintained to organize metadata and make it useful across different databases. The National Information Standards Organization (NISO) is accredited by the American National Standards Institute develops technical standards for data management. NISO (2004) describes three types of metadata: descriptive, structural, and administrative.

Descriptive Metadata

Descriptive metadata describes each data element to be captured and processed by information technology. This is the most common form of metadata and is that which is typically documented in a data dictionary. In 2006, AHIMA developed "Guidelines for Developing a Data Dictionary" and describes the purpose of a data dictionary as a means to "standardize definitions and ensure consistency of use." Data dictionaries are typically maintained in a database themselves, because they can become very large. A data dictionary contains the following:

- Names of entities, tables, and major categories of data elements

- Descriptions of data attributes (Chidley 1998; Martin and Fuller 1998), including:

  - Logical name (the name that would be presented to the user when displayed as a variable for data collection)

  - Physical name/field code name/label (a mnemonic or other code recognized by the computer)

  - Synonyms (aliases, if used)

  - Definition/description (ideally a standardized definition from a standard reference; otherwise the organization or vendor's definition)

  - Reference (source of the definition)

  - Source of data (person [and potentially qualifications] or medical device, and through which system application)

- Format type (alpha, numeric, alphanumeric; calculated or free text; position of characters [for example, mmddyyyy]; and so on)

- Length (number of characters allowed, if applicable)

- Allowable range, if any (for example, fixed, variable; number of decimal places)

- Valid values, if applicable (for which nonvalid entry would trigger an alert)

- Lexicon, if applicable (coding scheme and/or controlled vocabulary)

- Data restrictions/edits (for example, do not use hyphens)

- Access restrictions (keyed to organization's security access controls)

- Authority to change (for example, system administrator)

- Processing rules (usually recorded as a key to the rules retained in a separate database)

- Relationships among entities or classes (from a data model)

- Keys (links to data model)

Figure 10.12 is an example of a part of an entry in a data dictionary illustrating the metadata for the data element "Temperature, Oral."

Structural Metadata

Structural metadata describes how the data for each data element are captured, processed, stored, and displayed. A data model is generally used to describe these characteristics. Structural metadata not only helps with software development but also can be used to troubleshoot issues with data entry, processing, or information generation after implementation of the software. Structural metadata provides a roadmap to structured data requirements to perform various processes in an EHR and other types of health IT (Dolezel 2015).

Administrative Metadata

Administrative metadata is metadata programmed into software to be generated by the IT itself. This type of metadata provides information about how and when data were created and used. It is

Figure 10.12.   Example of a data dictionary entry

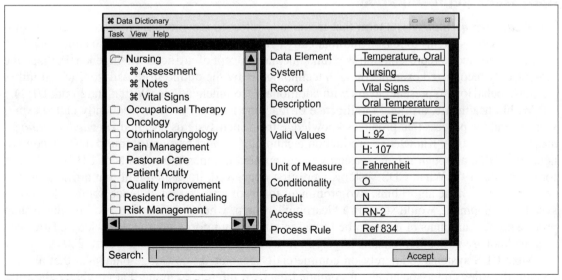

also a record of the instructions given to users about actions to be taken with the IT and what the user response was.

An audit log is an example of administrative metadata. Audit logs are records of actions taken on data within IT. The content of audit logs range from basic, such as only identifying who accessed what component of an EHR or other type of health IT, to complex, such as recording who accessed what data when and what process (for example, view, copy, enter, delete) was performed on the data. Audit logs are often used as a security control, but they may also help determine how a data entry error was made, when it was corrected, and who may have further accessed information about the error. Audit logs are sometimes used to evaluate the timeliness of actions performed, such as what time a drug was actually administered. Information system activity review logs (as required by the HIPAA Security Rule) document the events that impact information technology, such as attempted hacks or system crashes.

Another example of administrative metadata is decision support rules. Decision support rules are programmed into software to recognize various combinations of data that are being captured and to generate various types of actions by the technology according to the rule requirements. For instance, a data element is defined in the data dictionary as required to be entered. If a user does not enter data in this field, the software recognizes this omission because of the rule specifying this requirement and displays an alert to the user to enter data into this field. In health information systems, there are many types of decision support, including clinical decision support in an EHR.

Data provenance is another type of administrative metadata and refers to where data originated and where data may have moved between databases. This type of metadata is becoming increasingly important as the healthcare industry shares data across many different stakeholders. For example, a physician may want to know whether certain information in the EHR came from the patient's personal health record or another provider's EHR (Viola and Mookencherry 2012; Fountain 2014).

Legal Issues Related to Metadata

Although metadata is generally not considered part of the legal health record, it may be subject to compulsory discovery in a court of law under the Amendments to Federal Rules of Civil Procedure and Uniform Rules Relating to Discovery of Electronically Stored Information (referred to as *e-discovery*). It is important to understand what metadata exist within the health information system, to establish policies for their retention and about who may have access to them, and to ensure that these policies are being followed (Haugen et al. 2011).

Knowledge Representation

Knowledge representation is a term that technically refers to the encoding of knowledge on computers to enable systems to reason automatically (Van Harmellen et al. 2007). Also called *machine learning,* knowledge representation is a fundamental concept of artificial intelligence. Perhaps the most widely recognized example of such technology is by the online store Amazon, which mines purchase behaviors to present buyers with additional recommendations (Witten and Frank 2011).

Within healthcare, artificial intelligence or machine learning is more frequently called *expert systems* and the process that produces knowledge from such systems is called *knowledge management* (Koenig 2012). Knowledge production technology is most frequently found in CDS components of EHRs, although it is increasingly being applied in other components of EHRs and other forms of health IT. When CDS systems were first conceived, it was thought that artificial neural networks and genetic algorithms, two prominent forms of artificial intelligence applicable to such system development, would support a "learning" system, where what is "learned" by the system processing vast amounts of data can be turned into not only information but knowledge. However, such technology utilization remains largely in research applications (Boxwala et al. 2009).

Most CDS systems today rely on commercially generated knowledge databases that already contain the rules and associations of compiled data, an inference engine that combines the rules from the knowledge base with the patient's data, and a communication mechanism that allows the system to show the results of the combination of information to the user (Berner 2007; Berner 2009). Greenes suggests there are two key reasons why learning systems are not more widely available in healthcare (2007, 228). First, healthcare data still are not available or structured enough to allow knowledge to be "learned" from them. Second, while any single EHR may have a large amount of data, the data generally are not sufficient in volume or diversity to produce valid and reliable knowledge. Furthermore, the collection of sufficient data and information can be accumulated in typical healthcare environments takes too long, such that any generation of knowledge from them could be out-of-date. To accumulate sufficient data and information in a timely manner, population level data and information must be rapidly processed via sophisticated means and fed back to the user in a manner that is most relevant. Volume, velocity (speed), and variety (diversity) are the hallmarks of big data, and are covered in chapter 20.

Ontology

Ontology is a concept that is often discussed in the context of clinical knowledge representation and the ability to create robust CDS systems. In computer science, **ontology** is a structural framework or representation of knowledge within a given domain (Gruber 2009). Ontology specifies the concepts, relationships, and other distinctions that are relevant for modeling knowledge. The specification takes the form of *classes* (of concepts that comprise various objects), *attributes* (that is, properties or features of classes and their objects), *relations* (that is, how classes relate to each other), *restrictions and rules* (describing logical inferences that may be drawn from an assertion relating to the class or its objects), *events* (that is, how attributes or relations may change), and so on. This framework then is able to be adopted by developers of artificial intelligence/expert systems and in nonstructured information retrieval, extraction, and classification (Roma-Ferri and Palomar 2008). An example of the use of ontology is in the development of a medical error ontology (Mokkarala et al. 2008). In this project, 8 taxonomies used to describe medical errors are merged to create a reference ontology consisting of 12 multidimensional axes that encompass all aspects of a medical error event. The goal of the project is to use the ontology to identify strategies for preventing future adverse events in healthcare.

Data, Information, and Knowledge Governance

Governance is "the establishment of policies and the continual monitoring of their proper implementation for managing organization assets to enhance the prosperity and viability of the organization" (Business Dictionary n.d.). Key assets for all organizations and especially healthcare are data, information, and knowledge (Johns 2015). As previously defined, data are the raw facts and figures that by themselves need to adhere to principles of data quality set forth in the AHIMA Data Quality Management Model (Davoudi et al. 2015), but they generally do not provide value until they are processed into information and, in many cases, have experience applied to the information. Such processing may be performed entirely in the minds of the people collecting the data, or it may be aided by information technology.

At each step in the DIKW continuum, a number of governance processes are needed. Data governance ensures that the policies and continual monitoring of their proper implementation results in quality data collection. Quality data collection in an EHR and health IT environment is directly influenced by the quality of data modeling that contributes to software development that ultimately yields an easy-to-use user interface for data collection. Data collection strategies (technical and policy) need to be created, their use monitored, and improvements made as necessary. Information governance ensures that the policies and continual monitoring of their proper implementation results in retrieval strategies that provide value from the data (Kloss 2015). Knowledge governance similarly ensures that the various forms of experience when integrated with the information result in valued knowledge and ultimately contribute to best practices—which also must adhere to the systems development life cycle (SDLC) to make certain that they remain current and relevant (Foss and Michailova 2009). The technology that supports data collection (including data quality management), information retrieval, and knowledge generation and use) is described in chapter 11.

Check Your Understanding 10.4

Match the terms with the appropriate descriptions:

1. Audit log

2. Data dictionary

3. Data governance

4. Data management

5. Data modeling

6. Data provenance

7. Metadata

8. Knowledge representation

A. Tasks of managing databases, configuring systems, and assuring quality, confidentiality, and integrity of data

B. Record of where data originated and have moved

C. Machine learning

D. Database that stores results of data modeling

E. Administration of policies for quality data collection

F. Record of actions taken on data in information systems

G. Representation of data structures for a database

H. Describes characteristics of data elements

References and Resources

3M Health Information Systems (3M). 2013. 3M ICD-10 modeling and code translation services. http://solutions.3m.com/wps/portal/3M/en_US/Health-Information-Systems/HIS/Products-and-Services/ICD-10-Solutions-and-Services.

3M Health Information Systems (3M). 2014. 3M terminology consulting services: Bridge your data islands. http://solutions.3m.com/wps/portal/3M/en_US/Health-Information-Systems/HIS/Products-and-Services/Products-List-A-Z/Terminology-Consulting-Services.

42 CFR 412, 413, and 495. 2012 (September 4). Medicare and Medicaid Programs; Electronic Health Record Incentive Program—Stage 2; health information technology: Standards, implementation specifications, and certification criteria for electronic health record technology, 2014 edition; Revisions to the permanent certification program for health information technology; final rules.

42 CFR 425. 2011 (November 2). Medicare Program; Medicare Shared Savings Program: Accountable care organizations; final rule.

45 CFR 170(b). 2010 (July 28). Health information technology: Standards, implementation specifications, and certification criteria for electronic health records technology, final rule.

ABC Coding Solutions. 2016. About us. https://www.abccodes.com/about-us.

Alavi, M., et al. 2010. IT-enabled knowledge management in healthcare delivery: The case of emergency care. *ICIS 2010 Proceedings.* Paper 124. AIS Electronic Library. http://aisel.aisnet.org/icis2010_submissions/124.

Amatayakul, M., and M. Cohen. 2008 (May). Rewiring the brain. *ADVANCE for Health Information Executives.*

Ambler, S.W. 2006. Data modeling 101. Techniques for successful evolutionary/agile database development. http://agiledata.org/essays/dataModeling101.html.

American Academy of Dermatology (AAD). n.d. AAD Measurement Tools. http://www.aad.org/education-and-quality-care/performance-measurement-and-quality-reporting/aad-measurement-tools.

American Health Information Management Association (AHIMA) eHIM Workgroup on Core Data Sets for the Physician Practice Electronic Health Record. 2003 (October). Practice brief: Core data sets for the physician practice electronic health record. *Journal of AHIMA.* 74(10).

American Health Information Management Association (AHIMA). 2012. Managing a data dictionary. *Journal of AHIMA.* 83(1):48–52.

American Health Information Management Association (AHIMA). 2013 (May). Putting the ICD-10-CM/PCS GEMs into practice. AHIMA HIM Body of Knowledge.

American Medical Association. 2008. *Health Care Provider Taxonomy,* version 8.0. Chicago: American Medical Association.

American Nurses Association (ANA). 2012 (June 4). ANA recognized terminologies that support nursing practice. http://www.nursingworld.org/MainMenuCategories/Tools/Recognized-Nursing-Practice-Terminologies.pdf.

American Psychiatric Association (APA). 2015. *Essential Guides to DSM-5.* Arlington, VA: APA.

Assar, S. 2013 (February 5). How a terminology platform can support an EHR. Health Language blog. http://blog.healthlanguage.com/blog/bid/216980/How-a-Terminology-Server-Can-Support-an-EHR.

ASTM International. 2012. ASTM E2369-12 standard specification for continuity of care record (CCR). http://www.astm.org/Standards/E2369.htm.

Bali, R., and A. Dwivedi, eds. 2007. *Healthcare Knowledge Management.* London: Springer Science+Business Media.

Bellinger, G. 2004. Knowledge management—Emerging perspectives. *Knowledge Management Toolkit.* W3J.

Bellinger, G., et al. 2004. Data, information, knowledge, and wisdom. *Knowledge Management Toolkit.* W3J.

Berner, E.S. 2007. *Clinical Decision Support Systems: Theory and Practice.* New York: Springer Science+Business Media.

Berner, E.S. 2009. *Clinical Decision Support Systems: State of the Art.* Rockville, MD: Agency for Healthcare Research and Quality, publication no. 1 09-0069-EF. https://healthit.ahrq.gov/sites/default/files/docs/page/09-0069-EF_1.pdf.

Booker, L.D., et al. 2008. The relevance of knowledge management and intellectual capital. *Knowledge and Process Management.* 15(4):235–246.

Bowman, S. 2005. Coordinating SNOMED-CT and ICD-10: Getting the most out of electronic health record systems. *Journal of AHIMA* 76(7): 60-61

Boxwala, A., et al. 2009. Multilayered knowledge representation as a means to disseminating knowledge for use in clinical decision-support systems. American Medical Informatics Association 2009 Spring Congress.

Bronnert J, J. Clark, J. Cook, S. Fenton, R. Scichilone, M. Williams, P. Wilson P. 2011. Data mapping best practices. *Journal of AHIMA.* 82(4):46–52.

Brown, S.H., et al. 2007. Direct comparison of MEDCIN® and SNOMED CT® for representation of a general medical evaluation template. *AMIA Annual Symposium Proceedings 2007.*

Browsers, T. 2006. Appendix B: Terminology services and tools. In *Healthcare Terminologies and Classifications: An Action Agenda for the U.S.* AMIA and AHIMA Terminology and Classification Policy Task Force.

Burke, J. 2013 (March 11). Health analytics vs. business intelligence. http://www.jasonburke.us/health-analytics-vs-business-intelligence.Business Dictionary. n.d. Governance. www .businessdictionary.com/definition/governance.html.

Campbell, J.R., and M. Imel. 2005 (October). The function of rule-based mapping within integrated terminology management. *AHIMA's 77th National Convention and Exhibit Proceedings*. http://bok.ahima.org/doc?oid=61602#. V64IuJgrI2w.

Catuogno, G. 2010. HITECH Act Promises EMR Funding to Clinicians with "Meaningful Use." https://www.scribd. com/document/19197644/Article-Transcription-Impact-on-Meaningful-Use.

Cella, G. 2015 (June 16). Personal Connected Health Alliance, HIMSS and Games for Health announce strategic partnership (press release). https://gamesforhealth.org/2015/06/16/ personal-connected-health-alliance-himss-and-games-for-health-announce-strategic-partnership.

Centers for Disease Control and Prevention. n.d. National Program of Cancer Registries. http://www.cdc.gov/cancer/ npcr.

Centers for Medicare and Medicaid Services (CMS). 2015-2016. Fact sheets and FAQs: Quality Measures, Measures Management System, CMS Quality Measure Development Plan Supporting the Transition to the Merit-based Incentive Payment System (MIPS) and Alternative Payment Models (APMs). http://www.cms.hhs.gov.

Chidley, E. 1998 (June). Data dictionaries: What are they and why. *For the Record,* 14–18.

Crawford, M. 2013 (July). Truth about computer-assisted coding: A consultant, HIM professional, and vendor weigh in on the real CAC impact. *Journal of AHIMA*. 84(7):24–27.

Cuthbert, G. 2011 (September 1). What's the difference between a data mart and a cube? Quora. https://www.quora. com/Whats-the-difference-between-a-data-mart-and-a-cube.

Davoudi S., J.A. Dooling, B. Glondys, T.L. Jones, L. Kadlec, S.M. Overgaard, K. Ruben, and A. Wendicke. 2015. Data quality management model (updated). *Journal of AHIMA*. 86(10):62–65.

Delbanco, S. 2014 (July 2). The payment reform landscape: bundled payment. HealthAffairs blog. http://healthaffairs. org/blog/2014/07/02/the-payment-reform-landscape-bundled-payment.

Dolezel, D. 2015. Metadata offers roadmap to structured data. *Journal of AHIMA*. 86(2):44–46.

Dougherty, M., et al. 2013. Study reveals hard facts on CAC. *Journal of AHIMA*. 84(7): 54–56.

Dunkleberger, C. 2003. *Testing of ABC Codes Approved for Complementary and Alternative Medicine and Nursing.* Washington, DC: Alternative Link and the Foundation for Integrative Healthcare.

ECRI Institute. 2011. Universal medical device nomenclature system. https://www.ecri.org/Products/Pages/UMDNS. aspx.

ER/Studio Data Architect. 2015 (April 16). Data modeling concepts. ER/Studio wiki. http://docwiki.embarcadero.com/ ERStudioDA/XE7/en/Data_Modeling_Concepts.

Fea, R. 2016 (January 5). Specialty clinics still using paper? Get that data into your EMR! Extract Healthy Data blog. http://blog.extractsystems.com/blog/specialty-clinics-still-using-paper-get-that-data-into-your-emr.

Fenton, S.H. 2002. Clinical classifications and terminologies. In *Health Information Management: Concepts, Principles, and Practice.* Edited by LaTour, K.M., and S. Eichenwald. Chicago: AHIMA.

Food and Drug Administration (FDA). 2015–2016. Fact Sheets: Medication Errors, National Drug Code Directory, Unique Device Identification—UDI. http://www.fda.gov.

Foss, N.J., and S. Michailova. 2009. *Knowledge Governance: Processes and Perspectives.* New York: Oxford University Press.

Fountain, V. 2014. Using data provenance to manage patient-generated health data. *Journal of AHIMA*. 85(11):28–30.

Fowles, J.B., et al. 2008 (May). Performance measures using electronic health records: Five case studies. The Commonwealth Fund. http://www.commonwealthfund.org/publications/fund-reports/2008/may/ performance-measures-using-electronic-health-records--five-case-studies.

Fridsma, D. 2013 (January 31). EHR interoperability: The Structured Data Capture initiative. HealthITBuzz. http://www.healthit.gov/buzz-blog/electronic-health-and-medical-records/ ehr-interoperability-structured-data-capture-initiative.

Fung, K.W., et al. 2010. The UMLS-CORE project: A study of the problem list terminologies used in large healthcare institutions. *Journal of the American Medical Informatics Association.* 17:675–680.

Gao, S. 2010. Data modeling in systems analysis. Information System Analysis, University of Missouri–St. Louis. http://www.umsl.edu/~sauterv/analysis/Fall2010Papers/Gao.

Garshol, L.M. 2004 (October 26). Metadata? Thesauri? Taxonomies? Topic maps! Making sense of it all. Ontopia. http://www.ontopia.net/topicmaps/materials/tm-vs-thesauri.html.

Gonzalez, C. et al. 2011. Ontology-based framework for electronic health records interoperability. *Studies in Health Technology & Informatics.* 169:694–698.

Greenes, R.A. 2007. *Clinical Decision Support: The Road Ahead.* London: Elsevier.

Gruber, T. 2009. Ontology. In *Encyclopedia of Database Systems.* Edited by Liu, L., and M.T. Ozsu. New York: Springer-Verlag.

Haugen M.B., A. Tegen, and D. Warner D. 2011. Fundamentals of the legal health record and designated record set. *Journal of AHIMA.* 82(2):44–49.

Hazelwood, A. 2003. ICD-9-CM to ICD-10-CM: Implementation issues and challenges. *AHIMA's 75th Anniversary National Convention and Exhibit Proceedings.* http://library.ahima.org/doc?oid=59978#. V64AJpgrI2w.

Health Level Seven (HL7). n.d.(a). HL7/ASTM implementation guide for CDA R2-Continuity of Care Document (CCD) release 1. http://www.hl7.org/implement/standards/product_brief.cfm?product_id=6.

Health Level Seven (HL7). n.d.(b). HL7 version 3 specification: Data Elements for Emergency Department Systems (DEEDS), release 1. http://www.hl7.org/implement/standards/product_brief.cfm?product_id=326.

Institute for Safe Medication Practices (ISMP). 2010. ISMP's guidelines for standard order sets: 1. http://www.ismp. org/tools/guidelines/standardordersets.pdf.

International Health Terminology Standards Development Organisation (IHTSDO). 2016. SNOMED CT starter guide. http://snomed.org/sg.

International Organization for Standardization/International Electrotechnical Commission (ISO/IEC). 2010. ISO/IEC JTC1 SC32 WG3 Development/Maintenance. ISO/IEC 11179. Information technology—Metadata registries (MDR).

Johns, M.L. 2015. *Enterprise Health Information Management and Data Governance.* Chicago: AHIMA.

Kim, T.Y. et al. 2011 (October 22). Representation of nursing terminologies in UMLS. *AMIA Annual Symposium Proceedings 2011.*

Kloss, L. 2015. *Implementing Health Information Governance: Lessons from the Field.* Chicago: AHIMA.

Koenig, M.E.D. 2012 (May 4). What is KM? Knowledge management explained. *KMWorld.* http://www.kmworld.com/ Articles/Editorial/What-Is-.../What-is-KM-Knowledge-Management-Explained-82405.aspx.

Larsson, S. et al. 2011. Use of 13 disease registries in 5 countries demonstrates the potential to use outcome data to improve health care's value. *Health Affairs.* http://content.healthaffairs.org/content/early/2011/12/06/hlthaff.2011.0762. abstract.

LOINC from Regenstrief . 2010. LOINC background. http://loinc.org/background.

LOINC from Regenstrief. 2015 (December 21). Using LOINC in HIPAA transactions. https://loinc .org/attachments.

Manyika, J., et al. 2011 (May). Big data: The next frontier for innovation, competition, and productivity. McKinsey Global Institute. http://www.mckinsey.com/insights/mgi/research/technology_and_innovation/big_data_the_next_frontier_for_innovation.

Martin, T., and S. Fuller. 1998. Components of the EHR: An overview. *Journal of AHIMA*. 69(9):58–64.

MedDRA. 2015 (September). Welcome to the ICH MedDRA website. http://www.meddra.org/how-to-use/support-documentation/english.

Microsoft Dynamics. 2012. Microsoft Dynamics CRM: healthcare providers. http://crm.dynamics.com/en-us/healthcare-providers.

Mokkarala, P., et al. 2008 (August). Development of a comprehensive medical error ontology. In *Advances in Patient Safety: New Directions and Alternative Approaches,* volume 1: *Assessment.* Edited by Henriksen K., et al. Rockville, MD: Agency for Healthcare Research and Quality.

Mon, D.T. 2003. Relational database management: What you need to know. *Journal of AHIMA*. 74(10): 40–50.

Mostashari, F. 2011 (February 15). Information needs for the learning healthcare system. President's Council of Advisors on Science and Technology (PCAST) Work Group. PCAST Report.

MSNBC. 2004 (October 6). Report: Vioxx linked to thousands of deaths. http://www.msnbc.msn.com/id/6192603/ns/health-arthritis/t/report-vioxx-linked-thousands-deaths.

National Cancer Institute, National Institutes of Health. n.d. SEER data and software for researchers. http://seer.cancer.gov/resources.

National Committee for Quality Assurance (NCQA). 2016. What is HEDIS? HEDIS and Quality Compass. http://www.ncqa.org/hedis-quality-measurement/what-is-hedis.

National Committee on Vital and Health Statistics (NCVHS). 2003 (November 5). Letter to the Honorable Tommy G. Thompson. http://www.ncvhs.dhhs.gov.

National Coordinating Council for Medication Error Reporting and Prevention (NCC MERP). 2005. The National Coordinating Council for Medication Error Reporting and Prevention: The first ten years. http://www.nccmerp.org/tenYearReportExecSummary.html.

National Information Standards Organization (NISO). 2004. *Understanding Metadata.* Bethesda, MD: NISO Press. http://www.niso.org/publications/press/UnderstandingMetadata.pdf.

National Library of Medicine (NLM). 2013–2016. Fact sheets: 2015AA UMLS MEDCIN Source Information, MedDRA Source Information, 2016 MEDLINEFact Sheet, 2015AA UMLS UMDNS Source Information, Unified Medical Language System, UMLS Metathesaurus, Medical Subject Headings (MeSH), RxNorm, Meaningful Use Quality Performance Measures Benefit from New SNOMED CT "Public Good" Use Policy, The CORE Problem List Subset of SNOMED CT, Supporting Interoperability—Terminology, Subsets and Other Resources from NLM. http://www.nlm.nih.gov/pubs/factsheets.

Reese, S. 2008 (September 1). Disease registries have flown under clinicians' radar screens. *Managed Healthcare Executive.* http://managedhealthcareexecutive.modernmedicine.com/managed-healthcare-executive/content/disease-registries-have-flown-under-clinicians-radar-screens.

Rodriguez, G. 2009 (January 10). *What Are the Most Common Types of Databases?* Prentice Hall.

Roma-Ferri, M.T., and M. Palomar. 2008. Analysis of health terminologies for use as ontologies in healthcare information systems. *Gaceta Sanitaria.* 22(5):421–433.

Rouse. M. 2010. Data modeling definition. http://searchnetworking.techtarget.com/definition/data modeling.

Sagence. 2014 (December 12). The future of health care: NLP enables analytics and improves patient outcomes. Sagence Connection blog. http://info.sagenceconsulting.com/blog/the-future-of-health-care-using-nlp-to-enable-analytics-and-improve-patient-outcomes.

Schnitzer, G.L. 2000. Natural language processing: A coding professional's perspective. *Journal of AHIMA*. 71(9):95–98.

Schwartz, D. (2015 (June 16). Why do you need to have CureMD discrete reportable transcription service? CureMD blog. http://blog.curemd.com/why-you-need-curemds-discrete-reportable-transcription-service.

Sharma, T. 2011 (December 4). What's the difference between a data mart and a cube? Quora. https://www.quora.com/Whats-the-difference-between-a-data-mart-and-a-cube.

Singh, H., et al. 2009. Prescription errors and outcomes related to inconsistent information transmitted through computerized order entry. *Archives of Internal Medicine.* 169(10):982–989.

Spillman, A. 2013 (April). New handwriting recognition study compares usage and performance of OCR, ICR, and manual data entry. Captricity blog. https://captricity.com/blog/handwriting-recognition-study-on-ocr-icr-manual-data-entry.

Standards and Interoperability Framework (S&I Framework). n.d. What is the S&I Framework? http://www.siframework.org/whatis.html.

Stephens, R., and R. Plew. 2001. *Database Design.* Indianapolis, IN: Sams.

Thede, LQ, and P.M. Schwirian. 2014. Informatics: The standardized nursing terminologies: A national survey of nurses' experience and attitudes—Survey II: Participants' perception of the helpfulness of standardized nursing terminologies in clinical care. *OJIN: The Online Journal of Issues in Nursing.* 20(1). http://www.nursingworld.org/MainMenuCategories/ANAMarketplace/ANAPeriodicals/OJIN/Columns/Informatics/Perception-of-the-Helpfulness-of-Standardized-Nursing-Terminologies.html.

University of Chicago School of Medicine. n.d. MODY/Neonatal Diabetes Registry. http://monogenicdiabetes.uchicago.edu/our-research/registration/mody-registry.

Van Harmellen, F., et al. 2007. *Handbook of Knowledge Representation.* Amsterdam: Elsevier.

Viola, A., and S. Mookencherry. 2012 (February). Metadata and meaningful use. *Journal of AHIMA.* 83(2):32–39.

Weinberger, D. 2010 (February 2). The problem with the data-information-knowledge-wisdom hierarchy. *Harvard Business Review.* http://blogs.hbr.org/cs/2010/02/data_is_to_info_as_info_is_not.html.

Wickramsinghe, N., et al. 2009. *Healthcare Knowledge Management Primer.* New York: Routledge.

Witten, I.H., and E. Frank. 2011. *Data Mining: Practical Machine Learning Tools and Techniques*, 3rd ed. Burlington, MA: Morgan Kaufman.

World Health Organization (WHO). 2015. Classifications: International Classification of Functioning, Disability and Health (ICF). http://www.who.int/classifications/icf/en.

Zafar, A. 2008 (March 27). Presentation on HIE architectures. National HIT Audioconference on HIE Architectures..

Zikopoulos, P.C., et al. 2012. *Understanding Big Data Analytics for Enterprise Class Hadoop and Streaming Data.* New York: McGraw-Hill.

Chapter 11
Information Technology

IEEE

IEEE 802.11

Intranet

Mainframe

Mobile devices

MUMPS

Navigational devices

Net neutrality

On-demand computing

Open-source software

Open systems interconnection (OSI) model

Operating system (OS)

Processor

Protocol

Redundant array of independent (or inexpensive) disks (RAID)

Resolution

SAFER

Screen real estate

Scripting language

Secondary storage

Service-oriented architecture (SOA)

Source code

Storage network

Terminal

Thin client

Throughput

Topology

Uninterruptible power supply (UPS)

Universal serial bus (USB)

Virtualization

Virtual private network (VPN)

Web services architecture (WSA)

Workstation

Workstation on wheels (WOW)

Learning Objectives

- Discuss the scope of health IT system architecture.

- Identify the input/output, storage, primary processing, network, and other hardware associated with health IT systems.

- Identify the types of software that support health IT systems.

- Recommend improvements to usability and data quality in health IT use for data collection, retrieval, and sharing of information, documentation strategies, and generation and use of knowledge.

- Evaluate strategies for addressing emerging technologies.

The technology used in an electronic health record (EHR) or other type of health information technology (health IT) is by no means simple in its technical infrastructure, but the use of such technology should seem simple to the user. Unfortunately, many clinicians think today's data entry and retrieval strategies are anything but simple. The goal for information technology (IT) should be to ensure that hardware and software work together to deliver functionality to users. IT in general and health IT in particular are constantly changing, and so the primary goal of this chapter is to serve as a technical primer that points the reader in the right direction to continually monitor emerging technology trends. As an organization proceeds to fully adopt the components of an EHR and other health IT, it will want to assess its technical infrastructure and make applicable upgrades.

Scope of System Architecture in Health IT

When applied to the overall health IT system, **architecture** refers to the technical building blocks that support the functions of the health IT. The inputs, processes, and outputs of information systems must be carefully constructed. Just as a house or other building has a structural design, so must an information system have a structural design, or architecture.

Hardware Architecture

Every computer system operates with hardware, or equipment, that serves to capture data (input), save and manipulate the data (process), and present it to the user (output).

Input/Output Devices

Input/output (I/O) devices include keyboards (for entering text); display screens (for viewing); navigational devices (for selecting objects), such as a mouse, touch pad, light pen, and so on; speech recognition; optical character recognition (for handwriting recognition); optical scanners (for document imaging); bar code scanners; radio frequency identification (RFID) devices; picture archiving (for images); voice input (for navigational commands); voice output; video output; speakers; printers; and more. Because many of these devices serve both input and output functions, they are typically described together, although obviously some only serve input (for example, a keyboard) or output (for example, a printer).

In general, even if I/O devices are built into the computer's casing, they are considered peripheral devices because they are separate from the computer's **central processing unit** (**CPU**), which is the circuitry of the computer that causes the electronic components to function. For example, **mobile devices**, including notebooks, laptop computers, tablets, and personal digital assistants (PDAs), such as smartphones, have a keyboard, display screen, and navigational device physically in the same casing as the CPU.

The terms **workstation** and **human-computer interface** are often used as collective terms to encompass all potential I/O devices. Another term whose definition was blurred in the past but is becoming clearer is *desktop*. Originally, desktop computers were considered to be less powerful computers than workstations, but now the term *desktop* is generally used to distinguish between a computer that remains on a desk and is generally not portable and mobile devices.

Determining what type of I/O device(s) should be acquired for use in health IT is a critical component of the overall system architecture. Although one size does not fit all, too many different types of devices can be a nightmare for the IT department to appropriately manage and maintain. There are definitely economies of scale that must be considered. Still, because of the variety of work performed and the multiplicity of device types in casual use today, the IT department must inevitably support a variety of devices (Saran 2015). When determining what devices to support, the healthcare organization will need a bring your own device (BYOD) policy regarding whether users may be allowed to use their personal devices (such as smartphones) for work purposes. BYOD has been a burden on IT staff, and there are security concerns (see chapter 12). However, it will be increasingly difficult to prohibit BYOD for some users and/or some types of devices; therefore, a workable policy must be adopted.

Some of the considerations for selecting I/O devices include their source of power, network connectivity, portability, screen size and resolution, and navigational devices.

Source of Power

Power supply is a critical issue. Although most desktop computers are connected directly to a power supply, portable devices require a battery, which is perhaps one of their main drawbacks for use in a 24/7 environment, or even in an 8-hour shift. Some organizations address this issue by supplying each location where the portable device may be used with a power cable. Hospitals may use wheeled carts on which a portable computer is mounted. The cart can carry a more powerful battery pack as well as other peripheral computer equipment, such as bar code readers for medication administration, and medical devices, such as medication dispensing drawers. Moreover, there is an added measure of security for the computer devices when secured to such carts. Carts with computers, however, are not without their problems, as described later in this chapter.

Network Connectivity

Network connectivity is another issue. Again, a desktop computer generally has a hardwire connection to the organization's network, even if it is mounted to a wall or ceiling and even if the facility has wireless connectivity. However, portable devices also need a connection to the network to access data. It is possible to dock a portable device to a network station to download all the information needed for the day, or shift, and then dock it again to upload new information, but this practice is not satisfactory for robust clinical decision support processing. Clinical decision support processing demands more data than what would be downloaded for a day's work. As a result, many healthcare organizations use wireless network technology. Special considerations must be made to the building architecture to identify potential dead zones where the wireless network does not work. In addition, wireless technology tends to be a bit slower than wired technology, although this problem is being addressed by wireless standards organizations.

Portability

Portability is especially important when a clinician needs his or her hands free to care for a patient. Considerations include the weight of the I/O device, hot spots on tablet computers, ability to balance the device while attempting to use a keyboard, and where to put the device when examining the patient. All these considerations help explain why many hospitals have migrated to computers on wheeled carts.

Carts with computers were previously dubbed "computers on wheels," but it is now more common to refer to these as wireless on wheels or **workstations on wheels (WOWs)**. WOWs are not without their portability problems. Their battery packs must be recharged. Because the devices are fairly large and hospitals generally have not been built with "parking lots" or charging stations for such devices, putting them in hallways may be a fire code violation. In some hospitals, carts may be unwieldy to maneuver in small rooms, and so have to be temporarily parked in hallways, disrupting traffic flow. WOWs can also become too heavy to be pushed around, especially once they carry a large battery pack, medication dispensing drawer, and other devices.

An alternative to using a WOW is to carry a tablet. However, the user will require some place to put the device when administering to a patient and tablets could more easily get dropped or, worse, misplaced, lost, or stolen, especially because the user likely needs to carry other items simultaneously. Some nurses have begun to wear slings that hold a tablet, but these can be cumbersome as well.

Still, many hospitals find it is necessary to use either a WOW or tablet because the alternative to these is to either have a device beside each bed or use a device at a stationary location (between two rooms, at the nurses' station, or in a corner work area), which does not support point-of-care (POC) use. POC use of an EHR is necessary to take advantage of the alerts and reminders that provide the enhanced utility an EHR brings to direct patient care.

WOWs are not as frequently found in clinics, which have their own distinctive environmental challenges. For example, clinics need special shelving or pullout drawers for keyboards and swing arms on which to mount monitors (although physical safety must be evaluated or people will bump into the equipment). Many clinic physicians who thought they would like a tablet for its portability find that the battery life is not sufficient, the wireless connection is slower than wired access, and there is risk of dropping them. However, many physicians like to use tablets because they do not have to log on and log off at every workstation in multiple exam rooms.

Screen Size and Resolution

Monitors come in a variety of sizes, forms, and resolutions. The size of the screen is often referred to as **screen real estate**. One reason for the popularity of tablets is that the screen is nearly the same size as a sheet of paper. The screen real estate on PDAs is often considered too small to be useful except for occasional reference purposes or very focused applications.

The amount of resolution in a monitor determines the ability to clearly view the content. **Resolution** is measured by megapixels (MP). Generally, there are two categories of monitor resolution: medical grade and nonmedical grade. A good way to understand their difference is in reference to the ability to see detail on an x-ray. Medical-grade resolution generally refers to 3 MP, 4 MP, or 5 MP. Most radiologists report that this resolution is sufficient for diagnostic purposes, and the ability to rotate, zoom, and create a three-dimensional image enhances diagnostics even more. The Food and Drug Administration (FDA) requires 5 MP resolution for mammography viewing (FDA 2014). Nonmedical grade monitors are perfectly suitable for EHR and other health IT uses.

Navigational Devices

Workstations have a variety of **navigational devices**, such as keyboards, handwriting recognition pads and pens (or styluses), and voice recognition microphones associated with them for data entry and retrieval as well as various token slots, biometrics, and other devices for security. Anything that can be separated from the device is subject to loss. Many organizations find they need to either tether pens and portable microphones to the devices, or keep an extra supply on hand.

Storage Devices, Media, Architectures, and Management

Storage devices are peripherals in the same manner as I/O devices. Although there is some storage in the same "box" as the CPU, the amount of storage acquired in computers for widespread use within healthcare facilities may be minimal, as most organizations are moving to "thin clients" where data are almost always stored separately. EHR systems, with their large quantities of data to be shared across many applications and used by many persons, require "mass storage" devices, which are frequently separate units and may be separate networks. In addition to the main storage, back-up storage and remote disaster recovery capability must also be considered.

Storage Devices and Media

Memory in the CPU is considered primary storage and holds the permanent machine instructions. Peripheral devices for storing data can be referred to as **secondary storage** because they hold the data and software to be used in an application. Secondary storage may be available continuously (online) to the CPU for real-time access to data or maintained offline and require loading to be available for online use. The term *drive* is often used to describe the device that runs the secondary storage medium.

Secondary storage media are usually magnetic or optical, although solid state media are becoming more popular. The following are media commonly found in healthcare applications:

- *Magnetic tape* is an older storage medium that can be used for offline storage for back-up and archival purposes, although it is not currently used as frequently as in the past. It can store a fairly large amount of data, but access to data is sequential, so the time to access a particular data element on magnetic tape is relatively slow. Magnetic tape is removable from the tape drive.

- *Magnetic disks,* often called *hard disks,* come in a variety of forms. A computer's hard disk is a magnetic disk encased in a protective material and placed within the system unit, forming the hard drive. Hard drives are used in computers, including servers, as the primary source of continuous online data and programs. External hard drives are used for system back-up. Magnetic disks are frequently used where speed of access is essential. For the foreseeable future, hard disks will likely continue to be the mainstay form of storage for mass storage, and hard disk technology is an area of rapid improvement and cost reductions (Goodwins 2015).

- *Optical disks* are a newer alternative to magnetic disks. Write-once, read-many optical disks and erasable ones are both available. Optical disks are particularly well suited for storing multimedia information, including images, sound, and motion (video). The first optical disks used in healthcare, such as **computer output to laser disks (COLD)**, were used to store images of documents. Optical disks may come in a compact disc (CD) or digital versatile disk (DVD) form and be used for offline storage. CDs and DVDs can be recordable or re-recordable. They are often used in write-only format to give patients copies of their health records. Third- and fourth-generation optical disks include Blu-ray and holographic DVDs, which have capacity to display three-dimensional images and much greater storage capacity than CDs and older DVDs.

- *Solid state devices* contain computer circuitry for storing data. They come in different sizes and types. A flash drive or **universal serial bus (USB)** drive is a small, highly portable device that is inserted into a USB port on a computing device. Because of security concerns, many organizations are disabling the USB port on their computers. Although most EHR applications are written to prevent direct download capability to such a local drive, there are concerns that screen prints or cut-and-paste functionality can be used to copy data onto local storage media, and the small size of USB drives makes it easier to discreetly copy and carry away the data. Solid state drives are increasingly replacing hard drives *within* computers where they provide low to moderate storage capacity (relative to mass storage devices) and are not subject to removal by a user (Barnatt 2012).

Although not a form of media per se, configuration of media is an important part of storage. One configuration that is commonly used is called **redundant arrays of inexpensive (or independent) disks (RAID)**. RAID storage uses multiple disk drives so that data can be divided up and replicated throughout multiple drives, which contributes to reliability and performance of accessing the data. The number of drives does not have a direct correlation with the number of levels at which data are stored. There are typically from 2 to 10 levels across any number of drives. Usually, the first level uses multiple drives to increase **throughput**, or the ability of data to be read more rapidly. The second level is called **disk mirroring**, which means that each set is composed of two disks that are exact duplicates of each other. Thus, if one disk breaks down, the other can take its place. This level of RAID should be considered the minimum requirement for an EHR system. The highest level of RAID uses sets of three disks to address some of the shortcomings in lower-level RAID devices and is preferred in EHR systems that are truly paperless.

Storage Architectures and Management

Storage and back-up for mission-critical functions, such as the EHR, should be planned carefully. Although the storage media and devices are getting less expensive, managing storage is becoming much more expensive. Entire **storage networks** comprised of multiple types of storage devices connected to one another and to central servers are being created to manage data storage. Storage architecture options include:

- *Direct-attached storage (DAS)* is a storage device that is directly attached to a server or workstation. There is no network involved, although multiple computers can share the storage device through multiple ports on the device. Such storage would generally be used in small physician practices or in the home environment.

- *Storage area network (SAN)* is a dedicated network that provides access from storage devices to servers. SANs are generally their own network and not accessible directly by individual workstations. A SAN alone provides only block-level access to data, which enables it to provide high-speed access to databases and high-usage file servers that store structured data. As a result, they are popular in healthcare for the online transaction processing (OLTP) demanded in EHRs. A SAN also enables efficient disaster recovery because servers can boot directly to the SAN (Asaro 2005).

- *Network-attached storage (NAS)* is the converse of SAN because NAS provides file-level storage and access to clients. File-level storage is unstructured data, such as document and medical images. Healthcare organizations today have a tremendous amount of such images, which use a lot of storage space and are difficult to move around and back up (Hardy 2010). Because NAS provides both storage and a file system, it is widely used for electronic document management system storage.

- *SAN-NAS hybrid storage* constructs file systems on top of SANs to achieve both storage types for a single environment. Hospitals will likely use this kind of storage in the future because a large proportion of EHR data is structured but both document and medical images are essential parts of the information infrastructure.

- *Content-addressable storage (CAS)* is another storage option that enables retrieval of information based on content, not storage location. This option is suitable for long-term storage of information that does not change often, such as medical images (Marks 2008).

The various forms of storage structures connect to servers and clients via storage interfaces. These interfaces follow standard protocols. In general, a **protocol** is a system of rules that explain the correct procedures to be followed in specific situations; in computer technology, a protocol is standard set of regulations and requirements that allow two electronic items to connect to and exchange information with one another. The standard protocols for health IT storage interfaces are generic—that is, they are not unique to healthcare but specific to the components of the storage system being adopted. Examples of such standards include SCSI (Small Computer System Interface), ATA (Advanced Technology Attachment), SAS (Serial Attached SCSI), and SATA (Serial Attached ATA).

Processors

The CPU, sometimes called the **processor**, is the area of the computer where data in machine-readable form are processed according to specific instructions (software) that also are in machine-readable form. Processors are made of semiconductor material etched on a small electronic device called a (silicon) *chip* or an integrated circuit. Chips may contain from 100 to more than 1 million components. Data and instructions for their processing are converted into binary form, representing the two states of electrical pulses: on/off, the combination of which is what machines can read. The two states are commonly represented as 0 and 1 and are called *bits*. Sequences of bits, called *bytes*, are used to represent each character in any language. When describing the size of any component of a computer, reference is made to the number of bytes that can be stored or processed in the component. Sizes may be expressed in kilobytes ([KB], roughly 1,000 bytes); megabytes ([MB] roughly 1 million bytes); gigabytes ([GB] roughly 1 billion bytes); or terabytes ([TB] roughly 1 trillion bytes).

When a computer is first turned on, internal functions are activated ("booted") and diagnostics are performed to check for potential problems. The special instructions that perform these functions are kept in a section of the CPU called read-only memory (ROM). When the computer is turned off, the contents of ROM are retained. ROM does not have to be large, the size depending on the size of random access memory (RAM), number of processors, and processing speed.

RAM is sometimes just called *memory* or *central memory*. The memory section of the CPU houses the data and instructions being processed at any point in time. It is volatile, meaning that when the computer is turned off, anything in RAM is lost. The size of RAM relates to the amount of data that can be processed at one time and contributes to the speed with which processing of data can take place. CPU speeds are getting faster and faster. A *megahertz* (MHz) is 1 million cycles per second. Many CPUs can process cycles of instructions at *gigahertz* (GHz) speeds. One GHz is equal to 1,000 MHz.

The arithmetic-logic unit (ALU) is the location in the CPU that performs the actual processing of the data held in memory. The ALU also may be referred to as *registers*. As the name implies, the ALU is where addition, subtraction, multiplication, comparisons, and so on are performed.

The CPU also may contain cache (pronounced *cash*) memory, which is used to accelerate transfer of data and instructions between the registers and central memory. A memory cache is made of high-speed static RAM instead of the slower dynamic RAM used for main memory. Memory **caching** is a process wherein data and instructions that are used repeatedly are temporarily stored to speed up access. Disk caching is a similar concept, but it uses conventional main memory. The most recently accessed data from an application is retained in the disk cache. When a program needs to access data, it first checks the disk cache to see if the data are there. (If the needed data are not in the disk cache, the program needs to go to the hard disk or a special computer called a *storage server*.) Disk caching makes data retrieval faster when the most recent data are needed repeatedly. Because of disk caching, however, portable devices that connect to a network for only short periods of time and then are used elsewhere should have the data stored in cache erased as a security measure in the event the device is lost or stolen. Wireless devices provide this erasing capability when the device is moved a certain distance away from a wireless access point.

The CPU components are connected by tiny wires through which the data and instructions are passed. The collection of wires is often called a *bus*.

Finally, because the CPU is called on to perform so many tasks, seemingly simultaneously, many organizations buy computers with dual processors, or even dual-core or multicore processors. **Dual processor** refers to two separate physical computer processors, running in parallel. **Dual-core or multicore processors** combine two processors (dual-core) or more (multicore) onto a single integrated circuit. Such technology boosts the computer's multitasking capability.

Computer Categories

Although every computer operates in much the same way as described earlier, there are some significant differently types of computers, including the following:

- A supercomputer is a very fast, very high–capacity computer, usually dedicated to the performance of specialized applications that require an enormous amount of computation.

- A **mainframe** computer is a single large computer with many **terminals** connected to it; these terminals can be used to enter and retrieve data and share the resources of the single computer. When first introduced, mainframe terminals had no processing capability of their own. Mainframe computers are no longer common in healthcare delivery organizations (although they still are very prevalent in insurance companies, banks, and other industries).

- A personal computer (PC) is a standalone computer system. The term was coined by IBM and adopted by vendors who made similar machines, although computer purists would quickly point out that such computers also may be patterned after the Apple Macintosh. Some PCs have been beefed up to serve as powerful computers supporting other computers as servers in client/server network architecture. Other PCs have been stripped down to serve almost as if they were terminals in a mainframe environment (in which case they may be called *dumb terminals*).

- Mobile devices, such as notebook computers, laptops, or tablets, are smaller in size but may be as powerful as a PC. Handheld computers, or PDAs, are small enough to be carried in a pocket, purse, or briefcase. Smartphones combine the functionality of PDAs with cell phones (and other technologies).

- *Network computers* (NCs), also called **thin clients** (discussed under client/server network in the next section), are low-cost PCs with minimal processing capability of their own.

Communications and Network Architecture

Whenever two or more computers need to communicate with each other, a network is needed. Whether a computer is connected to the biggest network of all, the Internet, or simply to one other computer in a local area network (LAN), many of the same principles of network architecture apply. Networks have different configurations, or architectures, and an entire set of hardware devices, cabling, and protocols associated with them.

Two primary types of architectures currently are used to communicate among computers in a healthcare organization: client/server and web-services architectures.

Client/Server Architecture

Client/server architecture is the predominant form of computer architecture used in healthcare organizations today. In client/server architecture, certain computers (servers) have been configured to perform most of the processing and resource-intensive tasks, and other computers (clients), which are generally less powerful, capture, view, and perform limited processes on data.

The cost of a server can range from as little as $500 to more than $100,000. It is generally dedicated to providing a specific service to client computers on a network. For example, servers provide database services, application services, file-sharing services, print-sharing services, fax services, email services, and many other specialized services such as authentication. They may be centralized in one location or distributed throughout a network. When grouped together, the collection of servers is sometimes called a *server farm*. Blade servers are a newer configuration, where a number of server computers, or blades, occupy the space typically occupied by a single server.

Servers have their own operating systems, which may be Windows-based, a variety of UNIX and Linux versions, a Mac operating system (OS) version, or one of the more technical OSs provided by other vendors.

Client computers may be desktops or portable devices. They generally need, and have, considerably less power—and cost less—because they derive their functionality from the server. When client computers are stripped of most of their processing and storage capabilities, they are called *thin clients* or *NCs*. Although thin clients may be attractive because of their cost and security, some EHR applications will not run on them or will not run as well because of the intense processing and response time requirements of such applications.

Service-Oriented Architecture

Service-oriented architecture (SOA) is a logical way of designing software in modular and flexible components, called *services*. Very frequently, services are deployed so they meet web services standards for interoperability, in which case the architecture may be referred to as **web services architecture (WSA)** (W3C 2004). Web services use XML-based messages (discussed in more detail later in the chapter) conveyed by Internet protocols. Although WSA is the latest form of computer architecture, it is still not widely used for EHR systems because so many source applications that contribute data to an EHR are not developed using such protocols. In addition, there are concerns about the speed and reliability for OLTP when offered in a software as a service (SaaS) model (Sliwa 2009). Such a model, however, is increasingly being used for other types of applications in healthcare, such as electronic document management, back-up and disaster recovery, and data warehousing (Raffo 2010).

Virtualization and Cloud Computing

Although virtualization and cloud computing are not architectures in the same sense as client/server and SOA, they are important utilizations of Internet technology. Virtualization and cloud computing are distinct from each other, but related.

The National Institute for Standards and Technology (NIST) defines **virtualization** as "the simulation of the software and/or hardware upon which other software runs" (Scarfone et al. 2011). NIST observes that the simulated environment is called a *virtual machine*. Virtualization essentially creates a second "something." For example, computer hardware can be emulated within a software platform (for example, operations in a Windows-based PC can be made to look like the operations of a Mac). One computer can be made to operate like two computers when the actual hard disk is partitioned to hold data in one location and software in another. Such partitioning is essentially virtualization—creating two hard disks from one through a software process (Blokdijk 2010). The benefit of virtualization is that it allows resource sharing across multiple environments. It is considered "green computing" because it is less wasteful of computing resources. Virtualization can be applied to operating systems, servers, storage devices, or network resources (Davis 2009a). It is a building block for cloud computing (EMA 2009).

Cloud computing, according to NIST, is "a model for enabling ubiquitous, convenient, on-demand network access to a shared pool of configurable computing resources (e.g., networks, servers, storage, applications, and services) that can be rapidly provisioned and released with minimal management effort or service provider interaction" (Mell and Grance 2011). Cloud computing is also called **on-demand computing** because server time and network storage is paid for per use (that is, it is a "measured service," similar to gas or electric utilities). This payment method makes cloud computing a less expensive way to acquire computing resources.

According to NIST, cloud computing is delivered as a service in three different forms (Mell and Grance 2011). In all forms, the consumer does not manage or control the underlying cloud infrastructure. The first form is infrastructure as a service (IaaS). With IaaS, the consumer has the most control, including control of the OS, storage, deployed applications, and possibly limited control of certain networking components, such as host firewalls. In the platform as a service (PaaS) model (the second form of cloud computing), the consumer has control of the deployed applications and possibly application hosting environment configurations. In the SaaS form (the third type), the consumer has the least control—user control is limited to user-specific application configuration settings. The SaaS form is used for very low-cost EHRs. Finally, NIST also describes different deployment models of cloud computing (Mell and Grance 2011). A private cloud is operated solely for an organization; a community cloud is shared by several organizations and by a community with common interests; a public cloud is made available to the general public or a large industry group; and a hybrid cloud combines two or more forms of clouds (such as for load balancing between clouds).

Thin Client Support

With today's multiplicity of user devices for computing, security concerns, and desire for ubiquitous access to applications, it is important to create a thin client environment where any device, anywhere, can access applications as if they were directly on the device, even though they are not on the device. Two primary software tools provide such thin client support. Microsoft Remote Desktop Services (formerly called Windows Terminal Services) and Citrix HDX both deliver applications to users at their fingertips. The two products are very similar, but not necessarily duplicative (Chang 2015).

Network Configuration

Networks may be configured in a variety of ways, depending on what systems need to be included. Figure 11.1 displays a diagram of some of the concepts described in this section. For healthcare organizations, the most typical private network configurations are as follows:

- *Local area network (LAN)* refers to a group of computers typically connected within a relatively small geographic area, such as an office, building, or campus. Connectivity is generally achieved through dedicated cable.

- *Wide area network (WAN)* describes a group of computers that connect across greater geographical distances or where dedicated cable is cost-prohibitive. A WAN uses telephone or cable services for connectivity.

- *Wireless network* refers to group of wireless devices that connect via radio waves (wireless LAN) or mobile telecommunications cellular network (wireless WAN).

- **Virtual private network (VPN)** uses a "secure tunnel" through a public network (usually the Internet) to connect remote sites or users. VPNs are designed to reduce the cost of using leased lines through a WAN while maintaining security (Healthcare Practice IT 2011). Security procedures include firewalls, encryption, and server authentication. Tunneling protocols are primarily Internet Protocol Security (IPSec), Secure Sockets Layer (SSL), or SSL's newer counterpart, Transport Layer Security (TLS). IPSec requires third-party hardware and/or software and set up at all sites, whereas SSL/TLS does not (Bradley 2009). There remains controversy over the level of security each affords. Some security experts contend that IPSec is more secure—partly because its complexity and limitation of site-to-site connectivity lends greater control and because it operates at a deeper level of the OSI stack (see next section). Others, however, believe that SSL/TLS affords greater security because of its stronger encryption controls and support for certificate authentication.

Figure 11.1.   Diagram of concepts

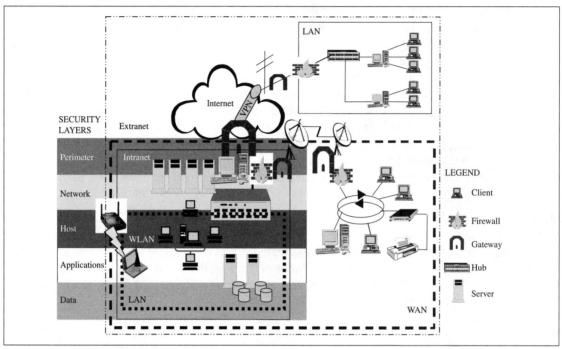

However, the latest version of SSL (3.0) cannot be validated under FIPS 140-2, the level of encryption required by the meaningful use (MU) incentive program criteria; TLS 1.0 should be used for the strongest form of such tunneling (NIST 2011).

In addition to the geographic reach and medium through which data are exchanged, networks may also be categorized according to who is permitted access to them. An **intranet** is a network located within an organization that uses Internet technologies to enable users to find, use, and share documents and web pages. Intranets use traditional Internet protocols to transfer data but reside behind a firewall (special hardware or software that provides a security barrier between networks and the Internet) for security so they are accessible only to authorized users. **Extranets** are networks that connect a given organization to its customers and business partners or suppliers (business associates in healthcare). Although extranets send information over public networks, requiring a greater level of security, access to them is still restricted to the services and persons authorized. The Internet is obviously the third type of network, and there is no limitation to access except as may be provided through an extranet service.

Topology

Topology refers to the arrangement of the network. There are two types of topology: physical and logical.

Physical Topology

A physical topology is the way network devices are connected. Networks are generally arranged in one of three physical topologies (Durkin and Just 2008):

- *Bus topology* is the simplest network topology, connecting one device to another along a "backbone." In a bus network, all computers on the network receive the same message at the same time. However, only one computer at a time can transfer information; thus, if one segment of the network goes down, the entire network is affected.

- *Star topology* connects individual computers through a central hub that serves as a "traffic cop" for the data. (This is illustrated in figure 11.1 within the LAN.) It is also easy to add a computer to the network, if needed.

- *Ring topology* connects computers via a cable arranged in a ring. Information is sent through the ring to get from one computer to another, and special kinds of signals are required to direct the data. (This is illustrated in figure 11.1 within the WAN.) It is difficult to add a computer to the network using ring topology because the ring would have to be redone to do so.

Logical Topology

A logical topology describes how data are transmitted through the physical devices. An Ethernet is the family of frame-based computer networking technologies that currently is the most widely used topology for LANs. It defines the wiring and signaling standards for the physical transmission of data. Ethernet is standardized as IEEE 802.3 (pronounced *eye-triple-E*). **IEEE** is the acronym for the Institute of Electrical and Electronics Engineers, the leading developer of international standards that underpin many current telecommunications, IT, and power generation products and services.

IEEE also creates standards for WLANs. **IEEE 802.11** standards are collectively referred to as *Wi-Fi technologies*. Different versions of the standards have evolved over time. The newest version is 802.11ac, which was standardized by IEEE in 2014. Today, version 802.11ac has the fastest maximum speed, best signal range, and provides interoperability among devices, but it is more expensive to use, and there are some infrastructure changes that can also add cost but will improve reliability. Version 802.11ac is backward-compatible with version 802.11n, so an organization may not need to purchase 802.11ac access points for an entire facility in order to achieve its benefits (Sessoms 2014).

Other WLAN standards also exist. Bluetooth is probably the most notable. It only supports a short range and relatively low bandwidth, but it is cost-effective for networking PDAs, cell phones, and medical devices that are used in close proximity to the devices to which they must connect. The WLAN standard IEEE 802.16 (WiMax) is designed for long-range networking.

Network Components

Every network must have at least three components to operate: a network operating system (NOS), a network interface card (NIC) or other form of adapter, and cabling or some other form of transmission medium (Derfler and Freed 2005).

Network Operating System

A NOS is a family of programs that run the networked computers. The most common NOS currently in use in healthcare are Windows- or UNIX-based, although a few EHR vendors have created their own OSs. (See the discussion of OS software later in this chapter.)

Network Interface Card and Other Adapters

A NIC, LAN adapter, or wireless access card creates the connection between a computer and the transmission medium. NICs create packages of data that enhance the strength of low-powered digital signals inside a computer to enable the packages to travel through a transmission medium.

Transmission Media

Transmission media carry data through a network and vary by cost, type of service, amount of potential interference and signal degradation, and bandwidth (the maximum speed at which a given device can transmit data).

Wired transmission media include coaxial cable, which carries electric current at radio frequencies; twisted pair cable (unshielded or shielded), which also carry electric current but are generally faster than coaxial cable; and fiber optic cable, which uses light signals to transfer information through a core of glass or plastic and is capable of very fast transmission speeds. Fiber optic cable is expensive and often reserved for the main cable, or backbone, of a network.

Wireless transmissions include radio waves, which can be local in origin or via satellite. As noted earlier, Bluetooth is a form of radio wave for very short distances. Wi-Fi uses radio waves for local access to the Internet, and cellular transmissions use them for longer distance access to the Internet (Stoffels 2012). Other types of wireless transmissions are microwaves, which can be used for relatively short distances when objects do not obstruct their path, and infrared waves, which are used in remote controls and in devices that need to communicate over very short clear/empty distances (Freeman 2014; CCM 2015).

For a WAN, transmission media are often included under the domain of telecommunications, which is defined as communication over long distances and includes telephone, radio, telegraphy, television, voice over Internet protocol (VoIP), cellular service, data communications, and computer networking. For constructing a WAN in the healthcare environment, the most common media remain different forms of phone service, such as plain old telephone services (POTS), digital subscriber lines (DSL), and, especially, trunk lines (T-lines). T-lines are the backbone of long-distance network transmission that transmits data in digital form. There are a variety of speeds, with the fastest being the most expensive.

Internet Access

Most of the LAN and WAN discussion above refers to transmission of information within a business and between a business and its suppliers, customers, and others external to it. However, access to the Internet is essential for most healthcare organizations. Two issues with respect to Internet access relate to broadband accessibility and, to a somewhat lesser extent for healthcare, net neutrality.

Broadband is a term that refers to high-speed telecommunication transmissions using a variety of network, types, including cable, DSL, Wi-Fi, and satellite. In early 2015, the Federal Communications Commission (FCC) redefined the minimum broadband speed at 25 Mbps (megabyte per second) download and 3 Mbps upload (from 4 Mbps download and 1 Mbps upload). As a result, more parts of the United States have access to broadband connectivity, although an estimated 10 percent of Americans lack such access, especially in rural areas, tribal lands, and some inner city areas (Mediati 2016).

Net neutrality is the principle that the Internet should give consumers access to all legal content and applications on an equal basis, without favoring some sources or blocking others. It prohibits Internet Service Providers (ISPs) such as AT&T, Verizon, Comcast, and others, from charging content providers (for example, Netflix or Amazon) for speedier delivery of their content on "fast lanes" and deliberately slowing the content from content providers that may compete with ISPs (Snider et al. 2015).

Other Network Devices

In addition to the three main components of a network, a variety of other devices may be used to serve various other purposes in the network. The device used depends on the network topology, the transmission medium, and the standards to which the device manufacturer adheres (Derfler and Freed 2005). These devices include the following:

- *Hub:* The central location where cables on a network come together.

- *Bridge:* Enables computers on individual networks or separate parts of a network to exchange information.

- *Routers:* Connectors used to link different networks together. These devices can automatically determine the best route for information given the amount of traffic on a network.

- *Switch:* Similar to a hub, but a newer type of device. It is applied to networks that have many users. The switch is beginning to take the place of bridges and routers.

- *Gateway:* The device that links two different network types together.

- *Multiplexor:* The device traditionally used to divide a long-distance, high-speed telecommunications line so that it can be shared by many users. High-end routers that can interface directly with wide-area communication services are reducing the need for multiplexors.

- *Modems:* Devices that enable computers on a network to exchange information across telephone lines by translating the information from digital form to analog form.

Network Protocols

Network protocols are the rules for sending and receiving data across a network. Whereas the physical topology of a network is the base of the network and the logical topology is how data are transmitted through the base, network protocols establish rules of communication.

The rules are based on a standard called the **open systems interconnection (OSI) model**, developed by the International Standardization Organization (ISO). The OSI model consists of seven layers, each of which is responsible for a particular aspect of communication. For example, one layer may be used to specify how information is addressed, and another checks for errors during transfer.

When data are transferred over a network, theoretically they must pass through each layer of the OSI model. As this happens, information is added to the data to help ensure consistency of communication. When the data reach their destination, they again must pass through the layers of the OSI model so that the information previously applied can be removed at each level (Petri 2009). Figure 11.2 shows the layers of the OSI model and their purposes. Although this is a theoretical model, it is a handy reference for network administrations troubleshooting network problems (Davis 2009b).

Figure 11.2.   OSI model

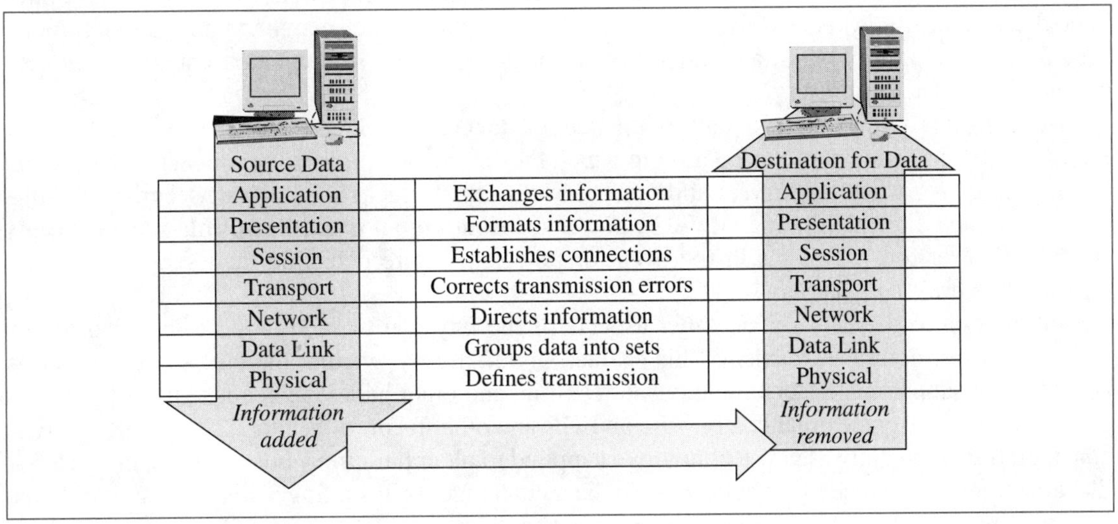

Source Data			Destination for Data	
Application	Exchanges information		Application	
Presentation	Formats information		Presentation	
Session	Establishes connections		Session	
Transport	Corrects transmission errors		Transport	
Network	Directs information		Network	
Data Link	Groups data into sets		Data Link	
Physical	Defines transmission		Physical	
Information added			*Information removed*	

Protocols, in this context, are the actual hardware or software components that carry out the OSI model guidelines for transferring information on a network. Most of the protocols are generic across the industries using them and specific only to the different OSs and network architectures employed.

TCP/IP is a collection of protocols used to allow the communication as described in the OSI model to occur among networks with different types of computer systems. It also is what is used on the Internet. The collection of protocols in TCP/IP include the following, among others:

- *Transmission control protocol (TCP):* Used to transfer information between two devices on a network

- *Internet protocol (IP):* Responsible for addressing information

- *File transfer protocol (FTP):* Used to transfer documents between different types of computers; sFTP refers to secure FTP where users must be credentialed prior to use

- *Hypertext transfer protocol (HTTP):* Used to transfer information from web servers to web browsers

At the application level of the OSI model, industries often create their own standard protocols for communicating (sending messages/exchanging data) between applications. (See the applications integration/interface section in this chapter.)

Physical Plant

In technical infrastructure planning for an EHR or other type of health IT, the most important part of the physical plant is often the **data center**, the location where computers and their components are housed. Whether or not the organization already has a lot of information technology, it can be helpful to assess the data center to ensure that it truly represents a mission-critical environment. Organizations should apply best practices to designing this facility to protect the equipment that remain local and evaluate remote locations for back-up and disaster recovery (Bell 2005). A hospital may need to renovate an older data center to house a greater number of servers and other devices, a "war room" in which to perform system configuration and maintenance, and a more robust and permanent training area, and to address other needs. Some hospitals have historically relied on their hospital information system vendor to support their data center needs, but with the EHR, these organizations may find that they have increasing numbers of devices and services that must be addressed locally. Alternatively, the maintenance of a data center may become too much for an organization adopting an EHR and other types of health IT, and it may decide to outsource or seek hosting for its data center services.

Very small providers may not have a full-fledged data center and may want to consider enhancing the space and features of the location in which they store their servers, or consider outsourcing/hosting. Even so, whatever servers and other devices remain local need proper security; heating, ventilation, and air conditioning (HVAC); power distribution; an **uninterruptible power supply (UPS)** to power down systems in the event of power loss, fire detection, and suppression; and potentially a back-up generator.

In addition to the data center, other aspects of the physical plant should be included in any technical infrastructure assessment. This evaluation determines whether the building construction is capable of supporting the electrical power, cabling, and other hardware needs that become more dispersed throughout the organization with an EHR and other forms of health IT. This is not a trivial consideration, especially as new technology is applied to older buildings. For example, the fortress-like construction of some older buildings can be a challenge for installing a wireless network. Historically, many IT departments were located in a remote corner of the hospital basement. As traffic to these departments is now exploding because many more business associates and clinical staff need access to them, organizations are moving their IT departments to a more accessible location, while enhancing security.

Software That Supports EHRs and Other Health IT

Software refers to the instructions, or programs, that direct the processing of data in computers. While organizations evaluating EHR systems or some other forms of health IT generally do not have access to source code (that is, the underlying software running the hardware or applications), a particular organization may have software preferences based on connecting home-grown systems, ease of writing interfaces in-house, or system maintenance. There are two primary types of software: OS software and application software. The nature of the OS and application software language will help determine much of the ability to program and thus support various functions of the EHR or other type of health IT. For example, if an EHR vendor does not use a **scripting language** designed for writing programs to be executed on the Internet, it will be difficult to incorporate intranet technology with the EHR system. However, it is not necessary to confine system selection to systems written with the same language. Frequently, developers use more than one language based on the task intended to be performed. In addition, new virtualization strategies allow different types of OSs and other computer resources to be used in combination with one another.

Operating System Software

Operating system (OS) software is considered the instructions that cause application programs to work. The OS performs basic tasks such as recognizing input from the keyboard, sending output to the display screen, keeping track of files and directories on a disk, and controlling peripheral devices such as disk drives and printers. The OS acts as a traffic cop, ensuring that different programs running at the same time do not interfere with each other. In addition, the OS is responsible for many security functions. An OS may be proprietary (developed by one vendor for its equipment and applications) or nonproprietary (intended to be used by many vendors).

An example of a nonproprietary (open) OS is UNIX. UNIX is the trademark name for OS software originally designed for mainframe computer systems. Because it was written in the nonproprietary programming language called C, it operates well on many different types of computers, although it lacks a graphical user interface (GUI). Linux is a newer version of UNIX available free on the web or through some low-cost distributors who add tools to enrich utilization. UNIX was fairly popular in healthcare computing platforms; Linux is becoming more popular as it becomes more stable and better supported.

Individual computers have OSs that permit just the one computer to use various application programs. When computers are networked, the OS must support multiple users, tasks, and processes. NOSs support such activities. Various Windows versions for networks are popular OSs for client/server environments. Macintosh computers have their own OS, although the latest Macs use Intel processors that now support both the Mac OS and Windows OSs.

MUMPS (Massachusetts General Hospital Utility Multi-Programming System) was an OS created in 1965 specifically for medical information systems. Revisions are still being used in some applications under the name of M Technology because it is an excellent source for structuring clinical decision support systems.

Application Software

Application (or high-level) software makes applications perform their functions. The language in which this software is written provides the algorithms, which are rules or instructions that define a path that guides a process to a logical end point. A variety of application programming languages are currently used in EHRs and other types of health IT. Java, Visual Basic (VB), C, C++, and MUMPS (also known as M) are the most common ones used in EHRs (Carter 2008, 62–67). Databases also require programming, and database management systems use languages such as SQL, Oracle, and others.

A central theme in this book and for the Office of the National Coordinator for Health Information Technology (ONC) is how well types of application software work together. The ability of two or more systems or components to exchange information and use the information that has been exchanged is termed *interoperability*. Chapter 13 covers interoperability in depth.

Source Code and Open Source Software

The actual application software that is written in any language to serve a specific purpose, such as EHR or other type of health IT, is called **source code** because it is the source of instructions for the application. Generally, the developer of the software owns the source code. By owning the code, the developer can sell the program to multiple consumers. However, healthcare organizations sometimes want to have a copy of the source code. For example, if the developer goes out of business, it may be difficult for the customer to maintain the application without this source code. Some healthcare organizations, particularly academic and other large institutions, want to customize an EHR system or other health IT extensively and often have the staff and expertise to make modifications in the source code.

Organizations that want the source code may find it difficult to acquire. Some are able to buy rights to a copy of the source code so they can maintain and enhance it themselves; others codevelop the code with a vendor and maintain interest in it. When the consumer obtains a copy of the source code, vendors may no longer support it when it does not function properly or when upgrades or patches do not work on it. However, many vendors will agree to put the source code for their products into an escrow account from which it may be withdrawn in the event the company goes out of business. This agreement should be guaranteed in the contract, especially if the vendor is small or just starting up. (See chapter 7 for more information on contract negotiation.)

As the name implies, **open-source software** is software that is freely distributed (referring to the fact that complicated licensure agreements are not required) and open to access. Open-source software may be desirable when organizations want to do unique customizations because the source code is available to the acquirer, who may make modifications to it. The open-access advantage, however, is also the greatest disadvantage of open-source software because the result is frequently lack of interoperability with other applications. The Open Source Initiative (version 1.9) provides criteria that open-source software should address. Open-source software should not require a royalty or other fee for use, but it may be embedded in products that are sold. **Free software** has been defined by the Free Software Foundation (version 1.92) as being software for which no fee is charged for its use. The definition is close to, but not precisely the same as, open-source software; with the primary difference being that free software may not be open to access. Free-and-open-source software combines the attributes of open-source and free software. While there are many excellent applications using such software, healthcare organizations should be aware that the quality of the software is highly variable due to the fact that there are no quality or security testing requirements for its distribution. It is wise to adopt a policy on whether such software may be permitted to be used, and if so under what circumstances.

Check Your Understanding 11.1

Choose the best answer:

1. The general trend in health IT input device technology is to:

    a. Allow all users to use any device they wish

    b. Consolidate on a single type

    c. Exclude all devices that do not conform to MU incentive program requirements

    d. Move to a controlled variety of devices

2. Which form of secondary storage is most common in healthcare?

    a. Magnetic disk

    b. Magnetic tape

    c. Optical disk

    d. Portable USB drive

3. Which form of storage architecture is most amendable to electronic document storage?

    a. Direct attached

    b. Network attached

    c. Storage area

    d. Storage network

4. When an input device has full processing capability, it is called:

    a. Mainframe

    b. Network computer

    c. Personal computer (PC)

    d. Thin client

5. Which of the following is an architecture that builds software in components?

    a. Cloud computing

    b. On demand

    c. Service-oriented architecture

    d. Web services architecture

6. Technology that enables sharing computing resources across multiple environments is:

    a. Cloud computing

    b. Interoperability

    c. Service-oriented architecture

    d. Virtualization

7. Technology that enables secure messaging through the Internet is:

a. Firewall

b. Intranet

c. Local area network

d. Virtual private network

8. Which of the following types of software is supplied at no cost from the developer?

a. Free software

b. Open-source software

c. Operating system

d. Source code

Usability and Data Quality in Data Retrieval and Documentation

Implementing the right hardware is the backbone for any information technology endeavor. However, finding the right software, configuring it to meet the needs of the organization, and implementing the software in a manner that users can successfully use to achieve value are what gives the technology life. For the EHR and other types of health IT, usability and data quality are probably the two most important factors today that must be addressed to assure success with these systems.

Usability

Usability from a vendor selection perspective was addressed in chapter 7. The Healthcare Information and Management Systems Society (HIMSS) usability maturity model was offered as functionality to be included in a functional specification (HIMSS 2011). Groups calling for more usability in EHRs acknowledge that not all usability issues are directly related to software—for example, some result from institutional policies, regulations, and suboptimal implementation and training (AMA 2014a). Nevertheless, technology solutions can make EHRs more usable (Mace 2015).

The National Institute of Standards and Technology (NIST) has done considerable work on health IT usability, including human factors modeling, workflow analysis, user interface design, and exception handling. It has conducted a technical evaluation of EHRs and offers guidelines for standardization (Lowry et al. 2015). In its work, NIST defines *usability* as "the extent to which a product can be used by specified users to achieve specified goals with effectiveness, efficiency, and satisfaction in a specified context of use." It goes on to suggest that without usable systems, clinicians and even consumers and other users "cannot gain the potential benefits of features and functions of EHR systems."

Frustrated by the fact that the traditional design of EHR and other types of health IT technology is embedded in legacy systems, some providers have created their own usability solutions. However, these provider-created solutions, as well as those offered by vendors, must be applied carefully as needed for the situation, or they could make the problem worse. One size does not fit all.

For example, some vendors have applied overlays and additional pop-up screens to their systems—only to find that they are destructive to workflow and thought processes (that is, *thoughtflow*, which discussed in chapter 5), and contribute to eyestrain and carpal tunnel injuries for clinicians. On the other hand, thoughtful overlays that are tailored to the type of practice and the practice environment can be helpful. Templates and macros need to be developed within specialty domains and with attention to the distinctive needs of physicians, nurses, and other users (Staggers and Rodney 2012).

Another conundrum has been in the use of voice recognition (including systems with natural language processing [NLP]). As noted earlier in this chapter, clinicians use a multiplicity of devices as they perform their work. Many speech-input technologies require a stored voice profile to be present at the point of speech. However, such a profile is not always available when a clinician shifts from one device to another.

Working on multiple devices has implications for the use of other systems as well. Not all devices are enabled to act as a thin client. Such set up can be time-consuming and tricky for an end user, and it is not necessarily desirable. For example, in an emergency, a physician at a dinner party may find it necessary to write a prescription through the e-prescribing network from a smartphone borrowed from a friend. He or she may be able to authenticate directly to the e-prescribing network but not have simultaneous access the office EHR. Voice recognition also will not work in that situation. Setting up remote desktop services or a Citrix solution would make no sense. The result could well be that the physician reverts to a series of telephone calls, all of which introduce risk the e-prescribing system is designed to avoid.

Saving drafts of lengthy structured notes is another example of a usability solution that has strengths and weaknesses. Saving work for later is a standard practice in medicine, but structured data entry is designed to capture data at the point of care when the patient is present and can be queried or examined. The alerts and reminders programmed into structured data entry are intended to be considered during the process of diagnosing and determining a treatment regimen. Therefore, saving a draft and finishing it after the patient goes home and diagnosis and treatment planning are believed to be complete can be a patient safety risk, because the alerts and reminders will not be reviewed at the point of care. Still, workflow in a given specialty or in a given environment may lend itself to use of such a feature. The note initiated on a mobile device may be easier to complete on a desktop.

As shown in table 11.1, the American Medical Association (AMA) has identified eight top challenges and solutions for making EHRs usable (AMA 2014b). The association urges vendors to find ways to seamlessly integrate technology into medical practice that is based on workflow needs. In considering these solution statements, the one factor the AMA has not addressed is the "how." Achieving the AMA's usability goals will take considerable work by vendors, clinicians, healthcare organizations, and policy makers. The ONC (2015) has defined "a shared nationwide interoperability roadmap," which emphasizes that the responsibility for a change of the magnitude being envisioned must be shared. Vendors will need to partner with clinicians of all types who are willing to systematically articulate their workflows (a characteristic not common to knowledge workers), and the developers will then need to take what they learn from the clinicians to create flexible products. The proposed solutions require a degree of flexibility and interoperability that are not currently part of the healthcare system. Realization of the proposed solutions therefore depends on a transformation of the culture and politics of the healthcare

Table 11.1.   AMA eight top solutions for making EHRs usable

- Enhance physicians' ability to provide high-quality patient care.
- Support team-based care.
- Promote care coordination.
- Offer product modularity and configurability.
- Reduce cognitive work load.
- Promote interoperability and data exchange.
- Facilitate digital patient engagement.
- Expedite user input into product design and post-implementation feedback.

Source: AMA 2014b.

delivery system. A longitudinal record for a patient means overcoming both clinical and organizational silos, but it is a critical ingredient for patient safety. The AMA cites then president-elect Steven J. Stack, MD, as saying "physicians believe it a national imperative to reframe policy around the desired future capabilities of this technology and emphasize clinical care improvements as the primary focus."

Data Quality

Usability must ensure that the data collected, used, and shared are as accessible, accurate, consistent, current, comprehensive, defined, granular, relevant, precise, and timely as possible. These characteristics of data must be well managed. The American Health Information Management Association (AHIMA) Data Quality Management Model (figure 11.3) establishes principles for managing the quality of health data in their collection, analysis, application, and warehousing (2015).

Interestingly, although quality data are necessary to support care delivery and measure the quality of care, little has been written about health data quality management as a process outside of the health information management (HIM) profession. However, there is an expanding body of knowledge about data quality management in other fields. For example, in "Data Quality Management: The Most Critical Initiative You Can Implement," Geiger observes that corporations have increasingly come to realize that customer and business data are important corporate assets (2004). Herin recounts that chief financial officers at a conference of the Financial Executives International identified data quality/information integrity as the top technology issue for two years in a

Figure 11.3.   AHIMA's Data Quality Model

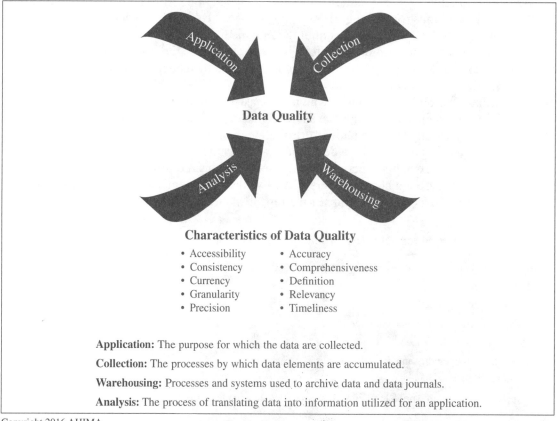

Characteristics of Data Quality

- Accessibility
- Consistency
- Currency
- Granularity
- Precision

- Accuracy
- Comprehensiveness
- Definition
- Relevancy
- Timeliness

Application: The purpose for which the data are collected.

Collection: The processes by which data elements are accumulated.

Warehousing: Processes and systems used to archive data and data journals.

Analysis: The process of translating data into information utilized for an application.

row (2008). *DM Review Magazine* estimated that the cost of poor data quality to U.S. businesses exceeds $600 billion each year (Loshin 2004).

The challenges in healthcare data quality are somewhat different than in general industry. Data quality for healthcare data must look to clinical data standards (Fenton et al. 2007), data content definitions (Kallem et al. 2007), and processes to verify that the data *values* as they are entered into an EHR or other type of health IT meet the principles outlined in AHIMA's Data Quality Management Model. In 2009, the National Committee on Vital and Health Statistics (NCVHS) included data quality in its stewardship framework (Baird and Carr 2009).

Today, companies are developing software to better manage data quality in customer databases. Such software can be used to profile, monitor, and actively manage the quality of enterprise data. Applications can integrate and standardize data across multiple systems and business units. Data correction rules can be defined that are organization-specific and used to cleanse and standardize data. In healthcare, evaluation of data validity, reliability, completeness, and timeliness may be accomplished through a combination of human and machine processes, although the subjective nature of some data makes even this effort difficult.

For example, data editing rules can be established that validate data entries into the EHR. If the value for a data element is to be between 1 and 10, a value of 11 entered by the user would be flagged for action. However, if a value of 4 is entered, there is no way to know with certainty that it is correct. In fact, if the variable for which this data was being entered was a pain scale, 4 could have been considered a severe pain (on a categorical pain scale of 1, none, to 4, severe) that would likely have triggered administration of pain medication such as morphine, or only a moderate pain (on a numerical scale of 1 to 10) that might have triggered only an extra-strength aspirin. Without correlating other information that may or may not have been documented in the record and appreciating the professional judgment of the clinicians involved, it would be impossible for anyone to judge the accuracy of this information after the fact, despite the importance of monitoring and attending to patients' pain (Haig 2007).

Data integrity is another tool that can be used to evaluate data quality. This term refers to whether the representation of the data in electronic systems is improperly altered after it is entered. Data integrity is obviously a critical component of the technical design of an EHR as well other forms of health IT. For example, suppose a data edit rule is for the data to be between 0.01 and 0.10. The user enters 0.1, but the equipment somehow alters the representation of the entry to 1.0—this error is as critical as if the user had entered the invalid value. It might even be more critical because the data-editing rules will not catch a machine error. As a result, data integrity controls must be in place to ensure that data are not altered after they are entered. Data integrity problems can arise from poor data integration, where data from multiple systems are not properly synchronized. Programming errors can contribute to data integrity issues where processes can produce erroneous data. Human error in keystroking can produce unintended commands that alter data. Exposure of equipment and media to excessive heat, strong magnetic fields, or other mechanical problems may corrupt data. Finally, viruses and other malicious codes are the biggest threat to data integrity (Ackerman 2013).

Data Retrieval Strategies

As usability and data quality are incorporated into the design and redesign of EHRs and other health IT, there are some key principles to consider. The model shown in figure 11.4 was introduced a number of years ago to describe clinical decision making in general and was based on a model created even earlier for basic information processing (Elson et al. 1997). Its relevance to current data retrieval and documentation strategies design is astounding. It shows that because of system constraints in external memory (primarily paper-based records but also knowledge sources such as literature and consultants), there is increased reliance on the clinician's long-term memory. Human

Figure 11.4.   Model of impact of system constraints on clinical decision making

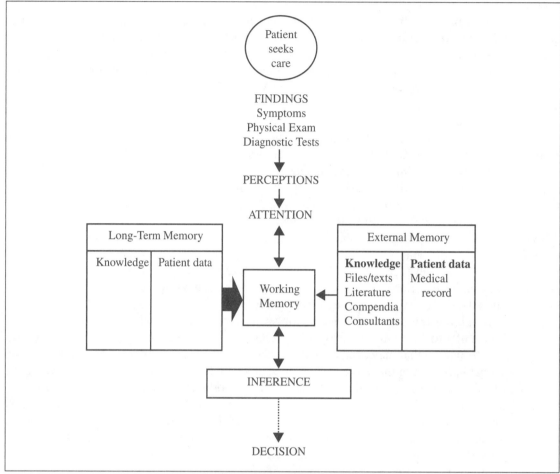

memory has significant failings; therefore, it is important to build a system that will enhance access to external memory for improved decision making. Key to that is an intuitive workstation that can be integrated into clinical workflow.

In using "external memory" support, clinicians can do the following:

- Scan data rapidly to obtain a quick overview and understanding of a new patient.

- Retrieve data to refamiliarize themselves with a former patient's history.

- Search data for specific facts relative to a current patient.

- Review a range of data to solve a problem relative to a current patient.

Each of these processes is accompanied by several levels of text processing, ranging from reading all the words in a paragraph to skipping a paragraph altogether. Workstation and screen design features must reflect how clinicians use information. Even within paper-based documents, graphic, textual, and positional features of the data, logically related and controlled, are essential for orientation, navigation, and effective limitation of search space. With this in mind, is it any wonder that clinicians complain about having to navigate through too many screens or having a limited amount of data on one screen?

There are many considerations relative to data retrieval and the functionality sought in developing functional specifications for an EHR system or other type of health IT. These include screen density, size of device, search capability, positioning of content and navigational support, consistency of design and flexibility, graphics, and use of color and icons. Moreover, attention must be paid to matching these characteristics to the applications they serve (Britto 2005).

Screen Density

Screen density refers to the amount of data on a single screen. In fact, data retrieval is enhanced by greater screen density. This assertion may seem counterintuitive, and many clinicians involved in the EHR selection process look for screens that are highly streamlined. But the Regenstrief Institute for Health Care, a privately endowed healthcare research organization founded in 1969, has conducted numerous studies on how people use components of the EHR. In studies of eye movements of EHR users, they determined that the denser the screen, the better it is for data retrieval purposes. To ensure dense screens are readable without eyestrain, screen resolution must as high as possible.

Size of Device

Size of device is a consideration closely related to screen density. Many clinicians want to be mobile with their computing and are using different types of devices depending on where they are at any given point in their daily work. Designs intended for a large monitor may not work on a smaller device, especially if it has a lower-resolution display screen. (As noted previously, the size of a screen is often referred to as *screen real estate*.) If EHR systems are being designed for use at both PC workstations and handheld device workstations, consideration must be given to how data can be displayed effectively on both types of device and whether the data will look the same across all devices.

Smaller screens generally make it more difficult to rapidly scan large volumes of data to obtain a quick overview and understanding of a new patient or to refamiliarize oneself with a former patient's history. However, creative ways are being found to overcome these issues. Figure 11.5

Figure 11.5.   Sample patient summary screen

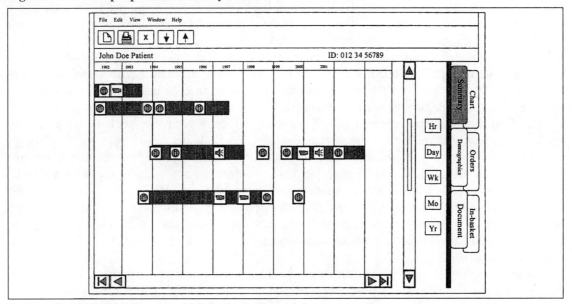

provides a sample patient summary screen that identifies the number of times the patient has been seen over time. The icons can characterize whether each event was an office visit, laboratory test, admission, and so on, and serve as a launching pad to information about that event. Ideally, this structure or a similar one should enable the user to access a longitudinal record encompassing multiple provider records and the patient's personal health record. Additionally, there should be search capability to use when a particular factor is being sought within the patient's healthcare history.

Search Capability

Search capability and the number of levels to drill down are important considerations for all data retrieval strategies. However, they are especially critical for viewing specific patient facts on a small screen or viewing a range of data to solve a current problem. The EHR and some other types of health IT need to permit users to make highly structured queries from one screen. Web browser experience shows that users who must go through multiple layers are more likely to lose the thread of meaning they are looking for in the data. In fact, this is one reason browser-based advanced search capability technology is needed for EHR systems.

Navigational Support and Content Positioning

Navigational support and content positioning are critical to helping clinicians retrieve data. Navigational support with respect to the display screen refers to the ability to move from one screen to another, drill down to retrieve further detail about something, access knowledge bases, or request a graph or other form of display. Navigation is made easy with options arranged in pull-down menus, buttons, radio dials, and slide bars, all of which can be selected with a navigational device, such as a keyboard, mouse, touch pad, trackball, track point, touch screen, and, to some extent, handwriting recognition and voice commands using speech recognition.

Although designs in paper record systems are not standardized, the application of certain design conventions for form construction helps clinicians navigate through the paper chart. For example, patient-identifying information typically is put at the top left or top right of each form. Sheets are colored or have color bars on them. There may be tabs, especially for inpatient charts at the nursing station.

Likewise, there are no standards for system display designs for health IT, and design conventions are not yet established. Some EHR vendors have attempted to make the EHR look like a paper record, with tabs and colors. Other vendors design screens to look like screens in Microsoft Windows applications. To some extent, the position of content and navigational support is a matter of personal preference. However, the extent to which such designs can be standardized helps clinicians who may have to use multiple applications or even multiple EHRs at different locations. Mace (2015) notes that there is a tension that runs through EHR usability improvement. He observes that some people push for totally standardized user interfaces and workflows for reasons ranging from simplicity of training and help-desk support to larger issues such as implementing quality measures. Alternatively, others want flexibility in EHR display options so the displays can conform to established workflows in an organization or personal preferences and distinctive professional priorities. He notes, for example, that a neurologist and a nephrologist have significantly different needs with respect to information; one who is heavily numbers-driven and one who is examination- and imaging-driven. It might therefore be best to set up different templates for these areas of practice, even though the fundamental data elements common to all patient care (such as, patient identification, authentication mechanisms, date recording) would still benefit from standardization.

When migrating to an EHR, an early step should be to take a forms inventory, reduce redundancy in present forms, evaluate how necessary redundancy in today's forms can be reduced further with the EHR, and plan how the presentation of the legal health record will be achieved in the electronic environment (Quinsey 2007). Many hospitals believe they have to replicate their paper record in the electronic record. Careful planning, however, can streamline even this presentation. For instance, in a paper environment, nurses often have to complete as many as a dozen forms with considerable repetition of data entry on each. An electronic documentation system would enable the repetitive data to be prepopulated on each form, saving time and also ensuring consistency. However, the hospital should assess whether it is necessary to retain all dozen forms. Because access to the data is now available across the hospital, the need for different forms to go to different destinations is no longer necessary. It may be more important to address what specific views are needed and ensure that each view can be captured for the legal health record.

Consistency of Design and Flexibility

Consistency of design and flexibility may seem to be opposing considerations, but both have an important relationship to data retrieval. Although it may not be feasible or even desirable to control the design of different vendor products, the placement of data and navigational devices ought to be consistent within a given system and there should be standards that cut across all systems where feasible. Within a given product, screens should essentially all have the same look and feel for ease of scanning the information and physically navigating through it. However, as already noted, to some extent, how screens should look and navigate is a matter of personal preference. Therefore, an ideal feature might be to have the flexibility to create unique user designs.

Some experts suggest that flexibility is critical to clinician adoption; others suggest that it may actually hinder adoption because it is not always possible to design a system to exact specifications. Furthermore, they argue that the sooner clinicians learn to be flexible rather than demanding flexibility in health IT products, the better off they will be. As with most debates, the truth is probably somewhere in the middle.

Graphics

Graphics is one of the unique features of retrieving data from an EHR system. Current **graphical user interface (GUI)** technology permits not only straight text and the ability to import images but also the ability to convert text into graphics. The Windows OS also permits many views of different data displayed at one time. Hence, drug dosages and laboratory results can be plotted on a graph while the clinician is viewing an x-ray image and seeing a textual reminder. Graphics can be zoomed in and out for better viewing.

Color and Icons

The use of color and icons is another important consideration when speaking of data retrieval and functionality. Color can be effective, but it should be accompanied by some other form of indicator. Some people are color blind, so relying totally on color to guide navigation may not work. In addition, different types of display screens display color differently. A lovely shade of green on one screen may look putrid on another.

Icons are popular indicators, and some can be made to flash when they represent an alarm or special form of alert. They can be popular in guiding a clinician through a list. For example, in figure 11.5, icons are used in the sample patient summary timelines to indicate the type of information. The icon representing sound signals that the user can listen to dictation. The camera icon represents an image that can be viewed. Most icons are relatively self-explanatory. Many are spinoffs from road signs or are conventionally used in many other applications. However, some designers can become creative, and their icons may not be universally understood.

Documentation Strategies

In addition to the strategies described for data retrieval, data capture for documentation must consider the various forms of data entry and creation, including free-text entry, structured data entry from pick lists or pull-down menus, template-based entry, and NLP.

Free Text

Free text is the entry of narrative data, primarily via keyboarding, although dictation, voice recognition, and handwriting recognition are possible. Free text entry can be facilitated by various input features, such as copy and paste, macros, and even "low-tech" solutions such as using scribes (see chapter 4). The result of free text entry is unstructured data, which may be more difficult to process than structured data, although new technologies are improving the processing of unstructured data (see chapter 10).

Data entry aids can be helpful, but they can also put an organization at risk for documentation compliance. **Copy and paste**, wherein a clinician literally copies an entry from a previous note or a different patient's record and pastes it into the new entry is one of the most commonly used data-entry aids—and one that poses considerable risk. Although **data reuse** is a common data entry strategy in computer applications, clinicians must be extremely cautious to ensure that the copied material is entirely applicable for the new entry. Inadvertently copying a reference to a different patient or a different time can nullify an entry and cause the entire record to be suspect. The copy-and-paste process is designed to speed data entry, but the clinician who works too quickly may not notice additional or missing data. Consequently, the entry misrepresents the case and potentially results in submitting a fraudulent claim for reimbursement (Dimick 2008). The data entry error could also result in harm to the patient and might be a sentinel event that must be reported to the Joint Commission (Joint Commission 2015). Because copy-and-paste functionality is prevalent in EHR products, every organization must evaluate how it might be used and develop solid application rules to ensure accurate use (AHIMA 2014). Many suggest that use of the functionality be prohibited. Although this policy may be desirable, the key to not permitting such functionality is making it unavailable. If such a function is available, policy alone is generally insufficient to prevent its use.

Another issue with free text is the potential for it to be inconsistent with structured data that are entered elsewhere or at another time. For example in one hospital, physician use of a comments field for medication orders in a CPOE system did not permit the clinical decision support system of the CPOE to operate, and the entries with comments caused extra work for nurses, who had to track down physicians to enter the orders correctly or take a telephone order. After this workaround, the comments and entry in CPOE were often somewhat different if not contradictory (Reynolds et al. 2005).

Data Entry from Pick Lists or Pull-Down Menus

Structured data entry from pick lists or pull-down menus is an important data capture technique. Most EHR systems use a combination of structured data entry and free text. When using structured data entry, it is important that the data options be clearly defined, comprehensive, and up to date. Ideally, the data should be drawn from a controlled vocabulary and encoded by the EHR system for use in processing. Structured data are essential to ultimately drive clinical decision support.

Structured data entry should be easier and quicker to use than keyboarding, even for experienced typists. However, the user must go through a learning curve and the system must be well designed, where underlying logic drives the menu options. For example, a structured data entry physical examination for an infant should not contain physical examination components relating only to adults. To be most effective, structured data entry should be highly tailored to the type of patient. This requires considerable work up front, especially when the setting includes unusual specialties. This is one reason many physicians prefer to buy EHRs related to their specialty, which come with many premade structured data entry menus.

Another consideration in structured data entry relates to **defaults**. Structured data entry should be designed so that rules are strictly followed relative to the absence of a response. It is not good documentation to have the default to an unanswered selection be "normal." If there is no response to an item, there should be a prompt to obtain a response for critical items, or the default should be "not recorded." Systems that are designed to prompt for a required response should permit the user to proceed, but the entry should be marked incomplete until a response is generated.

A final feature related to structured data entry is the ability to derive narrative from structured data. For example, after a physician responds to each item on a structured physical examination, some systems embed the responses into a narrative that makes the final output look as though it was dictated or keyed in. For example, if one element is "chief complaint" and the response is "shortness of breath," the EHR system could create this statement: "The patient complains of shortness of breath."

Template-based Entry

Template-based entry is something of a cross between free text and structured data entry. Because many notes follow a repeated structure and include similar types of data, templates may be developed wherein the clinician need only add variable data. Macros that provide phrases or sentences to complete the variable portions of templates can further speed the use of automated templates.

An example of a data capture screen that includes both pull-down menus for structured data and the results of macros is displayed in figure 11.6.

Natural Language Processing

Deriving structure from unstructured text refers to NLP. This endeavor is one of the biggest remaining challenges currently faced by computer scientists today. NLP is a technical process in which highly sophisticated computer programs "read" strings of free text and separate the words or

Figure 11.6. Example of structured data-entry template with macros

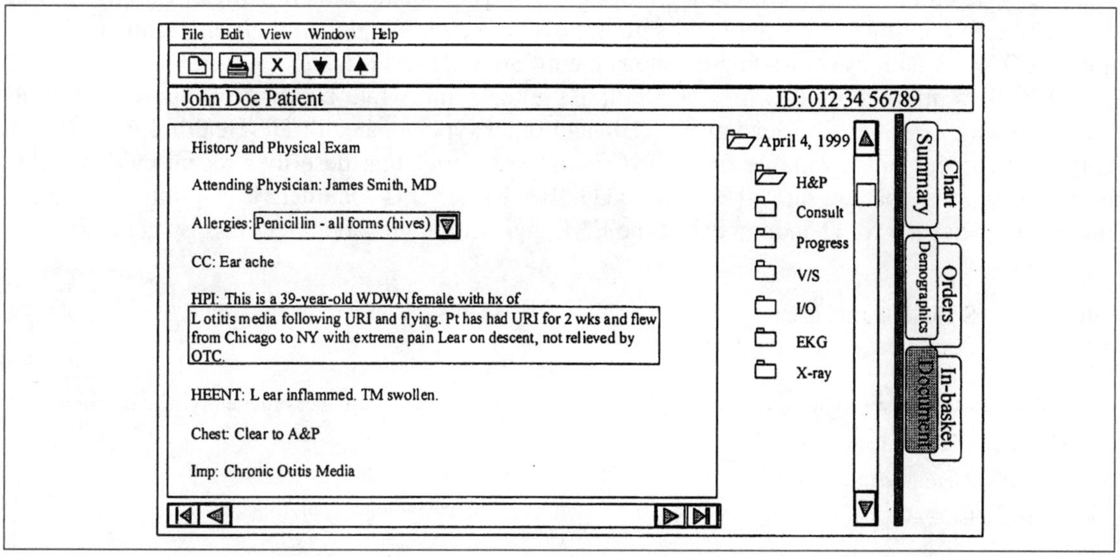

phrases into little packets (called *parsing*). The programs then assign computer codes to the individual packets, thereby codifying the text for storage, analysis, and later retrieval. NLP is increasingly being studied and refined. For example, to solve a problem similar to that described earlier in which doctors used comment fields to indicate medication orders, researchers were able to extract and normalize drug data stored in free text fields of an anesthesia EHR by comparing the entries to RxNorm. As a result, free text fields with their errors in spelling, abbreviations, and jargon could be used once NLP was applied (Levin et al. 2007). Still, the confined vocabulary of anesthesia drugs made this process easier than it would be for the entire medical vocabulary.

Progress on SAFER Systems for Patient Safety

While the many calls for improvements in EHRs may seem disheartening because they point to deficiencies in current health IT, it is important to point out that such calls would not be made if EHRs and other types of health IT had no potential to improve patient care and patient safety. There is evidence that EHRs have already led to patient safety improvements.

Improving the usability of EHRs and other forms of health IT and achieving better patient outcomes through their use are not just technological challenges. As discussed in chapter 6, the success of EHRs and other health IT is, at least in part, a function of change management. In introducing the SAFER Guides (described below) to its members, AHIMA published a document by Sittig and colleagues, who observe the following:

> EHR-related safety risks emanate not just from the features and functions of the technology itself, but also from the sociotechnical context and culture in which these systems are implemented and used. Sociotechnical context means that it is not just the hardware and software required to run the EHR application that factor into creating and maintaining an up-to-date, accurate medical record, but also the workflow processes, people, policies, and other social and organizational factors. (Sittig et al. 2014)

Figure 1.5 in chapter 1 echoes this sentiment.

In July 2013, the ONC published the Health IT Patient Safety Action and Surveillance Plan and established the Health IT Safety Program to coordinate activities related to the plan (ONC 2013). The tenets of the plan are to learn, improve, and lead. One of the initiatives from this plan is the issuance of **SAFER** (Safety Assurance Factors for EHR Resilience) Guides for EHRs and other health IT (HealthIT.gov 2014b). These guides are self-assessment tools that organizations can use to evaluate and optimize the safety and safe use of these technologies in their environment. There are nine SAFER Guides addressing the areas identified in table 11.2.

ONC also offers a number of other toolkits, guides, and white papers to support their goals for improving, learning, and leading in EHR and other types of health IT (HealthIT.gov 2014a). Among the documents available from ONC is an issue brief that describes recent evidence that health IT improves patient safety (Banger and Graber 2015). This document is inspirational reading for times when calls for abandonment of the EHR and complaints about technology get too loud.

Table 11.2   SAFER guide areas

• High priority practices	• Patient identification
• Organizational responsibilities	• Computerized provider order entry with decision support
• Contingency planning	
• System configuration	• Test results reporting and follow-up
• System interfaces	• Clinician communication

Check Your Understanding 11.2

Choose the best answer:

1. Alteration of the representation of data in electronic systems is:

    a. Data quality

    b. Data integrity

    c. Security

    d. Stewardship

2. The best way to afford usability in an EHR system is to:

    a. Buy new browser-based products

    b. Help users integrate their workflows into the technology

    c. Redesign user workflows to meet system requirements

    d. Retrain users

3. Which of the following data entry aids put an organization at risk for nullifying the content of the entire health record?

    a. Copy and paste

    b. Pick lists

    c. Saving drafts of structured notes

    d. Voice recognition

4. Which of the following tensions must be addressed in health IT to ensure its success?

    a. Achieving consistency and flexibility

    b. Gaining value without structured data

    c. Requiring vendors to improve products at no cost to organizations

    d. Hardware obsolescence versus software development

5. A data entry aid that can be misunderstood or not understood at all is:

    a. Drop-down menu

    b. Comment field

    c. Icon

    d. Template

Emerging Technologies

Obviously, technologies and their uses are rapidly evolving. Moore's law states that "technology changes every 18 months" (Yoffie 2010), although some suggest that this pace of change is not sustainable (Peckham 2012). Understanding trends in emerging technologies is critical to making the right choices about what new technologies to adopt and when.

New technologies for healthcare are not unique to information systems. In fact, healthcare often adopts new technologies more rapidly in the clinical arena than in the information systems arena. New clinical technologies include smart bandages that can differentiate among bacteria, new contamination-detection technology that can alert someone that his or her hands are not clean enough, RFID tags that can be implanted under the skin, digital pens, and radiosurgical technology to enhance radiography and radiation therapy.

Monitoring publications and websites is critical in the development and use of EHR systems. Even if the organization already has an EHR system, understanding what new technology is being created can help health IT decision makers anticipate upgrades, push for adoption of new technologies from vendors, and respond to challenges from those who want to adopt new technology the organization does not have yet.

By monitoring emerging technology, organizations can plan for new technology that serves the organization's mission and vision. Many healthcare providers have bought system components from a single vendor in a best-of-fit strategy because the components were well integrated. But as information systems capabilities have expanded, some of these vendors did not support some of the newer functionality or MU requirements, and in some cases, purchased functionality from other companies that were not as interoperable. This type of scenario leads many providers to consider their options: Do they wait for their vendor to support new technology for their older systems? Do they buy new clinical applications from another vendor or several vendors? Do they rip out and replace their aging systems? Obviously, there is no one right answer. However, to the extent that new or replacement systems are being acquired, it behooves the organization to buy as openly architected systems as possible so they can plug and play with many new technology components to come and to plan for obsolescence.

References and Resources

Ackerman, R.K. 2013 (July 31). Blog: Data integrity is the biggest threat in cyberspace. *Signal*. Armed Forces Communications and Electronics Association. http://www.afcea.org/content/?q=data-integrity-biggest-threat-cyberspace.

American Health Information Management Association (AHIMA). 2014 (March 17). Appropriate use of the copy and paste functionality in electronic health records. http://bok.ahima.org/PdfView?oid=300306.

American Medical Association (AMA). 2014a (September 16). Press Release. AMA calls for design overhaul of electronic health records to improve usability. http://www.ama-assn.org/ama/pub/news/news/2014/2014-09-16-solutions-to-ehr-systems.page.

American Medical Association (AMA). 2014b (September 16). 8 top challenges and solutions for making EHRs usable. *AMA Wire*. http://www.ama-assn.org/ama/ama-wire/post/8-top-challenges-solutions-making-ehrs-usable.

Asaro, T. 2005 (July). The athlete or the geek? Block vs. file storage. TechTarget Search Storage. http://searchstorage.techtarget.com/news/1103644/The-athlete-or-the-geek-Block-vs-file-storage.

Baird, S., and J.M. Carr. 2009 Health data stewardship: what, why, who, how—an NCVHS primer. National Committee on Vital and Health Statistics (NCVHS). http://www.ncvhs.hhs.gov/wp-content/uploads/2014/05/090930lt.pdf.

Banger, A., and M.L. Graber 2015 (February). *Recent Evidence that Health IT Improves Patient Safety*. Issue brief prepared for Office of the National Coordinator for Health Information Technology. https://www.healthit.gov/sites/default/files/brief_1_final_feb11t.pdf.

Barnatt, C.A. 2012 (September 13) Computer storage. ExplainingComputers.com Guide to Computing. http://explainingcomputers.com/storage.html.

Bell, M.A. 2005 (April 22). *Use Best Practices to Design Data Center Facilities*. Gartner Research ID no. G00127434. https://www.gartner.com/doc/476880/use-best-practices-design-data.

Blokdijk, G. 2010. *Virtualization—The Complete Cornerstone Guide to Virtualization Best Practices*, 2nd ed. Brisbane, Australia: Emereo.

Bradley, T. 2009 (August 7). VPN's: IPSec vs. SSL. Essential Computer Security. http://www.tonybradley.com/2009/08/vpsn-ipsec-vs-ssl.

Britto, J. 2005. Technologies that improve the clinical process. *ADVANCE for Health Information Executives*. 9(12):21–24, 73.

Carter, J. 2008. *Electronic Health Records: A Guide for Clinicians and Administrators*, 2nd ed. Philadelphia: ACP Press.

CCM Forum. 2015 (November). What is Wi-Fi and how does it work? CCM Benchmark Group. http://ccm.net/faq/298-what-is-wi-fi-and-how-does-it-work.

Chang, J. 2015 (December 17). 5 reasons to consider RDS over HDX. Workspot, Inc. blog. http://blog.workspot.com/5-reasons-rds-over-hdx.

Davis, D. 2009a (January 8). Server virtualization, network virtualization & storage virtualization explained. Petri IT Knowledgebase. https://www.petri.com/server-virtualization-network-virtualization-storage-virtualization.

Davis, D. 2009b (January 7). How to use the OSI Model to troubleshoot networks. Petri IT Knowledgebase. https://www.petri.com/csc_how_to_use_the_osi_model_to_troubleshoot_networks.

Davoudi, S, J. Dooling, B. Glondys, T. Jones, L. Kadlec, S. Overgaard, K. Ruben, and A. Wendicke. 2015. Data Quality Management model (2015 Update). *Journal of AHIMA* 86(10): expanded web version.

Derfler, F.J., and L. Freed. 2005. *How Networks Work*, 7th ed. Indianapolis, IN: Que Corporation.

Dimick, C. 2008. Documentation bad habits, shortcuts in electronic records pose risk. *Journal of AHIMA*. 79(6):40–43.

Durkin, S., and B. Just. 2008. An IT primer for health information exchange. *Journal of AHIMA*. 79(1):38–42.

Elson, R.B., J.G. Faughnan, and D.P. Connelly. 1997. An industrial process view of information delivery to support clinical decision making: Implications for system design and process measures. *Journal of the American Medical Informatics Association*. 4(4):266–278.

Enterprise Management Associates (EMA). 2009 (December). *The Building Blocks for Private Cloud: Automation, Virtualization, and Cloud Management Services*. Boulder, CO: EMA.

Fenton, S.H., et al. 2007. Data standards, data quality, and interoperability. *Journal of AHIMA* 78(2).

Food and Drug Administration (FDA). 2014 (October 29). Mammography Quality Standards Act regulations. http://www.fda.gov/Radiation-EmittingProducts/MammographyQualityStandardsActandProgram/Regulations/ucm110906.htm.

Freeman, A. 2013 (January 9). Networks & Transmission Media. http://nettran1.blogspot.com.

Geiger, J.G., Intelligent Solutions. 2004 (May). Data Quality Management: The Most Critical Initiative You Can Implement. http://www2.sas.com/proceedings/sugi29/098-29.pdf.

Goodwins, R. 2015 (January 1). The future of storage: 2015 and beyond. ZDNet. http://www.zdnet.com/article/the-future-of-storage-2015-and-beyond.

Haig, S. 2007 (February 20). How real is your pain? *Time Magazine*.

Hardy, K. 2010 (May 19). Data storage of top concern to healthcare providers. *Healthcare IT News*. http://www.healthcareitnews.com/news/data-storage-top-concern-healthcare-providers.

Healthcare Information and Management Systems Society (HIMSS). 2011(February). *Promoting Usability in Health Organizations: Initial Steps and Progress Toward a Healthcare Usability Maturity Model*. Chicago, IL: Healthcare Information Management Systems Society.

Healthcare Practice IT. 2011 (March 7). Virtual private networks—Do you need one? Healthcare Practice IT blog. http://www.healthcarepracticeit.com/2011/03/virtual-private-networks%E2%80%94do-you-need-one.

HealthIT.gov. 2014a (September 19). Policymaking, regulation, & strategy: Health IT and safety (launchpad). https://www.healthit.gov/policy-researchers-implementers/health-it-and-safety.

HealthIT.gov. 2014b (January). SAFER Guides. https://www.healthit.gov/safer/safer-guides.

Herin, J., Computer Sciences Corporation. 2008 (May 6). Chief financial officers cite data quality/information integrity as top technology issue for second year. *PR Newswire*.

http://www.himss.org/promoting-usability-health-organizations-initial-steps-and-progress-toward-healthcare-usability?ItemNumber=10910

Institute of Electrical and Electronics Engineers (IEEE). 2011. IEEE 802.11 wireless local area networks, Working Group for WLAN Standards. http://www.ieee802.org/11.

Joint Commission. 2015 (February). Preventing copy-and-paste errors in EHRs. *Quick Safety Advisory*, issue 10. http://www.jointcommission.org/assets/1/23/quick_safety_issue_10.pdf.

Kallem, C., et al. 2007 (July). Data content for EHR documentation. *Journal of AHIMA* 78(7):73–76.

Levin, M.A., et al. 2007. Extraction and mapping of drug names from free text to a standardized nomenclature. *AMIA Annual Symposium Proceedings*. 438.

Loshin, D. 2004 (April). Issues and opportunities in data quality management coordination. *DM Review Magazine*.

Lowry, S.Z., M. Ramaiah, E.S. Patterson, S.S. Prettyman, D. Simmons, D. Brick, L.A. Paul, M.C. Gibbons, and S.L. Taylor. 2015 (October 7). *Technical Evaluation, Testing, and Validation of the Usability of Electronic Health Records: Empirically Based Use Cases for Validating Safety—Enhanced Usability and Guidelines for Standardization*. National Institute of Standards and Technology. NIST interagency/internal report (NISTIR) 7804-1. https://www2.nist.gov/node/764686.

Mace, S. 2015 (June). How providers are achieving EHR usability. *HealthLeaders*, http://healthleadersmedia.com/content/TEC-321127/How-Providers-are-Achieving-EHR-Usability##.

Marks, H. 2008 (February 25). Long-term storage & compliance: CAS vs. locked NAS. *Network Computing*. http://www.networkcomputing.com/unified-communications/long-term-storage-compliance-cas-vs-locked-nas/1663316193.

Mediati, N. 2016. FCC: 10 percent of Americans still lack access to proper broadband. *PC World*. http://www.networkworld.com/article/3020578/internet/fcc-10-percent-of-americans-still-lack-access-to-proper-broadband.html

Mell, P., and T. Grance. 2011 (September). The NIST Definition of Cloud Computing: Recommendations of the National Institute of Standards and Technology. NIST special publication 800-145. http://nvlpubs.nist.gov/nistpubs/Legacy/SP/nistspecialpublication800-145.pdf.

National Institute of Standards and Technology (NIST). 2011 (March 3). Implementation Guidance for FIPS PUB 140-2 and the Cryptographic Module Validation Program. http://csrc.nist.gov/groups/STM/cmvp/documents/fips140-2/FIPS1402IG.pdf.

Office of the National Coordinator for Health Information Technology (ONC). 2013 (July). ONC Health IT Safety Program—Progress on Health IT Patient Safety Action and Surveillance Plan. https://www.healthit.gov/sites/default/files/ONC_HIT_SafetyProgramReport_9-9-14_.pdf.

Office of the National Coordinator for Health Information Technology (ONC). 2015. Connecting health and care for the nation: A shared nationwide interoperability roadmap final version 1.0. https://www.healthit.gov/sites/default/files/hie-interoperability/nationwide-interoperability-roadmap-final-version-1.0.pdf.

Peckham, M. 2012 (May 1). The collapse of Moore's Law: Physicist says it's already happening. *Time Magazine*. http://techland.time.com/2012/05/01/the-collapse-of-moores-law-physicist-says-its-already-happening.

Petri, D. 2009 (January 8). OSI model concepts. Petri IT Knowledgebase. https://www.petri.com/osi_concepts.

Quinsey, C.A. 2007. Managing forms in the legal health record. *Journal of AHIMA*. 78(7):58–59.

Raffo, D. 2010 (February 19). Healthcare system rolls its own data storage "cloud" for researchers. SearchStorage.com. http://searchstorage.techtarget.com/news/1389746/Health-care-system-rolls-its-own-data-storage-cloud-for-researchers.

Reynolds, K., et al. 2005. The impact on patient safety of free-text entry of nursing orders into an electronic medical record in an integrated delivery network. *AMIA Annual Symposium Proceedings*. 1095.

Saran, C. 2015 (March). What will office desktop computing look like in 2020? ComputerWeekly.com. http://www.computerweekly.com/feature/What-will-office-desktop-computing-look-like-in-2020.

Scarfone, K., et al. 2011 (January). *Guide to Security for Full Virtualization Technologies*. National Institute of Standards and Technology (NIST) special publication 800-125. http://csrc.nist.gov/publications/nistpubs/800-125/SP800-125-final.pdf.

Sessoms, D. 2014. 11 myths About 802.11ac on hospital wireless networks. SecureEdge Networks blog. http://www.securedgenetworks.com/blog/11-Myths-About-802-11ac-on-Hospital-Wireless-Networks.

Sittig, D.F., et al. 2014. ONC issues guides for SAFER EHRs. *Journal of AHIMA*, 85(4):50–52.

Sliwa, C. 2009 (February 10). Storage explained: Cloud storage defined. SearchStorage.com. http://searchstorage.techtarget.com/news/1347466/Storage-Explained-Cloud-storage-defined.

Snider, M, et al. 2015 (February 27). What is net neutrality and what does it mean to me? *USA Today*. http://www.usatoday.com/story/tech/2015/02/24/net-neutrality-what-is-it-guide/23237737.

Staggers, N., and M.R. Rodney. 2012 (June 23). Promoting usability in organizations with a new health usability model: implications for nursing informatics. *Nursing Informatics*. http://www.ncbi.nlm.nih.gov/pmc/articles/PMC3799150.

Stoffels, B. 2012 (February). Wi-Fi and cellular. *OSP Magazine*. http://www.ospmag.com/issue/article/022012-Stoffels.

World Wide Web Consortium (W3C) Working Group. 2004 (February). Note 11: Web Services architecture. http://www.w3.org/TR/ws-arch.

Yoffie, D.B. 2010 (March 18). Innovations changing the world: New technologies, Harvard, and China. Presentation at Harvard and China: A Research Symposium. http://projects.iq.harvard.edu/harvardcentershanghai/opening-events.

Chapter 12
Health IT Privacy and Security

Key Terms

Accountability
Agent
Alteration
Authentication
Availability
Certificate authority (CA)
Confidentiality
Corrective action
Cyberspace
Cyber threat
Designated record set
Destruction
Digital certificate
Digital signature
Disclosure
Electronic signature
Encryption
Event
Failover
Full redundancy
Identity proofing
Incidental uses and disclosures
Informed consent
Integrity

Medical identity theft

Minimum necessary

Mobile device management (MDM)

Nonrepudiation

Payment Card Industry Data Security Standard (PCI-DSS)

Privacy

Protected health information

Public-key infrastructure (PKI)

Red Flags Rule

Registration authority (RA)

Reliability

Resolution amount

Risk analysis

Security

Settlement agreement

Storage management program

Storage virtualization

Target

Threat

Threat intelligence

TPO

Triggered review

Trust

Unified threat management (UTM)

Vulnerability

X.509

Learning Objectives

- Explain the federal privacy and security standardization efforts.

- Describe technology and other solutions that can help support privacy and security management.

- Discuss the steps necessary to manage a breach of protected health information.

- Describe the possible applicability of the Red Flags Rule and the Payment Card Industry Data Measure in certain organizations.

- Summarize key administrative and physical factors that can contribute to reducing risks to privacy and security in a health IT environment.

- Identify emerging privacy and security threats and suggests strategies for addressing them.

Although healthcare has always been concerned with patient privacy and the confidentiality of health information, there were no relevant national standards prior to the adoption of the Health Insurance Portability and Accountability Act (HIPAA) of 1996 and its subsequent regulations. HIPAA's Administrative Simplification provisions include important privacy and security standards for covered entities (health plans, healthcare clearinghouses, and providers that conduct administrative and financial transactions in electronic form) and other entities with which they do business. The Health Information Technology for Economic and Clinical Health (HITECH) Act of 2009 called for updating the HIPAA Privacy, Security and Enforcement Rules and the addition of a Breach Notification Rule from the US Department of Health and Human Services (HHS) and a similar Breach Notification Rule from the Federal Trade Commission (FTC) relating to breaches from vended personal health records. The Omnibus Rule, as a composite of several rules finalized in 2013, contributed further to addressing the privacy enhancements called for under HITECH (although there are still some remaining privacy standards yet to be updated per HITECH). Other laws and the regulations derived from them have also addressed specialized aspects of health-related privacy and security.

These federally adopted standards are currently overseen by the HHS Office for Civil Rights (OCR) with technology guidance from the HHS Office of the National Coordinator for Health Information Technology (ONC) and the US Department of Commerce National Institute of Standards and Technology (NIST). Many guidance documents, toolkits, and educational materials on the topic of security have been distributed by these agencies as well as many professional associations and vendors, and the OCR has undertaken a number of enforcement activities. Nevertheless, privacy and security issues continue to be pressing problems in healthcare—as they have been in other industries.

HIPAA Privacy and Security Rules

Privacy has been a basic tenet of medicine since Hippocrates, and information security has always been a good business practice. In recent decades in the United States, HIPAA has become the primary source of privacy and security requirements for healthcare. As noted in the introduction to this chapter, additional legislation, regulation, and guidance documents have enhanced HIPAA since it was enacted in 1996. It is important that people working with health information technology (health IT) and the electronic health record (EHR) understand the definitions of terms associated with privacy and security in general, recognize who is affected by the HIPAA regulations, and be familiar with the business case for addressing privacy and security in a context where the sharing of health data can be considered beneficial for healthcare organizations and patients.

Definitions of Terms

One of the best-known sources of definitions associated with privacy and confidentiality is a document referred to as the Belmont Report (HHS 1979), which provides the ethical principles and guidelines for the protection of human subjects of research. While the report's focus is research and it was created nearly four decades ago, it serves as the underpinnings for much of the US approach to privacy policy in healthcare.

Privacy is the right of an individual to be left alone. In healthcare, it has come to mean the right to control the uses and disclosures of protected health information (PHI), and for individuals to be assured of certain rights in their health information.

Security measures complement privacy and also afford certain legal and usability assurance. Security provides **confidentiality**, which pertains to the treatment of information that an individual has disclosed in a relationship of trust and with the expectation that it will not be divulged to others in ways that are inconsistent with the understanding of the original disclosure unless the individual grants permission. Security also affords **integrity**, which—as related to data—refers to the accuracy and validity of data over its lifecycle. The third function of security is to afford **availability**, generally meaning that data continue to be able to be provided to authorized users at a required level of performance in situations ranging from normal through disastrous. These three functions of security are sometimes described as "the CIA of security."

Each security function has a specific risk associated with it. The risk of insufficient security for confidentiality is wrongful **disclosure**. Threats to data integrity result in improper data **alteration** or **destruction**, and threats to data availability result in many types of potential business harm that come from not having data when needed. The relationships between these terms are illustrated in figure 12.1.

Additional important terms are defined within the HIPAA privacy and security rules. A few of these terms and their definitions as they are used in this chapter are provided in figure 12.2.

HIPAA Enforcement Rule

Another important aspect of changes to the Privacy and Security Rule under HITECH is that of enforcement. On October 30, 2009, HHS issued an update to the existing HIPAA Enforcement Rule, which increased the civil monetary penalty amounts of violations considerably; clarified that individuals—not just organizations—were subject to civil and criminal penalties; authorized state attorneys general to take enforcement action against HIPAA violators; and enabled penalty money to be returned to OCR for both further enforcement and to be shared with harmed individuals. Perhaps most important, the HITECH enforcement changes also made it a requirement for OCR

Figure 12.1.   Privacy and security principles and relationships

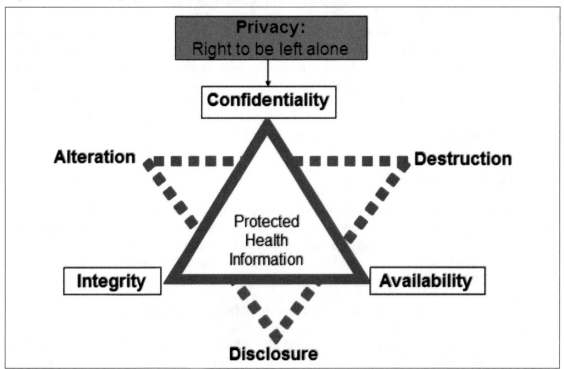

Figure 12.2.   Key privacy and security terms and definitions

- Protected health information (PHI): Individually identifiable health information transmitted by electronic media, maintained in electronic media, or transmitted or maintained in any other form or medium (including paper, voice, image, and other).
- Covered entity: A health plan, healthcare clearinghouse, or healthcare provider who transmits any health information in electronic form in connection with a transaction covered by HIPAA (referring to transactions such as health insurance eligibility, claims submission, remittance advice, and other financial/administrative processes standardized under HIPAA). It should be noted that Medicare requires electronic submission of claims from providers who accept reimbursement under Medicare; therefore, all Medicare providers are covered entities; however, any provider who does not accept Medicare could potentially not be a covered entity under HIPAA.
- Business associate: A person who creates, receives, maintains, or transmits PHI on behalf of a covered entity or who provides services for a covered entity that involve the disclosure of PHI. A business associate contract, or agreement, is required between covered entities and business associates to carry out such functions and assure the privacy and security of the PHI. It is noteworthy that, in 2013, HIPAA was amended under HITECH in a set of rules referred to as the Omnibus Rule to make business associates and their agents liable for civil money penalties (a punitive fine imposed by a civil court) for a violation of the HIPAA Security Rule and certain parts of the Privacy Rule based on the act or omission of any agent of the business associate.
- TPO (treatment, payment, and operations): The three core types of healthcare activities for which covered entities are permitted to use and disclose PHI (except when an authorization or prohibition is explicitly required by the Privacy Rule). Examples of TPO include conducting quality assessment, reviewing staff competency, underwriting health insurance, business planning and management.
- Disclosure: The release, transfer, provision of access to, or divulging in any other manner of information outside of the entity holding the information.
- Use: The sharing, employment, application, utilization, examination, or analysis of PHI within an entity that maintains such information.
- Authorization: The giving of permission. In the Security Rule, authorization refers to granting credentials for staff to access PHI. In the Privacy Rule, authorization refers to a detailed document that gives covered entities permission to use PHI for specified purposes other than TPO (which do not require such permission) (HHS n.d.[a]).
- Consent: Another term for the giving of permission. The meaning of consent may be nuanced by various regulations or best practices. The HIPAA Privacy Rule does not require that a covered entity voluntarily obtain patient consent for TPO and explicitly states that a voluntary consent is not sufficient to permit a use or disclosure of PHI when an authorization is required. Some states have pre-empted HIPAA and require consent in certain circumstances, which vary by state. Informed consent in healthcare refers to permission to perform a treatment (often governed by state law [ACS 2014]) or engage an individual in a clinical trial or research study. Informed consent in trials and studies is governed by the Common Rule, the federal policy for the protection of human subjects that regulates a wide variety of governmental agencies and departments (HHS 2016a). In 2015, these agencies, including the Department of Homeland Security (DHS), HHS, and 15 others, came together and developed proposed revisions to their respective regulations to modernize, strengthen, and make more effective the Common Rule (DHS et al. 2015).

Source: As specified above or 45 CFR 160, 162, 164.

to issue civil monetary penalties (CMPs) for noncompliance due to willful neglect. In the 2013 Omnibus Rule expanded and clarified the Enforcement Rule as it relates to determining the amount of any CMPs, including consideration for the following:

- The nature and extent of the violation, including number of individuals affected and duration of violation
- The nature and extent of any individual's resulting physical, financial, or reputational harm, including hindrance to the individual's ability to obtain health care
- History of prior noncompliance, including similar prior indications of noncompliance and the offending party's response to them

- Financial condition of the offending party, including difficulties that could have affected compliance or that could cause a CMP to jeopardize the future provision of health care

The OCR website provides a graphic that tracks the number of complaints received each year, which have increased from the first full year (2004) with 6,534 complaints to the last reported year (2014) as of the updating of this book with 17,779 complaints (OCR 2014a). Thus, it is clear that many issues with Privacy and Security Rule compliance persist. (Many privacy complaints have security components to them, and most attacks on security vulnerabilities have privacy ramifications.)

As of October 31, 2015, the OCR website notes that more than 123,000 complaints were made and almost 24,000 cases required **corrective actions** (for example, implementation of solutions to mitigate risk and reporting to OCR on outcomes for a period of three years) by HIPAA-covered entities and/or their business associates. OCR also reports that it has settled 26 cases requiring a **settlement agreement** (a resolution agreement signed by HHS and a covered entity or business associate in which the covered entity or business associate agrees to perform certain obligations and make reports to HHS, generally for a period of three years; and often with a **resolution amount** intended to cover the government costs of the investigation and subsequent monitoring). A settlement agreement may arise out of an investigation of a complaint or a breach (see section on Breach Notification Rule in this chapter). As of October 31, 2015, $22,874,400 was paid in resolution amounts. In another 10,865 cases, OCR determined that no violation had occurred. Finally, 70,695 cases were closed because OCR lacks jurisdiction under HIPAA (for example, the alleged violation was conducted by a noncovered entity or business associate), the complaint was untimely or withdrawn by the filer, or it was determined that the activity described does not violate HIPAA, such as where a covered entity was permitted to make a disclosure (OCR 2015a).

The amount of the settlement agreement is not the total amount the covered entity or business associate must pay to address a complaint. The Ponemon Institute (2015a) has been tracking breaches across industries for several years, and each year it calculates their actual cost, considering legal fees, consultant fees, replacement of equipment, retraining costs, labor costs, and others. Across all industries in the United States, the average cost per record was $217. For the US healthcare industry, the average cost was estimated at $363 per record. The number of individual records in any given breach varies considerably. OCR provides a breach portal where breaches affecting 500 or more records must be reported (OCR n.d.). As of October 31, 2015, there were 1,437 breaches of this size. A running total of the number of records breached is not provided in the portal, but they range from 500 to more than 1 million. As an example of the magnitude of the cost of a breach, a breach involving 10,000 records could cost a covered entity or business associate $3.6 million—not including a resolution amount or CMPs. Finally, the impact to those harmed in healthcare is virtually unmeasurable. The Ponemon Institute notes that, with a credit card breach, the period between the breach and mitigation is relatively short when compared to a breach of a person's health record, which could result in medical identity theft (see below) lasting many years or even impact a person's physical and mental health for the rest of that person's life (2015a). Recent contributors to *The Journal of the American Health Information Management Association* (AHIMA) have called medical identity theft the "crime that can kill" (McNabb and Rhodes 2014) and offer medical identity theft patient flags for the EHR (Bowe 2013).

The Privacy Rule

HIPAA's Privacy Rule, which became effective April 14, 2003, addresses the uses and disclosures of PHI, including uses and disclosures that are **minimum necessary** (that is, a use or disclosure should be limited to that necessary to satisfy a particular purpose or carry out a specific function), those requiring an authorization, and those using de-identified data.

HIPAA's Privacy Rule also addresses individuals' rights to their PHI, including the right to a notice of privacy practices, access to their health information stored in a **designated record set** (which is the medical and billing records used to make decisions about individuals), and the right to request amendments, restrictions and confidential communications, and accounting for disclosures.

Finally, the Privacy Rule has administrative standards that require the designation of an information privacy official (IPO), the provision of training, the handling of complaints, and the application of appropriate sanctions against members of the workforce who fail to comply with privacy requirements. The rule also requires the entities covered under HIPAA to mitigate the harmful effects of a use or disclosure violation; refrain from retaliation; and have in place policies and procedures, as well as documentation that provides evidence of compliance (such documentation must be retained for six years from date of creation or when last in effect).

The administrative standards of the Privacy Rule include a requirement for administrative, technical, and physical safeguards to protect the privacy of PHI. This same standard addresses the need to reasonably safeguard PHI to limit **incidental uses** or **disclosures** (which are those made pursuant to an otherwise permitted or required use or disclosure). An example of an incidental disclosure is where one patient may see the name of another patient on a doctor's office sign-in sheet. Incidental disclosures have been the subject of a number of frequently asked questions (FAQs) posted on the OCR website, as they are often misunderstood and misinterpreted. This standard on administrative, technical, and physical safeguards is sometimes referred to as the "mini-security rule" because it predated the issuance of the final Security Rule.

It is important to recognize that state law preempts HIPAA where state law is more stringent than the HIPAA Privacy Rule. This rule is particularly applicable in the area of consents and authorizations for uses and disclosures. As noted in figure 12.2, the Privacy Rule permits—but does not require—consent for use or disclosure of PHI to carry out TPO. Many states, especially when setting up requirements for health information exchange (HIE), have incorporated a consent requirement for participation.

Technology and Other Solutions for Privacy Rule Management

Privacy is critical in an electronic environment. With one keystroke or one hack attack, millions of health records could possibly end up on the Internet, completely open to public view. Despite the number of breaches and records involved, this catastrophe has not happened—but there certainly have been many other intolerable consequences. As a result, technology and policy solutions are being developed and implemented to help mitigate privacy concerns and reduce untoward events. Table 12.1 describes some recently developed solutions. New solutions are expected to emerge, especially as the focus turns to increased sharing of PHI across the continuum of care and for quality improvement, health reform initiatives, clinical research, and, in some cases, monetization of data (that is, generating revenue from data).

Check Your Understanding 12.1

Match the terms with the appropriate descriptions:

    A. Authorization

    B. Consent

    C. Civil monetary penalty

    D. Data segmentation

Table 12.1.   Solutions for privacy assurance

Solution	Description
Patient identification and matching	Despite the requirement in HIPAA for a healthcare person identifier, Congress, citing privacy concerns, has blocked such development in every relevant appropriations bill since 1999 (Ritz 2013). The College of Healthcare Information Management Executives (CHIME) is pressuring Congress to allow person identifiers by issuing a $1 million challenge to developers to create a universal matching process (Hagland 2015). The ONC commissioned a study on patient identification and matching that recommends standardized patient identifying attributes for all relevant exchange transactions (Morris et al. 2014) and has included patient identification in its SAFER Guides (see chapter 11). The Joint Commission's National Patient Safety Goals (2015) include "improving the accuracy of patient identification" and requires at least two patient identifiers when providing care; the Joint Commission has also provided extensive guidance to nursing staff on patient identifiers.
Master person index (MPI)	An MPI is not a requirement in HIPAA, but virtually every provider and most health plans have some form of MPI. From creating an entry in an MPI at the time a patient is first registered in a healthcare environment (of any kind) to maintaining the integrity of the MPI with subsequent patient care events, the MPI has long been the mainstay of person identification in healthcare. MPI management is more necessary now than ever before in the health information exchange (HIE) and other health data–sharing environments, as duplicate records and comingling of patient data are privacy, healthcare, and payment issues. AHIMA provides practical tools for MPI clean-up (AHIMA 2009), has issued a resolution on MPI integrity (Demster et al. 2012), and updated its guidance on managing the integrity of patient identity in HIE (Dooling et al. 2014).
Health record integration	Healthcare organizations must ensure accurate patient identification when health records are integrated as that is the only way to yield a single record that is truly related to only one person and thereby avoid privacy violations and healthcare delivery issues related to patient misidentification. Health record integration is important in HIE when health data from multiple providers are made accessible. However, *health record integration* usually refers to the integration of personal health record (PHR) data (potentially from multiple PHRs) into a health record compiled by a provider. Concerns about data integrity with respect to patient identification need to be addressed (although there are additional, unrelated concerns, including provider concerns about the accuracy of patient-generated data [see chapter 17]). Technologies that can help overcome privacy concerns include patient authentication, provision of proxy access, and data provenance (see chapter 10) (Snell 2015a).
De-identification	De-identification is a requirement in the HIPAA Privacy Rule that has been troublesome to implement. An international study on the state of data sharing for healthcare analytics conducted by Privacy Analytics (2015) looked at secondary uses of PHI, defined as uses for other than direct patient care, such as data analysis, research, safety measurement, public health, payment, provider certification, or marketing. The study found that healthcare organizations lack maturity in how they use such data, but that data analytics was growing considerably—stymied only by concerns for privacy, the lack of expertise in healthcare organizations to properly de-identify data, and cost of such processes. These findings highlight that the predominant form of privacy protection for such shared data is a data sharing agreement, followed by masking (which is not a form of de-identification per the HIPAA Privacy Rule). On November 26, 2012, OCR issued Guidance Regarding Methods for De-Identification of PHI in Accordance with the HIPAA Privacy Rule. The Privacy Analytics study found that the HIPAA Safe Harbor method of removing 18 types of identifiers was the third most common form of de-identification and that the HIPAA statistical process of anonymization or expert de-identification followed. Finally, 33 percent of respondents stated that none of the measures identified were applied when they shared data. This study also highlights that those who are not familiar with advanced statistical methods of de-identifying data may be releasing information that has been stripped of its usefulness.

(continued)

Table 12.1.   Solutions for privacy assurance (Continued)

Solution	Description
Data sharing agreements	A data use agreement is required under HIPAA for use of a limited data set, which includes PHI from which most—but not all—of the safe harbor de-identification requirements are applied. (*Safe harbor* describes a provision that affords protection from liability under specified circumstances.) HHS (n.d.[b]) provides a Data Use Agreement template. Data sharing agreements differ from data use agreements in that data sharing agreements have more expansive data governance requirements, often including certification and recertification of the de-identification of data being used and, where applicable, usage fees (Allen et al. 2014). Medicare offers a voluntary data sharing agreement (VDSA) to coordinate healthcare benefit payments between employers, their agents, and Medicare (CMS 2016). A data use and reciprocal support agreement (DURSA) is required for use of the eHealth Exchange (the national HIE) (Sequoia Project 2014).
Genomic Data Sharing and GINA	The Genetic Information Nondiscrimination Act (GINA) of 2008, which became effective on May 22, 2009, prohibits discrimination in health coverage and employment based on genetic information (NHGRI 2009). Genomic data sharing is increasing as researchers seek to combine genomic information with clinical care data to learn more about cancer and other conditions. De-identification and enhanced security measures must also be taken to protect this information.
Privacy and trust principles for precision medicine	Precision medicine, as previously noted in chapter 4, is defined by the National Library of Medicine (NLM) as "an emerging approach for disease treatment and prevention that takes into account individual variability in genes, environment, and lifestyle for each person" (NLM 2016). In supporting the Precision Medicine Initiative (PMI) and integrating such a variety of information, the White House issued privacy and trust principles that address governance; transparency; respect for participant preferences; empowerment of participants through access to information; ensuring appropriate data sharing, access, and use; and maintaining data quality and integrity (Handelsman and Patil 2015). The principles require multiple tiers of data access according to user qualifications. They also require privacy-preserving methods to maintain a link to participant identifiers in order to link participant data obtained from different sources and to return appropriate information to the patient and provider. Participants in this form of medicine must be able to access their own information, easily report any inaccuracies, and request that they be addressed in PMI records. Educational resources must also be made available to participants to help them understand their information (Snell 2015b).
Emergency uses of PHI	The Privacy Rule allows for PHI disclosures for public health purposes, but healthcare organizations are not always prepared to address all forms of potential disclosures in certain situations, such as the Ebola virus outbreak in 2014. The OCR (2015b) has developed a decision tool to help determine how the Privacy Rule applies to disclosures for public health purposes. The Privacy Rule also allows for disclosures when there is a threat to the health or safety. Misunderstandings relating to that aspect of the rule during the 2013 mass shootings in Newtown, CT, and Aurora, CO, led the director of OCR to send a message to healthcare providers to remind them of the need to balance privacy protections and the good of persons' health, such as arose when a patient may have put others in harm's way (Rodriguez 2013).
Criminal background checks	The Privacy Rule allows uses and disclosures for specialized government functions. To ensure that accurate but limited information is reported to the National Instant Criminal Background Check System (NICS), a modification to the Privacy Rule (at 45 CFR 164.512[k]7) was made on January 4, 2016. The modification, which applies to only a small number of state agencies or others designated to report to the NICS, permits limited demographic and certain other information to be disclosed to NICS, but it explicitly excludes diagnostic or clinical information for such purposes, an exclusion that is especially important to maintain the patient-provider relationship and encourage individuals who may need treatment to seek it.

(continued)

Table 12.1.   Solutions for privacy assurance (Continued)

Solution	Description
Right of access	Individuals have the right under HIPAA to access their PHI. However, OCR has found that right to access is consistently among the top three complaints made with respect to the Privacy Rule (OCR 2015a). As there is increasing emphasis on patient engagement in their health care and integrating records from multiple sources, it is becoming increasingly important for patients to access their records. On January 7, 2016, HHS released a fact sheet that provides a set of FAQs designed to improve access to medical records, billing and payment records, insurance information, laboratory test and x-ray results, wellness and disease management information, clinical case notes, and other information used to make decisions about individuals. The fact sheet makes no modifications to the HIPAA Privacy Rule surrounding right of access, but it aims to clarify and encourage support for such access (HHS 2016b). Helpful technology such as patient portals and personal health records may need to be enhanced with interactive, visualization, and integration tools.
Clarification of mental/ behavioral health record sharing	A number of factors surrounding mental health services have heightened attention on how sharing information relating to mental health may be improved. The American Hospital Association (AHA) points out that highly prevalent behavioral health disorders have a significant economic and social impact. Behavioral health disorders and medical conditions often co-occur and lead to the risk of suboptimal outcomes. Behavioral health provider shortages and fragmented care delivery—with behavioral health services often needing to be provided by ill-equipped primary care providers—impede effective treatment for behavioral health conditions (AHA 2012). Recognizing this constellation of concerns over the past several years, OCR, ONC, and the Substance Abuse and Mental Health Services Administration (SAMHSA) have considered modifications to the Privacy Rule and/or 42 CFR 2: Confidentiality of Alcohol and Drug Abuse Patient Records (which have yet been made, although there have been bills before Congress to do so [Robeznieks 2015]), and have issued periodic guidance documents. The most recent such guidance from HHS on HIPAA Privacy Rule and sharing information related to mental health provides a set of FAQs to help providers address a number of the communication issues surrounding mental health (HHS 2014b).
Data segmentation for privacy (DS4P)	Categorization of information that requires a higher degree of security may be needed to ensure the privacy of sensitive, or high-risk, information in EHRs and other types of health IT. AHIMA proposed that such technology include role-based access controls, VIP status indicators, alias assignment to mask patient identity, the ability to restrict access to patient information to only those who are providers of record (mandatory access control), the ability to block access to specific data such as a progress note or laboratory test and/or its result, and the ability to track versioning or mask sensitive entries for release of information (Barbera et al. 2008). As technology has evolved, data segmentation ("the process of sequestering from capture, access, or view certain data elements that are perceived by a legal entity, institution, organization, or individual as being undesirable to share" [Goldstein and Rein 2010]) has become technologically feasible. ONC has created a DS4P initiative utilizing ONC's Standards and Interoperability (S&I) Framework to do so, which has included pilot tests with the US Department of Veterans Affairs and SAMHSA and others. Building on the results of this work, the Health Level Seven (HL7) standards development organization produced the *HL7 Implementation Guide: Data Segmentation for Privacy,* which includes the application of metadata to the HL7 Clinical Document Architecture (see chapter 10) and inclusion in the Direct and Exchange Transport Profiles for exchanging health information in the nationwide health information network. Additional HL7 DS4P products include a privacy and security classification system, labeling service, privacy and security ontology, and the Fast Healthcare Interoperability Resources (FHIR) security for web services (see chapter 13). A launchpad for these resources is available on the healthIT.gov website (2014).

E.   Disclosure

F.   Health record integration

G.   Patient matching

H.   Resolution amount

I.   Safe harbor

J.   Use

1.   Compensation for investigation and monitoring of an enforcement action

2.   Release of information external to the holder of the information

3.   Provision that protects against liability

4.   Process of separating information

5.   Combining of health and personal records

6.   General form of permission

7.   Access to information within an organization that created the information

8.   Special form of permission

9.   Combining data to identify a person

10.   Financial penalty

The Security Rule

The HIPAA Security Rule, to which both covered entities and business associates are fully liable, includes standards for administrative, physical, and technical safeguards, as well as requirements for policies, procedures, and documentation.

Risk Basis of HIPAA Security Rule

The HIPAA Security Rule is risk-based. In other words, the standards provide general requirements for security safeguards, but each organization must decide for itself, through a risk analysis, what specific controls will afford those safeguards.

A **risk analysis** is a process in which the organization analyzes its **vulnerabilities** (weaknesses in security controls) and **threats** (actions that might exploit vulnerabilities, including acts of nature, human acts ranging from errors to theft, and environmental issues such as power outages) with respect to all locations where PHI is stored, received, maintained, or transmitted. Controls to thwart threats to vulnerabilities should consider the size, complexity, and capabilities of the organization; the organization's technical infrastructure; the costs of security measures; and the probability and criticality of potential risks to PHI (Walsh 2013). Various types of controls serve to prevent, deter, detect, react to, and/or recover from a threat action. Figure 12.3 illustrates the risk analysis process at a high level.

Threats typically involve agents, targets, and events. A threat **agent** is usually an individual with the motivation and resources to carry out a threat (for example, a computer-savvy disgruntled employee or a cybercriminal). Threat **targets** are the objects of a threat. HIPAA identifies data

Figure 12.3. Overview of risk analysis

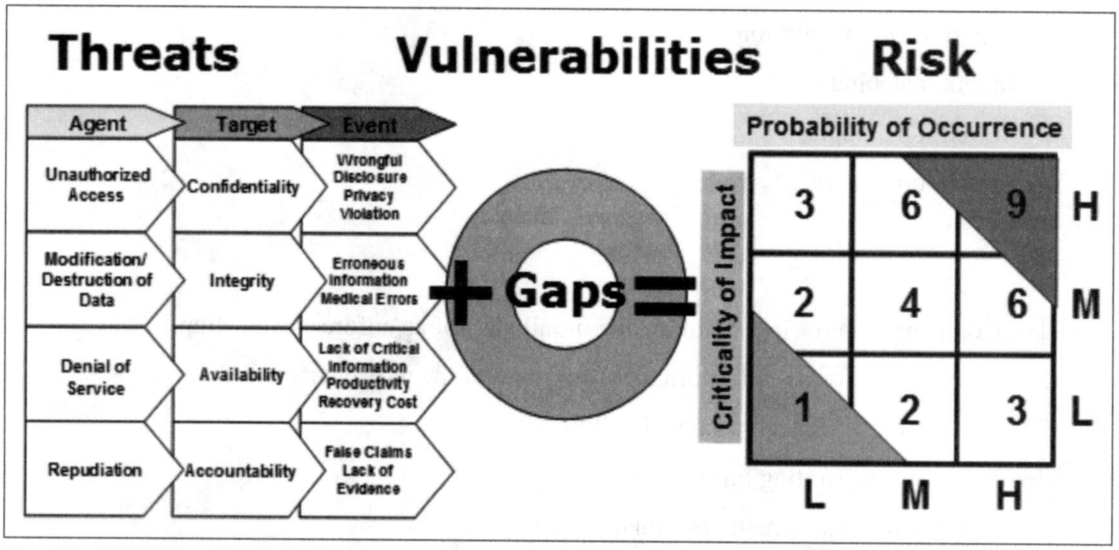

confidentiality, integrity, and availability as the objects to be concerned about. Many add **accountability** (the property that ensures that the actions of an entity can be traced solely to this entity) to this list of objects. Threat **events** are the results of the threat. In general, four types of events can occur (and each is related to one of the types of targets):

- Unauthorized access and disclosure are a threat to confidentiality in which data are accessed inappropriately or revealed to an unauthorized person.

- Modification, alteration, or destruction of data causes a data integrity problem and often a data availability problem as well.

- Denial-of-service attacks prevent the system from performing its functions and may render data unavailable.

- Repudiation is a situation in which a user or system denies having performed some action, such as modification of information. There is no accountability for the action.

Vulnerabilities are weaknesses, or gaps, that occur in administrative processes, the physical facility, and the technical infrastructure. Lack of policy or policy enforcement is a common vulnerability. In healthcare, a wide open campus with unguarded doors may be a vulnerability. Viruses and other malicious software can attack any computer system, but as computers become more networked and use the Internet for communications, they are more vulnerable to all forms of attack.

HIPAA Security Rule Standards

Table 12.2 summarizes the HIPAA Security Rule standards. All federal regulations are filed in the Code of Federal Regulations (CFR) by section number. In addition to the standards, the Security Rule includes implementation specifications that are either required (R) or addressable (A). Required implementation specifications must be implemented. Addressable implementation specifications must be implemented or an alternative measure should be implemented, if reasonable and appropriate. Any deviation from implementing the specification must have an explanation documented.

Table 12.2.   Summary of the HIPAA Security Rule standards

Security Standards	CFR Sections	Security Implementation Specifications (R) = Required, (A) = Addressable
Administrative Safeguards		
Security Management Process	§164.308(a)(1)	Risk Analysis (R) Risk Management (R) Sanction Policy (R) Information System Activity Review (R)
Assigned Security Responsibility	§164.308(a)(2)	(R)
Workforce Security	§164.308(a)(3)	Authorization and/or Supervision (A) Workforce Clearance Procedure (A) Termination Procedures (A)
Information Access Management	§164.308(a)(4)	Isolating Health Care Clearinghouse Function (R) Access Authorization (A) Access Establishment and Modification (A)
Security Awareness and Training	§164.308(a)(5)	Security Reminders (A) Protection from Malicious Software (A) Log-in Monitoring (A) Password Management (A)
Security Incident Procedures	§164.308(a)(6)	Response and Reporting (R)
Contingency Plan	§164.308(a)(7)	Data Backup Plan (R) Disaster Recovery Plan (R) Emergency Mode Operation Plan (R) Testing and Revision Procedure (A) Applications and Data Criticality Analysis (A)
Evaluation	§164.308(a)(8)	(R)
Business Associate Contracts and Other Arrangements	§164.308(b)(1)	(R)
Physical Safeguards		
Facility Access Controls	§164.310(a)(1)	Contingency Operations (A) Facility Security Plan (A) Access Control and Validation Procedures (A) Maintenance Records (A)
Workstation Use	§164.310(b)	(R)
Workstation Security	§164.310(c)	(R)
Device and Media Controls	§164.310(d)(1)	Disposal (R) Media Re-use (R) Accountability (A) Data Backup and Storage (A)
Technical Safeguards		
Access Controls	§164.312(a)	Unique User Identification (R) Emergency Access Procedure (R) Automatic Logoff (A) Encryption and Decryption (A)
Audit Controls	§164.312(b)	(R)
Integrity	§164.312(c)(1)	Mechanism to Authenticate ePHI (A)
Person or Entity Authentication	§164.312(d)	(R)
Transmission Security	§164.312(e)(1)	Integrity Controls (A) Encryption (A)

Source: 45 CFR 164 appendix A, Security Standards: Matrix.

Technology and Other Solutions for Security Management

Several technical standards in the Security Rule should prompt regular review by HIPAA-covered entities and business associates as security threats increase (in all industries). Requirements for authentication, access controls, audit logs, encryption for both data at rest and data in transit, and device security must be understood and enhanced regularly.

Authentication Requirements

The HIPAA Security Rule requires user identification, makes encryption and decryption addressable for access control, and requires person or entity authentication, but the rule does not specify the **authentication**, or signature, requirements a healthcare organization should use. A signature serves three main purposes: (1) it is a symbol that signifies intent to approve terms, confirmation of review, and approval of content, or authorship; (2) it identifies the person providing the signature; and (3) it guards the integrity of the document against repudiation (that is, the signer claiming the entry is invalid) or alteration.

Electronic signature is a generic, technology-neutral term for the various ways an electronic record can be signed. The Electronic Signatures in Global and National Commerce Act (ESIGN), which was signed into law in June 2000 defines an electronic signature as "an electronic sound, symbol, or process, attached to or logically associated with a contract or other record and executed or adopted by the person with the intent to sign the record." There are three general types of electronic signatures:

- Level 1: Digitized signatures are representations of a wet signature made by a person signing onto a signature pad, the scanned image of which is stored in the information system in association with the information that is signed. Although this is generally considered a weak form of signature in information systems, it is acceptable ESIGN. Such a signature is widely used in retail stores. In healthcare, digitized signatures are used to capture patient signatures on authorization forms, consents, and other documents when presented electronically.

- Level 2: A personal identification number (PIN), password, biometric, or token is the second form of electronic signature and may use any one or some combination of PIN, password, biometric, or token to create a logical manifestation of a signature. The stronger the component and the more components used, the stronger the authentication becomes. For example, a password—irrespective of its strength—is not as strong as a biometric; a password and biometric or token together is even stronger. Two-factor authentication refers to the use of two components together. A recent study conducted for ONC found that nearly half of all healthcare organizations are using two-factor authentication. Those that use it tend to be larger and urban facilities over small and rural facilities (Gabriel et al. 2015). Password strength continues to be important to data security. It is generally recommended that passwords include at least 6 and preferably 8 characters, and include a combination of uppercase and lowercase letters and at least one special character (such as a punctuation mark). Many systems today include processes for enforcing the use of strong passwords. Passwords should be easy for the user to remember but difficult to guess. For example, "0$acuC" could be remembered as "Oh (zero) say ($a) can (c) you (u) see (C)." There are cautions, however, that certain substitutions, such as "$" for "s", "@" for "a", "1" for "l," are easier to guess than others (Lee 2014). It also is important to not use a publicly available online password checker to check the strength of a password, as the site could be a rogue one used to collect passwords and associate them with the IP address of the computer. Passwords should not be incrementally changed, and many password checkers today enforce this rule.

- A user ID is technically not part of authentication, but it is used to identify the user for purposes of triggering access controls. The electronic signature may be invoked when the user logs on to the system with the user ID and whatever components of electronic signature are required. For example, in signing a transcribed document, the system may require that the user log on, but the document will not be considered signed until the end of the document is reached and the user clicks an icon signifying acceptance of the document. At present, the electronic signature is the most commonly used means to authenticate information electronically in health record applications.

- Level 3: **Digital signature** is the term reserved to describe a process of encryption and non-repudiation. *Encryption* is a form of cryptography where an algorithm is used to scramble the content so that only an equivalent algorithm can be used to decrypt the message. It provides the means to protect the content of a message from being revealed (whether the message is a signature only or content and signature). **Nonrepudiation** is substantial evidence of the identity of the signer of a message and of message integrity, sufficient to prevent a party from successfully denying the origin, submission, or delivery of the message and the integrity of its contents. Many mathematical algorithms have been used to create various forms of digital signature. NIST has a Digital Signature Standard that has become a Federal Information Processing Standard (FIPS 186-4). This standard enables the use of the RSA (Rivest-Shamir-Adleman) digital signature algorithm or the DSA (Digital Signature Algorithm) to digitally sign messages. RSA is the most popular form of digital signature, used in many web browsers and with the SSL protocol. This type of signature is often accomplished by logging in to an applicable website and "signing" your name by typing in your name or clicking on an icon that indicates your intent to authenticate. When integrity of the data within the message is required, the Secure Hash Algorithm (SHA-1) can be added. *Hash,* also called a *message digest,* is a number generated from a string of text. It is substantially smaller than the text itself, and is generated by a formula in such a way that it is extremely unlikely that some other text will produce the same hash value (Barron et al. 2009; Downing 2013).

Public Key Infrastructure

Public key infrastructure (PKI) is the set of policies, procedures, standards, and practices that enable use of a digital signature. PKI consists of a **certificate authority (CA)** that issues and verifies a **digital certificate** that identifies the individual. It also identifies a **registration authority (RA)** that acts as the verifier for the CA before a digital certificate is issued to an individual, one or more directories where the certificate and their public keys are held, and a certificate management system that stores certificates and saves encrypted private keys in a certificate database for disaster recovery purposes (Lawton 2015). A federally approved credential service provider or certification authority must issue a digital certificate that affords **identity proofing** (to verify that a person is who he or she claims to be) where one may be required for use in healthcare. Digital certificates are standardized under the **X.509** standard. The process of digital signature works with a combination of public key and private key cryptography, as illustrated in table 12.3.

Table 12.3. How PKI works

To do this . . .	Use
Send an encrypted message	Receiver's public key
Send an encrypted signature	Sender's private key
Decrypt an encrypted message	Receiver's private key
Decrypt an encrypted signature (and authenticate the sender)	Sender's public key

Requirements for Digital Signature/Digital Certificate/Encryption

Under eprescribing requirements issued by the Drug Enforcement Administration (DEA), the use of eprescribing for controlled substances (EPCS) requires a digital certificate, identity proofing at NIST SP 800-63-1 Electronic Authentication Guidelines Level 3, and other requirements (21 CFR 1300 1304, 1306, 1311 2010). The National Council for Prescription Drug Programs (NCPDP), which establishes the standards for e-prescribing, provides electronic signature guidance (2014). Each state board of pharmacy may also describe requirements for identity proofing, issuing authentication credentials, and configuring logical access controls that exceed the DEA minimum requirements (CHCF 2013).

There currently is no requirement within HIPAA for use of a digital signature. However, that may change with new operating rules (CAQH CORE 2015), which are currently available for voluntary use by willing trading partners but may be adopted by federal regulation at some point in the future. The Council for Affordable Quality Healthcare (CAQH) Committee on Operating Rules for Information Exchange (CORE) phase IV operating rules for processing the HIPAA electronic claims and prior authorization transactions as a document described by the Web Services Definition Language (WSDL) using the Simple Object Access Protocol (SOAP) messaging protocol requires that a health plan must use an X.509 digital certificate when requested to do so by a provider.

The federal government's meaningful use (MU) incentive program requires that an encryption algorithm be used whenever electronic health information is created, modified, accessed, or deleted in order to record the date, time, patient identification, user identification, and indication of what action(s) occurred and by whom. This algorithm must be one identified in Annex A of the FIPS Publication 140-2, Security Requirements for Cryptographic Modules. It also requires the use of a hashing algorithm with a security strength equal to or greater than SHA-1 as specified in the FIPS Publication 180-3, Secure Hash Standard (subsequently updated as FIPS Publication 180-4) to verify that electronic health information has not been altered in transit.

Access Controls

Access control is a security technique that regulates who or what (for example, other computer systems) can use or disclose what resources, and under what circumstances in a computing environment. The HIPAA Security Rule does not specify the nature of the access controls to be used, except that they must conform to the applicable requirements in the Privacy Rule. Based on the preamble to the privacy final rule (HHS 2002), the applicable requirements in the Privacy Rule are described at 45 CFR 164.514(d): Minimum necessary requirements. They require that a covered entity must identify the following:

- Those persons or classes of persons in its workforce who need access to PHI to carry out their duties; and

- For each such person or class of persons, the category or categories of PHI to which access is needed and any conditions appropriate to such access. Conditions appropriate to such access are not described in the Privacy Rule but may include time of day, location in facility, types of patients, certain applications, certain views within applications, and privileges such as view only, view and write, authenticate, delete from active view, and system administration functions such as allow access.

In translating the minimum necessary requirements into access controls, covered entities must consider the choices of access controls available to them. Table 12.4 presents the most common forms of controls, their strengths and weaknesses, and how they might relate to the Privacy Rule minimum necessary requirements.

Table 12.4. Access controls

Privacy Rule Minimum Necessary Standard	Common Access Control Types in the Industry	Strengths and Weaknesses of Access Control Type
Persons or classes of persons Example 1: Mary Example 2: Nurse	Discretionary access control (least restrictive)	Restricts access based on identity of user or membership in group. Allows changes to access by owner of resource.
Categories of PHI Example 3: Emergency department nurse	Role-based access control	Access based on individuals' roles and responsibilities within the organization. Does not address conditions appropriate to access and does not allow for multiple roles simultaneously.
Conditions appropriate to access Example 4: Emergency department nurse, midnight to 7 a.m. shift	Rule-based access control	Affords ability to dynamically assign roles to users based on criteria. Can be resource-intensive.
	Mandatory access control (most restrictive)	Access controls established by the owner or custodian of the data (in healthcare these may be called *providers of record*— those who have documented care delivery in the record).
	Attribute access control (newer model; second most restrictive.) (Hu et al. 2014)	Access control associated with a set of rules expressed on measurable parameters for users who can prove compliance with the rules

Source: Content based on analysis of HIPAA rules as well as OWASP (2015).

By definition, access controls are restrictive, which is not always desirable in a healthcare environment where emergency situations can require access that is not pre-established, Therefore, whatever type of access control is used in a healthcare organization, it should be extended with "break-the-glass" functionality. Much like breaking the glass on a fire alarm to pull the alarm, break-the-glass functionality enables a person to gain access to computing resources quickly. There are a variety of ways to establish this type of functionality (Brucker and Petritsch 2009). In most healthcare environments using break-the-glass technology, a set of potential reasons are displayed to the person denied access (such as "emergency," "curbside consultation," and others). Selection of one of the reasons then enables access. A special audit log is created that can be used to later investigate the legitimacy of the access. In some cases, a notification of access is sent to the data owner (for example, person who wrote the content being accessed). Break-the-glass functionality has proven to be a strong deterrent to any person who might try to casually access information (for example, someone snooping on a relative or a celebrity patient).

Audit Logs

The Security Rule requires audit controls that record and examine activity in information systems that contain or use electronic PHI. Ideally, audit logs should provide metadata as to who did what to which information at what date and time and from what location. Audit logs, however, can only be as specific as the access controls permit. Hence, if access controls only authenticate a user at the system level, the audit log cannot be specific to the levels other than the system level, such as the application level, record level, or data level. When audit logs are weak or not available, these problems can have implications for investigations of security incidents (such as inappropriate access to PHI) and lawsuits involving health record documentation.

Audit logs produce massive amounts of data that need to be stored for the six-year retention period required by HIPAA. Audit logs need to be retained in a database that can be searched on each of the available parameters Examples of relevant queries include "What did this user ID do at this time?" and "Which users ever accessed these data?" If audit logs are not stored in a searchable database, it is difficult and time-consuming to prove the details regarding actions taken on data. Most organizations aim to analyze the audit logs on a periodic basis, at least for certain types of potential problems, such as access to records of celebrity patients or employees' relatives and other common concerns. Even when there is some nondigital suggestion of a problem that could steer the analysis, evaluation of audit logs is still a very difficult task. For example, one hospital's maternity ward saw an increase in traffic by a certain new group of pediatricians. Curious, the hospital checked the audit logs and found that the pediatricians were accessing a list of births and mothers who delivered each day from the hospital and using that information to introduce themselves to the mothers who might then be inclined to adopt those pediatricians as providers for their newborns. Event log management software and other comparable tools that deploy pattern analysis and artificial intelligence are available to support such analysis, but the process requires a skilled analyst and the support of the information privacy official to cull out false positives and false negatives.

Encryption

Encryption was defined in the previous discussion of the digital signature and explained within the context of PKI. It was also observed in chapter 10 that encryption was used in virtual private networks (VPNs) to create a secure tunnel through which data could flow. Encryption is only an addressable specification within the HIPAA Security Rule, but guidance associated with the Breach Notification Rule identifies that encryption is a safe harbor for breach notification. In other words, an attack on PHI would not succeed if both the PHI and the system holding the PHI (such as a laptop that is stolen or lost) or the transmission mechanism transporting the PHI (such as the VPN) are encrypted.

The number of breaches and cyber threats in all industries is rising. **Cyber threats** are malicious activity that can occur through **cyberspace**, the virtual environment created by computer systems (White House 2015). NIST (2014) has created a framework for improving critical infrastructure cybersecurity that enables organizations to apply best practices of risk management while incorporating privacy and civil liberties as part of a comprehensive cybersecurity framework for all industries. At the end of 2015, Congress passed the Cybersecurity Information Sharing Act (Brandom 2015), which improves information sharing on cyber threats so that organizations can be more prepared to address such threats. ONC has released guidance on understanding electronic health records, the HIPAA security rule, and cybersecurity (ONC 2015). Although small providers may believe they will not be attacked due to their small size, ONC notes that new attacks are often aimed at small to midsize organizations, which are more vulnerable to such attacks.

In healthcare, there have been two primary concerns surrounding encryption. First is the cost and complexity to implement. Cost is a consideration, but EHR technology certified for MU is required to be able to encrypt PHI, so that cost is part of the cost of the overall EHR package. Source systems and other types of health IT that contribute to the EHR also should be encrypted. Poorly implemented encryption can be worse than no encryption. For example, improperly implemented encryption can blind software that monitors outbound data movement (commonly referred to as *data loss prevention [DLP] software*). The second issue is that encryption makes access to data more burdensome for legitimate users. For example, if a physician must wait 10 minutes to access an encrypted x-ray image, the physician might find it quicker to repeat the test. The latest encryption software has very little latency, but it still must be implemented properly to not affect performance. File-level encryption in particular can seem burdensome. Most organizations implement full-disk encryption, encrypting everything on their hard drives. This level of encryption requires users to only authenticate once to the system. However, if an attacker does obtain user credentials, full-disk encryption will provide access to everything. File-level encryption is more secure because it limits access to a particular file; however, if users must access multiple files, each access requires a separate authentication.

Solutions to some of the encryption issues do exist. Using thin clients (see chapter 11) is a good approach. Because the thin client has no data on the device, no data can be accessed without both a user's credentials and access to the user's network. Using two-factor authentication also reduces the risk of a hacker gaining access to credentials. This measure is not foolproof because a hacker might be able to obtain a password through phishing (luring users to reveal their password on a fake website), inserting malware onto a device, using visual hacking (for example, cell phone photography) or malware keystroke analysis, or by stealing credentials stored on the device (Heath 2015a; Heath 2015b). Another solution is to combine data segmentation (the division of data into multiple "containers") with security controls to block attempts to move data from one container to another. Firewalls, anti-malware software, enforcement of strong authentication mechanisms, and other security controls are not substitutes for encryption, but their use may allow organizations to use encryption in less onerous ways (Terry 2015).

Devices

Device and media control is a HIPAA Security Rule standard that is included in the Physical Safeguards section, which requires that attributes of the physical surroundings of a specific workstation are secured. This area of the HIPAA Security Rule may need updating, because devices are ubiquitous and often not totally under the control of the organization that is most concerned about their use. Devices that store PHI are also increasing not only in number, but type.

Medical devices (ranging from portable ultrasound devices to huge magnetic resonance imaging devices and including pacemakers and other devices implanted into patients) increasingly store PHI and therefore are increasingly at risk for attack (Healey et al. 2015). Historically, medical devices usually stored only the data from the last use of the device; however, now that much more data can be stored on very small devices, medical devices are storing more and more data. Such data may be used as part of the device's quality control mechanisms or to provide baseline data for comparisons that can provide an alert that there is a defect in the device or a patient complication. Many medical devices are also being connected to local and wide area networks, including potentially the cloud. In addition to standard HIPAA security standards, medical device security standards are available from the International Electrotechnical Commission (IEC), which is recognized by the Food and Drug Administration (FDA) as foundational standards for medical device security (Coderre and Surber 2015).

Mobile computing devices are described in chapter 11. These devices are increasingly being used by both providers and patients. **Mobile device management (MDM)** is the term currently being used to describe mobile device administration. Stein (2012) describes the following four phases of such administration:

- Phase 1 is provisioning of the mobile device(s), which involves the distribution of such devices and the establishment of bring your own device (BYOD) policies to regulate the use of personal mobile devices for work purposes.

- Phase 2 is policy configuration, which involves establishing what resources the device may access, configuring the device to gain such access, and setting other policies, such as encryption requirements, what other uses may be made of the device other than those intended by the provisioning organization, and others. Policy configuration literally "bakes" the policies onto the device itself. In fact, one of the first considerations for BYOD is whether users will allow such configuration (if they will not, there must be controls on the organization side to disallow access to resources from personal devices).

- Phase 3 is the creation of a mobile device application library. For all mobile devices that the organization will provision and for those BYOD devices that it will allow to be used, the organization develops and retains a standard protocol regarding the maintenance and updating of applications, as well as their reuse on other similar devices. For example, the organization needs protocols about how to configure smartphones with different types of operating systems.

- Phase 4 is the continuation of the MDM software life cycle, including decommissioning devices when people leave the organization and remotely wiping devices in the event of loss or theft.

Security procedures for mobile device computing must include education for users about mobile device use that is not under control of the organization. For example, many providers now use short messaging service (SMS) text messaging on their personal smartphones with no connection to the healthcare facility's resources. A message to a patient or another provider might include PHI. Most users of mobile messaging do not realize that these transmissions are not secure. Secure messaging apps are available and should be part of the provider organization's MDM program (Heath 2015c). Health apps used by patients, however, cannot be controlled in this manner, and, in fact, the HHS guidance on individuals' rights under HIPAA to access their information does not have specifications for mobile device security but does state that "individuals have the right . . . to have copies of their PHI transferred or transmitted to them in the manner they request, even if the requested mode of transfer or transmission is unsecure" (HHS 2016b).

Breach Notification Rule

As data breaches of all kinds increased in all industries, many states passed breach notification laws either for health information specifically or for all personal information that would include financial and other sensitive data. HITECH required HHS to adopt a federal breach notification process. On September 23, 2009, an interim final rule (45 CFR 160, 164) was published, and on January 25, 2013, under the Omnibus Rule, modifications were made to the risk assessment that determines whether a disclosure is a breach. The HHS Breach Notification Rule has required reporting of breaches to HHS since February 18, 2010. Breaches involving more than 500 records must be reported essentially as they occur and become a matter of public record (posted on an HHS website). Figures 12.4 and 12.5 summarize the breach discovery and notification processes as outlined in the rule and subsequently modified. Breaches involving fewer than 500 records may be reported annually and are not posted to the HHS website.

OCR (2009) has published guidance specifying the technologies and methodologies that render PHI unusable, unreadable, or indecipherable to unauthorized individuals, which includes directions to use encryption processes for both data at rest (that is, stored on a server or in a storage device) and data in motion (that is, as data are transmitted through a network). The encryption technologies are those specified by NIST (see discussion earlier in the chapter).

In addition to breaches of PHI, breach notification for personal health information held in standalone personal health records was mandated by HITECH. On August 25, 2009, the FTC issued the Health Breach Notification final rule (16 CFR 318), which required full compliance by February 22, 2010.

Figure 12.4.   Breach notification discovery process

1. A breach is the acquisition, access, use, or disclosure of PHI in a manner not permitted under the Privacy Rule that compromises the security or privacy of PHI.

2. Breach discovery starts a 60-day clock for notification. The first day is the day the breach is known or, by exercising reasonable diligence would have been known, to a workforce member of the covered entity (CE) or an agent of the CE.

3. A business associate (BA) must notify the CE of breaches as provided in business associate contract (BAC) and in no case later than 60 days after discovery.

4. Breach *excludes*:

   a. Unintentional acquisition, access, or use by member of the CE or BA workforce if the member's actions were made in good faith and within scope of authority and do not result in further unpermitted use or disclosure.

   b. Inadvertent disclosure to a person at the same CE or BA if no further use or disclosure in violation of Privacy Rule is made.

   c. Disclosure where the CE or BA believes the unauthorized recipient would be unable to retain the PHI.

5. To assess risk that PHI has been compromised, consider following:

   a. The nature and extent of PHI involved, including types of identifiers and likelihood of re-identification. (PHI that has been de-identified in accordance with Privacy Rule is no longer PHI. See HHS Guidance on De-Identification, November 26, 2012.)

   b. The unauthorized person who used PHI or to whom disclosure was made.

   c. Whether PHI was actually acquired or viewed.

   d. The extent to which risk to PHI has been mitigated.

6. Safe harbor: Refer to HHS guidance specifying technologies and methodologies that render phi unusable, unreadable, or indecipherable to unauthorized individuals for breach notification (April 27, 2009).

   a. Encryption:

      1. Data at rest consistent with NIST SP 800-111

      2. Data in motion consistent with FIPS 140-2, referencing NIST SP 800-52 [TLS], 800-77 [IPsec VPN], or 800-113 [SSL VPN])

   b. Destruction:

      1. Paper, film, or other media shredded or destroyed so that PHI cannot be reconstructed); or

      2. Electronic media consistent with NIST SP 800-88 (Media Sanitization)

Source: Summarized from Breach Notification Rule, 45 CFR 164.400–414.

Identity Theft Controls

According to the FTC, identity theft is one of the fastest growing crimes in the United States (FTC 2010). In the past, misuse of credit cards accounted for the majority of such theft, but this type of theft is decreasing as card processing requirements are tightened via the **Payment Card Industry Data Security Standard (PCI-DSS)** and electronic chip cards that encrypt personal information on the card. Healthcare organizations that accept credit cards for payment must be aware of the PCI-DSS requirements. The regulations are complex and require significant reporting to guarantee the privacy and integrity of customer data.

Because the credit card industry has added greater security controls, hackers are now looking for easier targets and targets that may offer greater value. The American Medical Association (AMA) has warned physicians of identity theft issues in general and medical identity theft in particular—especially because such theft is often an "inside job." Cited in an AMA newsletter was a report from the World Privacy Forum, a nonprofit research and consumer education organization,

Figure 12.5.   Breach notification process

---

1. Delay breach notification if law enforcement agencies have requested delay because notification may hinder investigation.

2. Determine whether breach may result in imminent misuse of unsecured PHI, in which case the covered entity (CE) should notify individuals by telephone or other means in addition to written notice.

   a. Send written notice via first-class mail within 60 days of breach discovery.

   b. Electronic notice may be used if the individual agrees.

   c. If the individual is known to be deceased, send notice to the next of kin or personal representative, if known.

   d. Substitute notice can take the following forms for individuals with out-of-date contact information:

      1. If fewer than 10 individuals, provide notice by an alternative written form of communication, telephone, or other means.

      2. If more than 10 individuals, post notice on the home page of the CE's website or in major print or broadcast media in geographic areas where individuals affected likely reside. Include a toll-free phone number for individuals to learn whether their PHI is included in breach (the phone number should be active for at least 90 days).

      3. If 500 or more individuals live within one state, notify major media outlets in that state.

3. Notice must be in plain language and include the following:

   a. A description of the breach, the date of the breach, and the date of discovery

   b. A description of the types of PHI breached (such as full names, Social Security numbers, dates of birth, home addresses, account numbers, diagnoses, or disability codes)

   c. Steps individuals should take to protect themselves from potential harm

   d. A description of what the CE is doing to mitigate harm and protect against further breaches

   e. Contact procedures for individuals to ask questions, including a toll-free number, e-mail address, website address, or postal address

4. Record breach in a log and report it to HHS:

   a. If fewer than 500 individuals are affected, report the breach to HHS not later than 60 days after the end of each calendar year.

   b. If 500 or more individuals are affected, notify HHS contemporaneously with the notice to individuals.

Source: Summarized from Breach Notification Rule, 45 CFR 164.400–414.

about an employee of a provider organization who pled guilty to selling information involving more than 1,000 patients, a crime that resulted in $7 million in Medicare fraud—despite the organization having browser controls to limit the number of records employees could view (Wilson 2008).

In June 2008, ONC awarded a contract for the assessment and evaluation of the scope of medical identity theft in the United States (HDM 2008). **Medical identity theft** is the inappropriate or unauthorized misrepresentation of individually identifiable health information for the purpose of obtaining access to property or services, which may result in long-lasting harm to an individual interacting with the healthcare continuum. Medical identity information has greater value than credit card information and easier to carry out, especially in small and medium-sized facilities which generally do not implement strong controls. Examples of medical identity theft include situations wherein an individual accesses medical services in another individual's name to obtain benefits for which the first individual is not eligible, obtains services for which the individual will not pay, or perpetuates other fraud or illegal activity, such as erroneous billings or drug-seeking behavior for personal use or illegal distribution. Medical identity theft is extremely serious, with the potential for patient harm when records get comingled.

To thwart identity theft in general, the FTC issued the **Red Flags Rule** that became effective January 1, 2008. The rule seems to have contributed to decreased credit card fraud. In the Red Flags

Rule, organizations that extend credit to their clients must develop and implement written identity theft prevention programs that help identify, detect, and respond to patterns, practices, or specific activities, known as *red flags,* which could indicate identity theft. Although this rule is certainly valid, many healthcare groups were opposed to having to adopt yet another administratively burdensome process and argued that general security requirements in the HIPAA Security Rule and the PCI-DSS (if applicable to them) were sufficient. After considerable lobbying and a number of delays in implementing the rule for healthcare organizations, physicians, attorneys, and many hospitals (that is, those that do not regularly request credit reports when they extend credit to patients) were exempted from the rule (Anderson 2010). However, many healthcare organizations find the recommendations for deterring or identifying potential identity theft situations in the Red Flags rule useful. For example, healthcare organizations may seek electronic verification of insurance eligibility or require that patients show a government-issued photo ID at the start of an encounter.

Administrative and Physical Factors to Reduce Privacy and Security Risk

When it comes to reducing privacy and security risks, administrative and physical factors are at least as important as technical ones. To fully understand an organization's security needs and invest wisely in security controls overall, it is important to not only consider HIPAA's requirements to identify threats and vulnerabilities but also understand how likely these problems are to occur and what impact they will have, and plan a layered approach that reinforces each set of controls as threats reach deeper to the core of EHR and health IT.

Technical tools are not the only, or necessarily the most effective, way to control patient data. The strongest possible authentication measures and audit logs may exist in the organization, but if management does not support sanctions for misuse of privileges, the technology cannot be effective. OCR has not done many proactive audits to date, focusing instead on complaint and breach investigations. ONC has conducted audits of the MU program, which requires that a risk analysis and technical security controls to be in place. Both agencies have repeatedly identified two major areas of noncompliance: First, risk analysis is absent, old, or incomplete. Second, policies and procedures are nonexistent or not tailored to the organization's risk analysis.

Risk Analysis

The lifecycle of risk analysis follows the systems development life cycle (SDLC). Monitoring, auditing, and triggered reviews should be enabled by the organization so that the current state of risk is known and appropriate controls can be put into place. Figure 12.6 illustrates the SDLC as applied to information security.

Risk analysis documentation proves that such analysis has been performed and can serve as a plan for implementing and monitoring controls. Figure 12.7 provides a structure for risk analysis documentation. This structure utilizes a spreadsheet to capture observations that may be identified through ongoing risk monitoring, periodic auditing, or triggered reviews. A **triggered review** occurs when a monitoring system identifies an event that could be a potential risk. That event then leads to a more comprehensive investigation. Observations may be rated according to their probability for occurrence and criticality of their impact. A risk score can be calculated (see figure 12.3). The observations are keyed to the Security Rule standards and to the organization's policies, procedures, and documentation. The structure shown in figure 12.7 is not required by HIPAA, but it is a common structure used by consultants and auditors. It may also be used to conduct an audit for assessing an organization's compliance with the Privacy Rule, in which case the criticality and probability of a threat exploiting a vulnerability would not be included. This structure ensures that

Figure 12.6.   SDLC for security

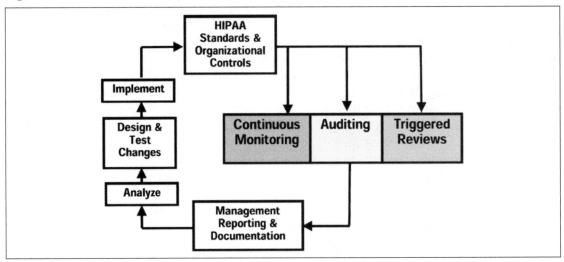

every Security Rule and Privacy Rule standard is addressed and has associated policy, procedure, and documentation.

Policies and procedures (and documentation if desired) may also be documented on a separate worksheet (as shown in Figure 12.8). This worksheet is constructed as a reference checklist wherein every policy, procedure, and documentation associated with Security Rule or Privacy Rule

Figure 12.7.   Risk analysis documentation structure

		Vulnerabilities					Potential Threats			Risk Management
HIPAA Security Assessment										
Security Standard 45 CFR (Required/ Addressable)	Policy, Procedure, Documentary Evidence	Guiding Questions (This guidance is drawn from NIST, CMS, and other security standards in the absence of further guidance from HIPAA)	Interview	Survey Results / Level of Risk		Observed Practice	Criticality	Description of potential threats	Probability / Risk Score	Recommended Control
ADMINISTRATIVE SAFEGUARDS										
1. Security Management Process §164.308(a)(1)										
1.1 Risk Analysis		Has executive management's risk position/level of residual risk tolerance with respect to information security been determined?	ISO RM Exec							
		Have threat sources for all aspects of information security been identified?	ISO							
		Is there intelligence available concerning known information security vulnerabilities of all types maintained?	ISO							
		Is executive management engaged in contributing to an ongoing program of information security risk management?	ISO Exec							
1.2 Risk Management (R)		Is there a process to enable ongoing risk analysis that describes the business case and residual risk associated with existing information security controls?	ISO	25						
		Is there an effective and timely process for reporting new vulnerabilities and threats that leads to prompt remedial action?	ISO							
		Does a configuration management/change control process exist to ensure there are documented approvals for modifications to security policy, physical plant, additions or changes to I.T./I.S. (e.g., version control, s/w discipline)?	ISO IT							

Cover / TOC / Privacy Assmt / Privacy Doc Inventory / Privacy Risk Scoring \ Security Assmt / Security Doc Inventory / Security Risk Scoring / Perce

Figure 12.8. Policy and procedure inventory structure

HIPAA Privacy Policy & Procedure Inventory															
Yes	Meets HIPAA compliance requirements														
No	Addresses topic, but not w/respect to HIPAA														
Part	Partially addresses HIPAA requirement														
Policy & Procedure Number	Title	Last Revised & Rev #	1. U&D General	2. Minimum Necessary	3. Subject to Restriction Rqstd by Individual	4. De-identified PHI	5. Disclosures to BA	6. Deceased Individuals	7. Personal Representatives	8. Confidential Communications	9. U&D Consistent w/NOPP	10. Disclosures to Whistleblowers	11. U&D Organizational Reqmts	13. BA Contract

Privacy standards have been numbered for ease of reference.

compliance is listed and its contents described by its association to the applicable standard in the Rules. Many policies and procedures address multiple standards; therefore, this type of worksheet helps the organization cross-check that all standards are addressed in some policy and procedure. Maintaining a list of the type of documentation and/or location of documentation can also be helpful to assess whether updates are needed and to be able to quickly locate such documentation in the event of an external audit or investigation. For example, in many information technology (IT) departments, the help desks use help desk software to track requests and reports of problems. This system may be used to also document issue resolution. However, not all necessary documentation would be retained in such a system. For example, an analysis of audit logs would not trigger a call to a help desk. Not all organizations have a help desk or such software, instead relying on exchange of e-mail and retention of the e-mail messages. Having a system that enables documentation of retention that is easy to locate and relate to each of the Security Rule and Privacy Rule standards is good preparation for an inevitable audit or other circumstance requiring documentary evidence of action by the organization.

Finally, the risk analysis documentation structure in figure 12.7 identifies technical controls that may be used in risk management. Many organizations use their risk analysis spreadsheet as a project plan, extending the columns to track who is responsible for implementing controls and that the controls have, in fact, been implemented. Table 12.5 lists some of the controls that can assist in monitoring security (Schultz 2011; CORE Security Technologies 2011). Other technical security controls, such as access controls, encryption, device management, and others are described earlier in this chapter.

Physical Controls

Physical controls are as important as technical controls in managing information security, and are increasingly becoming technical in nature. For example, table 12.5 lists 24/7 perimeter sensor monitoring and secure entry tools that should be used to afford physical security for data centers and, in many cases, for the entire organization campus. Other vital physical controls include data backup, contingency planning and disaster recovery.

Many organizations recognize the need for a comprehensive **storage management program**, with experts who can identify the appropriate storage media for different types of data, information, knowledge, and content (documents and images), and manage various retention requirements,

Table 12.5.   Technical monitoring tools

24/7 perimeter sensor monitoring
Secure entry tools
Intrusion detection system
Intrusion prevention system
Data loss prevention
Threat intelligence
Treat management response
Anti-malware protection
Audit/event log management
Patching
File integrity monitoring
Security information and event management
Mobile device management
Vulnerability assessment
Ethical hacking/penetration testing

retrieval strategies, and storage costs. New technologies for storage can lower cost and improve retrieval rates. For example, **storage virtualization** is a process that creates a virtual version of an operating system, server, storage device, or network resources by decoupling these applications from their host resources—reducing the number of devices required and using less energy and maintenance (Daly 2012). Cloud storage may use storage virtualization, but it is a service not a physical infrastructure. Data deduplication and compression techniques are also used for storage management. Each type of storage management, however, requires a full appreciation of their technical management requirements and security needs. Many healthcare organizations are considering cloud computing, previously defined in chapter 10, but are concerned about security. A white paper prepared by ClearData (2014) describes seven essential layers of secure cloud computing to "defend the castle" (see also discussion later in this chapter). A layered approach to defending a castle involves a wide moat, a strong building structure, look-out towers, a fleet of defenders, and tunnels to escape through. This is a good analogy for cloud computing because many healthcare organizations only consider the transmission of data to and from the cloud and may not fully investigate the cloud storage company's administrative and physical security controls as well as its own processes and controls.

Physical controls must also address reliability of services. **Reliability** refers to the ability of a system to perform its functions without errors, crashes, or performance problems. Errors may occur because of system performance issues or attacks that alter data and/or software. Performance issues relate to how well an organization structures its services, performs maintenance, and assures availability. Crashes are caused by many of the same system performance issues or security threats that cause errors, but rather than produce an error, crashes cause the system to stop functioning altogether (that is, experience downtime). Reliability is particularly important in cloud computing, where a provider organization is dependent on the cloud vendor to provide much of these services but is also reliant on an Internet Service Provider (ISP) to maintain connectivity. In some communities, there is only one ISP, which increases the risk of system unavailability and has nothing to do with either the provider or the cloud vendor. In a mission-critical information system, such as the EHR and certain other types of health IT, full redundancy must be in place to ensure the system operates 24 hours a day, 7 days a week. **Full redundancy** entails at least two of every mission-critical device, network, power supply, and so on. These redundant components should work simultaneously, so that if one component fails, there is automatic **failover** to the remaining system. If a healthcare organization uses a remote vendor to support its applications, lack of network redundancy at the organization's local site can wipe out any redundancy the remote site provides. Full redundancy, therefore, does not negate the need for backup, disaster recovery planning, and emergency mode operations procedures/business continuity (collectively referred to as *contingency planning*) because a fully redundant system is intended only to serve in the event of emergency.

Layered Approach to Security Administration

A layered approach to security aids in securing information resources. Many security experts compare layered security to the layers of an onion, where each layer protects the next layer in. The Security Rule itself is structured in a layered approach, first addressing administrative security requirements, then physical, then technical. In a layered approach, there is an entire system of security in which:

- A solid base of management support understands and can articulate its risk posture, which establishes the level of controls desired.

- A thorough applications and data criticality analysis, as well as a vulnerability assessment, has been performed and supports the organization's understanding of a potential threat's impact.

- Executive management has approved policies that reflect the organization's risk posture and are available to all members of the workforce, and procedures that provide detailed instruction for carrying out controls (some of which may involve sensitive information that should be safeguarded to the same or even greater extent than PHI).

- Responsibility for security is part of everyone's job, but the organization also needs to designate an information security officer (ISO) to provide oversight.

- Administrative, operational, and physical controls support technical controls, and these all have been appropriately implemented and tested, and changes managed effectively.

- Users have been thoroughly trained on security, with follow-up provided via ongoing awareness building and reminders.

- An ongoing auditing and monitoring process serves continuously as a feedback loop to enhance controls, where necessary.

Multiple levels of security protection have also been described as zones of trust (Tipton and Nozaki 2012). Trust is a concept that is widely related to privacy and security. Patients need confidence that their health information is held in confidence and secured. Providers need to be able to trust the information in EHRs and other types of health IT, especially where it is coming from multiple sources. Business associates must garner trust in their clients by offering cost-effective solutions for them to succeed in business. In the context of privacy and security, Braunstein (2014) proposes a working definition of **trust** as the means by which the recipient or sender of information knows that the people and organizations involved in the electronic interaction are who they say they are.

Emerging Threats

Monitoring the complaints reported to OCR and monitoring breaches reported to HHS are good ways to identify how threats are changing. For example, in 2015, many more breaches related to an external hack attack were reported than in previous years (the external hacks also increased the size of each breach) (Landi 2015). However, data from other sources reveal that internal actions (malicious or not) still account for a substantial percentage of data breaches (Widup 2015). Internal actions that resulted in lost or stolen devices and improper destruction of paper or electronic data continue to rank high in causes of breach (Widup 2015). Although some believe that inadequate security precautions taken by business associates are an increasing threat (ISMG 2015), actual causes of breaches are significantly more prevalent from external sources (nearly 60%) and internal sources (nearly 35%) as compared to partner (business associate) sources (5%) (Widup 2015).

A variety of resources can be used to monitor emerging privacy and security threats. Such regular monitoring has been called **threat intelligence**, which is the active use of reliable sources to monitor trends and implement appropriate controls. The Ponemon Institute (2015b) identifies that 80 percent of companies having experienced a cyberattack have concluded that they could have prevented or minimized the consequences of the attack if they had ensured that their anti-virus/anti-malware solutions were up to date, monitored intrusion detection systems, and used next-general firewalls or a **unified threat management (UTM)** program. Because threat intelligence can be delivered through a subscription service from a variety of companies, this same report emphasized the need for human analysis of the threat intelligence to ensure it is timely, relevant, and trustworthy and offers clear guidance on how to resolve the threat.

Check Your Understanding 12.2

Match the terms with the appropriate descriptions:

   A. Accountability

   B. Authentication

   C. Digital certificate

   D. Digital signature

   E. Electronic signature

   F. Minimum necessary

   G. Nonrepudiation

   H. Public key infrastructure

   I. Reliability

   J. User ID

   K. Vulnerability

   L   X.509

   1. Supplies the basis for defining access controls

   2. Standard for identifying a person in a digital signature

   3. Set of policies that enable a digital signature

   4. A process of conveying approval or authorship

   5. Ability of a system to perform its functions correctly

   6. A process that digitally verifies the identity of an individual

7. Property that traces an action to its entity

8. Process of encryption and nonrepudiation in authentication

9. Computing action that triggers access

10. Process by which an electronic record can be signed

11. Evidence of message integrity

12. Weakness in security controls

References and Resources

16 CFR 318. 2009 (August 25). Federal Trade Commission. Health breach notification rule: final rule.

21 CFR 1300, 1304, 1306, 1311. 2010 (March 31). Drug Enforcement Administration. Electronic prescriptions for controlled substances: final rule.

45 CFR 160. 2009 (October 30). HIPAA administrative simplification: Enforcement: interim final rule.

45 CFR 160, 164. 2009 (August 24). Department of Health and Human Services. Breach notification for unsecured protected health information: interim final rule.

45 CFR 160, 164. 2013 (January 25). Department of Health and Human Services. Modifications to the HIPAA privacy, security, enforcement, and breach notification rules under the Health Information Technology for Economic and Clinical Health Act and the Genetic Information Nondiscrimination Act; other modifications to the HIPAA Rules: final rule. (Also known as the *Omnibus Rule*.)

45 CFR 160, 162, 164. 2003 (February 20). Department of Health and Human Services. Health insurance reform: Security standards: final rule. Appendix A. Security standards matrix.

45 CFR 2. 2010. Department of Health and Human Services, Substance Abuse and Mental Health Services Administration. Substance abuse confidentiality regulations (revised).

Allen, C., et al. 2014. Data governance and data sharing agreements for community-wide health information exchange: Lessons from the Beacon Communities. *eGEMS (Generating Evidence and Methods to Improve Patient Outcomes)*. 2(1):1057. https://www.ncbi.nlm.nih.gov/pmc/articles/PMC4371395.

American Cancer Society (ACS). 2014 (July 28). What are the legal requirements of informed consent? http://www.cancer.org/treatment/findingandpayingfortreatment/understandingfinancialandlegalmatters/informedconsent/informed-consent-legal-requirements-of-consent.

American Health Information Management Association (AHIMA). 2009 (July 21). MPI Clean Up: It's a Must (webinar). http://campus.ahima.org/audio/2009/RB072109.pdf.

American Hospital Association (AHA). 2012 (January). Bringing behavioral health into the care continuum: Opportunities to improve quality, costs and outcomes. *AHA TrendWatch*. http://www.aha.org/research/reports/tw/12jan-tw-behavhealth.pdf.

Anderson H. 2010 (December 20). Obama signs Red Flags exemptions bill. GovInfoSecurity blog. Information Security Media Group. http://www.govinfosecurity.com/articles.php?art_id=3197.

Barbera L., et al.; American Health Information Management Association (AHIMA) e-HIM Work Group on Security of Personal Health Information. 2008. Ensuring security of high-risk information in EHRs. *Journal of AHIMA*. 79(9):67–71.

Barron, D., et al.; AHIMA eHIM Workgroup on Best Practices for Electronic Signature and Attestation. 2009. Electronic signature, attestation, and authorship (updated). *Journal of AHIMA*. 80(11): expanded online edition.

Bowe, R. 2013. Identity crisis: Organizations are implementing medical identity theft teams to combat rising incidents. *Journal of AHIMA*. 84(1):38–42.

Brandom, R. 2015 (December 18). Congress passes controversial cybersecurity bill attached to omnibus budget. *The Verge*. http://www.theverge.com/2015/12/18/10582446/congress-passes-cisa-surveillance-cybersecurity.

Braunstein, M.L. 2014. *Contemporary Health Informatics*. Chicago, IL: AHIMA.

Brucker, A.D., and H. Petritsch. 2009. Extending access control models with break-glass. *Proceedings of the 14th ACM Symposium on Access Control Models and Technologies*. Association for Computing Machinery.

California Healthcare Foundation (CHCF). 2013 (November 24). Guidelines for the Electronic Prescribing of Controlled Substances: Identity Proofing, Issuing Authentication Credentials, and Configuring Logical Access Controls. http://www.chcf.org/~/media/MEDIA%20LIBRARY%20Files/PDF/PDF%20G/PDF%20GuidelinesEPCS.pdf.

Centers for Medicare and Medicaid Services (CMS). 2016 (April 7). Voluntary data sharing agreement. https://www.cms.gov/Medicare/Coordination-of-Benefits-and-Recovery/EmployerServices/Voluntary-Data-Sharing-Agreement.html.

ClearData. 2014 (December). *The 7 Essential Layers of Secure Cloud Computing*. https://www.cleardata.com/wp-content/uploads/2014/12/SET-MKTG-7-Essential-Layers.pdf.

Coderre, M., and D. Surber. 2015 (August). Standard security framework for medical device technologies: A work in progress. *Medical Design Briefs*. http://www.medicaldesignbriefs.com/component/content/article/mdb/features/22579.

CORE Security Technologies. 2011. Putting NIST Guidelines for Information Security Continuous Monitoring into Practice. http://www.coresecurity.com/system/files/attachments/2013/12/Core%20and%20NIST%20-%20Putting%20NIST%20Guidelines%20for%20Info%20Security%20into%20Practice.pdf

Council for Affordable Quality Healthcare Committee on Operating Rules for Information Exchange (CAQH CORE). 2015. CAQH CORE phase IV operating rules. http://www.caqh.org/core/caqh-core-phase-iv-operating-rules.

Daly, J. 2012 (October 8). What is virtualization? *Ed Tech Magazine*. http://www.edtechmagazine.com/higher/article/2012/10/what-virtualization.

Demster B., L. Fernandes, S. Torzewski, M. Nabers, and V. Wheatley; AHIMA MPI Taskforce. 2012. *Managing the Master Patient Index in a Healthcare Environment Resolution*. http://library.ahima.org/xpedio/groups/public/documents/ahima/bok1_049789.hcsp?dDocName=bok1_049789.

Dooling, J.A., S. Durkin, L. Fernandes, B. Just, S. Kotyk, E.S. Karl, and K. Westhafer. 2014. Managing the integrity of patient identity in health information exchange (updated). *Journal of AHIMA*. 85(5):60–65.

Downing, Kathy. 2013. Electronic Signature, Attestation, and Authorship (2013 update) AHIMA Practice Brief. http://bok.ahima.org/doc?oid=107151#.V9xWMPkrK70

Federal Trade Commission (FTC). 2010 (February). *Consumer Sentinel Network Data Book for January–December 2009*. https://www.ftc.gov/reports/consumer-sentinel-network-data-book-january-december-2009.

Gabriel, M. et al. 2015 (November). State and national trends of two-factor authentication for non-federal acute care hospitals. ONC Data Brief no. 32. https://www.healthit.gov/sites/default/files/briefs/oncdatabrief32_two-factor_authent_trends.pdf.

Goldstein, M.M., and A.L. Rein. 2010 (September 29). Data segmentation in electronic health information exchange: Policy considerations and analysis. Prepared for Office of the National Coordinator for Health Information Technology. https://www.healthit.gov/sites/default/files/privacy-security/gwu-data-segmentation-final-cover-letter.pdf.

Hagland, M. 2015 (July 15). CHIME moves forward on a challenge-based approach to developing a national patient ID. *Healthcare Informatics*. http://www.healthcare-informatics.com/article/chime-moves-forward-challenge-based-approach-developing-national-patient-id.

Handelsman, J., and Patil D.J. 2015 (November 9). Building trust and protecting privacy: Progress on the president's Precision Medicine Initiative. White House blog. https://www.whitehouse.gov/blog/2015/11/09/releasing-privacy-and-trust-principles-precision-medicine-initiative.

Healey, J., N. Pollard, and B. Woods. 2015 (March 18). The healthcare Internet of things: Rewards and risks. Atlantic Council. http://www.atlanticcouncil.org/publications/reports/the-healthcare-internet-of-things-rewards-and-risks.

Health Data Management (HDM). 2008 (June 12). Medical identity theft study launched. *HDM Breaking News*. http://www.healthdatamanagement.com/news.

HealthIT.gov. 2014 (September 15). Enabling privacy: Data segmentation: DS4P Initiative. https://www.healthit.gov/providers-professionals/ds4p-initiative.

Heath, S. 2015a (December 16). Visual hacking poses a new healthcare data security threat. *HealthIT Security*. http://healthitsecurity.com/news/visual-hacking-poses-a-new-healthcare-data-security-threat.

Heath, S. 2015b (November 17). Keystroke logger leads to health data breach at KY hospital. *HealthIT Security*. http://healthitsecurity.com/news/keystroke-logger-leads-to-health-data-breach-at-ky-hospital.

Heath, S. 2015c (November 9). Most physician secure messaging apps not HIPAA compliant. *HealthIT Security*. http://healthitsecurity.com/news/most-physician-secure-messaging-apps-not-hipaa-compliant.

Hu, V.C. et al. 2014 (January 8). Guide to attribute based access control (ABAC) definition and considerations. National Institute of Standards and Technology (NIST) special publication 800-162. http://nvlpubs.nist.gov/nistpubs/specialpublications/NIST.sp.800-162.pdf.

Information Security Media Group (ISMG). 2015.Healthcare information security today—2015 survey analysis: Evolving threats and health info security efforts. http://www.databreachtoday.com/whitepapers/2015-survey-analysis-evolving-threats-health-info-security-efforts-w-2065.

Joint Commission. 2015. National Patient Safety Goals Effective January 1, 2015. Hospital Accreditation Program goal 1. Improve the accuracy of patient identification. http://www.jointcommission.org/assets/1/6/2015_npsg_hap.pdf.

Landi, H. 2015 (September 9). Healthcare hacks account for most data breaches in 2015. *Healthcare Informatics*. http://www.healthcare-informatics.com/news-item/healthcare-hacks-account-most-data-breaches-2015.

Lawton, S. 2015 (March 17). Introduction to public key infrastructure (PKI). *Tom's IT Pro*. http://www.tomsitpro.com/articles/public-key-infrastructure-introduction,2-884.html.

Lee, K. 2014 (July 8). Four methods to create a secure password you'll actually remember. LifeHacker.com. http://lifehacker.com/four-methods-to-create-a-secure-password-youll-actually-1601854240.

McNabb, J., and H.B. Rhodes. 2014. Combating the privacy crime that can kill. *Journal of AHIMA*. 85(4):26–29.

Morris, G., G. Farnum, S. Afzal, C. Robinson, J. Greene, and C. Coughlin. 2014 (February 7). *Patient Identification and Matching*. Report prepared for the Office of the National Coordinator for Health IT. https://www.healthit.gov/sites/default/files/patient_identification_matching_final_report.pdf.

National Council for Prescription Drug Programs (NCPDP). 2014 (February). *Electronic Signature Guidance, Version 1.0*. https://www.ncpdp.org/NCPDP/media/pdf/wp/NCPDPElectronicSignatureGuidanceFinal.pdf.

National Human Genome Research Institute (NHGRI). 2009 (April 6). *The Genetic Information Nondiscrimination Act of 2009: Information for Researchers and Healthcare Professionals*. https://www.genome.gov/Pages/PolicyEthics/GeneticDiscrimination/GINAInfoDoc.pdf.

National Institute of Standards and Technology (NIST). 2014 (February 12). *Framework for Improving Critical Infrastructure Cybersecurity: Version 1.0*. http://www.nist.gov/cyberframework/upload/cybersecurity-framework-021214-final.pdf.

National Library of Medicine (NLM). 2016 (January 11). What is precision medicine? *Genetics Home Reference*. http://ghr.nlm.nih.gov/handbook/precisionmedicine/definition.

Office for Civil Rights (OCR). n.d. Breach portal. https://ocrportal.hhs.gov/ocr/breach/breach_report.jsf.

Office for Civil Rights (OCR). 2009. HHS guidance specifying technologies and methodologies that render PHI unusable, unreadable, or indecipherable to unauthorized individuals for breach notification. http://www.hhs.gov/hipaa/for-professionals/breach-notification/guidance/index.html.

Office for Civil Rights (OCR). 2012 (November 26). Guidance regarding methods for de-identification of protected health information in accordance with the Health Insurance Portability and Accountability Act (HIPAA) Privacy Rule. http://www.hhs.gov/hipaa/for-professionals/privacy/special-topics/de-identification/index.html.

Office for Civil Rights (OCR). 2014a. Enforcement results by calendar year. http://www.hhs.gov/hipaa/for-professionals/compliance-enforcement/data/complaints-received-by-calendar-year/index.html.

Office for Civil Rights (OCR). 2014b (February 20). HIPAA Privacy Rule and sharing of information related to mental health. http://www.hhs.gov/hipaa/for-professionals/special-topics/mental-health/index.html.

Office for Civil Rights (OCR). 2015a. Enforcement highlights. http://www.hhs.gov/hipaa/for-professionals/compliance-enforcement/data/enforcement-highlights/index.html.

Office for Civil Rights (OCR). 2015b. Disclosures for emergency preparedness—a decision tool: Overview. http://www.hhs.gov/hipaa/for-professionals/special-topics/emergency-preparedness/decision-tool-overview/index.html.

Office of the National Coordinator for Health Information Technology (ONC). 2014 (January 29). *SAFER Guides: Patient Identification*. https://www.healthit.gov/safer/sites/safer/files/guides/safer_patientidentification_sg006_form.pdf.

Office of the National Coordinator for Health Information Technology (ONC). 2015. Understanding electronic health records, the HIPAA Security Rule, and cybersecurity. Chapter 4 in *Guide to Privacy and Security of Electronic Health Information*. https://www.healthit.gov/sites/default/files/pdf/privacy/privacy-and-security-guide-chapter-4.pdf.

Open Web Application Security Project (OWASP). 2015. Access control cheat sheet. https://www.owasp.org/index.php/Access_Control_Cheat_Sheet.

Ponemon Institute. 2015a (May). *2015 Cost of Data Breach Study: Global Analysis*. Benchmark research sponsored by IBM. http://www-01.ibm.com/common/ssi/cgi-bin/ssialias?subtype=WH&infotype=SA&htmlfid=SEW03053WWEN&attachment=SEW03053WWEN.PDF.

Ponemon Institute. 2015b. Importance of cyber threat intelligence to a strong security posture. Research sponsored by WebRoot. http://www.webroot.com/shared/pdf/CyberThreatIntelligenceReport2015.pdf.

Privacy Analytics. 2015 (December 2). *The State of Data Sharing for Healthcare Analytics 2015–2016: Change, Challenges and Choice*. http://www.privacy-analytics.com/de-id-university/white-papers/the-state-of-data-sharing-for-healthcare-analytics.

Ritz, D. 2013 (July 11). Opinion: It's time for a national patient identifier. *HIMSS News*. http://www.himss.org/News/NewsDetail.aspx?ItemNumber=21464.

Robeznieks, A. 2015 (June 10). Bill aims to clarify mental health record-sharing under HIPAA. *Modern Healthcare*. http://www.modernhealthcare.com/article/20150610/NEWS/150619992.

Rodriguez L. 2013 (January 15). Director, Office for Civil Rights, US Department of Health and Human Services: Message to our nation's health care providers. https://www.hhs.gov/sites/default/files/ocr/office/lettertonationhcp.pdf.

Schultz, E. 2011. Continuous monitoring: What it is, why it is needed, and how to use it. SANS Institute InfoSec Reading Room. https://www.sans.org/reading-room/whitepapers/analyst/continuous-monitoring-is-needed-35030.

Sequoia Project. 2014 (September 13). Data use and reciprocal support agreement (DURSA). http://sequoiaproject.org/ehealth-exchange/onboarding/dursa.

Snell, E. 2015a (November 14). Is HIE security affected with health record integration? *HealthIT Security.* http://healthitsecurity.com/news/is-hie-security-affected-with-health-record-integration.

Snell, E. 2015b (December 1). Maintaining healthcare data security in genomic data sharing. *HealthIT Security*. http://healthitsecurity.com/news/maintaining-healthcare-data-security-in-genomic-data-sharing.

Stein, A. 2012 (February 13). How does mobile device management (MDM) work? Meeting mobile IT's need for securing apps, policies and permissions across the multi-OS smart device enterprise. *Network World*. http://www.networkworld.com/article/2185771/tech-primers/how-does-mobile-device-management--mdm--work-.html.

Terry, K. 2015 (March 16). EHR security: To encrypt or not to encrypt. *iHealth Beat*. http://www.ihealthbeat.org/insight/2015/ehr-security-to-encrypt-or-not-to-encrypt.

Tipton, H.F., and M.K. Nozaki. 2012. *Information Security Management Handbook*, 6th ed. Boca Raton, FL: CRC Press.

US Department of Health and Human Services (HHS). n.d.(a). HIPAA FAQs for Professionals, FAQ 264: What is the difference between "consent" and "authorization" under the HIPAA Privacy Rule? http://www.hhs.gov/hipaa/for-professionals/faq/264/what-is-the-difference-between-consent-and-authorization/index.html.

US Department of Health and Human Services (HHS). n.d.(b). Enterprise Performance Life Cycle Framework. *Data Use Agreement Practices Guide*. http://www.hhs.gov/ocio/eplc/EPLC%20Archive%20Documents/55-Data%20Use%20Agreement%20(DUA)/eplc_dua_practices_guide.pdf.

US Department of Health and Human Services (HHS). 1979 (April 18). The Belmont Report. http://www.hhs.gov/ohrp/humansubjects/guidance/belmont.html.

US Department of Health and Human Services (HHS). 2002 (August 14). Preamble to the privacy final rule. *Federal Register.* 67(157):53194. https://www.gpo.gov/fdsys/pkg/FR-2002-08-14/pdf/FR-2002-08-14.pdf.

US Department of Health and Human Services. 2016a (March 18). Federal policy for the protection of human subjects ("Common Rule"). Office for Human Research Protections. http://www.hhs.gov/ohrp/humansubjects/commonrule.

US Department of Health and Human Services (HHS). 2016b. Individuals' right under HIPAA to access their health information 45 CFR § 164.524. http://www.hhs.gov/hipaa/for-professionals/privacy/guidance/access/index.html.

US Department of Homeland Security (DHS), et al. 2015 (September 8). Federal policy for the protection of human subjects: Notice of proposed rulemaking. *Federal Register.* 80(173):2015–21756. https://www.gpo.gov/fdsys/pkg/FR-2015-09-08/pdf/2015-21756.pdf.

Walsh T. 2013. Security risk analysis and management: An overview (updated). *Journal of AHIMA.* 84(11): expanded web version. http://bok.ahima.org/doc?oid=300266#.V7IJHJgrI2w.

Weinstein S., and I. Singureanu. n.d. Data segmentation for privacy. S&I Framework wiki post. http://wiki.siframework.org/Data+Segmentation+for+Privacy+Paper#top.

White House. 2015 (February 15). Fact sheet: White House Summit on Cybersecurity and Consumer Protection. https://www.whitehouse.gov/the-press-office/2015/02/13/fact-sheet-white-house-summit-cybersecurity-and-consumer-protection.

Widup S., et al. 2015 (December 17). 2015 Protected health information data breach report. Verizon Enterprise Solutions. http://www.verizonenterprise.com/resources/reports/rp_2015-protected-health-information-data-breach-report_en_xg.pdf.

Wilson, B. 2008 (March 3). Medical identity theft is often an "inside job." *American Medical News.* http://www.amednews.com/article/20080303/profession/303039962/7.

Chapter 13
Interoperability and Health Information Exchange

Key Terms

Agile Modeling

American National Standards Institute (ANSI)

ANSI Standards Committee (ASC) X12

Application Programming Interface (API)

ASTM International

Blue Button

Certificate Authority (CA)

Clinical Documents for Payers (CDP)

Consent management

Consolidated architecture

Consolidated Clinical Document Architecture (C-CDA)

Consumer-mediated exchange

Continuity of Care Record (CCR)

Continuity of Care Document (CCD)

Council for Affordable Quality Healthcare, Committee on Operating Rules
for Information Exchange (CAQH CORE)

Data normalization

Data stewardship

Data Use and Reciprocal Services Agreement (DURSA)

Decision Support Services (DSS)

Digital Imaging and Communications in Medicine (DICOM)

Direct

Directed exchange

Directory

Direct Project
Direct Trust
eHealth Exchange
Electronic data interchange (EDI)
Electronic Healthcare Network Accreditation Commission (EHNAC)
Extensible Markup Language (XML)
Fast Healthcare Interoperability Resources (FHIR)
Federated architecture
Health data stewardship
Health Information Service Provider (HISP)
Health Level Seven (HL7)
HIE Data Sharing Agreement
HIE Participation Agreement
Human-computer interface
Hybrid architecture
Identity management
Identity matching
Information model
Integrated
Integrating the Healthcare Enterprise (IHE)
Integration profiles
Interface
Interface engine
Interoperability
Interoperability Standards Advisory
Message format standards
National Association for Trust Exchange (NATE)
National Council for Prescription Drug Programs (NCPDP)
Operating rules
Opt in
Optionality
Opt out
Person identification
Process interoperability
Pull technology
Push technology
Query-based exchange
Record locator service (RLS)
Reference Information Model (RIM)
Registration Authority (RA)
Registry service

Representational State Transfer (REST)

Scalable normalization

Semantic interoperability

Semantic normalization

Sequoia Project

Simple Object Access Protocol (SOAP)

Situational

Standard message protocols

Standards and Interoperability (S&I) Framework

Standards development organization (SDO)

State Health Information Exchange Cooperative Agreement Program

State-Level Health Information Exchange Consensus Project

Stewardship

Syntactic interoperability

Technical interoperability

Trust Agents

Trust Bundle

Unified Modeling Language (UML)

Virtual Medical Record (vMR)

Workgroup on Electronic Data Interchange (WEDI)

Learning Objectives

- Describe the continuum of interoperability maturity.

- Describe technical standards for interoperability.

- Explain the role of semantic interoperability.

- Understand standard messaging protocols.

- Assess the importance of process interoperability.

- Discuss the impetus for health information exchange in the United States.

- Describe the status and basic forms of health information exchange organization structures, architectures, and services.

- Describe the nationwide health information exchange, called eHealth Exchange, and explain how providers share data over this network.

Information system **interoperability** is the ability of two or more systems or components to exchange information and use the information that has been exchanged (NAHIT 2008). Heath information exchange is the electronic movement of health-related information among organizations according to nationally recognized (interoperability) standards (NAHIT 2008). In its *Connecting Health and Care for the Nation: A Shared Nationwide Interoperability Roadmap,* the Office of the National Coordinator for Health Information Technology (ONC) observes that "the nation needs an interoperable health system that empowers individuals to use their electronic health information to the fullest extent; enables providers and communities to deliver smarter, safer, and more efficient care; and promotes innovation at all levels" (ONC 2015). In the world of the Internet and browsers, it may seem like interoperability should be a simple matter. Unfortunately, interoperability in the healthcare environment is very difficult to achieve. Over the years, providers have invested not only a tremendous amount of money but human capital in systems based on client/server technology that does not operate in the same manner as the Internet and browsers are used. Conversion of these systems to what has been described as third platform technology using web services is an expensive undertaking. Most established electronic health record (EHR) vendors whose initial EHR offerings were built on second platform technology are moving gradually to third platform services, but they cannot outpace the ability of their clients to replace legacy source systems. In some respects, this is more of an economic dilemma than a technical one. It is, however, a challenge that many vendors, standards development organizations, and others in the industry are working on and an issue that the federal government views as critical over the next decade to address.

Continuum of Interoperability Maturity

A continuum of interoperable maturity has been described (HIMSS 2013). This is illustrated in figure 13.1.

The continuum begins with **technical interoperability**—the ability of two or more systems or components to exchange information without error. According to the European Telecommunications Standards Institute, technical interoperability may be considered to be comprised of two parts (Kubicek et al. 2011). One part relates to computer hardware having the basic connection points, and the other part relates to data being structured in a manner that enables exchange between two software applications. The later form of interoperability is sometimes referred to as **syntactic interoperability**. The standards that ensure basic connectivity are not specific to healthcare computing, but to computer use in general. The standards that ensure the data are structured the same way for the two applications exchanging the data are often referred to as **message format**

Figure 13.1.   Continuum of interoperability

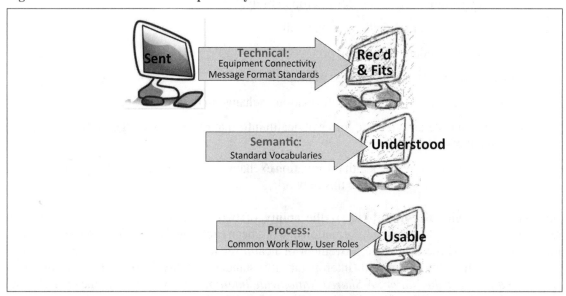

standards. When two separate applications are not compatible with one another, special software, called an **interface**, must be written to exchange the data between the two applications. This is largely where health information technology (health IT) is today.

Semantic interoperability enables interpretation and therefore more effective use of information that is exchanged. Semantic interoperability is being aided by the meaningful use (MU) incentive requirements that call for standardized terminologies to be used for certain data. Significantly more needs to be done to achieve full semantic interoperability.

Finally, **process interoperability** is the degree to which the integrity of workflow can be maintained between systems and includes maintaining and conveying information such as user roles, data protection, and system service quality between systems (Open HIT Labs 2011). Today, process interoperability is the most challenging form of interoperability to achieve in healthcare because there is so little standardization and very few federal requirements addressing such. Perhaps the best example of where there is beginning to be some successful adoption of agreement on process is in the Health Insurance Portability and Accountability Act (HIPAA) operating rules for financial and administrative transactions of claims, eligibility verification, and others. Operating rules describe the business processes necessary to exchange such transactions, such as response time, turnaround time, acknowledgement of receipt, and others. One of the biggest challenges in exchanging protected health information (PHI) across US organizations has been related to requirements for patient authorization for disclosures, which vary in each of the 50 states. Access permissions can be equally troublesome where there is lack of trust between two healthcare organizations because one has policies that are much more liberal than the other's. Security levels, such as whether encryption is required and, if so, at what technical specification, are another example of what should be included in process interoperability.

Technical Interoperability

For purposes of health IT interoperability, the most basic form of technical interoperability, which is associated with the ability to make a connection between two computers, exists. The fundamental need for health IT, then, is to ensure that the message being sent from one system cannot only be received but also is received in a manner that "fits" into the software application's processing capability. When different applications have software that enables them to be designed together and work together with no required intervention, those applications are said to be **integrated**. Integrated applications should exchange data seamlessly. Perhaps the best example of this is the Microsoft Office suite of programs. Word, Excel, Access, PowerPoint, Outlook, and other Office components all look the same and exchange data easily (although, even in this case, the programs do not work absolutely exactly the same).

When application programs are written independently of one another, they do not have the same look and feel and may not have the same data-formatting requirements. For example, systems in the United States most commonly structure dates in the format mm/dd/yy. Alternatively, other countries often format dates as dd/mm/yy. When a date needs to be sent from one system to another, instructions need to be developed to translate one format to the other. In other words, an interface must be written. An **interface** is a software application that is written to tell one application how another application structures its data so that the receiving application can put the data in the structure necessary for it to process the data. An interface for sending a date formatted as mm/dd/yy to a system that needs to have the date structured as dd/mm/yy must be written to explain that the first two characters, *mm,* should be put into the second field of the receiving system's date fields.

A further complication might be if the sending application formats the date in only one field, as mmddyy, and the receiving application then needs to parse the single data element into three separate data elements to accommodate the fact that the receiving system has three fields: one for dd, a second for mm, and a third for yy. It is further noted that this interface is unidirectional. If the receiving system later needs to send a date to the sending system, another interface needs to be written. If both systems need to share dates back and forth, a bidirectional interface must be written.

Creating an interface can be expensive and time-consuming, and the interface may never work as well as a fully integrated system. In addition, if an organization has many systems that need to exchange data, multiple interfaces need to be written. When any one system is updated by its vendor, the interfaces written to exchange data between that system and the others need to be checked to determine whether the interfaces also need to be updated. In purchasing systems that require interfacing, the organization must consider the tradeoff between a less than completely smooth connection and the advantages of the newly introduced system. Vendors are becoming more experienced in writing interfaces, and **interface engines**, which are software tools that manage multiple interfaces, are helping as well. Still, interfacing can be an arduous process.

Because health IT has expanded to virtually every area needing information, many vendors have been unable to keep up the development pace and address all information system needs. In many cases, vendors have bought companies and tried to integrate their respective products to round out the company's product lines, or companies partner with other vendors to supply certain applications. In these cases, the vendors typically hardwire interfaces into the products so that a separate interface is not needed. However, though, if an entirely new product is introduced into the mix and needs to exchange data, these vendors must modify their built-in interfaces. Some of these efforts have been more successful than others. Not only must the systems be able to exchange data, but also the **human-computer interface**—that is, the look and feel of the applications—should also be as similar as possible. Some use the term *human-computer interface* only to describe the device (such as PC or tablet) the user uses to enter and retrieve data. But there are many more considerations than just the device. Many users need to interact with multiple applications and find it difficult to use them if, for example, one application puts patient-identifying information in one location and another puts it in a different location.

One important consideration in buying health IT products is how well they will work with the rest of the organization's applications. One way to ensure more integrated data is to use a data repository, to which data can be sent and integrated for retrieval by each of the EHR or other health IT applications (Dunbrack and Holland 2008). (Data repositories are discussed in chapter 10.) New web-based products using extensible markup language (XML) can achieve data access that simulates integration, although many of the analytical processes for clinical decision support are unavailable without a repository. These new technologies must be integrated with existing core systems for them to reach their full potential (Managed Healthcare Executive 2008).

Standard Messaging Protocols and Related Work

The ability to interface systems depends on **standard message protocols**, which are sometimes called *message standards, interoperability standards,* or *data exchange standards*. Standard message protocols provide the tools to map proprietary formats to one another and more easily accomplish the exchange of data. However, because the standard protocols developed to date have often had a lot of optionality, full interoperability is still not completely ensured.

Standards development organizations (SDOs) bring together all the stakeholders to a standards arena and, through an open and voluntary, consensus-based process, create standards for their industry. SDOs often seek accreditation under the **American National Standards Institute (ANSI)**, which is a way of validating that they are representative of industry stakeholders and have produced standards that are not biased to any one group of the stakeholders they are attempting to represent. ANSI accreditation also affords a voice in the international standards-setting community—an important element for companies selling products abroad. When the US federal government seeks to adopt standards, it prefers standards from an ANSI-accredited SDO.

In healthcare, there are several SDOs that have emerged focusing on technical, semantic, and process interoperability. Figure 13.2 provides examples of the different types of messaging standards used in healthcare, which are discussed next.

It is important to understand that a standard generally reflects the lowest common denominator with respect to the requirements for the protocol being addressed. This is because standards are consensus-based, where each stakeholder may have had to give up something to get something else. For example, these stakeholders may be vendors arguing against a data element being required because their provider clients do not want to enter too much structured data or the data element requires a code set for which there is a fee that the vendor does not want to have pay. This results in standards having considerable **optionality**, where a data element or associated process may be used at the discretion of the vendor in developing software using the protocol. In some cases, data can also be **situational data**, required only when the situation (such as purpose or nature of other data) calls for the data. For example, in using software to generate a claim, a flag may be set only if an attachment will accompany the claim transactions. Both optionality and situational data essentially set up a chain reaction that begins with vendors that adopt the standards in different ways. Some vendors may adopt them very strictly, whereas others may adopt only the required components and only some or none of the optional components. The resultant products, then, are less than fully compliant with the standards, and hence less than fully interoperable. The American Hospital Association (AHA) recently highlighted this issue in a report on "Why Interoperability Matters," describing events such as data in critical fields being missing, a value documented in the wrong section of a laboratory report, and others (AHA 2015). Figure 13.3 provides an example of one line from an interface written (using the Health Level 7 [HL7] V2.3.1 standard) to exchange data between a provider and an immunization registry. Each data element is separated from another by an indicator (|). In this case, the use of the double indicator (||) denotes that a data element could be placed at the point in the line of programming code, but was not—for whatever reason.

Health Level Seven

Health Level 7 (HL7) is the most common healthcare application level standard that helps ensure data exchange across health information systems. HL7 is the name of both the ANSI-accredited SDO and many of the standards the SDO produces. The standards consist of protocols (that is,

Figure 13.2.   Messaging standards

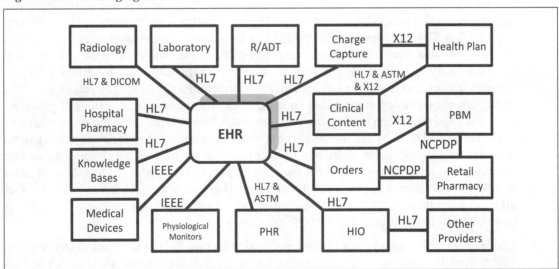

Figure 13.3.   Line of interface example illustrating optionality

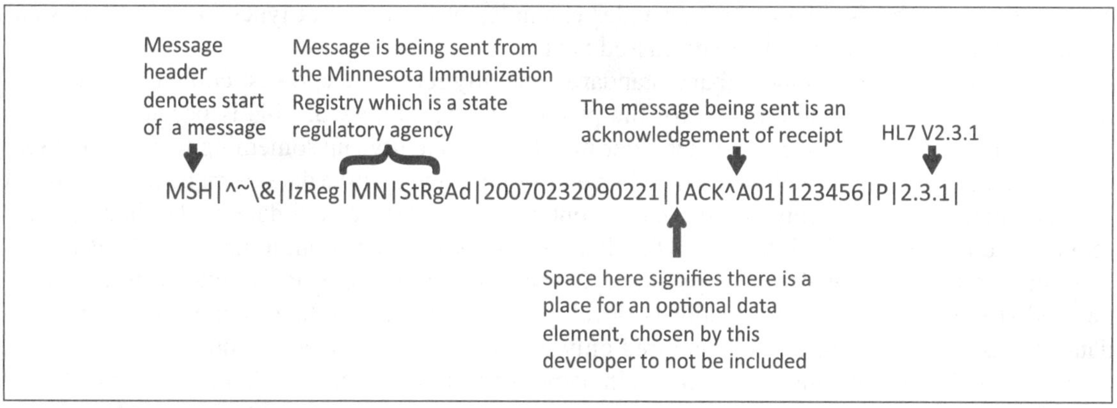

agreed-upon ways) for structuring and transmitting a wide variety of data among many different types of applications. Originally HL7 standards were limited to use in applications that supported exchange of data among applications within an organization. Increasingly, HL7 is used by health information exchange (HIE) organizations to share data with other providers.

HL7 maintains two major versions of standards, HL7 V2.x and HL7 V3. HL7 V2.x (for example, V2.3, V2.4, and V2.5) are used in point-to-point data exchanges—in other words, in traditional second platform data exchange. HL7 V3 was initiated in 1999 and adopted an XML schema for use in a WSA. Unfortunately, HL7 V3 is not backward-compatible with the HL7 V2.x, and so few vendors for the US market have incorporated it in their product development. However, it has been widely adopted by other countries who were newer to health IT, and by US vendors selling products internationally.

HL7 work on V3, however, has delivered benefits to the US market, and HL7 is working to help the United States make the transition from second platform to third platform technology via HL7 standards. The benefits from HL7 V3 and transitional strategies include the following:

- Development of the HL7 **Reference Information Model (RIM)**, which provides the grammar for HL7 messages, specifying the basic building blocks of the language and their permitted relationships. The RIM is also associated with a data type specification and a vocabulary specification. Together, these enable the RIM to depict every conceivable relationship where information must flow—from a generic perspective. For example, an "observation" may be a laboratory test result, an x-ray report, a vital sign, or subjective information from a patient's history and physical examination. Data modeling was discussed in chapter 10, and its importance cannot be emphasized enough. Modeling creates visualizations of programming code and other form implementation that sustain the programming through creation of many versions. The RIM and the data type specification ensure that, for every data element collected in an application, there are all necessary associations—that the users and uses are defined in a way that ensures that they can be accurately handled in a system. In other words, no data element exists without a purpose. There are no "black holes." The fact that all terms must be designated with a vocabulary specification also means there are no terms permitted that have obscure meanings (Shakir 2014).

- The HL7 V3 also created a clinical document architecture (CDA) standard, which was the first nationally certified **extensible markup language (XML)**–based standard for healthcare (Dolin et al. 2006). XML is a meta-language, or series of tags for describing markup languages, used in exchanging documents on the web. It has been at the forefront of incorporating healthcare semantics into healthcare message content. HL7 teamed up with ASTM International, which had created the **continuity of care record (CCR)** standard (discussed later in this chapter), to produce the **continuity of care document (CCD)**. Subsequently, HL7 developed a suite of templates for different types of health documents, including the CCD, and that suite is collectively called the **consolidated-clinical document architecture (C-CDA)**. For each document, there is a document type specified using the Logical Observations Identifiers Names and Codes (LOINC) data type codes (see chapter 10). A CDA may be transmitted with an HL7 V3 message, but it can also be sent as an attachment to an HL7 V2.x message, as illustrated in figure 13.4. In this example, "OBX" designates that the message contains an observation, with one page, that in this case is an emergency department (ED) report. The ability for providers to produce documents rendered using the C-CDA standard and exchange them with others providers is one of the requirements of the MU incentive program. More recently, the HL7 created the first set of **clinical documents for payers (CDP)** version 1 (CDP1). These are intended to be used for claims attachments or supporting documentation for prior authorization for referrals and other services needing approval from a payer for reimbursement. The CDP1 uses the CDA standard, the C-CDA implementation guide, and LOINC attachment type codes to transmit the CDP1 as part of an ASC X12 message (discussed later in this chapter) in much the same way as the CDA can be referenced as an attachment in the HL7 V.2 message shown in figure 13.4 (Day 2015).

- HL7's **Fast Healthcare Interoperability Resources (FHIR)** (pronounced "fire") addresses the transition from HL7 V2.x and second platform technology to HL7 V3 and third platform technology. FHIR recognizes the need to not only share views of documents (as made possible by the CDA) but also have structured and standardized data from these documents that can to be exchanged so that the recipient of any such data can incorporate the data into their own EHRs, data repositories, or data warehouses. FHIR uses web-based **RESTful (Representational State Transfer) Application Programming Interfaces (APIs)**, which are programs that allow internal functions to operate outside of their internal structure in a limited way (Raths 2014). Adopting the web services REST standard for transport replaces using the **Simple Object Access Protocol (SOAP)** for transport over the web, which can be cumbersome and slow. A good example of how an RESTful API works is when a website

Figure 13.4.   Transmission of CDA via HL7 V2 or V3

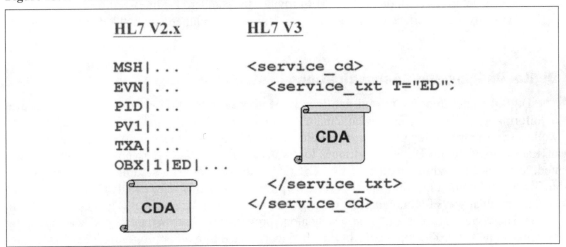

for a restaurant creates a website with an embedded map to show potential diners where it is located. For healthcare, certain structured data elements in an EHR, such as a patient's laboratory test results (referred to as a *resource*) can be shared (with an authorized recipient) via the resource's own Uniform Resource Locator (URL).

- **Blue Button** functionality affords the ability to click the Blue Button logo and view online and download personal health records. In the first version of Blue Button, these records were either in plain text or portable document format (PDF), which were easy for patients to read but could not be uploaded into another provider's EHR. Blue Button functionality was first used in 2010 by the Departments of Defense (DoD), Health and Human Services (HHS), and Veterans Affairs (VA) for their beneficiaries (Manos 2012). In 2014, the ONC Standards and Interoperability (S&I) Framework (discussed later in this chapter) initiated efforts to standardize content formats and transport mechanisms for Blue Button data to make it more interoperable. In 2012, HL7 C-CDA was used to improve interoperability for what became known as Blue Button + (Brull 2013). Now, HL7 FHIR is contributing to further interoperability for the Blue Button initiative (Scrimshire 2016). See also chapter 17.

- HL7 **Decision Support Service (DSS)** standard specifies a standardized interface for providing clinical decision support (CDS) as a software service. As will be described further in chapter 14, there are three technological components necessary to provide CDS. One is a knowledge base of information. For example, for a drug-drug interaction alert, there must be information that one drug is contraindicated when another, specific drug is being taken by the patient. There must also be a rules engine, sometimes referred to as an *intelligent filter,* that translates the knowledge into "if-then" rules. So, if a patient is taking X and the provider is ordering Y, the rules engine checks this combination of drugs against the knowledge base of information and, finding this contraindication, alerts the physician. The user interface is the manner in which this alert is presented to the user. For example, the system may flash a warning, pop up a notification box, not allow the order to be accepted until the alert is actively acknowledged, or all of the above. The DSS standard specifies the descriptive traits, data requirements, and semantic requirements in support of making CDS more uniform and interoperable (Murugesan et al. 2014).

- HL7 **Virtual Medical Record (vMR)** standard is a data model for representing the data that are analyzed or produced by CDS rules engines. The vMR works with the DSS to produce an interoperable package of functionality for CDS. Whereas the DSS provides the standard for the interface component, the vMR provides the standard for interfacing any rules engine with any user interface to take advantage of multiple, commercial knowledge-base products (Kawamoto 2012).

Digital Imaging and Communications in Medicine

The **Digital Imaging and Communications in Medicine (DICOM)** standard supports retrieval of information from imaging devices and equipment to diagnostic and review workstations as well as short-term and long-term storage systems. Originally developed by the American College of Radiology/National Electrical Manufacturers Association, DICOM is now an ANSI-accredited, independent, and international SDO. DICOM is the de facto standard in virtually all picture archiving and communication systems (PACS) products. For this reason, DICOM viewers have become popular ways for clinicians from any location to view PACS images (Hoyt and Yoshihashi 2014). These viewers are available as a standalone programs for both Windows and Mac operating systems, or as ActiveX components that can be incorporated into other programs. The "I Do Imaging" website provides free, open-source viewers (2014). DICOM works collaboratively with HL7 in incorporating the CDA into its protocol for encoding, transmitting, and storing the diagnostic report with the image (Noumeir 2006). However, when standards such as DICOM and HL7 are used in products, there are often ambiguities and conflicting interpretations. As a result, DICOM (and HL7) have been very active in Integrating the Healthcare Enterprise (IHE), with integration protocols for diagnostic imaging being among the strongest collaborations (Leontiev and Parisot 2003; Indrajit and Verma 2007).

Integrating the Healthcare Enterprise

Although not an SDO, **Integrating the Healthcare Enterprise (IHE)** is an example of one of the initiatives helping rein in the standardization of standards. IHE was formed by healthcare professionals and industry leaders to improve the way that computer systems in healthcare share information. IHE promotes the coordinated use of established standards, such as DICOM and HL7, to address specific clinical needs in support of optimal patient care. IHE develops **integration profiles** to provide a reliable way of specifying a level of compliance to existing standards that is sufficient to achieve truly efficient interoperability. Integration profiles include those for anatomic pathology, cardiology, eye care, radiation oncology, and radiology, and also for IT infrastructure, laboratory, patient care coordination, and patient care devices. These integration profiles help ensure strong adherence to standards for tasks such as synchronization for consistent time stamps, audit trails, cross-enterprise document sharing, personnel white pages (for providing directory information on workforce members), sharing laboratory reports, basic patient privacy consents, preprocedural history and physical, and many others. IHE's profiles associated with document sharing are very commonly used. Examples include the following (Brull 2012):

- *Cross-enterprise Document Medial Interchange* (XDM) for transferring documents and their metadata using compact disks (CDs), universal serial bus (USB) memory, or e-mail attachments

- *Cross-enterprise Document Reliable Interchange* (XDR) for exchanging documents using a web-based, point-to-point push-enabling direct interchange between EHRs, personal health records (PHRs), and other systems without the need for a data repository

- *Patient Demographics Query* (PDQ) for requesting patient identifications (IDs) based on demographic data from a central patient information server (such as might be used in a health information exchange organization [HIO])

- *Patient Identifier Cross Referencing* (PIX) for cross-referencing multiple local patient IDs between hospitals, HIOs, and others when the local patient IDs have been registered with a PIX manager

Standards and Interoperability (S&I) Framework

Also not an SDO but a process that has made significant contributions to helping existing standards work better—especially when used for HIE—the **S&I Framework** is an open, collaborative community made up of stakeholders from the public and private sectors. The community's mission is to find technical solutions to facilitate standardized, interoperable health information exchange. It is supported by the ONC with project management, subject matter experts, coordination tools, and other resources. To do its work, the S&I Framework uses a well-defined process similar to that required by ANSI for SDOs. Some of its currently active projects include defining data provenance needs for transport and security, identifying semantic standards and content standards for clinical quality measures, integration of Blue Button + and health IT, and structured data capture standards, architectures, and services. Earlier initiatives have included projects relating to laboratory test result interfaces, public health data sharing, longitudinal coordination of care, esMD (electronic submission of Medical Documents from providers to Centers for Medicare and Medicaid Services [CMS] auditors), data segmentation for privacy (DS4P), and the transitions of care (ToC) companion guide to the C-CDA (ONC 2014). See chapter 12 for more information on DS4P.

National Council for Prescription Drug Programs

National Council for Prescription Drug Programs (NCPDP) is an ANSI-accredited SDO whose standards are widely adopted by pharmacies and payers for exchange of retail pharmacy payment information. The NCPDP Telecommunication Standard Implementation Guide, version 5, release 1, and the equivalent NCPDP Batch Standard Batch Implementation Guide, version 1, release 0, were specified in the HIPAA Transactions and Code Sets regulation for use for retail pharmacy claims, eligibility verification, and payment and remittance advice. These guides have been updated to versions D.0 and 1.2, respectively, as have medical claims and other HIPAA transactions (see X12) that are required by CMS and were effective on January 1, 2012 (CMS 2009).

The NCPDP also provides a standard for e-prescribing, called SCRIPT. This standard communicates prescription information (including new prescriptions, refill requests, fill status notifications, and cancellation notifications) between prescribers and pharmacies and has been regulated for use under the Medicare Modernization Act (MMA) of 2003, Medicare Part D e-prescribing. It should be noted that MMA does not require eprescribing but does require use of the NCPDP standard if e-prescribing is used (NCPDP 2010). The MU incentive program requires e-prescribing for those physicians wishing to participate in the program. (See also chapter 15.)

ANSI-Accredited Standards Committee X12

Although ANSI is an accrediting body and not itself an SDO, it occasionally designates groups for certain standards-setting activities, especially where the standards may cross industries. The **Accredited Standards Committee X12 (ASC X12)** is one such SDO, and it develops messaging standards for **electronic data interchange (EDI)** of financial and administrative transactions. These transaction standards can and are being used by several industries. An insurance subcommittee of X12 is responsible for developing and maintaining standards for insurance transactions, including for healthcare institutional (837I), professional (837P), and dental (837D) claims; coordination of benefits (837); eligibility inquiry and response (270/271); claims status inquiry and response (276/277); payment and remittance advice (835); and referral certification and authorization (278). Version 4010A1 was required for adoption by those using electronic transactions under HIPAA. An upgrade to v.5010 was adopted in 2009 and becomes effective on January 1, 2012 (CMS 2009).

Another set of X12N standards (277/275) is under development for health plans to request, and providers to send, claims attachments electronically. X12N 275 was designed to embed an HL7 message containing electronic content, either as discrete data using LOINC codes (discussed in chapter 10) to encode the message, or in CDA format. Currently available are messages for ambulance services, rehabilitation services, medications, laboratory test results, clinical reports, and emergency department services. A small pilot of the claims attachments was conducted by Empire Medicare Services in 2005, under the auspices of the **Workgroup on Electronic Data Interchange (WEDI)**, a national association of payers, providers, and vendors, to work through information technology (IT) challenges facing healthcare with respect to the privacy and security of transactions, identifiers, and related needs. As no progress has made in adopting this standard, the Affordable Care Act (ACA) called for a review and regulation of the claims attachment standard (and associated operating rules), which is still under consideration (2010).

Council for Affordable Quality Healthcare, Committee on Operating Rules for Information Exchange

The Council for Affordable Quality Healthcare (CAQH) is an alliance of health plans and trade associations. It serves as a catalyst for industry collaboration on initiatives that seek to simplify healthcare administration. CAQH's Committee on Operating Rules for Information Exchange (CORE), which has expanded its participants to also include providers and vendors, is building consensus-based **operating rules** that enhance interoperability between providers and payers, streamline the use of the X12 transactions, and reduce the amount of time and resources providers spend on administrative functions. CAQH CORE has been designated by the Secretary of HHS as the operating rules authoring entity for the HIPAA transaction standards, which have been and continue to be adopted in regulations as they are developed (CAQH CORE 2012). So far, there have been mandated operating rules for the eligibility, claims status, remittance advice, and electronic funds transfer HIPAA transactions (see also Chapter 19). CAQH CORE is also undertaking projects focused on simplifying administrative functions associated with alternative payment models being adopted to reform healthcare reimbursement into a value-based construct (CAQH CORE 2016).

ASTM International

One other SDO of note for healthcare is ASTM International. Formerly known as the American Society for Testing and Materials, this organization is not ANSI-accredited, but its history predates ANSI and it follows the ANSI-prescribed SDO processes. It has been developing standards since 1899 and may be best known in other industries for standardizing materials—ranging from basic infrastructure requirements. such as the width of railroad ties and the size of sewer pipes, to the toxicity of ink in colored markers. (Look for the ASTM D4236 designation of nontoxic on such markers.) Several ASTM committees developed standards (but not message format standards) for laboratory instruments that are used in clinical laboratories. ASTM Committee E31 has developed standards for healthcare data management, security, confidentiality, and privacy; information capture and documentation; and data analysis. These standards have not been adopted by federal regulators for health IT.

ASTM E31 also worked with the American Academy of Family Physicians, the Massachusetts Medical Society, and Health Information Management and Systems Society (HIMSS) to create the Standard Specification for Continuity of Care Record (CCR) (ASTM E2369-12). An IHE XSD File-SML Schema for the CCR is also available from ASTM. The CCR was developed in response to the need to organize and make transportable a set of basic patient information comprising the most relevant and timely facts about a patient's condition. As noted above in the discussion of HL7, the CCR has been incorporated with the HL7 CDA as the CCD and enhanced with multiple document types in the C-CDA. The CCR standard was not intended to be a standard for all of the EHR but, rather, to provide a minimum data set for making patient referrals, transferring the care of patients to other providers, ensuring that discharge information (such as from an emergency department or urgent care center) goes to a primary care physician, and serving as a PHR (Ferranti et al. 2006).

Institute of Electrical and Electronics Engineers (IEEE)

Institute of Electrical and Electronics Engineers (IEEE) is an ANSI-accredited SDO, although its focus is broader than healthcare alone. IEEE 1073 is a set of medical device communications standards, which is also promulgated by the International Organization for Standardization (ISO) and known as ISO 11073. These standards communicate patient data from medical devices such as patient monitors, ventilators, infusion pumps, and so on. IEEE also has wireless networking standards (IEEE 802.11), although these standards are not unique to healthcare. (See chapter 11.)

National Institute of Standards and Technology

In addition to private sector standards development, the federal government may create standards and regulate their use. The National Institute of Standards and Technology (NIST), a nonregulatory agency of the Department of Commerce, creates standards for many different technologies in many different industries—from automated teller machines to semiconductors. It promotes performance excellence among US institutions through its Baldrige Performance Excellence Program, which started in 1988 and began including healthcare institutions in 2002. NIST laboratories conduct research that advances the nation's technology infrastructure and its products and services. ONC used NIST to develop an accreditation program for organizations to be accredited to test health IT starting in 2012 (45 CFR 170[e] 2011) under the MU incentive program. By developing technical evaluation, texting, and validation guidelines and use cases NIST has also contributed to the national discussion on ways that EHR usability can be assessed (Lowry et al. 2015). NIST urges vendors and other developers of EHRs to focus on three key risk areas that NIST identifies as highly frustrating to clinicians and areas where they frequently use workarounds such as paper shadow charts or whiteboards. The areas identified to improve usability and assure patient safety include the following (Lowry et al. 2015):

- Consistently displaying information critical to patient identification in a reserved area to avoid wrong patient errors

- Providing cues to reduce the risk of entering information and writing orders in the wrong patient's chart

- Supporting efficient and easy identification of inaccurate, outdated, or inappropriate items in lists of grouped information by having that data presented clearly and in a well-organized manner

NIST also has contributed significantly to information processing standards. It is the federal government's SDO for Federal Information Processing Standards (FIPS) and it has contributed to the HIPAA Security Rule and subsequent guidance on securing health information technology. Its encryption standards are required for use in certified EHR technology (CEHRT) under the MU incentive program. Its Computer Security Resource Center produces special publications that provide excellent information on topics from covering how to conduct a security risk analysis to implementing various forms of encryption that render data unreadable without special access provisions (NIST 2016).

Check Your Understanding 13.1

Match the terms with the appropriate descriptions:

A. ANSI

B. ASTM

C. CAQH CORE

D. DICOM

E. HL7

F. IEEE

G. IHE

H. NCPDP

I. NIST

J. S&I Framework

1. Standards development organization for the federal government

2. Message format standards for HIPAA transactions

3. Creates integration profiles for use with healthcare standards

4. Standards development organization for radiological image display and transport

5. Predominant message format standard used in healthcare

6. Creates operating rules for use with HIPAA transaction standards

7. Body that accredits standards development organization

8. Creates standards for exchange of retail pharmacy data

9. Community that helps standards adoption in HIE

10. Creates standards for wireless networking

Semantic Interoperability: Conveying Meaning

Semantic interoperability addresses shared data types, terminologies, and coding. It ensures that not only does a message reach its destination and can be used by an appropriate application (technical interoperability) but also the data can be interpreted in the same manner as the sender intended. Semantic interoperability begins with use of a vocabulary specified in a message. For example, the HL7 message format standard applying semantic interoperability would require each data element to be associated with a specific vocabulary standard, such as International Classification of Diseases (ICD), Systematized Nomenclature of Medicine—Clinical Terms (SNOMED-CT), LOINC, RxNorm, and others—including language, such as English, French, and so on. Chapter 10 identified the major clinical vocabularies currently in use in the United States.

To achieve full semantic interoperability, however, it is not enough to just specify a vocabulary when transmitting a message. Data types must be known, generally derived from data models (see chapter 10). The relationship of datum to one another must also be understood. This requires information modeling. As HIE matures and providers take in data from other sources, data normalization, including semantic normalization, becomes very important to ensure a single source of truth about a patient, as do identifiers. As massive amounts of data may be both exchanged and analyzed, scalable semantic computing has become an emerging focus of semantic interoperability.

Data Types

The types of data shared include not only medical terms, but numbers, dates, and others. It is necessary to describe the type of data as reflecting the many different levels of exchange capability. Types of data may include messaging formats, which may be simple, such as ASCII or HTML (text-based), or extensible, such as XML. Data type codes from LOINC are used in exchanging CDA-structured documents. Data types also relate to the underlying programming language used in the application and how the data are able to be produced, such as in integer form, a string of data, and others.

Types of terminologies refer to adoption of a standard terminology for the exchange of information where clear meaning is enabled. SNOMED CT, for instance, enables very precise definition of the meaning associated with the concepts being described. These were discussed in chapter 10.

Shared coding refers to establishing standardized codes to be shared among systems. This includes not only the codes typically considered in healthcare, such as ICD and Current Procedural Terminology (CPT), but software programming functions. Also included in shared coding is the need for shared data and information models.

Information Modeling

Information models are used to describe how types of data (often referred to as *objects*) may be used together to provide value (consider the data-information-knowledge-wisdom [DIKW] continuum). Information models are not as detailed as data models, which focus on the details surrounding a specific data element. Instead, information models are somewhat abstract but provide enough of a picture to allow understanding of how data operate together ("relationships"), when they may or may not operate together ("rules'), and what "constraints," or circumstances may require or preclude their use. Figure 13.5 illustrates the relationship between an information model and data models (Schonwalder 2014).

There are several information modeling languages that may be used to depict the information model. Entity relationship diagrams were the first and are the oldest way to depict such relationships (illustrated in chapter 10). **Unified Modeling Language (UML)** arose out of newer object-oriented programming languages. UML provides a standard that can help modelers share their work with others and enables models to be used across different programming situations. UML 2.x is an enhancement of the first version of the UML standard and is actually a suite of tools, including activity diagrams, use cases, and others, all of which help document the various aspects of an information model (Ambler 2014a). **Agile modeling** was developed to support the need for more agile (flexible) information modeling as computing environments change so rapidly. It is a methodology for information modeling that is based on best practices, and it uses UML 2.x to envision a project, brainstorm through details, prioritize requirements, engage all stakeholders (including users), and produce an information model that is sufficient to develop software (Ambler 2014b).

Figure 13.5.   Information models and data models

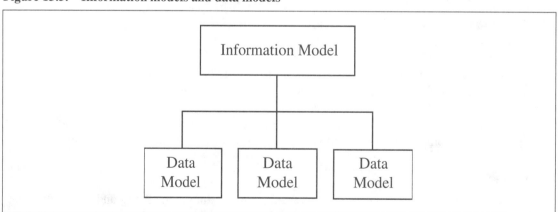

Source: Summarized from Schonwalder, J. 2013 (March 14). Information Models, Data Models, and YANG, Presentation at IETF 86, Orlando

In healthcare, HL7 has used UML to produce the RIM (discussed earlier). The RIM serves as an overarching information model for use in determining what types of messages exist in all of healthcare. Any given information system designer will also use an information model to describe the overarching nature of the database needed to produce the desired information.

Data Normalization

Data normalization was introduced in chapter 10 as an important practice in data repositories, although not necessarily in data warehouses. **Data normalization** is the ability to reconcile data elements so that there is no redundancy in the data repository. As a simple example, if a physician asks a patient about past medical history and is told about breast cancer in the right breast, and then the physician also receives health information about that patient from another provider that also identifies breast cancer (in the right breast), it would be redundant to store data indicating cancer in the right breast twice for this patient—in fact, storing the data twice could potentially create confusion. However, if the current provider determines that there is now cancer in the left breast, this new finding would be a separate data point. To ensure data are truly redundant, however, it may be necessary to associate them with other information. For example, if the documentation of history of cancer of the right breast diagnosed in 2010 for this current patient was paired with a record of the earlier provider's 2010 diagnosis of cancer of the right breast, one could assume these data were one and the same for the same patient. Even without the laterality afforded by ICD-10-CM, a new diagnosis of breast cancer in 2016 would be assumed to be a second data point and not redundant. However, *assume* is the operative word, and it is best not to assume in healthcare. As such, the process of data normalization can be quite complex. In fact, data normalization has come to refer to the ability for an organization to reconcile medical terminology across disparate healthcare systems to eliminate semantic ambiguity (Levy 2014).

As the amount of data from multiple providers ultimately may come together in HIE and for the purposes of analytics that may help promote a better understanding of each individual's health history in a longitudinal manner and also support knowledge generation, data normalization becomes increasingly important, and semantic normalization also becomes important. **Semantic normalization** refers to translation among different terminology standards. (As suggested in chapter 10, this is also referred to as *data mapping*.) This mapping is not just to transition from ICD-9-CM to ICD-10-CM but also to enable understanding between, for example, a physician office CPT code and a hospital ICD-10-CM code used to describe a health condition for a given patient. Similarly, there is increasing interest in understanding more about the continuum of care and ensuring care continuity. The ability to map CPT codes to and from ICD-10-CM codes may be appropriate for longitudinal studies evaluating the quality of care as the patient moves from physician office to hospital to physician office (Wolfson 2014). Mapping diagnoses coded in ICD-10-CM to SNOMED-CT and laboratory test results coded in LOINC to SNOMED-CT normalizes the coded data so they can be used together, such as in software to generate an alert that a patient may have a hospital acquired infection. In analyzing large amounts of such data, there must also be **scalable normalization** across distributed networked systems (Sundvall 2013; Hench et al. 2008).

Identifiers

Semantic interoperability must also include the use of standard identifiers. The original HIPAA legislation required adoption of four types of identifiers, for employers, providers, health plans, and individuals.

The *Employer Identification Number* (EIN) issued by the Internal Revenue Service was adopted by CMS as the identifier for employers because EINs may be referenced by health plans and providers in their exchange of insurance and sponsor information (CMS 2016).

According to regulations adopted in 2004, all providers, health plans, and healthcare clearing-houses must a *National Provider Identifier* (NPI) in the HIPAA administrative and financial trans-actions (CMS 2004). A National Plan and Provider Enumeration System (NPPES) was created to assign the NPI to providers. It also provides a registry of NPIs.

A *Health Plan Identifier* (HPID) is in the process of being adopted, under an ACA mandate, with a proposed rule published in April 2012.

A unique healthcare identifier for individuals has been put on hold, with Congress not permit-ting federal funds to be used for investigation or regulation until a federal privacy law is enacted. (Remember, the HIPAA Privacy Rule is a regulation, not a law—this is perhaps only a minor distinction with respect to compliance, but it is a major consideration at the public policy level.)

Process Interoperability

Process interoperability originated in the early 1990s with electronic commerce in business, where business rules were developed to enable end-to-end processing. Healthcare has just begun to address process interoperability because of the operating rules for HIPAA financial and administra-tive transactions. Otherwise, process interoperability remains as a frequently identified requirement for totally successful interoperabilityin healthcare, but it has not gained much traction. In fact, HL7 conducted an analysis of interoperability in 2007 and noted that only in leading-edge organizations in the United States and in other countries was process interoperability given any credence (Gib-bons et al. 2007). A further review of the literature provides an interesting example from Australia, which has adopted a process interoperability framework for its government to enable seamless ser-vice delivery. In the Australian framework, "business process interoperability" is considered first, rather than last, when constructing a roadmap for improving customer service, ensuring compli-ance, and reducing costs (Australian Government 2007).

In the US healthcare system, process interoperability was first identified as important in a report titled *Building a Better Delivery System: A New Engineering/Health Care Partnership*, released in 2005 by the Institute of Medicine (IOM), now known as Health and Medicine Division (HMD) of the National Academies of Sciences, Engineering, and Medicine. The report begins with the observation that "American medicine defines the cutting edge in most fields of clinical research, training, and practice worldwide, and U.S.-based manufacturers of drugs, medical devices, and medical equipment are among the most innovative and competitive in the world." It then goes on to state that, "at the same, time relatively little technical talent or material resources have been devoted to improving or optimizing the operations or measuring the quality and productivity of the overall U.S. healthcare system. The costs of the collective inattention and the failure to take advantage of the tools, knowledge, and infrastructure that have yielded quality and productivity revolutions in many other sectors of the American economy have been enormous."

HL7 includes the following factors that would optimally achieve integration of computer sys-tems into actual work settings:

- Explicit user role specification

- Useful, friendly, and efficient human-machine interface

- Data presentation/flow supports work setting

- Engineered work design

- Proven effectiveness in actual use

HL7 also observes that process interoperability not only optimizes the communication of infor-mation but also does so in a time-, event-, or sequence-oriented manner to coordinate the work processes of the care team. "Key documentation as well as safety and quality reminders can automatically enhance human interventions to assure that the care team can access information to treat the patient in the most effective, efficient, and safe way possible" (Gibbons et al. 2007). In its "Nationwide Interoperability Roadmap," ONC refers to process interoperability in discussing the need for technical and *policy* conformance among networks, technical systems, and their components (ONC 2015).

Interoperability Standards Advisory

In 2015, ONC initiated a process by which it would identify, assess, and determine the "best available" interoperability standards and implementation specifications for the healthcare industry to use to fulfill specific clinical health IT interoperability needs. ONC issued its first **Interoperability Standards Advisory** in 2015. The 2016 advisory categorizes the interoperability standards, including those in the advisory, as the following types:

- Vocabulary/code sets/terminology (that is, semantics)

- Content/structure (that is, syntax)

- Services (that is, the infrastructure components deployed and used to fulfill specific interoperability needs)

ONC notes that standards for "low-level transport" were excluded from the Interoperability Standards Advisory because they were considered common to all computer systems and networks; however, some higher level transport standards are included in standards for services. Much of the services section of the advisory addresses services associated with using the nationwide health information network, although some of these could certainly be considered elements for process interoperability for electronic "commerce" in healthcare.

Check Your Understanding 13.2

Match the type or types of interoperability to the related items:

A. Technical interoperability

B. Semantic interoperability

C. Process interoperability

1. Workflow improvements

2. Message format standards

3. Data normalization

4. UML

5. Data types

6. Usability

Importance of Interoperability and Health Information Exchange

A number of events in the past decade have highlighted the need to be able to better share health information not only among applications, such as was the original goal for interoperability, but across the continuum of care as well. The IOM report *To Err Is Human* (1999) has been cited as the wake-up call that raised the nation's collective consciousness concerning patient safety and the need to recognize that the healthcare delivery *system* was not engaging in HIE. The IOM believed that HIE would help reconcile medications across care providers, reduce unnecessary tests that are not only costly but potentially harmful to the patient, and address other system-related issues. Subsequent events, such as the hurricane disasters of 2005, where individuals were left unable to access prescription information, let alone their actual medications, reemphasized the need for the transportability and ubiquity of health information (McIlwain and Lassetter 2009).

Another key factor contributing to the emphasis on HIE is the fact that many indicators suggest the need for significant improvements in the quality, cost, and experience of care afforded by the US healthcare system. For example, according to the Organisation for Economic Cooperation and Development (OECD), the United States ranked first in 2015 in per capita healthcare expenditures in a comparison of 30 industrialized countries and in the lowest third in physicians per capita. The United States ranked at the bottom third in obesity in adults and children and middle third in alcohol consumption, although the United States was fifth-best in smoking in adults. The United States ranked in the bottom third in performance on life expectancy for men and women at birth and the middle third for mortality from cardiovascular diseases. OECD also looked at experience of care factors, such as physicians spending enough time with patients, patients given an opportunity to ask physicians questions, and patients participating in shared decision-making, where the United States ranked in the lowest third on all measures (OECD 2015). Earlier data from the *New England Journal of Medicine* reveal that there are also "dramatic variations among regions and racial or ethnic groups in the rates of death from preventable causes" (Murray and Frenk 2010).

There is always controversy over exact numbers and their meaning. But it should be clear from the constellation of indicators that the quality of outcomes for the level of spending (that is, value) is generally poor in the United States. Identifying causality for healthcare outcomes and then instituting corrective action is certainly very difficult, but many believe that technology—including the EHR, other types of health IT, and HIE—can contribute substantially to improvement. Health reform initiatives that focus on paying for value (that is, positive outcomes) rather than volume of patient services are also being looked at very closely for this reason, and these initiatives will require technological improvements to provide information for managing healthcare in such an environment.

Challenges to Interoperability and Health Information Exchange

As has been discussed throughout this book, many factors are related to the slow adoption of health IT. As Swensen and colleagues have observed in a perspective published in the *New England Journal of Medicine*, one factor relating to HIE in particular is that the US healthcare system remains a cottage industry despite its level of spending (Swensen et al. 2010). These authors, who included a recent CMS administrator, note:

> Growing evidence highlights the dangers of continuing to operate in a cottage-industry mode. Fragmentation of care has led to suboptimal performance. The gap between established science and current practice is wide. It is well documented that U.S. patients receive only about half of scientifically advisable care; many unnecessary procedures are performed, leading to avoidable complications and costs; safety problems abound; and there are tremendous regional variations in the quality and quantity of care delivered. Moreover, fragmentation makes it more difficult to transform the industry—for example, through the adoption of health information technology.

Many providers, whether they are solo practitioners, practice in a group, or are employed by a healthcare organization, view themselves as independent of other providers in how they work and what they do. In a study of discretionary decision making by primary care physicians and the cost of US healthcare, the Sirovich and colleagues concluded that efforts to improve the value of US healthcare have focused largely on fostering physician adherence to evidence-based guidelines (Sirovich et al. 2008). Use of evidence-based guidelines, fostered through the use of health IT, is important with respect to outcomes but not necessarily important to cost control. Physicians often use their discretionary bent to order tests or perform other interventions irrespective of cost. In fact, a Massachusetts Medical Society survey found widespread distrust and lack of knowledge in the use of evidence-based guidelines to manage quality and cost (2005).

Information systems also have focused on individual functions and the operations of only their respective departments or users. Indeed, the definition of EHR includes recognition of the need to collect data from multiple sources for use in clinical decision making at the point of care—and across care settings for continuity of care. Although providers recognize the need for data from across disparate sources, and may often be frustrated by the lack of such data, the fact remains that, until recently. little has been done to support the seamless exchange of health information. It is almost as if providers understand that they need access to data to treat patients, but they nevertheless are unwilling to share their own data.

Further complicating the ability to streamline and seamlessly enable HIE is the long-held view by many physicians in particular that information is the property exclusively of the provider, and this perspective has often translated into frequent denials or obstacles for patients seeking to access their information. Providers still hold to the notion that providing information to the patient is bad and continue to refuse access. In fact, being denied access to records, especially by private practices, consistently ranks third in the top five complaints filed with HHS Office for Civil Rights (OCR) under the HIPAA Privacy Rule.

Clearly, a major theme of the federal government has been interoperability across entities. "Data exchange," "data sharing," and HIE are terms that have been consistently used in every one of the nation's health IT strategic plans. As the first National Coordinator for Health Information Technology, David Brailer stressed that the importance of interoperability is "an essential factor in using HIT to improve the quality and efficiency of care in the US." He observed that "interoperability and health information exchange are techno-speak jargon for health care information that is treated as a required element of diagnosis and therapy, albeit one that jealously guards patients' privacy and confidentiality." It could be observed that Brailer, who is both a physician and an economist as well as founder of one of the first health information exchanges (in Santa Barbara County, CA), may be suggesting that market demand has not done enough to overcome the lack of interoperability:

> Without interoperability and health information exchange, health information will remain in proprietary silos, in which the health care enterprise hopes to gain competitive advantage by imposing high costs on consumer switchover and by exercising market leverage over small niche players such as solo physicians and community hospitals.

Finally, Brailer concluded that "interoperability and HIE are best understood as business concepts rather than technical concepts," with a need for uniform business processes, uniform privacy laws, uniform patient identification, controlled medical terminology, and commonly accepted business transaction definitions (HHS 2005).

Status of Health Information Organizations

A *health information organization* (HIO) is an organization that oversees and governs the exchange of health-related information among organizations according to nationally recognized standards (NAHIT 2008). In 2004 the eHealth Initiative, a nonprofit organization with a mission to drive improvement in the quality, safety, and efficiency of healthcare through information and information technology, started tracking HIO development and funding. The eHealth Initiative identified nine operational HIOs in 2005. In early 2010, it described various stages of HIO development, as illustrated in figure 13.6, and identified 145 HIOs across the stages. In general, it considered those HIOs in stages 5, 6, and 7 to be operational—and less than half of the HIOs met the criteria in 2009 (eHealth Initiative 2010). In a webinar later in 2010, Matthews discussed that the eHealth Initiative was tracking 234 HIOs, with at least 73 of those being operational.

Although the eHealth Initiative stopped tracking status of HIOs in 2010, others have reported various assessments of their status over time, including a significant increase and then a significant drop off, yet all reports reflecting continuing difficulty in their ability to thrive. For example, the Agency for Healthcare Research and Quality (AHRQ) estimated that in 2014 there were more than 280 HIOs and that over 50 percent of the nation's hospitals were actively participating in HIOs (AHRQ 2014). In 2015, the Robert Wood Johnson Foundation reported that there were only 158 HIE efforts, of which about 80 percent were operational and 20 percent were in planning phases. Furthermore, of these HIE efforts, 50 percent were HIOs, another 25 percent were state-based HIEs, and the remaining 25 percent were a mix of integrated delivery networks, community-based organizations, public health departments, technology vendors, state Medicaid agencies, academic institutions, and other state governmental agency (Robert Wood Johnson Foundation 2015).

It has always been difficult to track exact numbers of HIOs because there are many different models and many organizations that have come and gone. Federal grants for HIO startup have been significantly cut back, and some state-based HIOs, while still operational, have taken on various other services to sustain themselves. New technology is also enabling HIE to occur more readily without a formal HIO infrastructure.

The **State HIE Cooperative Agreement Program** was enacted under the Health Information Technology for Economic and Clinical Health Act (HITECH) and provided federal support for states to promote HIE, especially as relating to the ability for hospitals and physicians to earn MU incentives. In 2010, $548 million was appropriated to 56 state-designated entities (SDEs) for a four-year project. After the first year, they were required to match part of the grant money. The AHIMA Foundation was funded by ONC to guide research and contribute to analysis and recommendations regarding HIO development across states through the **State-Level Health Information Exchange Consensus Project**.

As noted previously, state-based HIOs are continuing to serve their constituents. However, as federal funding has largely gone away, other forms of HIEs are developing proprietary HIE services and helping their constituents participate in the nationwide health information network, now referred to as the *eHealth Exchange*.

Figure 13.6.   eHealth Initiative stages of HIO development

Stage	# HIOs (2009)	
1. Recognition exists in state or region	9	
2. HIO getting organized	17	88
3. Developing business plan	26	
4. Implementing and/or piloting	36	
5. Operational, transmitting data	27	
6. Operational, transmitting data, sustainable business model	13	57
7. Operational, organization expanding	17	
Totals	145	145

Source: eHealth Initiative

HIE Architectures and Services

However, HIE may be performed, there are basic architectures and services that enable data sharing among disparate organizations.

HIE Architectures

There are primarily two architectures for exchanging HIE in a consolidated and federated HIO. These, along with the switch service, which is not an HIE, and the patient-managed HIE discussed in chapter 17, are illustrated in figure 13.7.

The earlier HIOs tended to be of the **consolidated** architectural type. In this model, data are contributed to a central data repository and managed centrally. As each entity participating in the HIO needed data, it could tap into the data repository by using the appropriate credentials and permissions. In most cases, however, the central data repository was logically partitioned into separate sections for each participant in the HIO. Much like a bank managing its safe deposit boxes, access to the data was highly controlled. Because of the centralized management, strong security controls were applied—and accepted by the users. However, as data became more integrated in these data repositories, separated only by logical (access) controls, the consolidated model became more of a concern with respect to privacy and security—and competitiveness issues. In a guidance document to public health agencies looking to participate in a HIO, these agencies were cautioned that "in a highly competitive market, healthcare institutions and providers are more likely to be concerned about losing control of their patient data or turning it over to a competitor" (Livingood et al. 2009).

The **federated** architectural type has become more prevalent for HIOs. There are two forms of this architecture. The *consistent* federated form is very similar to the consolidated architecture in which the data repository is partitioned but centrally managed. The consistent federated form, however, takes this one step further and physically separates the data but still offers centralized

Figure 13.7.   HIE architectural models

HIE Model	Illustration
Consolidated: multiple independent enterprises agree to share resources using a central repository	
Federated: • **Consistent databases:** multiple independent enterprises agree to connect and share specific information managed centrally but with independent repositories • **Inconsistent databases:** multiple independent enterprises agree to connect and share specific information in a point-to-point manner	
Switch: a service that enables the exchange of information across multiple independent enterprises that have unilateral agreements to exchange data and in which there is no access to personal health information	
Patient managed: patients "carry" their own electronic records or subscribe to a service that enables the patient to direct exchange of data	
Hybrid: (not illustrated) combination of any of these models	

management. Essentially, this is much like an application service provider (ASP) or software as a service (SaaS) model of acquiring software (see chapter 7). The *inconsistent* federated form is one in which each participant in the HIO maintains its own data in its own systems (locally or via an ASP or SaaS) and uses the HIO only to manage point-to-point connections that are processed individually.

As integrated delivery networks have started offering proprietary HIE services, there is now a more **hybrid** architecture form. A data warehouse often stores considerable data used for quality measurement and data analytics across the network, while many of the entities within the network also maintain their own data repositories.

HIE Services

For whatever architecture an HIO may have, there needs to be a way to identify participants, find records, provide security, manage patient consent, and provide data transport. The relationship among these services is illustrated in figure 13.8.

Identification of participants includes identification of individual providers, representatives of payer organizations, and patients/consumers, as well as organizational entities and their information systems. It is highly likely that some of the data to be exchanged through an HIO will not be triggered only by a person but also by the availability of data. For example, laboratory test results may not only be specifically requested by a provider but also returned directly to a provider's information

Figure 13.8.   HIE services

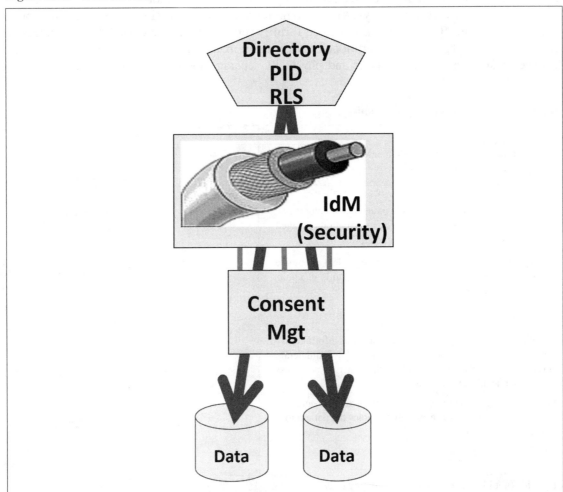

system when they become available and even directly to a person's PHR. A **registry service**, which is a process to qualify an identified participant, would keep an index, called a **directory** in most HIOs, of all users and systems. This directory is more than a master person index (MPI), as it must serve an entire HIO, and may, itself, be a system of registries, or federated directories.

Because, as noted previously, Congress currently prohibits the development or use of a unique patient identifier, ensuring that the HIO can identify the right person as it seeks to exchange information is a process of **identity matching**. This process can be anything from a basic comparison of data elements using an exact match of demographic information (for a very small, stable environment) to—much more commonly—the use of sophisticated mathematical or statistical algorithms (AHIMA 2009).

Once an individual's identity is confirmed, the HIO must next locate where there may be information. A **record locator service (RLS)** is used for this purpose. It is essentially a series of pointers. In a consolidated architecture, all individuals (users and patients) as well as all inbound data could be assigned an internal identifier that would then operate much as an MPI would. However, in the federated model, there must be the ability to identify the individual (user and patient) and where information may be located.

Identity management is a process that operates to ensure that individuals who have been identified are who they say they are, that they have authority to do what they want to do, and that their actions are tracked. This process essentially involves the typical security functions of authorization, authentication, access control, and audit control. In distinguishing between **person identification** and identity management, it should be noted that there is a difference between identify and identity. *Identify* is an action, in which one determines who people are and perhaps assigns them an identifier for future reference. *Identity* is a status. It is proof of who a person is, and in the case of HIE, what that person may do.

As part of ensuring the HIO has the right person, right location, and right record, identity management provides the assurance of right authority to access the HIE network and its functions. However, a special case of authority is being adopted by most HIE organizations. This is **consent management**, where not only is a user authorized to have specific access, but the individual patient/consumer also has the authority to provide specific consent directives. Hence, Dr. Smith may be authorized to use an HIE network, has authenticated herself to the network, and is granted access to clinical data where there is an identified treatment relationship with the individual. However, Mary Jones, the patient, may provide specific consent directives that indicate that Dr. Smith may access all of her medical information but none of her genetic information, and Dr. Smith has full access to medical information only if Mary is in the emergency department of a hospital.

The basic forms of consent directives include opt in and opt out, which are defined as follows:

- **Opt in:** Data may not be exchanged by default unless the individual consents.

- **Opt out:** Data may be exchanged by default unless restricted by the individual.

Although these basic forms of consent directive appear simple to deploy, they actually are not, and, in many cases, individuals seem to have a preference for a "quilted" form of consent, where a subset of data can be exchanged with individual consent based on institution, data user, data producer, and situation, such as in the example of Dr. Smith and Mary Jones. Despite this apparent preference, it seems that most HIOs choose to offer opt out, and, in at least one case study (Bass 2011), few patients actually do opt out. Patient education, however, is very important to enable patients to make informed consent choices (Warner 2011). In a research study conducted for ONC, Goldstein and Rein (2010) describe the following five consent models:

- *None,* which may be found in HIOs servicing states that require no additional provisions for HIE beyond the floor set by HIPAA (where PHI may be disclosed for treatment, payment, and operations without patient authorization).

- *Opt-out,* which is as previously described. It is observed that many HIOs not required by the states in which they provide services to have additional consent often adopt this approach as means to provide notice to patients about the HIO.

- *Opt-out with exceptions,* which enables patients to apply exceptions to their HIE. This model is technically and procedurally complex to administer and has been rarely implemented.

- *Opt-in,* which is as previously described. This is an all-or-nothing approach that does not permit any exceptions. This model is easier to manage technically and procedurally, but it could eventually put the patient's health at risk when much more reliance is put on HIOs for HIE.

- *Opt-in with restrictions.* In theory, this model enables clearly delineated patient consent rules. In practice however, Goldstein and Rein note that "there are as many choice model permutations as entities that participate in HIE." The level of granularity for consent may be by data type, by provider, by time range, and by purpose. It may even extend to giving providers participating in one HIO preferences in what consent options each provider offers its patients. Finally, this model will very likely require considerable patient education and flexibility to make changes as patients chose to modify their restrictions.

Obviously, a basic service provided by an HIO must be the actual transmission of the data. This is the technical networking service that provides appropriate bandwidth, latency, availability, ubiquity, and security.

Finally, all of the above services would be described in a formal **HIE data sharing agreement** or **HIO participation agreement**. These agreements would spell out in detail how data will be shared, including patient consent requirements and identity management requirements, as well as who the participants are, what services the organization will provide, how the organization will be structured, how the organization will be funded, and other legal matters of ownership, liability, risk mitigation, and so on. In addition, as HITECH has identified that HIOs are business associates of HIPAA-covered entities, a business associate agreement or contract would also be needed.

Data Governance in HIE

As with governing data in any given provider setting, data governance is equally important for HIE. In addition to the participation agreements, there need to be policies that ensure appropriate data handling and data stewardship. The American Health Information Management Association (AHIMA) offers a list of recommended data governance policies that HIOs should develop and implement. Included are:

- Data conversion planning policy

- Enterprise data integrity maintenance policy

- Policy on an integrated medical record

- Core patient identifiers and naming convention policy

- Medical record corrections policy

- Duplicate record validity determination policy

- Record search policy

- Data conversion testing policy

- Electronic record linking policy

- Maintenance of user and provider master records policy

- Patient involvement in medical record accuracy policy

- Legal medical record and eDiscovery policy

- Data ownership agreements and the **Data Use and Reciprocal Services Agreement (DURSA)** (required for participation in the nationwide health information network—see below).

- HIE opt in/opt out policy

- Red flag alert

- Data governance terms and definitions (AHIMA 2013).

Stewardship, in general, is personal responsibility for taking care of something one does not own. For example, a bank takes care of funds that individuals put into savings accounts. **Data stewardship** has become an important function in corporate America—where management of the corporation's data assets is critical for competitive advantage. In healthcare, the American Medical Informatics Association (AMIA) has defined **health data stewardship** as encompassing "the responsibilities and accountabilities associated with managing, collecting, viewing, storing, sharing, disclosing, or otherwise making use of personal health information" (AMIA 2007).

It should be observed that this definition extends beyond HIPAA's PHI to also include personal health information, such as health information that may be held by individuals themselves or in commercial PHR systems that are not subject to HIPAA but subject to the Federal Trade Commission's Health Breach Notification regulation. However, even AMIA's definition may not encompass all the data stewardship responsibilities and accountabilities that are necessary to support value-driven healthcare. For example, as data are collected and used to evaluate quality of care, provide MU incentives, and so on, there is a need not only to protect the privacy and security of those data but also to ensure the quality of the data and how well analytics are performed to draw conclusions about cost and quality. The general public has focused on privacy and security concerns but have not paid equal to attention to the issue of whether data are documented, collected, and used properly. The quality of the data and how well they are analyzed directly contributes to the knowledge that builds evidence-based guidelines. Data that do not adhere to a common data dictionary, that are incomplete, or that are not interpreted correctly can have a deleterious effect on an individual's health. Therefore, health data stewardship should do all the things AMIA defines, but there also needs to be respect for the data as "assets" that contribute to the well-being of individuals treated in the healthcare delivery system as well as the financial viability of the organizations established to provide such treatment.

In 2007, ONC was interested in identifying steps to enhance protections for what it called "secondary uses" of health data as it increasingly worked with large pools of data. In December 2007, the National Committee on Vital and Health Statistics (NCVHS) returned a set of recommendations, including that the term *secondary use* should not be used to describe the full range of uses of health data, as such terminology was believed to promote the idea that such uses were less important and potentially less in need of protection. NCVHS also called again for federal privacy legislation that would extend and enhance the requirements of HIPAA to all uses and users of personal health information. Specific recommendations also were made relating to the attributes in table 13.1. In 2008, ONC adopted the principles espoused by NCVHS in its Nationwide Privacy and Security Framework for Electronic Exchange of Individually Identifiable Health Information.

Table 13.1.   NCVHS health data stewardship

Data Stewardship Attributes	Summary of Recommendations
Accountability/Chain of Trust	Heighten attention on how business associates and their agents use health information, either in identifiable or deidentified form
Transparency	Achieve greater clarity in notices of privacy practices and other documents required for use in exchange of data
Individual Participation	Utilize HIPAA requirements for authorizations and consent appropriately, and ensure that the Federal Trade Commission exercises its authority over non-HIPAA covered entities in their use of privacy notices
HIPAA De-identification	Utilize the safe harbor or statistical process required by HIPAA to ensure proper deidentification of health information
Security Safeguards and Controls	Apply fully the HIPAA Security Rule requirements, especially with respect to auditing access logs, recognizing increased risk in an HIE and NHIN environment
Data Quality and Integrity	Apply principles of data quality and integrity to ensure precision, accuracy, reliability, completeness, and meaning to data collected
Oversight of Data Uses	Consider applying a joint oversight to uses of data for quality and research, as these uses blend into one another, yet have significantly different data protection requirements

Source: NCVHS

eHealth Exchange

A national health information infrastructure (NHII) was first described in 2001 by NCVHS, which viewed such an infrastructure as necessary to bring timely health information to, and aid communication among, those making health decisions for themselves, their families, their patients, and their communities. This vision remains valid for what then came to be called the *nationwide health information network* (with the change from *national* to *nationwide* made to emphasize that it was not to be a federally funded network).

Although many still refer to a nationwide health information network, this network is now referred to as the **eHealth Exchange**. Spanning all 50 states, it was incubated by ONC and transitioned to function as an independent initiative with private sector responsibility for the stewardship of the network. The **Sequoia Project** (formerly known as Healtheway) is providing support for the eHealth Exchange, which in 2016 served 40 percent of all US hospitals, 13,000 medical groups, 3,400 dialysis centers, 8,300 pharmacies, more than 100 million patients, and four federal agencies (DoD, VA, CMS, and Social Security Administration [SSA]) (HealthIT.gov). Figure 13.9 is an illustration of the eHealth Exchange.

The federal government has observed that the eHealth Exchange is not a physical network that runs on servers at HHS, nor is it a large network that stores patient records. This statement has been made to alleviate concerns that the government is creating a giant database. In fact, the federal government wants to ensure that any HIE network serves as a secure means to route data, and does not store data. HHS has provided supplementary funding to advance nationwide interoperable health IT standards harmonization, compliance certification, and privacy and security solutions. Participants in the eHealth Exchange pay an annual service fee based on their revenue that covers the cost to support participants who exchange data under the DURSA. This support includes ongoing maintenance of trust framework, specifications, service registry, certificate management, and so on. Two wikis are used to develop production-caliber interoperability specifications based upon existing industry standards and address policy and technical implications. In addition to the annual

Figure 13.9. eHealth exchange

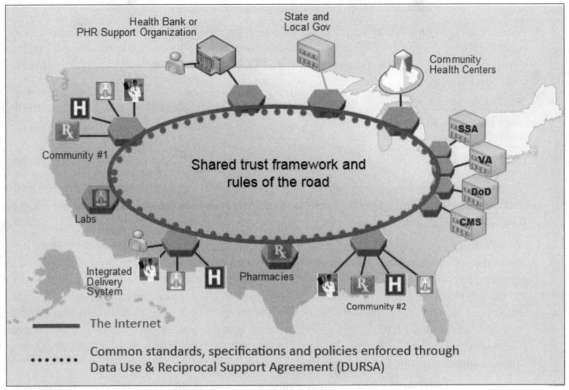

Source: Healtheway. Available at: http://slideplaycr.com/slide/3814212/

service fee, eHealth Exchange participants also pay testing fees paid during participant onboarding and product testing fees for vendors to validate their products.

Carequality is a community that the Sequoia Project uses to engage participants in the eHealth Exchange. It supplies the coordinating committee that provides governance for the eHealth Exchange. Its membership currently includes representatives from the American Medical Association, SSA, several of the major EHR and HIE vendors, Surescripts, and different types of providers. Its roles include:

- Determining whether to admit a new participant

- Maintaining a definitive list of all transaction patterns supported by each of the participants

- Developing and amending operating policies and procedures in accordance with the DURSA

- Receiving reports of breaches and acting upon such reports in accordance with the DURSA

- Suspending or terminating participants in accordance with the DURSA

- Resolving disputes between participants in accordance with the DURSA

- Managing the amendment of this agreement in accordance with the DURSA

- Evaluating, prioritizing and adopting new performance and service specifications, changes to existing performance and service specifications and the artifacts required by the validation plan in accordance with the DURSA

- Maintaining a process for managing versions of the performance and service specifications, including migration planning

- Evaluating requests for the introduction of emergent specifications into the production environment used by the participants to transact message content

- Coordinating with ONC to help ensure the interoperability of the performance and service specifications with other HIE initiatives including, but not limited to, providing input into the broader ONC specifications activities and ONC Standards and Interoperability Framework initiatives

- Fulfilling all other responsibilities delegated by the participants to the coordinating committee (The Sequoia Project 2016)

The federal government currently recognizes three key forms of HIE:

- **Directed exchange** is the ability to send and receive secure information electronically between care providers to support coordinated care. It is often referred to as a *push exchange* because it pushes information from one location to another location.

- **Query-based exchange** is the ability for providers to find and/or request information on a patient from other providers. This type of exchange is often used for unplanned care and is often referred to as a *pull exchange* because of the ability to send a request for information to the HIO and then receive any and all information that applies from whatever locations may have the applicable information. Query-based exchange can also be set up to provide notifications without having to make individual queries. For example, a primary care provider can be notified each time one of its patients is seen in an emergency department or is admitted to a hospital.

- **Consumer mediated exchange**, also called patient-managed HIE, is the ability for consumers to aggregate and control the use of their health information among their different providers. In some cases, this type of exchange may only be a process of providing consent for provider exchange of personal health information, but in other cases it may be the ability to direct information to a PHR.

Directed Exchange

The **Direct Project** was launched in March 2010 to establish a set of standards, policies, and services for Direct exchange. **Direct** is a simple, secure, scalable, standards-based way for participants to send authenticated, encrypted health information directly to known, trusted recipients over the Internet. Directed exchange was part of the stage 1 MU requirements for EHRs to communicate summary care records, referrals, discharge summaries, and other clinical documents in support of continuity of care and medication reconciliation, and communication of laboratory test results to providers. It is also being used for sending immunization data to public health organizations or to report quality measures to CMS.

The Direct Project is careful to point out that it focuses on the transport of health information, but it does not alone produce "interoperability." The Direct Project does not address the other two components necessary for interoperability: structure and format of exchanged content (for example, CCD) or terms used within the content (for example, SNOMED CT).

In some respect, Direct is similar to encrypted email, but requires a Direct Address for secure transport of email that is associated with a trust agent. The trust agent may be a **health information service provider (HISP)**, which can be, but is not necessarily, an HIO. The Direct protocol also provides technical specifications for directed exchange. There are four ways for a provider to start using Direct. A provider may subscribe to a Direct service through an HISP or HIO, use Direct through an EHR vendor, use the Direct protocol that has been embedded in the EHR, or use a Direct infrastructure that has been built within the provider's organization. While the Direct protocol provides the specifications for securing and transporting a directed exchange, there are best practices that should be followed when using Direct. The Direct Project (2010) provides a set of best practices for health information service providers to follow, including the following:

- Sender has obtained a patient's consent, as applicable, to send information.

- Sender ensures the patient's privacy preferences are being honored.

- Sender determines that it is clinically and legally appropriate to send information.

- Sender determines that the receiver's address is correct.

- Sender has communicated to the receiver the purpose for exchanging information.

- Sender and receiver do not require any common or prenegotiated person identifiers (which is required in a query-based exchange, as described in the next section of this chapter).

- Sender relies on the HISP for following best practice guidance for privacy, security, and transparency developed by the Direct Project.

Query-Based Exchange

Query-based exchange is used by providers to search and discover accessible clinical sources on a patient. Health IT.gov (2014) provides an example of an emergency department physician using query-based exchange to access a patient's current medications, recent radiology images, and problem lists before carrying out treatment plans to avoid adverse medication reactions or duplicative testing.

Query-based exchange uses an interface to reach the eHealth Exchange. The first such interface developed for reaching the nationwide health information network was CONNECT, which is free, open-source software. Initially, all query-based exchange was called CONNECT because of the first software used for this purpose. However, it is not necessary to use this particular software. Other companies have developed their own interfaces (Duck 2012).

Query-based exchange is different than Direct in several respects. First, Direct is considered **push technology** because a provider is pushing information to another provider known to need the information. For example, if a provider and commercial laboratory establish a Directed exchange, the laboratory will push laboratory test results to the provider using the directed exchange. Query-based exchange is considered **pull technology**. It is often not known in advance who may have information about the patient and so a query is released, usually to an HIO, that then uses its registry, patient ID matching, and record locator services to determine where information may be located. As a result, query-based exchange uses a much more robust trust fabric, including the operating procedures, DURSA (which is required in the directed exchange), and eHealth Exchange service interface specifications. Query-based exchange also uses more sophisticated security structures, including more comprehensive event and audit logging.

Consumer-Mediated Exchange

Consumer-mediated exchange provides patients with access to their health information so they, in turn, may provide other providers with their health information, identify and correct wrong or missing health information, identify and correct incorrect billing information, and track and monitor their own health. (HealthIT.gov 2014). Consumer-mediated exchange is not a formal process overseen by the federal government, but it has been promoted through the MU requirements, federal and commercial EHR vendor use of Blue Button technology (Pedulli 2015), and other promotional efforts of the federal government.

Certifications and Accreditations for HIE

Several organizations have formed to ensure that HIE is performed in a manner intended by the federal government, and to certify conformance with federal requirements.

The **Electronic Healthcare Network Accreditation Commission (EHNAC)** was founded in 1993 to "improve transactional quality, operational efficiency, and data security in healthcare" (EHNAC 2015a). Initially, it developed criteria for third-party review and accreditation primarily for healthcare clearinghouses, which helped the industry exchange HIPAA financial and administrative transactions, such as claims, remittance advice, and eligibility inquiry and response. Over the years, EHNAC—with its commission members from financial services firms, payers, and others—branched out into providing accreditation services for other outsourced service organizations, such as printing companies, document imaging companies, media storage services, call centers, data centers, and network administrators. More recently, it has collaborated with a number of security organizations, state regulators, physician organizations, consumer groups, and others to add accreditation for e-prescribing networks, accountable care organizations, practice management systems, and HIOs.

EHNAC and DirectTrust (see below) have collaborated to offer ONC-endorsed accreditation to HISPs (DirectTrust 2016). The accreditation program validates the technical, security, trust, and business practice conformance of trust agents involved in Direct. **Trust agents** are HISPs, **certificate authorities (CAs)** for issuing digital signatures, and **registration authorities (RAs)** for verifying the validity of the request for a digital signature to a CA (EHNAC 2015b).

DirectTrust is a collaborative nonprofit association of health IT vendors and provider organizations to support secure, interoperable HIE via the Direct message protocols. It has created a "trust framework" that extends use of Direct exchange to over 40,000 healthcare organizations and 760,000 Direct addresses. The trust framework supports provider-to-provider HIE and exchange between patients and their providers. More than 300 EHR and PHR vendors' products and over 50 HIOs participate in the DirectTrust network (DirectTrust 2016).

The **National Association for Trusted Exchange (NATE)** is a nonprofit organization that participates in projects to support HIE. It develops **Trust Bundles** that provide a common set of policies and procedures for different types of exchanges. For example, the NATE Blue Button for Consumers Trust Bundle (NBB4C) describes policies and procedures for exchanges between providers and patients. There are a number of other Trust Bundles, and any given organization can have more than one Trust Bundle depending on the types of exchanges the organization conducts. Trust Bundles also represent common practices, so that any organization may also choose to put other restrictions in place based on local policy preferences (for example, between providers) or requirements (for example, between providers using a state-based HIO) (NATE 2015).

Check Your Understanding 13.3

Choose the best answer:

1. Directed exchange is used to:

   a. Exchange structured data between applications in an EHR

   b. Push data to another provider or organization

   c. Pull data from another provider or organization

   d. Query an HIO for data

2. The HIE architecture most preferred for its privacy support is:

   a. Consolidated

   b. Cooperative

   c. Federated

   d. Hybrid

3. Responsibility for taking care of something is referred to as:

   a. Data governance

   b. Information governance

   c. Stewardship

   d. Transparency

4. Which of the following is required *only* in a query-based exchange?

   a. Honoring patient privacy preferences

   b. Patient consent as applicable

   c. Prenegotiated person identifier

   d. Receiver address verification

5. An organization that accredits HISPs is:

   a. Direct Trust

   b. EHNAC

   c. NATE

   d. ONC

6. An example of a Trust Bundle is:

   a. Certificate authority, HISP, registration authority

   b. Direct address

   c. Policies and procedure for each data exchange type

   d. Interface for exchange of data in the eHealth Exchange

7. Which of the following is *true* concerning the eHealth Exchange?

   a. It is funded by the federal government.

   b. It is privately managed.

   c. It requires use of semantic interoperability.

   d. Only state HIOs may use it.

References and Resources

45 CFR 160. 2009 (October 30). HIPAA administrative simplification: Enforcement: Interim final rule.

45 CFR 162. 2004 (January 23). Department of Health and Human Services. HIPAA administrative simplification: Standard unique health identifier for health care providers: Final rule.

45 CFR 162. 2009 (January 16). Department of Health and Human Services. Health insurance reform: Modifications to the Health Insurance Portability and Accountability Act (HIPAA): Final rule (X12 Version 5010 and NCPDP Version D.0 and Medicaid subrogation for pharmacy claims NCPDP Version 3.0).

45 CFR 170(e). 2011 (January 7). Department of Health and Human Services. Establishment of the permanent certification program for health information technology.

Agency for Healthcare Research and Quality (AHRQ). 2014 (March 26). Innovations Exchange. Trends in health information exchanges. https://innovations.ahrq.gov/perspectives/trends-health-information-exchanges.

AHIMA Foundation. n.d. State-Level Health Information Exchange Consensus Project. http://www.ahimafoundation.org/PolicyResearch/SLHIE.aspx.

Ambler, S.W. 2014a. Introduction to the diagrams of UML 2.X. Agile Modeling: Effective Practices for Modeling and Documentation. http://www.agilemodeling.com/essays/umlDiagrams.htm.

Ambler, S.W. 2014b.Home page. Agile Modeling: Effective Practices for Modeling and Documentation. http://www.agilemodeling.com.

American Health Information Management Association (AHIMA). 2009. Managing the integrity of patient identity in health information exchange. *Journal of AHIMA*. 80(7):62–69.

American Health Information Management Association (AHIMA). 2013. Understanding the HIE landscape. *Journal of AHIMA*. 84(1):56–63.

American Hospital Association (AHA). 2015 (October 6). *Why Interoperability Matters*. http://www.aha.org/content/15/interoperabilitymatters.pdf.

American Medical Informatics Association (AMIA). 2007 (July). Toward a national framework on secondary use of health data: Testimony to the National Committee on Vital and Health Statistics. http://www.amia.org/inside/initiatives/healthdata/2007/labkoffbloomrosenncvhssecondarydata.pdf.

ASTM International. 2012. ASTM E2369-12: Standard specification for continuity of care record (CCR). http://www.astm.org/Standards/E2369.htm.

Australian Government, Department of Finance and Administration. 2007 (July). *The Australian Government Business Process Interoperability Framework: Enabling Seamless Service Delivery*. https://www.finance.gov.au/sites/default/files/Business_Process_Interoeprabiltiy_Framework.pdf.

Bass, D. 2011. Opting for opt out: How one HIE manages patient consent. *Journal of AHIMA*. 82(5):34–36.

Brull, R. 2012 (January 31). What is integrating the healthcare enterprise (IHE)? Corepoint Health GENi blog. http://corepointhealth.com/geni/what-integrating-healthcare-enterprise-ihe.

Brull, R. 2013 (February 11). Blue Button+, a step forward. Health Standards blog. http://healthstandards.com/blog/2013/02/11/blue-button-a-step-forward.

Centers for Medicare and Medicaid Services (CMS). 2016 (June 21). EIN. https://www.cms.gov/Regulations-and-Guidance/Administrative-Simplification/Unique-Identifier/EIN.html.

Council for Affordable Quality Healthcare, Committee on Operating Rules for Information Exchange (CAQH CORE). 2012 (September 12). Letter from Kathleen Sebelius, Secretary of HHS to NCVH on designating CAQH CORE the operating rules authoring entity. http://www.caqh.org/sites/default/files/core/HHS%20Response%20to%20NCVHS%20RE%20Author%20for%20ACA%20Third%20Set%2009.12.12.pdf?token=QdUiHJ4r.

Council for Affordable Quality Healthcare, Committee on Operating Rules for Information Exchange (CAQH CORE).2016 (January 21). New phase IV CAQH CORE operating rules (webinar). http://www.caqh.org/sites/default/files/core/CORE%20Webinar%20-%20Phase%20IV%20-%201-21-16_Final_0.pdf?token=SUWNqy3M.

Day, D. 2015 (September 14). Cultivating EDI into E-Solutions. http://www.npag.org/uploaded_files/361/files/Day%20-%20HL7%20-Attachments.pdf

Direct Project. 2010. Best practices for HISPs. http://wiki.directproject.org/Best+Practices+for+HISPs.

DirectTrust. 2016. DirectTrust 101: A brief introduction to Direct, Direct Exchange, and DirectTrust, intended for both technical and non-technical audiences. https://www.directtrust.org/directtrust-101.

Dolin, R.H., et al. 2006 (January/February). HL7 clinical document architecture, release 2. *Journal of the American Medical Informatics Association.* 13(1):30–39.

Duck, B. 2012 (March 11). Hospitals and providers using NHIN (Nationwide Health Information Network) to connect and share medical records with the VA and DOD and even with each other. . Medical Quack blog. http://ducknetweb.blogspot.com/2012/03/hospitals-and-providers-using-nhin.html.

Dunbrack, L.A., and M. Holland. 2008 (August). The critical need for connected healthcare: Meeting today's integration challenge. *Health Industry Insights*, White Paper, HI212098.

eHealth Initiative. 2010 (March 17). 2009 eHealth Initiative survey, migrating toward meaningful use: The state of health information exchange. http://www.ehealthinitiative.org.

Electronic Healthcare Network Accreditation Commission (EHNAC). 2015a. EHNAC overview. https://www.ehnac.org/about.

Electronic Healthcare Network Accreditation Commission (EHNAC). 2015b. Direct Trusted Agents. https://www.ehnac.org/direct-trusted-agent.

Ferranti, J.M., et al. 2006. The clinical document architecture and the continuity of care record: A critical analysis. *Journal of the American Medical Informatics Association.* 13(3):245–252. http://www.ncbi.nlm.nih.gov/pmc/articles/PMC1513652.

Gibbons, P., et al.; Health Level Seven EHR Interoperability Work Group. 2007 (February 7). Coming to terms: Scoping interoperability for health care. https://www.hln.com/assets/pdf/Coming-to-Terms-February-2007.pdf.

Goldstein, M.M., and A.L. Rein. 2010 (March 23). Consumer consent options for electronic health information exchange: Policy considerations and analysis. Prepared for Office of the National Coordinator for Health Information Technology. http://www.himss.org/consumer-consent-options-electronic-health-information-exchange-policy-considerations-and-analysis.

Hagland, M.2013 (August 30). Health information exchange: Are we at an inflection point? *Healthcare Informatics.* http://www.healthcare-informatics.com/article/health-information-exchange-are-we-inflection-point.

Health Information Management and Systems Society (HIMSS). 2013 (April 5). Definition of interoperability. http://www.himss.org/library/interoperability-standards/what-is-interoperability.

Health IT.gov. 2011 (May 26). Approved state plans. https://www.healthit.gov/policy-researchers-implementers/approved-state-plans.

Health IT.gov. 2014 (July 15). What is HIE? https://www.healthit.gov/providers-professionals/health-information-exchange/what-hie.

Hench, G. et al. 2008 (August). A conceptual roadmap for scalable semantic computing. *Proceedings of the 2nd IEEE International Conference on Semantic Computing.* Santa Clara, CA: IEEE.

Hoyt, R.E., and A. Yoshihashi, eds. 2014. *Health Informatics: A Practical Guide for Healthcare and Information Technology Professionals*, 6th ed.. Informatics Education. http://www.informaticseducation.org.

I Do Imaging. 2014. Free Medical Imaging Software. www.idoimaging.com.

Indrajit, I.K., and B.S. Verma. 2007. DICOM, HL7 and IHE: A basic primer on healthcare standards for radiologists. *Indian Journal of Radiology and Imaging.* 17(2):66–68.

Institute of Medicine (IOM). 1999. *To Err Is Human: Building a Safer Health System,* edited by L.T. Kohn, J.M. Corrigan, and M.S. Donaldson. Washington, DC: National Academies Press.

Institute of Medicine (IOM). 2005. *Building a Better Delivery System: A New Engineering/Health Care Partnership.* Washington, DC: National Academies Press.

Kawamoto, K. 2012 (August 14). HL7 decision support service (DSS) and virtual medical record (vMR) standards, and OpenCDS open-source implementation. HL7 Ambassador Webinar. http://www.google.com/url?sa=t&rct=j&q=&esrc=s&frm=1&source=web&cd=1&ved=0ahUKEwjeoYvVvMPKAhUKTCYKHRb-BbYQFggeMAA&url=http%3A%2F%2Fwww.opencds.org%2FPortals%2F0%2FDownloads%2FReferences%2FKawamoto-HL7_DSS_and_vMR_Standards_and_OpenCDS_Open-Source_Implementation.ppt&usg=AFQjCNFftinz5Yj7o0dVojq8kL_k0G4kbA.

Kubicek, H., R. Cimander, and H.J. Scholl. 2011. *Organizational Interoperability in E-Government: Lessons from 77 European Good-Practice Cases.* Berlin: Springer-Verlag Berlin Heidelberg. http://www.springer.com/978-3-642-22501-7.

Leontiev, A., and C. Parisot. 2003. DICOM and integrating the healthcare enterprise: Five years of cooperation and mutual influence. National Electrical Manufacturers Association (NEMA) Workshop.

Levy, B. 2014. Health care's semantics challenge. *For the Record.* 26(5):26.

Livingood, W.C., et al. 2009. Public health & electronic health information exchange: A guide to local agency leadership. Institute for Public Health Informatics and Research, Duval County Health Department, Robert Wood Johnson Foundation. http://www.phii.org/sites/default/files/resource/pdfs/Public%20Health%20%26%20EHIE%20(DCHD)%20FINAL.pdf.

Lowry S.Z., et al. 2015 (September 28Technical evaluation, testing, and validation of the usability of electronic health records: empirically based use cases for validating safety—enhanced usability and guidelines for standardization. National Institute of Standards and Technology. NISTIR 7804-1. http://nvlpubs.nist.gov/nistpubs/ir/2015/NIST.IR.7804-1.pdf.

Matthews, T. 2010 (July 28). eHealth Initiative: HIEs nearing meaningful use. *Health Imaging.*

Managed Healthcare Executive. 2008 (October 1). State of the industry 2009: IT system integration. http://managedhealthcareexecutive.modernmedicine.com/managed-healthcare-executive/content/state-industry-2009-it-system-integration?page=full.

Manos, D. 2012 (January 10). The VA's hot Blue Button. *Healthcare IT News.* http://www.healthcareitnews.com/news/vas-hot-blue-button.

Massachusetts Medical Society. 2005 (October). *Transparency in Health Care Cost and Quality.* http://www.massmed.org/AM/Template.cfm?Section=Home&CONTENTID=14449&TEMPLATE=/CM/ContentDisplay.cfm#265,10,Q.8.

Mcllwain, J.S., and K. Lassetter. 2009. HIE: Decision support. Building sustainable HIEs. In the aftermath of Hurricane Katrina, the need for a true health information exchange in Mississippi cannot be denied. *Health Management Technology.* 30(2):8–11.

Murray, C.J.L., and J. Frenk. 2010. Ranking 37th—Measuring the performance of the U.S. health care system. Perspective. *New England Journal of Medicine.* 362(2):98–99.

Murugesan, P. et al. 2014. Clinical decision support systems. Computer Sciences Corporation white paper. http://www.csc.com/innovation/insights/109189-clinical_decision_support_systems.

National Alliance for Health Information Technology (NAHIT). 2008 (May). *Report to the Office of the National Coordinator for Health Information Technology on Defining Key Health Information Technology Terms.* http://www.himss.org/national-alliance-health-information-technology-report-office-national-coordinator-health.

National Association for Trusted Exchange (NATE). 2015. Understanding Trust Bundles. http://nate-trust.org/understanding-trust-bundles.

National Committee on Vital and Health Statistics (NCVHS). 2001 (November 15). Information for health: A strategy for building the national health information infrastructure. http://www.ncvhs.hhs.gov.

National Committee on Vital and Health Statistics (NCVHS). 2007 (December). Enhanced protections for uses of health data: A stewardship framework for "secondary uses" of electronically collected and transmitted health data. http://www.ncvhs.hhs.gov/wp-content/uploads/2014/05/071221lt.pdf..

National Council for Prescription Drug Programs (NCPDP). 2010 (August). What is electronic prescribing? http://www.ncpdp.org/eprescribing.aspx.

National Institute of Standards and Technology (NIST). 2016 (August 15). Computer Security Resource Center (CSCR). http://csrc.nist.gov.

Noumeir, R. 2006. Benefits of the DICOM structured report. *Journal of Digital Imaging.* 19(4):295–306.

Office of the National Coordinatorfor Health IT (ONC). 2014 (June 17). S&I Framework update. HIT Standards Committee. https://www.healthit.gov/facas/sites/faca/files/HITSC_SI_Initiatives_Update_2014-06-17.pdf.

Office of the National Coordinator for Health IT (ONC). 2015 (October 6). Connecting Health and Care for the Nation: A Shared Nationwide Interoperability Roadmap. Final version 1.0. https://www.healthit.gov/sites/default/files/hie-interoperability/nationwide-interoperability-roadmap-final-version-1.0.pdf.

Office of the National Coordinator for Health IT (ONC).2016. 2016 Interoperability Standards Advisory. https://www.healthit.gov/standards-advisory/2016.

Open HIT Labs. 2011. Healthcare interoperability standards. http://www.openhitlabs.org/healthcare-interoperability-standards.

Organisation for Economic Cooperation and Development (OECD). 2015 (November 4). Health at a glance 2015. http://www.oecd.org/health/health-systems/health-at-a-glance-19991312.htm

Pedulli, L. 2015 (February 3). NATE demonstrates trust bundle for patient-mediated exchange. Clinical Innovation + Technology. http://www.clinical-innovation.com/topics/interoperability/nate-demonstrates-trust-bundle-patient-mediated-exchange.

Raths, D. 2014 (February 19). Top ten tech trends: Catching FHIR. *Healthcare Informatics.* http://www.healthcare-informatics.com/article/top-ten-tech-trends-catching-fhir.

Robert Wood Johnson Foundation. 2015. Health information technology in the United States, 2015: Transition to a post-HITECH world. http://www.rwjf.org/content/dam/farm/reports/reports/2015/rwjf423440.

Schonwalder, J. 2013 (March 14). Information models, data models, and YANG. *Internet Engineering Task Force (IETF) 86 Proceedings.* https://www.ietf.org/proceedings/86/slides/slidcs-86-i2rs-3.pdf.

Scrimshire, M. 2016 (January). HL7 WGM Blue Button on FHIR. Blue Button on FHIR presentation to Attachments Work Group at HL7 Meeting, January 2016. http://www.slideshare.net/ekivemark/bluebutton-on-fhir-presentation-to-attachments-work-group-at-hl7-meeting-jan-2016.

Sequoia Project. 2016a. What is e-Health Exchange? http://sequoiaproject.org/ehealth-exchange.

Sequoia Project, 2016b. What is Carequality? http://sequoiaproject.org/carequality.

Shakir, A. 2014 (March 3). Health Level Seven Reference Information Model. HI3 Solutions. http://www.slideshare.net/AShakir/hl7-reference-information-model.

Sirovich, B., et al. 2008. Discretionary decision making by primary care physicians and the cost of U.S. health care. *Health Affairs.* 27(3):813–823.

Sundvall, E. 2013 (January 22). *Scalability and Semantic Sustainability in Electronic Health Record Systems* [dissertation]. Linköping. Sweden: Linköping University. http://liu.diva-portal.org/smash/get/diva2:599752/FULLTEXT03.pdf.

Swensen, S.J., et al. 2010. Cottage industry to postindustrial care—The revolution in health care delivery. Perspective. *New England Journal of Medicine.* 362(5):e12.

US Department of Health and Human Services (HHS). 2005 (October 6). Press Release. HHS awards contracts to advance nationwide interoperable health information technology. http://archive.hhs.gov/news/press/2005pres/20051006a.html.

Warner, D. 2011. HIE patient consent model options. *Journal of AHIMA.* 82(5):48–44.

Wolfson, J. 2014 (October 27). Data normalization for semantic translation. Becker's *Health IT & CIO Review.* http://www.beckershospitalreview.com/healthcare-information-technology/data-normalization-for-semantic-translation.html.

Chapter 14
Optimizing the Acute Care EHR

Key Terms

Active (CDS) advice

Adverse drug event

Adverse drug reaction

Alert fatigue

Automated informed consent system

Clinical Laboratory Improvement Amendments (CLIA)

Closed-loop medication management

Contingency plans

DailyMed

Data mining at the bedside

Data visualization

Diagnostic imaging reports

Digital images

Drug-drug interaction (DDI)

Five rights of medication administration

Inference engine

Knowledge base

Medication reconciliation

Nurse staffing by patient acuity

Optimization

Order communication

Passive (CDS) advice

Patient-flow management system

Point of care (POC) documentation

Quick read (QR) code

Real-time location system (RTLS)

Report wizard

Results management

Results review

Role-specific training

Rules engine

Smart bed

Supply chain management system

Unique Device Identification (UDI)

Units of measure

User interface

Learning Objectives

- Explain the importance of a critically constructed and maintained migration path that supports the hospital's journey to achieving the benefits of the EHR.

- Describe an overall optimization strategy for the EHR that helps improve results and user satisfaction.

- List results management issues associated with integration of data from ancillary source systems.

- Describe point of care (POC) documentation applications that address quality and productivity improvement.

- Explain medication management applications (computerized provider order entry [CPOE] and bar code medication administration record [BC-MAR]) and strategies to achieve patient safety.

- Characterize the inclusion of clinical decision support in a comprehensive EHR.

- Evaluate various types of reporting technology that should be included in or complementary to an EHR.

- Recognize various other components that have clinical as well as financial and administrative, operational, or educational impact for the hospital.

Hospital use of electronic health record (EHR) systems has increased tremendously as a result of the meaningful use (MU) incentive program. Data from the Office of the National Coordinator for Health Information Technology (ONC) show that in 2008 just about 10 percent of nonfederal acute care hospitals had a basic EHR. The number of hospitals using a basic EHR grew to nearly 30 percent in 2011; by that point, over 70 percent of hospitals had acquired an MU-certified EHR (although most of the systems were still in the implementation phases). By the end of 2014, basic use of EHR rose to 75 percent in hospitals, and 96 percent of hospitals had acquired a MU-certified EHR (Charles et al. 2015).

There have been many success stories about the implantation of EHRs in hospitals. The Commonwealth Fund examined nine hospitals and found that their systems facilitated patient safety and quality improvement through use of checklists, alerts, and predictive tools; embedded clinical guidelines that promote standardized, evidence-based practices; electronic prescribing and test order that reduce errors and redundancy; and discrete data that foster use of performance dashboards and compliance reports (Silow-Carroll et al. 2012). These hospitals found that faster, more accurate communication and streamlined processes through their health information technology (health IT) systems led to improved patient flow, fewer duplicative tests, faster responses to patient inquiries, redeployment of transcription and claims processing staff, and more complete capture of charges. The American Hospital Association has described technology as the "common fiber supporting patient engagement, team-based care, healthcare models, and care coordination" (Davis 2015).

Although the numbers, results of leading hospitals, and goals for health IT are impressive, concerns persist that EHRs are not sufficiently improving key measures of patient safety, that they are worsening productivity, and that they are not designed to support innovations in healthcare, such as changes in reimbursement associated with health reform. One of the key drivers for the MU incentive program was the Institute of Medicine (IOM) "wake up" call in its report *To Err is Human: Building a Safer Health System* (2000). In this report, IOM (now known as the Health and Medicine Division [HMD] of the National Academies of Sciences, Engineering, and Medicine) revealed that up to 98,000 Americans may die each year as a result of medical errors. Thirteen years later, an evidence-based estimate of patient harms associated with hospital care suggested the number of deaths associated with preventable harm in US hospitals was 210,000 at the lower limit and potentially 400,000 at the upper limit, especially if serious harm is included (James 2013). In testimony to Congress, Harvard University professor of health policy and management, Ashish Jha, MD, observed that "the potential [for improvement] is not going to be realized unless those [EHR] tools are really focused on improving patient safety." He then added that "the tools themselves won't automatically do it" (McCann 2014).

To achieve success with their EHRs, hospitals need to develop an optimization strategy that enables them to fully support their users in gaining benefits out of the EHR (National Learning Consortium 2013). Hospital planning, infrastructure preparation, selection, implementation, privacy and security assurance, and achieving interoperability have been covered in previous chapters. This chapter focuses on how to optimize use of an EHR overall, and for each of its core clinical components.

Constructing and Maintaining the EHR Migration Path for Hospitals

As described in chapter 1, the clinical components comprising an EHR include collecting and integrating source data, capturing and enabling use of data at the point of care, supporting clinical decision making, exchanging health information across the continuum of care, and measuring, reporting, and improving quality of healthcare. The MU incentive program largely laid out the requirements for sequencing implementation of these components, but hospitals often have additional health IT that must be fit into their migration path, and they need to have a plan to ensure that every component works and is being used optimally. As described in chapter 3, a migration path is a tool that can help focus the strategic initiative of using health IT to achieve the Triple Aim goals of improved health, healthcare, and experience of care. In fact, as the MU program winds down and hospitals are potentially left with disgruntled staff and physicians and questions about return on investment (ROI) for health IT, it is imperative that the migration path be reexamined with a new focus. **Optimization** refers to the fine-tuning of the hospital's EHR and other types of health IT in a systematic way, including assessment and improvement of the systems' hardware, software, people, policy, and process aspects, in order to improve its value (HCI Group 2014).

If a migration path was not constructed prior to implementing the EHR for the MU program, a first step in EHR optimization should be to document the existing health IT infrastructure, critically assess each component's strengths and weaknesses, and then design a strategy for achieving and celebrating better results over various phases. Figure 14.1 provides a template for such a migration path.

When using the migration path template, key stakeholders should be engaged to describe strengths and weaknesses. For example, it may be a strength that the computerized provider order entry (CPOE) has been fine-tuned with a limited set of critical clinical decision support (CDS) alerts relating to high-risk medications, unnecessary duplicative tests, and patient costs associated with discharge medications. It may be a weakness that the problem list is only generated from nursing diagnoses because structured documentation for physicians has not been implemented. Another weakness maybe that physicians would like to bring their own devices to use while making rounds but the organization does not have a bring your own device (BYOD) policy. Some weaknesses may be expressed as complaints until their root causes are studied. Expressions of strengths and weaknesses may also reflect both subjective perceptions and objective realities—but all should be listed at least in a first pass for further investigation. Subjective perceptions can strongly influence behavior and become self-fulfilling prophecies. As the hospital plans its optimization strategy, a key ingredient will be to establish metrics and a measurement system to quantify the key components (this point is expanded later n this chapter). As more becomes known about the hospital's health IT system strengths, weaknesses, and value, corrective actions, enhancements, updates, and new applications, technology, people, policy, and process elements can be plotted in phases to be accomplished.

Overarching Optimization Strategies for the EHR and Health IT

Superimposed on the sample migration path template in Figure 14.1 are the key steps in planning for optimization of the EHR or other health IT system. These steps reflect the systems development life cycle (SDLC) and include the following:

1. Engage all stakeholders in the process of assessing the strengths and weakness of the hospital's EHR and health IT. Provide regular feedback to stakeholders on how these strengths and weaknesses are being addressed.

2. Establish SMART goals, construct metrics, and measure goal achievement.

3. If goals are not being achieved, determine the root causes.

4. Take corrective action that addresses the root causes of issues to support goal achievement.

5. Report on all feedback, communicate the need for feedback and results, and celebrate large and small successes.

6. Continue refining goals, monitoring results, and finding innovative ways to make improvements.

Engage All Stakeholders

Despite the extensive amount of literature that supports the need for engaging stakeholders in every step of EHR planning and implementation, many hospitals found it challenging to do so, for a variety of reasons. Many physicians did not want to get involved. Some hospitals wanted to move quickly into the MU incentive program and did not want to take the time to engage stakeholders. Other hospitals could not spare clinical staff time. However, as the stakeholders are now required

Figure 14.1.   EHR and health IT migration path for optimal results

Current EHR and Health IT Infrastructure	Strengths	Weaknesses	Phase 1 Optimization	Phase N Optimization
Applications				
−Results management				
−POC documentation				
−Medication management +CPOE +BCMAR				
−Clinical decision support				
−Reporting +CQM +Registries +Business intelligence +Health intelligence +*Enumerate all others*				
Source systems −Financial +*Enumerate all* −Administrative +*Enumerate all* −Departmental clinical +*Enumerate all*				
Specialty clinical systems −*Enumerate all*				
Smart peripherals −*Enumerate all*				
Consumer-facing applications −Portals −Personal health records −Telehealth −Health monitoring −*Enumerate all others*				
Technology				
−Data architecture +Data repository +Data warehouse −Information infrastructure Supporting platform +Client/server or WSA +In-house/hosted +*Enumerate all other components* −Storage management				
−Devices and device management −Connectivity +Networking +Health information exchange +*Enumerate all other components* −Standards +Technical +Semantic +Process				

(continued)

Figure 14.1.   EHR and health IT migration path for optimal results (Continued)

Current EHR and Health IT Infrastructure	Strengths	Weaknesses	Phase 1 Optimization	Phase N Optimization
People				
−Executive leadership −Stakeholder engagement −Support staff −Patient advocates			−Engage stakeholders in health IT optimization	
Policy				
−Responsibility −Accountability −Transparency −Governance −Stewardship −Trust			−Determine root cause for not achieving goals −Provide feedback −Continuous improvement	
Process				
−SMART goals −Metrics and measurement +Patient safety +Outcomes +Return on investment +Productivity +User satisfaction +Patient satisfaction −Workflow −Physical layout −Process improvement −Documentation −Support			−Review and update or establish SMART goals −Measure and monitor value of health IT	

to use the systems and are gaining experience and understanding of what they like and do not like, it may be easier to get them engaged in optimization. Hospitals may also find that such investment will have more value.

Engaging stakeholders requires creative ways to gain vital input without returning to the previous issues of lack of time and little evidence of value in engagement, such as often occurs when there are only routine monthly meetings or newsletters. Many of the ways to engage stakeholders are the same approaches that are recommended to hospitals for monitoring. These include the following:

- Executives walking around to:

  - Make observations

  - Listen to complaints

  - Express appreciation

  - Ask questions

- Holding open-door events for people to gather to informally discuss EHR and health IT. Bagel breakfasts, pizza lunches, and milk-and-cookie breaks are tried and true methods for gaining invaluable feedback. It may be necessary to garner a few enthusiastic stakeholders to begin or reinstate this process. Follow-up by staff, however, must demonstrate that the hospital is actively taking feedback into consideration. As word spreads sufficiently that feedback sessions can make a difference, they will become more popular and productive.

- Piggybacking on existing formal meetings (department meetings, grand rounds, and so on) to gain feedback. An attendee may be asked to briefly introduce an issue and call for others to provide feedback. Showcasing such an issue in a balanced manner should identify particular strengths and weaknesses.

- Letting others collect the feedback. Encourage members of the IT help desk to not just report issues but also ask strategic follow-up questions to learn about the likes and dislikes of staff. Ask nurses to describe what they are hearing from other clinical staff, physicians, and patients.

- Using the technology to track and review adoption statistics, such as usage rates of printers, session time, staff working overtime, and other relevant data.

- Creating an environment in which people are willing to open up and participate in goal setting and strategizing about what solutions might work.

It is not possible to gain stakeholder feedback in a meaningful way if they are not given any feedback in the form of "mission accomplished." At this stage, it should be apparent to users that there are no magical solutions that can be implemented overnight. But they should also know that optimization is being undertaken. It may be necessary to first focus stakeholder input on certain areas already known to be at issue and for which there may be some viable solutions that will produce quick wins. One way to identify the potential for quick wins is to review the literature of best practices in EHR implementation and use. Organizations can consider how other hospitals have achieved positive outcomes in areas of concern and identify tactics to successfully follow in their paths.

Establish SMART Goals for Optimization

EHR and other health IT products do need to mature, and, in many cases, implementations could have been done better. On the other hand, part of the dissatisfaction being experienced today may well be due to unrealistic expectations. Unrealistic expectations can arise out of lack of goal setting. The process of goal setting often helps temper expectations by clarifying where the hospital is at the start of a project and establishing an appreciation of the efforts needed to realistically achieve the desired results in the time frame anticipated. SMART goals were described in chapter 4. If such goals were previously set in the hospital, the organization should review them and revise them as needed. If they were previously not established, the organization should set them now. SMART goals are essential for optimization.

The *M* in SMART stands for *measurable*. Sometimes, hospitals set goals, but they are not measurable. For example, "reduce medication errors" is not stated in a way that is measurable. For many hospitals, one challenge when attempting to set measurable goals is that the organization does not have metrics and baseline measurements to know what a realistic measure of improvement might be. Another issue is that technology may change how metrics are measured. For example, a hospital initially has a reported medication error rate of 5 percent, and when it implements a bar code medication administration record (BC-MAR) system, the reported error rate is 10 percent. Some might conclude that the rate is increasing or that the postimplementation measurement is in error. However, medication errors can be measured much more precisely by a BC-MAR. In fact, it might have been impossible to accurately measure the error rate in the paper environment, and so the rate actually may have gone down after implementation. Medication errors may also be defined differently in an automated environment than a paper-based environment. It may have been too cumbersome to measure all of the potential types of errors in the medication process performed manually, so some errors were never identified. Initially higher error rates may seem discouraging, but a lack of valid baseline data should not prevent hospitals from improving on their measurement process during optimization. As noted in chapter 5, a benchmarking study is another way to set metrics to measure outcomes. Dr. Jha, whose testimony before Congress was previously quoted, also points out, "If you don't have data and metrics, you don't know how you're doing; you don't know how you compare to anyone else, and you have no way to judge whether your efforts are making a difference or not" (McCann 2014).

Determine Root Causes if Desired Measures Are Not Met

One reason for measuring outcomes to be achieved from EHR and health IT is to determine if, in fact, there is an actual problem. Because the implementation of an EHR involves enormous changes for users, they may conclude that the new workflow processes are less productive or diminish the quality of care, but the evidence about outcomes may tell a different story.

Figure 14.2 is clip art that was found a number of years ago to illustrate a physician documenting in a patient's chart. In an EHR environment, many physicians complain that they are buried in the computer and cannot make eye contact with their patients. Many, however, probably do not realize the amount of time they spent not making eye contact with patients previously. This point is not meant to suggest that there is not room for improvement in physician-patient interactions—there is always such room. In fact, the use of an EHR or other health IT may actually provide new ways to make care feel more personal. For example, chapter 4 recounts how physicians at Mayo Clinic found that having patients enter their health history into an automated system prior to being seen by the physician increased patient engagement (among other benefits). This particular example may not apply to the hospital environment as well as it does in the ambulatory environment, but it is a good example of thinking "outside of the box" to find new solutions.

Root causes can be found by a variety of methods. A focused observation or process mapping is a good way to determine issues associated with patient communications. Physical layout and traffic pattern analysis can help with understanding productivity issues as well as the selection of input devices that may be easier to use in certain environments. A review of CDS rules, evidence-based

Figure 14.2.   Documentation practices

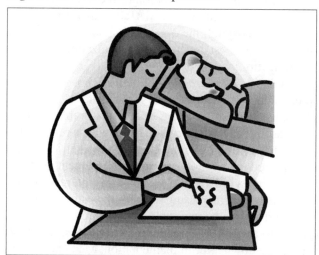

guidelines embedded in the EHR, and even the data model for a specific task can help pinpoint needs for system reconfiguration. Simulating or even attempting to replicate an issue in the system (in the nonproduction environment—see chapter 9) may be necessary to determine the root cause of why the system consistently produces an error state. Root cause analysis should be conducted on a variety of sample situations. For instance, if one nurse reports that an error state is occurring, do all nurses have the same issue? If not, there may be a data entry error, a training issue, or even a misunderstanding of a term by the one nurse that can easily be corrected with a brief explanation.

Finally, root cause analysis should consider where users are the process of learning the new system and the extent to which basic change is affecting the results of use. Communications may be at issue. In one facility, one nurse was not using the BC-MAR when it was first implemented, complaining that it was difficult to wand patients' wristbands. Very few other nurses had an issue with this task. When the troubled nurse was interviewed, he said that the first time he performed the new task, the patient stated it was like being a can of beans at the grocery store. Believing that all patients felt this way, the nurse immediately came to dislike the task. In this case, the nurse was given a script to help him explain to patients why the process was being performed and how patients benefited from this new approach. Other ways to help implement change can include role-playing or development of a use case (see chapter 5) as a simulation exercise.

Take Corrective Action

Once a problem and its root cause have been identified, steps obviously must be taken to make a change to improve the situation. Unfortunately, such actions are not always taken. It may be that the hospital cannot find any solution at all, or the solution may seem to be too expensive or unlikely to succeed for other reasons. Hospitals must commit to taking some form of corrective action, even if the action needs to be delayed until a vendor can resolve the issue or enhance the product, or until the next upgrade arrives. If the solution is related to workflows or training, the corrective action must be implemented in at least a staged manner.

Provide Feedback

Communication to users during the corrective action investigation and implementation is essential. Some form of corrective action is almost always feasible. Users should be informed of the corrective action(s) being taken, results should be monitored closely during initial go-live, and users should be given help to manage the change. If training was insufficient during the first go-live with a system, increased training on the corrective action should be conducted. If workflows and process improvements were not made initially but are being made now, users must be engaged in their development, implementation, and assessment to determine that the action does, in fact, result in improvement. Users are not the only ones from whom feedback is necessary. Management must also provide feedback in the form of transparent measurement and celebration of success. Appreciation for bearing with the hospital, commendation for raising the issue and helping find a solution, and even recognition for small steps toward improvement must be provided. If things are still not going well, the hospital must also acknowledge this challenge and continue to work with the users to find solutions. Change management strategies are very important to put into place. In fact, the hospital may find that it needs to change its culture to help improve results of significant changes. In those rare cases where corrective action cannot be taken, hospitals should be transparent about the lack of a solution and explain why.

Continuous Improvement

As optimization occurs, the hospital will likely find not only improved patient outcomes but also a change in the organizational culture toward being more supportive of the use of the EHR and other types of health IT. These are notable accomplishments, but there is more work to be done. EHRs and other health IT systems will continue to mature. The pace of enhancements should not be so fast that they are difficult to keep up with, but they should be anticipated and welcomed. Continuous improvement requires continuous monitoring, measurement, and feedback.

As optimization succeeds, users may become more amenable to additional innovative solutions. Some of these maybe changes they come up with themselves. If so, the hospital needs a formal means to share the change with others and have the new solution sanctioned, if necessary. Some proposed changes may be changes in personal workflows. Other users may benefit from learning such "tips" from their peers and having the opportunity to adopt them. Other possible changes, however, could be detrimental. Therefore, some method is necessary for collecting and reviewing all changes to determine whether they can be included in a hospital's best practices. This process should be supportive and transparent—and not viewed as stifling innovative thinking.

Check Your Understanding 14.1

Choose the best answer:

1. Optimization of EHR occurs:

   a. After initial use

   b. At go-live

   c. Before vendor selection

   d. During requirements specification

2. The *least* effective way to engage stakeholders in EHR optimization is likely to be:

   a. Informal communications

   b. Monthly meetings

   c. Open door gatherings

   d. Technology tracking of adoption rates

3. Process mapping conducted during EHR optimization is an example of:

   a. Executive management responsibility

   b. Measurement of adoption

   c. Root cause analysis

   d. Stakeholder input

4. If corrective action cannot be taken, the recommended next step is to:

   a. Explain why

   b. Ignore need

   c. Offer alternatives

   d. Plan to address in the future

5. If measurement finds more error *after* implementing corrective action, the most likely cause is:

   a. Baseline data were wrong

   b. Measurement is inaccurate

   c. Metrics were wrong

   d. Users may be sabotaging measurement

Optimization Strategies for EHR Components for Hospitals

Once an overall strategy for optimization is developed and announced, the migration path can be used to plot the course of the optimization across all areas of need. The following sections provide specific suggestions for best practices and ways to optimize use of the core clinical components that comprise the EHR. It should be recognized that, just as with the original development of the hospital's migration path, there will be dependencies between applications, technology, people, policy, and process. For example, optimal use of a given application may require use of a different input device or changing policy to allow users to bring their own devices. Workflow changes, retraining, and reinforcement on existing practices are frequently found to contribute to optimization.

Results Management

Clinical View

Access to laboratory test results is the most fundamental function clinicians want as they approach information system adoption. The American Clinical Laboratory Association has observed that laboratory test results influence more than 70 percent of clinical decisions (Roe 2008). Interest in better access to diagnostic studies results—including laboratory test results, anatomic pathology reports, radiology reports, and diagnostic study images—crosses all departments and users and provides the most immediate value to the clinician. Even if the results are presented in view-only mode, providers still get significant benefit from access. In the hospital, the function of making results accessible is typically called **results review**.

Comprehensive View

Going beyond results review is **results management**, which is typically defined as the presentation of results of diagnostic studies in an accurate, timely, accessible, interpretable, and targeted manner (Darcy and Kretzschmar 2010). Clinical laboratory results management requires results data to be in structured format so that results may be trended, graphed with other data, and used in CDS. To optimize results management, a hospital might upgrade its EHR to make the data more accessible on a mobile device or offer additional options for constructing and displaying graphics. **Data visualization** is a relatively new technique to actuate in information systems the human need for visual representations of information for easier understanding and improved retention (SAS n.d.) Data visualization often transforms text into a graphical display, but it can also wrap context around structured data (Few 2013). Most results management systems already have some such support in the form of using color or symbols to highlight a result that is out of normal range. Data visualization, however, can also be interactive, such as enabling a user to adjust the amount of data to be viewed simultaneously. For example, a user may only wish to see laboratory test results for a given patient for the past two days but then decide two weeks of data would be better. Adding data visualization to results management may be a feasible optimization opportunity, but it should be used with caution to ensure that the results change outcomes significantly.

Drug-lab checking, is a process of identifying whether a drug being ordered is suitable for the patient, especially evident from laboratory test results. For example, a number of medications are contraindicated for patients with liver disease. When such a drug is entered into the CPOE system, the system should check for a liver function study and advise the provider accordingly. Unfortunately, not all EHRs accommodate such functionality, which has not been a requirement of the MU incentive program. Integrating the data in a manner that supports clinical decision making generally requires a clinical data repository and a more sophisticated CDS rules engine than is presently found in some EHRs.

Anatomic pathology results are often provided in a dictated report but may also include some structured data. Blood banks are also often associated with laboratory systems and have unique requirements and applications as well. Radiology and other diagnostic study images stored in a picture archiving and communications system (PACS) should provide advanced visualization tools such as three-dimensional navigation and series mapping for the variety of modalities used by radiologists, cardiologists, orthopedists, ophthalmologists, and other specialists (for example, x-ray photos, computed tomography, magnetic resonance imaging, ultrasound, electrocardiograms, and many others).

Results management may be viewed more broadly than only from the clinical perspective. Results management begins with registration of the patient or an order placed for the study. Then, depending on the type of study, the process involves scheduling and performing the procedure or collecting, delivering, and processing the sample; analyzing the results; quality assurance; tracking results; reporting the results in a manner that can be managed as desired by the end-user clinician; capturing charges; and patient follow-up. Several different applications, crossing different types of standard protocols, are involved in the total results management workflow picture for both laboratory test results from the laboratory information system (LIS) and radiology results from the radiology information systems (RIS) and PACS (see figure 14.3).

Addressing Challenges in Results Management

Although some of the steps in the comprehensive view of the results management workflow are administrative, the accuracy and timeliness with which these steps are performed can also impact the quality of the clinical results management process. This is especially true for ordering, reporting results, updating and correcting results, and exchanging and integrating data across different care settings.

Design issues associated with CPOE systems are discussed later in this chapter. Suffice it to say that there are both technical designs and human factors that must ensure that the right order is written for the right patient and the results are directed to the right location. This challenge is especially compounded in laboratory testing and radiology (the latter is used here as a collective term to refer to all diagnostic imaging studies, whether performed by radiology, cardiology, or others). Many hospital laboratory and radiology departments serve not only the hospital's own inpatients but also its own outpatients and its physician offices' patients, and these departments may potentially as a reference site for other hospitals (in or out of the hospital's own integrated delivery network) and other physicians. Hospitals may also send laboratory test specimens to other commercial laboratories if they are understaffed or do not perform certain specialized tests. Hospitals will use reference laboratories to validate results for certain types of tests. "Night hawk" services are very common, in which diagnostic study images are sent electronically for reading to other parts of the world during "off hours." Therefore, getting patient demographics right during the registration process is a critical first step to ensuring that orders are placed and results are received correctly.

Another issue associated with CPOE and results management is test-naming conventions. Even in a closed environment, which rarely exists anymore, test names can change over time, and different users may use different terms for the same test. Physicians who went to medical school or previously practiced in a different part of the country or world may not use the same terms as the

Figure 14.3.   Results management

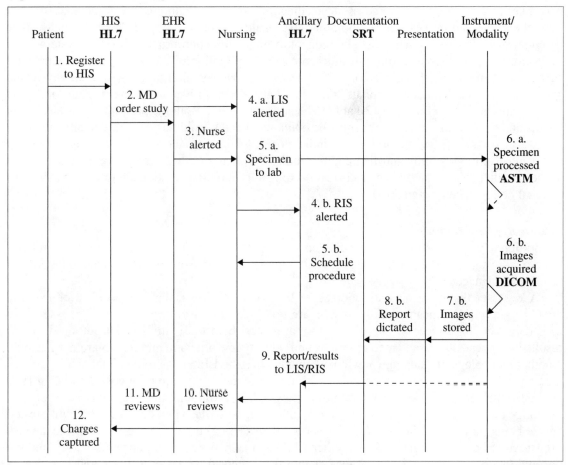

hospital in which they currently admit patients. Across different hospitals, naming conventions represent an exponentially larger challenge. One of the major commercial laboratories observed that it had stored as synonyms 21 different "names" (that is, spellings and abbreviations) for the very common test to measure blood sugar levels in people with diabetes. *Glycosylated hemoglobin* is technically the correct name for this test, but most people refer to it as hemoglobin A1c, which may also be written as HbA1c, HgA1c, A1c, "hemoglobin," and many other variations.

Workflows associated with carrying out orders are another challenge. Although workflow issues are not unique to an EHR environment, they sometimes can be exacerbated in an automated situation. For example, an order can be placed for a blood product where nursing has no order to transfuse; another example is the assumption that a laboratory test order was placed when the dose of a medication to be administered depends on laboratory test results. Diagnostic study procedures frequently have to be canceled because the patient was not prepped on time for various reasons, including ordering and resulting. A similar workflow issue relates to who will collect a laboratory test specimen and when. Will nursing always keep an eye on the computer to ensure timely completion of tasks? If the laboratory test order is simultaneously sent to nursing and the laboratory, will a phlebotomist appear to take the patient's blood within minutes of a nurse having drawn the blood? Other issues relate to whether special comments can be added to an order, such as "do not collect specimen from left arm" or "patient allergic to a specific contrast medium." Will laboratory test draws be timed in a manner consistent with medication administration issues? Will laboratory personnel and radiologists have access to medication orders and administration records to determine their potential impact on the laboratory test results or imaging study? There are many other potential workflow issues that should be thought through with appropriate policy and system build to ensure that the diagnostic study results represent the intention of the ordering provider. Many such issues can potentially be overcome through alerts; however, alert fatigue (for both physicians and nurses) is such that many hospitals "pick their battles" carefully to avoid overreliance on alerts.

Updates and corrections must be able to be accommodated. Both the preliminary or erroneous results and final or corrected results must be maintained and should be accessible to anyone needing to access them. There should be clear indication of who, what, and when any change occurs to any results (or reports of diagnostic imaging studies), with any further explanation in notes. Alerts to the fact that there is an update or correction to results should also be made in accordance with hospital policy (Wiedemann 2010).

Laboratory Test Results

In addition to the results-management challenges already described that are common to both laboratory test results and diagnostic imaging study reports; there are some issues unique to laboratory test results management.

A key issue that hospitals must address for the MU incentives is that many LISs produce only "flat" reports, which means that the results are provided only as a printer-ready file, essentially as if they were on a piece of paper. This format makes them look familiar, but putting data and results into a repository and creating graphs and other types of data manipulation are not feasible. Another technological challenge previously noted is that the LIS and automated laboratory instruments ("autoanalyzers") are not designed with the same data exchange protocol—LIS using HL7 and autoanalyzers using ASTM International (now CLSI). Although interfaces can be written to exchange these data, they are expensive and challenging to write. They must be thoroughly tested before being put into production. Interfaces (and their testing) are also necessary when exchanging structured data from one LIS to another LIS, such as between a reference laboratory and the hospital laboratory, although these types of interfaces tend to be easier to write and less expensive. Finally, laboratories and other parts of hospitals make extensive use of robots to transport specimens and load specimens into autoanalyzers. Although these robots are highly efficient and often very effective, they are still computer systems that also must be appropriately used (Lum and D'Amarino 2009).

Delivery of test results can be yet another source of potential safety issues. An example of a laboratory test results review screen is provided in figure 14.4.

Delivery of results includes addressing regulatory requirements of the **Clinical Laboratory Improvements Amendments (CLIA)**, display of results, identifying results as preliminary or final, flagging results as normal or abnormal, communication handoffs, updates and corrections, and integrating laboratory test data across performing laboratories. For example, the hospital's laboratory may send alert about an abnormal laboratory test result via a page to the ordering provider and include a red exclamation mark on the results themselves; another laboratory sending results to the hospital may not be able to page the provider and may use a different set of symbols (for example, "low" and "high," or down arrow and up arrow) to designate abnormal results. There may also be inconsistency between views of laboratory test results, such as those on the actual laboratory report and those transferred (electronically or manually) to a flow sheet. "Abnormal" is also subject to communication issues. Although it would seem that physicians should look at results themselves, such a review is not always convenient. However, if the physician asks a nurse for the result, the nurse may indicate it is normal. That could be an accurate statement of the current result, but the interval change between the current result and last result might be abnormal. There also may be comments from the laboratory that should be considered in light of the actual results. Units of

Figure 14.4.   Example of results review screen

	Last	Next		

MRI: 123-456   Name: Patient Name   DOB: 01/01/1940   Sex: M

Laboratory Results: 03/12   10:25:30

03/12/11	3 days ▼	All labs ▼	Display	Clear

Collected: 12/14	Iron/Iron Binding Capacity		Updated: 03/11	
Iron (Iron)		23	L	33–150	UG/DL
Iron Binding Capacity (IBC)		139	L	210–400	UG/DL
Collected: 06/02	Urea Nitrogen		Updated: 03/10	
Plasma Post Dialysis					
Urea Nitrogen (UN)		18		8–20	MG/DL

measure may also differ. Today, there are three different standard **units of measure** deployed by various laboratories (and imaging centers), including ANSI X3.50, ISO 2955, and the Unified Code for Units of Measure (Schadow 2009).

The MU incentives require that use of the Logical Observation Identifiers Names and Codes (LOINC) for laboratory tests. However, it should be recognized that LOINC only provides codes for names of tests, whereas other coding systems, such as Systematized Nomenclature of Medicine (SNOMED), provides codes for the results. LISs, however, must attach the LOINC code for the test to the result message to ensure proper matching that the result for a specific test ordered has been resulted (Darcy 2010).

Finally, a 2014 amendment to the CLIA regulations now permits patients to access their test results directly from a laboratory. Previously, CLIA required that all laboratory test results be sent to the ordering provider, which often delaying the reporting of results to the patient (HHS 2014).

While all of the potential issues with results management are real and documented here to draw attention to the need for careful planning and ongoing monitoring (Yackel and Embi 2010), it should be emphasized that there are many significant benefits of these systems—including both for patient care and cost reduction. Although some of the challenges in results management are certainly attributable to the technology itself, many are associated with human factors—systems that have not been fully configured to meet a specific hospital's needs, not fully tested after being configured, and not used by users as intended (Callen et al. 2011).

Diagnostic Imaging Reports

Diagnostic imaging reports are by nature different than laboratory test results and present some distinctive challenges, although, as previously described there are some common issues, too.

A key difference between laboratory data and diagnostic imaging results is that the latter are essentially in two parts: the report and the image itself. **Diagnostic imaging reports** are typically a dictated summary of findings with respect to the purpose of the study and the image. Today, however, there are several improvements on this traditional process. Speech recognition technology (SRT) is widely used by radiologists, who typically view images on one or more monitors and dictate while reviewing and correcting the report simultaneously on another monitor (see figure 14.5).

These reports are then electronically fed as documents into the EHR. Some of these SRT systems enable discrete reportable transcription (DRT) that embed data mining tools within them to produce structured data. There are also a number of companies that offer structured data entry templates—which may be used solely (Liu 2003) or in combination with SRT, as speech commands, as well as population of demographic and clinical information from connected systems (Lang 2009).

The Radiological Society of North America (RSNA) has been conducting a radiology reporting initiative to foster adoption of best-practices reporting methods in radiology and other imaging specialties (RSNA 2011). RSNA, in conjunction with the American College of Radiology (ACR), has also created a lexicon to organize and retrieve radiology information, replacing the ACR Index for Radiological Diagnoses and supplementing other lexicons and standards including SNOMED-CT and Digital Imaging and Communications in Medicine (DICOM) (Langlotz 2006).

Not surprisingly, the move to more structured data for reporting radiology and other imaging studies has its controversies and naysayers. Weiss and Langlotz (2008) have evaluated the pros and cons of structured data in radiology reporting. Benefits cited include retrievability and reuse of data, consistency in report organization, and standardized language. While recognizing the first two benefits as important, the main counterargument is that having to focus on the structured template interferes with the image interpretation process, especially as most imaging systems require constant use of two hands to manipulate various views of the images being studied. It is also argued that "point-and-click reporting" is impractical for complex cases and that even the natural language processing technology embedded in the DRT systems has limitations. In summarizing these positions, the authors suggest that there is probably a common ground where a blend of technology may be necessary, especially for different types of cases. Similarly, the American College of Cardiology and several other organizations have jointly issued a health policy statement on structured reporting in cardiovascular imaging and draw much the same conclusion that a balanced approach is preferred, not only in the technologies used but the scope of the report needing to be both complete and concise (Douglas 2008).

Figure 14.5.   RIS-PACS

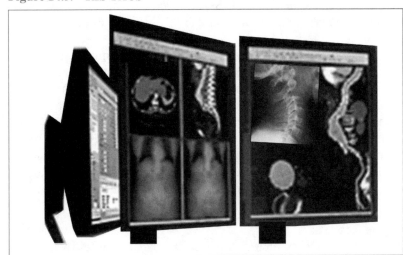

Copyright © 2016 Margret\A Consulting, LLC. Reprinted with permission.

Digital images managed in PACS are the second part of the imaging studies report. As of 2008, PACS had replaced film in 76 percent of US hospitals, and the rate of PACS use has been steadily rising since first deployed in the mid-1980s (Tieche et al. 2010). Although there were initial concerns about whether digital images could be of diagnostic quality, new technologies—including the ability to run PACS on personal computers (Diagnostic Imaging 2003), medical-grade high-resolution LCD monitors, and calibration sensors and software (Tyagi and Hagen 2006)—have enabled greater versatility with digital images than film could ever provide, as well as the benefits of economical storage, rapid retrieval, access to images acquired through multiple modalities, and simultaneous access at multiple sites. Many hospitals provide access to their PACS to their medical staff in their offices via a physician portal, but increasingly the images are being copied to CDs and given to patients to take with them as needed to other providers, who can then view them very successfully on more standard workstations (Cape Cod Health n.d.).

Some considerations in acquiring PACS include the fact that they are classified as medical devices and hence regulated by the Food and Drug Administration (FDA) (2016). Still, when planning optimization, adherence to DICOM standards and Integrating the Healthcare Enterprise profiles is essential (Boochever 2004). These standards help enable integration between RIS and PACS (Tomczak 2002) and PACS with modalities (Mack 2005). They also aid data migration as systems are upgraded (Massat 2008). Note that integration and data migration capabilities are qualified—to this day, integration issues remain due to optionality in standards and vendors applying proprietary tags or attempting to sell fully integrated RIS/PACS rather than enabling interfacing (Means 2009).

Point of Care (POC) Documentation

Whereas results management is fairly well advanced in many hospitals and viewed very favorably by clinicians, **point of care (POC) documentation**, which is clinician use of the EHR not only to view but to document, or chart, the clinician's findings and actions, is not as well liked. With the exception of special forms of documentation that essentially have their own applications—notably CPOE and BC-MAR—POC documentation has been a much harder sell to physicians and nurses alike.

Nursing Documentation

Nursing documentation currently is the primary focus of much POC documentation. Many hospitals start their POC documentation with documentation of nurse assessments and care planning. In many cases, the nursing documentation is further categorized into separate modules, where some hospitals may start with certain assessment templates, then add additional assessment templates, and finally add alerts and prompts associated with standard assessments. There are many different types of assessments, some of which are identified in table 14.1.

Each assessment includes a critical action point. Automating the alerts means the nurse does not have to remember each separate standard and its critical value. Instead, the nurse can focus on doing the assessment using clinical knowledge, with the computer tracking and monitoring for criticality. When standards change, which they often do, online systems can be updated. The assessments can be used further to generate orders for physician review and approval (Ligon and de los Reyes 2005).

Other nursing documentation that has been automated includes interdisciplinary consultations, vital signs, intake and output, plan of care, problem list, POC testing and specimen labeling, shift reports, and patient education. Hospitals also have found success with providing access to clinical reference tools and incorporating nurse staffing and patient acuity to automate nurse staffing by patient acuity functions (King et al. 2004). **Nurse staffing by patient acuity** refers to how many nurses are needed to treat the hospital's patients given the nature of their illnesses.

Table 14.1.   Examples of automated nursing assessment results and other prompts

Assessment	Action
Admission assessment	Orders for physician review and approval
Home medication order sheet	Orders for continued medications for physician review and approval
Functional status screens	Orders for physical therapy, speech therapy, or occupational therapy for physician review and approval
Body mass index calculations for obese surgical patients	Special treatment and preparation protocols
Alcohol-use screen	Alcohol withdrawal protocol
Smoking assessment	"Stop-smoking" patient education Nicotine withdrawal protocol
High risk for falls	Special alerts
History of congestive heart failure	Patient education
Multidisciplinary needs assessment	Automatic notification to chaplain, case management, nutrition services, enterostomy therapy, infection control
Immunization screening	Orders for pneumococcal and influenza vaccinations for physician review and approval
Lab test orders requiring fasting	"Hold tray" order
Radiology procedures requiring special patient preparation	Specific preparation information and timing information and/or alert

Source: Ligon and de los Reyes 2005.

Hospitals are further investigating the ability to manage an enterprise patient safety program through automated warnings when a patient's vital signs indicate an oncoming crisis or physical deterioration. This automation allows across-the-hospital surveillance of spikes in temperature, hemodynamic instability, potential adverse drug reactions, or dangerous blood glucose levels (Rogoski 2005).

Although there are many benefits of an EHR to nurses, many have been uncomfortable adopting their use—and frustration seems to be growing. In 2014, Miliard reported that hospital nurse retention and recruitment were being hindered by poorly implemented EHRs and a lack input from nurses into the EHR selection process. The latest data available show that 55 percent of the nursing workforce is age 50 years or older, and that annual turnover rates in hospitals of 14 percent do not make up for the 10 percent rate of growth in positions that is needed (AACN 2014). There are many factors for nurse attrition, but hospitals can ill afford to lose nurses as a result of technology that should improve rather than reduce productivity and job satisfaction (Miliard 2014a; 2014b).

A number of studies have been conducted on the impact of the EHR on nursing productivity and workflow, and the results are contradictory. Keenan (2008) conducted an extensive literature review and found that many surveys reported that nurses were dissatisfied with what they perceive as the time-consuming nature of recording (which varied by age and attitudes toward computers in general). A study by Moody and colleagues (2004) reported similar findings, but these authors also stated that 81 percent of nurses found that EHRs were more a help than a hindrance to care. Other studies also reported real benefits from EHRs for nursing documentation, especially in focused areas. For example, Gunningberg and colleagues (2009) found that EHRs improved the quality and comprehensiveness in nursing documentation of pressure ulcers. This documentation is also helping physicians attend to and better document their role in care for pressure ulcers, improving compliance with value-based purchasing initiatives, such as Medicare's Medicare Severity Diagnosis Related Group (MS-DRG) payment methodology (Hale 2009). Another focus area where improvements are evident is the accuracy of nurses' diagnoses (Lunney 2008), which can have broad-based implications, including for nurse scheduling based on acuity and support for creation of evidence-based care and practice guidelines.

Moody and colleagues also found less than optimal functionality in the nature of systems that nurses were expected to use. For instance, 61 percent of nurses reported having to log on to multiple documentation systems, and 61 percent reported software and system problems. More than half (54 percent) of the nurses surveyed indicated that they were using duplicate methods of clinical documentation—often using worksheets, scraps of paper, or paper towels to document at the bedside and then transcribing the results at the nursing unit. Their reasons for this type of documentation included a reluctance to use the computer in front of the patient or patient's family, an insufficient number of workstations or workstations not conducive to POC charting, or simply difficulty breaking old habits (Moody et al. 2004).

With regard to the questions of nurses' productivity, Keenan found that the number of studies in the literature review that concluded EHRs saved time in documentation was nearly equal to the number that found documentation time increased. Interestingly, chart audits consistently revealed an increase in the quality of nursing documentation, reduction in the variability of charting, and an increase in charting compliance. This same survey of the literature observed that time spent documenting patient care (even in a paper environment) is generally not regarded by nurses as being patient care, even though there is a Nursing Intervention Classification term for it. It was also noted that nurses regularly copied data from the health record and other documents to create personal records that guided their activities. A work sampling study found that nurses spent on average 15.8 percent of their shift time on some form of documentation, with 10.6 percent for entry on paper and 5.2 percent on the computer (Keenan 2008).

Some lessons learned for optimizing use of the EHR by nurses is to ensure that nurses are given general computer training, not just keyboarding skills. One hospital reported that although its system experienced virtually no downtime, the nurses were very concerned about access and availability of the computer (Barrameda 2011). Specific **contingency plans** for reverting to paper processes in the event of downtime were developed and practiced as part of disaster recovery drills. Even showing nurses how to clear printer jams seemed to be reassuring to them, even though this task is not necessarily something that should be part of their job. **Role-specific training** that addresses the unique needs of each of the users is vital. This same hospital created "one day in the life of a nurse" training materials that took nurses step by step through the workflow associated with using the EHR. Where physicians tend to want only minimal and one-on-one training, nurses usually prefer to learn in groups and seem to almost want to be overtrained to anticipate and be able to deal with virtually every contingency. Lunney (2008) describes the need to supply nurses with situational context and models of nurse-patient relationships. Finally, measurement and recognition of success are important to keep interest up and as motivation for ongoing use. Again, the hospital cited above took care to study and provide actual results about what was happening when the EHR was first introduced. Although focused on medication administration (discussed further below), the hospital did a time-in-motion study to evaluate how long it took nurses to use the BC-MAR in comparison to paper processes and found—actually to their surprise—that nurses using the BC-MAR were significantly faster with more complete documentation. Reporting this finding to nurses reassured them that what they may perceive as a longer process was actually shorter, often as a result of less rework (Barrameda 2011). A cautionary note, however, should be applied here. This finding could have had a negative effect if nurses felt they were being asked to speed up their processes or could have encouraged them to slow down if they felt the end result was more work. Expectations must be set so time savings accrue to professional nursing duties and caring more for patients.

Physician Documentation

Physician documentation done outside of the physician's own office of items other than orders in hospitals has been a considerable challenge—both because physicians are not always willing to cooperate in the use of the EHR and because designing suitable tools is difficult. In a report to the eHealth Initiative in 2008, Agarwal and colleagues observed that clinical documentation systems were beginning to take on a more prominent role in inpatient medical care but the documentation is not at the level envisioned even five years earlier. A study in the hospital system overseen by the Veterans Health Administration of the US Department of Veterans Affairs (VA) found improved documentation availability, legibility, and education opportunities, but the authors also found that the quality of the notes was not always satisfactory and workflow and communication actually suffered (Embi et al. 2004). Hirschtick (2006) described electronic documentation as "bloated and obfuscated," "awkward," and often wrong when physicians used the copy-and-paste functionality to overcome the often list-like nature of output from structured data entry.

Still, EHRs in general have benefits that physicians value, including the ability to access information anywhere. Health IT systems that allow the user to tap into enormous digital data sets are being deployed. Such tools are especially helpful to optimize differential diagnosis when physicians are confronted with an unusual constellation of signs and symptoms.

As people are living longer, they are experiencing a greater number of chronic conditions and taking an increasing number of drugs. Thus, it is often unclear whether a patient's signs and symptoms are attributable to one or more of the underlying conditions or related to an adverse reaction to one or more of the drugs (Ruscin and Linnebur 2014). "Symptom checkers" are available via physician apps, and, in some cases, are accessible to the public online (Gilchrist 2015). Integrating these tools into an EHR could optimize the EHR's value to physicians.

EHRs could also be further enhanced through the use of data visualization tools that can integrate text from multiple sources and present them in user-friendly analytical formats (Braunstein 2014). Having the ability to review a comprehensive set of information about the patient displayed in an easy-to-use format prior to seeing the patient can improve decision making and enhance efficiency. However, physicians need to use these tools with care and not neglect face time with patients. At one VA hospital, patients complained about not seeing their doctors because house staff members were able to perform so many functions via the EHR in the staff lounge (Embi et al. 2004).

The bottom line with respect to the value of POC documentation for physicians, however, is difficult to assess, as noted by Raimey, because so few hospitals have implemented a comprehensive electronic physician documentation system (2010). Many hospitals are using a blended approach of transcription and structured-data entry templates (Cannon and Lucci 2010), which, in fact, may continue to be the best approach for some time to come. Two physicians offer key points to consider in optimizing use of physician documentation:

- Lipsitz (2010) observes that "we physicians haven't been taught very much about documentation in medical school or training." Although Lipsitz is a medical reviewer for a denials management company who sees the "worst of the worst," she makes the point that poor documentation practices "can lead to erroneous coding, improper DRG calculations, denials, and difficulty filing appeals." She believes "most physicians don't understand the link between what they write in a medical record and what the hospital—and they—get paid. Nor do they understand the very real risks of fraud and abuse charges than can result from patterns of errors." Attorneys Romney and Hayward (2014) confirm this situation remains prevalent today.

- Essin (2011) urges his physician counterparts to "think clinical process, not automation." He asserts that, "in the future, medicine will be practiced in a way that information, encompassing discrete data elements, narrative, audio, video, etc. will be captured, stored and used as an integral part of delivering patient care." He believes, however, this type of practice is not possible today for several reasons—including the focus on "automating the chart" and not focusing on finding ways "to re-invent the clinical workflow in ways that a computer could be incorporated into the process without causing excessive disruption." He reminds hospital executives that clinicians perform "knowledge work" that "bears no relationship to a manufacturing production line."

The American College of Physicians (ACP) has adopted policy recommendations for optimizing clinical documentation in an EHR environment (Kuhn et al. 2015). ACP encourages its members to engage with their hospitals and practices to apply these recommendations throughout the continuum of care. The ACP recommendations are summarized below:

1. The primary purpose of clinical documentation should be to support patient care and improve clinical outcomes through enhanced communication.

2. Physicians working with their care delivery organizations, medical societies, and others should define professional standards for clinical documentation practices.

3. As value-based care and accountable care models grow, the primary purpose of the EHR should remain the facilitation of seamless patient care to improve outcomes while contributing to data collection that supports necessary analysis.

4. Structured data should be captured only where they are useful in care delivery or essential for quality assessment or reporting.

5. Prior authorizations, as well as other documents required by other entities [e.g., health plans and regulators] must no longer be unique in their data content and format requirements.

6. Patient access to progress notes, as well as the rest of their medical records, may offer a way to improve both patient engagement and quality of care.

7. Further research is needed to identify best practices, study authoring processes, understand ways to improve medical education for the growing use of information technology, and determine the most effective methods of disseminating professional standards of clinical documentation and best practices (Kuhn et al. 2015).

Steps are being taken to both better design physician documentation tools and analyze their impact on data integrity in the EHR (Bowman 2013) and quality of care. New technologies are also integrating different types of documentation in ways that can help achieve the best balance of structured data for CDS and research and unstructured data that describe the patient story. Physicians are not naturally opposed to technology, if they perceive that it improves their care of patients. Technological innovations with the potential to make physicians more willing to use EHRs for documentation include speech recognition tools (Chavis 2010), DRT (Cannon and Lucci 2010), and use of HL7's Clinical Document Architecture Release 2 (CDA-R2) standard to unlock transcribed notes that "support information flow between narrative notes and EHR systems" (Health Story Project 2009). Another new technology being adopted is the smart pen that integrates a digital audio recorder and handwriting recognition with an EHR (Shareableink. com 2011). These and other technologies, perhaps yet to be invented, should not only address the need for more readable documentation but reduce the risk of "template thinking," which seems to come from some uses of EHRs (Koriwchak 2011), where the EHR template may influence the physician's thought process in ways that preclude consideration for outlier diagnoses if a patient's condition does not fit the template. A blended approach that supports physicians' natural workflow and facilitates better physician adoption will likely achieve faster MU of EHR because it is "practical use," as suggested by one vendor (Webmedx n.d.).

Medication Management

As EHRs and other forms of health IT are developed and implemented, significant attention is being placed on **closed-loop medication management**, a process that integrates all components of medication ordering, verifying, dispensing, and administering in order to provide safe and effective patient care (Smaling and Holt 2005), because this process typically involves CPOE and BC-MAR systems, as well as **medication reconciliation** (the process of verifying medications at each point of patient transfer), automated drug dispensing equipment, and other related systems. Figure 14.6 illustrates the components of medication management, reflects the proportion of errors that have been made without automated assistance at each point, according to studies by Bates and colleagues (1997) and Santell (2005), and identifies information system applications intended to reduce errors and improve patient safety. A study by Farrell puts medication order

Figure 14.6.   Medication management

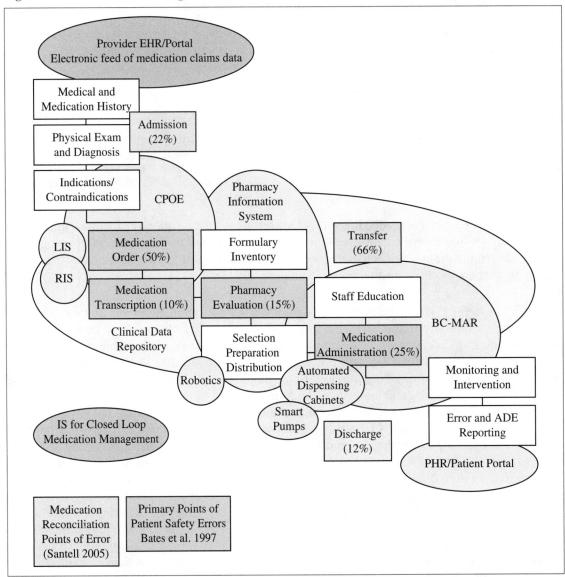

Source: Compiled from data published by Bates et al. 1997 and Santell 2005. Illustration copyright © 2016 Margret\A Consulting, LLC. Reprinted with permission.

errors at about 39 percent, medication transcription errors at 12 percent, pharmacy evaluation/dispensing errors at 11 percent, and medication administration errors at 38 percent, and observes that while "only" 50 percent of the first three sources of error reach the patient—the others being caught in subsequent processes—98 percent of the medication administration errors reach the patient 2008.

To improve patient safety, the EHR components of CPOE and BC-MAR have been required for earning incentives under the MU program and, prior to that, were part of other stimulus efforts by employer groups, the Joint Commission, and others seeking to reduce cost and improve quality. In light of continuing concerns, Meeks and colleagues (2014) conducted a study of medication incidents and found that 74 percent involved unsafe technology and the remaining involved unsafe use of the technology. Nontechnical dimensions of medication incidents included workflow, policy, and personnel interactions with technology. Technical dimensions included unmet data-display needs, software upgrades or modifications that were not implemented properly (often due to hidden dependencies between two or more systems), and data transmission issues between components of the EHR. The Veterans Health Administration has had an EHR for many years, and it is one of few organizations that have a dedicated Office of Informatics and Analysis, which is continuously monitoring opportunities for improvement and optimization in their system (Weston and Roberts 2013). VA hospitals have found significant benefits from their closed-loop medication management systems, and the Veterans Health Administration plans to deploy more of the components in outpatient VA facilities as well. However, in their 2014 study on medication incidents, in which the VA participated, Meeks and colleagues noted that a study of nontechnological factors such as user behaviors, clinical workflow demands, and organizational policies and procedures is needed. The study by Meeks and colleagues also observed that acute care settings are at higher risk than physician offices, especially for medication errors made in CPOE as opposed to e-prescribing systems, because of the complexity of care, time critical interventions, systems, staffing, and communications systems (Meeks 2014; Chapman 2014).

One of the outcomes of the study by Meeks and colleagues is a list of recommendations for mitigating EHR-related safety concerns within closed-loop medication management components. Table 14.2 lists these recommendations for each of the categories of concerns identified. Monitoring and measuring practices with a system-wide scope are necessary to track incidents, identify what is working, and continuously improve in areas needing attention.

Electronic/Bar Code Medication Administration Record Systems

A significant element of online documentation for nursing has been electronic medication administration records (EMAR). Some EMAR systems are essentially preprinted forms generated by the pharmacy system on which medication administration information is recorded in legible form and used by nurses to guide their actual administration. Documentation of the administration is still conducted on that paper form but is improved by making the medication information legible.

Table 14.2.   Suggested mitigating procedures for EHR-related safety concerns

Category of Concern	Examples of Mitigating Procedures
Unmet display needs	• Real world testing • Check visibility of data
Software modifications	• Test all modifications prior to go-live • Explore impact of changes on workflow
System to system interfaces	• Disallow partial transmission of information
Hidden dependencies among distributed systems	• Document ideal actions • Make dependencies explicit in software and workflows

Source: Summarized from Meeks, et al. 2014.

Another form of EMAR is sometimes referred to as *bedside medication verification*. In these applications, a computerized dispensing system is used at the bedside along with a computer that displays the medication administration record form. The computer enables the drug to be visually compared with a picture on the computer, is able to provide drug knowledge information to the nurse, and supports accurate and timely recording of the medication administration. See figure 14.7 for an example.

Positive patient identification via use of bar codes or radio frequency identification (RFID) has been added to many EMAR systems (then called BC-MAR systems). In this case, the entire medication administration record process is automated from the point of retrieving information on what medications are to be administered to documenting the actual administration or exception, as outlined in figure 14.8.

EMAR/BC-MAR Challenges

Hospitals should be aware that there are many challenges to implementing EMAR/BC-MAR systems, which are now required under the stage 2 MU incentive program:

- If the hospital is not yet fully using its CPOE system, the transcription into the pharmacy information systems and resultant EMAR/BC-MAR system still must take place manually, which has been found to be a source of error in itself.

- The BC-MAR system depends on the ability to have bar-coded unit doses available. The FDA has required that all human drug products and biological products have bar codes on the package that identifies the drug or biological (FDA 2004). However, this requirement relates only to the package, which may be the bottle of pills in the pharmacy. If the hospital does not purchase drugs in unit dose form, or does not have a unit dose packaging system and qualified staff to perform this function, the use of BC-MAR is not feasible. For small and rural hospitals, this can be a significant challenge. Purchasing drugs in unit dose form is generally more expensive. Not all small hospitals stock all the drugs being ordered, as some drugs may not be used frequently enough and their shelf life may be too short to warrant retaining in inventory. Many small and rural hospitals have to supplement their inventories with drugs from local retail pharmacies. It is possible to purchase a unit-dose drug packaging system, but this is yet another application that adds cost and time to the process.

Figure 14.7.   BC-MAR

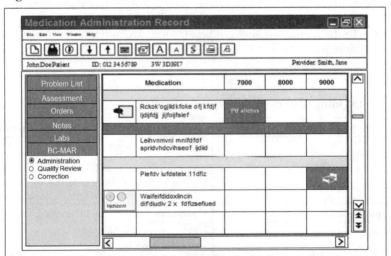

Figure 14.8.   BC-MAR process

1. On patient admission, the hospital gives the patient a bar-coded identification bracelet to link the patient to his or her EHR.

2. When ready to administer the medication, the nurse scans the patient's bar code, which causes the computer to retrieve the patient's EHR.

3. When the patient's EHR displays the medication to be administered, it is retrieved (as a unit dose prepackaged with its own bar code) and scanned.

4. The computer compares the drug that is scanned with the drug that is on the medication administration record. If it is a match, the nurse administers the medication or documents an exception. An exception may include patient refusal or patient not being present. (See step 5.) If it is not a match, the computer displays an error message (for example, wrong patient, wrong dose, wrong drug, or wrong time to administer drug). The nurse can then make the necessary adjustments.

5. Some systems also generate a computerized reminder about what medications patients are scheduled to take and when. This may be generated immediately after all medications are scheduled to be administered and alert nursing personnel that someone may have been missed. This may occur, for example, when the patient is not on the nursing unit at the time medications are normally passed because the patient is having a diagnostic study performed elsewhere in the hospital or is undergoing physical therapy. Some systems automatically advise the nurse when it is appropriate to administer the drug and in what dose so that drugs are not doubled up or skipped altogether.

Finally, not all drugs are easily bar coded. It can be challenging to apply unit dose bar codes to drugs administered through intravenous (IV) bags, especially in the intensive care unit when multiple bags are piggybacked onto a single IV stand, although some hospitals are acquiring their own label makers to tailor the information to the specific admixture (Wideman et al. 2005).

- Another challenge, and the reason to engage a pharmacist early in the implementation process, is that the naming conventions of the drugs used in the EMAR/BC-MAR may not be the same as the drug names in the pharmacy system. Pharmacy systems generally record drug names using the National Drug Code (NDC), which is a naming convention used in naming packages of drugs. The name of the manufacturer, brand name, serial number, and other such information all are elements embedded in this code. However, when providers enter medications into CPOE systems and when nurses record these medications on a medication administration record, they may use terminology that is more clinically relevant. In some cases, they may refer to a proprietary naming convention; in other cases, they may use the RxNorm that has been recommended by the federal government for use in EHRs. A closed-loop medication management system with CPOE, up-to-date pharmacy system, and BC-MAR would enable mapping to occur automatically so that there is equivalency between the naming conventions. If the systems are standalone or only generated from a pharmacy system without the mapping on the naming conventions, the result can be confusing.

Medication Errors

Another potential pitfall in gaining adoption of EMAR/BC-MAR systems is, as previously noted, they may increase errors, or appear to do so. For example, the administration of a drug at the wrong time has always been error, but such an error was often not documented in a paper-based system, especially if the timing was off by only a few minutes. A BC-MAR, however, is tireless in reporting every discrepancy. It is important to define terms associated with errors carefully and recognize that, although the new systems may report more errors than were previously documented, there are likely not more actual errors but potentially better reporting.

Reported errors should be classified by their type, including those that are not true errors, adverse reactions that may have been anticipated, and near misses. Different hospitals use different definitions for these concepts, often driven by differences in required reporting systems. The following definitions are supplied by the Agency for Healthcare Research and Quality (AHRQ):

- **Adverse drug event:** In some reporting systems, *adverse drug event* is a widely encompassing term referring to actual errors, near misses, and adverse drug reactions. In other reporting systems, *adverse drug event* refers solely to harm caused by an actual error in medication management. The derivation of the error may be from one or more sources, not only from medication administration. In implementing an EMAR/BC-MAR system, one of the most frequent increases in error is due to timing. Many of these systems identify a timing error as one with a narrow window. It is important to reach agreement on what an acceptable window of time is; if the window is smaller than previously due to other reporting requirements, workflow and processes should be studied to determine the impact of this change in definition. Because timing can be affected by many factors, including that the patient was not available at the time the medication was to be administered, at least one group of researchers has proposed a "missing dose day" as the quality summary measure of medication omission (FitzHenry et al. 2005).

- *Adverse event* is any injury caused by medical care—for example, postoperative wound infection and pneumothorax from central venous catheter.

- *Sentinel event* is an event in which death or serious harm to a patient has occurred; this term is usually used to refer to events that are not at all expected or acceptable, such as wrong-site surgery or administration of a drug to the wrong patient (Joint Commission 2006).

- *Near miss* is an event or situation that did not produce patient injury but only because of chance (also referred to as a *close call*). This good fortune might reflect robustness of the patient (for example, a patient with penicillin allergy receives penicillin but has no reaction) or be due to a fortuitous, timely intervention (for example, a nurse happens to realize that a physician wrote an order in the wrong chart). EMAR/BC-MAR systems may be able to identify some of these near misses when an alert or reminder is invoked in the CDS component of the application.

- **Adverse drug reaction** is used to describe an adverse effect produced by the use of a medication in the recommended manner. In many cases, these effects may be anticipated. These effects range from nuisance effects (for example, dry mouth with anticholinergic medications) to severe reactions (for example, anaphylaxis due to penicillin when the patient had never previously taken penicillin and therefore it was unknown that the patient was allergic) (AHRQ n.d.).

Workarounds

Another potential pitfall to consider regarding the use of EMAR/BC-MAR systems concerns adherence to procedures. As these systems become more sophisticated, and especially where they significantly change workflow, it is important to (1) engage nursing staff in all aspects of workflow and process changes prior to and during implementation, and (2) ensure that these changes are monitored either for adherence or for potential need to make adjustments. Sometimes, staff do not have input into or training in systems that change their workflow. As a result, staff members find workarounds to solve either real or perceived problems in workflow, which can put patient safety at risk or limit productivity. For example, some pharmacy dispensing systems require the nurse to unload the medications and stock them into the workstation on wheels (WOW) or kiosk for administration, thereby altering nursing workflow, increasing the time nurses need to administer medications, and potentially requiring nurses to assume a role typically played by pharmacy technicians. From the nurses' perspective, the preferred scenario would be that the pharmacy delivers trays for each WOW or kiosk.

Phillips and Berner (2004) identified a number of ways nurses have found to "beat the system" when they find issues, which were also identified in a number of VA medical centers (Mills et al. 2006). Koppel et al. (2008) also found a number of similar workarounds as they documented 15 different ways nurses failed to use the BC-MAR systems as intended, with as many as 31 types of causes. Workarounds included everything from affixing copies of patient identification bar codes to the nursing unit so they could "wand" the patient there instead of at the bedside to scanning a single medication package multiple times (similar to the method used at the grocery checkout counter where the purchase is for five of the same item). Reasons given for such workarounds were cited as unreadable medication bar codes, malfunctioning scanners, failing batteries on the WOWs, and so on.

It is important to plan thoroughly for EMAR/BC-MAR implementations. The American Hospital Association (AHA), Health Research and Educational Trust, and the Institute for Safe Medication Practices (ISMP) have compiled an excellent tool titled *Pathways for Medication Safety: Assessing Bedside Bar-coding Readiness* (2002) for this purpose. This readiness assessment considers learning curving; nurse resistance to change; lack of portability of equipment; technology problems relating to hardware, software, or wireless network capability; and definition of what results in a reportable medication error.

Swenson (2007) identifies the following recommendations for optimizing EMAR/BC-MAR systems:

- Think about the workflow for nurses as well as through the entire medication management process.

- Analyze product design, including not only the application but the human–computer interface device that is essential to preventing workarounds.

- Scrutinize software capabilities to ensure that the systems are simple to use, yet powerful in their support.

- Ensure one-to-one. Devices must be ubiquitous. A nurse who has to look for a device once may never do so again!

- Assess integration of systems. The idea is to avoid duplication of data entry, so considering the ability of the pharmacy information system and other applicable systems and devices to interface with the EMAR/BC-MAR is important.

- Allow for communication. Communications capabilities with physicians and pharmacists must be supported (likewise, both nurses and pharmacists should be involved in selecting and configuring these systems).

The Five Rights of Medication Administration

One final consideration relates to the goals set forth by the ISMP to promote patient safety through the **five rights of medication administration**: right medication, right dose, right time, right route, and right patient. Many experts have provided procedural details for each of these rights. For example, procedures to ensure that the right patient is identified include checking the name on the order and the patient, using two identifiers, asking the patient to identify him or herself, and, when available, using technology such as a barcode system. The AHRQ glossary suggests that strong policies and procedures surrounding these five rights be established by each healthcare organization (AHRQ n.d.). Experts have also added three more rights of medication administration to optimize the use of new technology: right documentation (including documenting medication administration *after* giving the ordered medication—not before, as is often the case), right reason (confirming the rationale for the ordered medication, especially using CDS tools where available) and right response (monitoring the patient's response and documenting this and interventions taken as applicable) (Dowding 2013; Bonsall 2011). As suggested by the discussion of workarounds, having a BC-MAR system does not, by itself, guarantee that it is used properly.

CPOE

CPOE is the process whereby providers directly enter orders, making them more accurate and legible, and receive back any alerts or reminders that they would act on in real time and that would help reduce errors, particularly medication errors. It was emphasized in chapter 4 that physicians and others authorized to write orders should perform this process through the CPOE system themselves rather than assign it to a scribe for entry in order to take advantage of the CDS embedded in the system. CPOE is not to be confused with **order communication**, which was a system used by the nursing service to transcribe orders handwritten by a provider authorized to write orders into a computer system for distribution to respective ancillary department systems.

Figure 14.9 illustrates an CPOE order-entry screen that includes an order check, which is basically a reminder or an alert. Reminders and alerts can be very specific, such as where a specific medication ordered might be contraindicated because of an allergy or another medication. The alert can also be more global, although still specific to the patient, such as the one illustrated in figure 14.9, which reminds the provider about the patient's current laboratory result status and number of medications already being taken. Types of alerts available through CPOE vary with the vendor. In

Figure 14.9.   CPOE

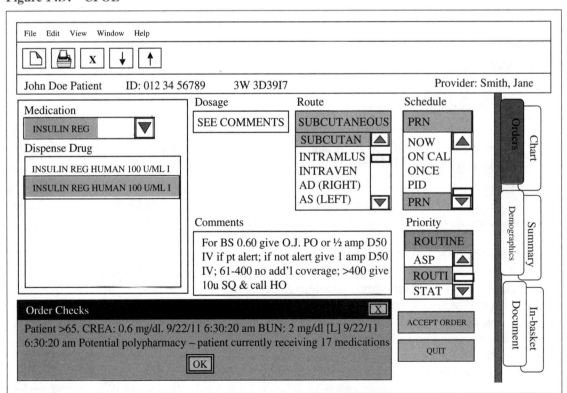

research on the use of alerts and their impact, CSC Healthcare researchers identified the following five alerts that most CPOE systems provide (Hagland 2010):

- Drug-allergy contraindication
- Inappropriate single dose
- Therapeutic duplication
- Drug-drug interaction
- Inappropriate route

These researchers also identified the following types of more advanced CDS capabilities that are available in only certain CPOE products:

- Inappropriate cumulative (daily) dose
- Inappropriate dosing per patient weight
- Age contraindication (all ages as applicable; Beers List in the elderly)
- Labs—creatinine
- Labs—other
- Drug-diagnosis contraindication
- Corollary orders (monitoring)

Alerts and reminders should be used judiciously in CPOE systems. In some cases, hospitals have implemented so many alerts and reminders that they appear with practically every order, and there may be multiple alerts with just one order. Many providers find reviewing and responding to numerous alerts to be annoying and time-consuming. The phenomenon is known as **alert fatigue**. In a study of alert fatigue using an expert panel, Phansalkar and colleagues (2013) cite studies reporting that up to 90 percent of **drug-drug interaction (DDI)** alerts are overridden. The expert panel recommended a list of 33 class-based low-priority DDIs that do not warrant being interruptive alerts in an EHR. Phansalkar and colleagues report that, in one hospital, these accounted for 36 percent of such DDIs.

Alerts and reminders in the CPOE must be configured for use in a manner that follows the hospital's business rules. For example, clinicians may be required to respond to some reminders but permitted to dismiss others. Hospitals might choose to establish audits on alerts that are dismissed or require documentation of the rationale for overriding an alert. Different hospitals approach this documentation differently; some consider alerting to be an immature science and a provider's review of an alert is no different than a provider reviewing a reference, a process that is typically is not documented. Alternatively, other hospitals documentation of responses to alerts helps all members of the care team understand what is happening and reduces calls and questions (Rollins 2005). In certain limited circumstances, hospitals may safely turn off frequently overridden drug-drug interaction alerts (Van der Sijs et al. 2008).

CPOE does not require an EHR, but the level of CDS that makes CPOE most effective generally is found when many of the components of an EHR exist; otherwise, providers may view performing order entry to be a clerical function. In addition, some CPOE systems have been implemented with little attention to existing processes that provide adequate control points. There is also a growing body of literature that is questioning the role of CPOE in potentially facilitating medication errors (Han et al. 2005; Koppel et al. 2005; Koppel et al. 2008; Slight et al. 2016).

Optimizing CPOE Systems

As suggested earlier, hospitals have had variable success with CPOE systems. Order entry is particularly challenging for physicians to adopt because it changes workflows substantially. In the CSC Healthcare research already cited, 81 US hospitals with eight different EHR products agreed to participate in a study between April and August 2008 on how their CPOE systems were used and their impact. The results revealed that there was largely no correlation between any particular vendor product and the rate at which orders detected potential adverse drug events, although the study did find that some variation in performance was correlated with vendor choice. The study concluded that the way a hospital implements CPOE has a tremendous influence on the success of that product (Hagland 2010). As part of optimization efforts surrounding both CPOE and BC-MAR, it is essential that physicians and nurses work together on configuring the types of alerts and how they will be presented. CPOE affects not only physicians' workflow at the point an order is input but also nurses' workflow as well with respect to the output of CPOE (Neal 2011).

CPOE optimization may focus on making order entry quicker and easier for physicians, who have sometimes found that, compared to paper ordering, entering some orders takes longer via CPOE and requires that they enter more information at the time the order. Short orders can take longer to enter than longer orders because longer orders often are enabled by standard order sets whereas the physician must enter all applicable parameters of the short order. In addition, physicians find entering orders into CPOE more time-consuming than paper orders because some elements required in the CPOE order may previously have been verbally communicated in-person to nurses and/or pharmacists or addressed in a follow-up phone call from the pharmacist or nurse. Although such conversations and calls also took time, physicians are often unaware of the cumulative effect of such communications on staff resources or patient care (the need for follow-up on written orders can delay treatment). Hospital policies on the discontinuance of certain types of orders, countersignature requirements, or adherence to a managed care formulary that may have been enforced only informally in a paper-ordering system now are enforced directly through the CPOE system, contributing to the time factor for physicians.

For CPOE to be successful, physicians must be involved in the process of designing the system to ensure that it meets their needs and to understand its benefits. Advice from those hospitals that have previously implemented CPOE (Briggs 2004; Feldbaum and Fuller 2007; Dixon and Zafar 2009; Oregon Patient Safety Commission 2015) repeatedly describe the following factors as contributing to optimization of CPOE by physicians:

- There is top-down commitment to mandating CPOE use in the hospital. The risks of maintaining dual systems are great, and physicians who resist using the CPOE rarely come around on their own. Top-down commitment also means executives commit to ongoing investment in CPOE optimization.

- Change leadership is assumed by all types of leaders—including the trustees or board of directors, medical staff, and administration. A mandated CPOE system must be fast, user-friendly, reliable, and stable before go-live. The information technology and clinical staff must work together to configure the system. In fact, the process of working together builds trust in the system.

- The hospital has planned for resistance. Even when a hospital tries to fully engage its medical staff, it will encounter some pushback. Clear policies, developed in concert with the medical staff, must be in place, and leadership must commit to supporting them. The legal department may need to review the CPOE policy to clearly delineate noncompliance issues from those of disruptive behavior. Dealing with unprofessional behavior is not the responsibility of the CPOE implementation/optimization team.

- The hospital has scrutinized workflow throughout the entire medication management process and from any location where providers may enter orders or be affected by order entry. In one hospital, implementation of CPOE involved the evaluation of between 2,000 and 3,000 types of workflow.

- Medical staff departments develop the order sets. Physician participation builds physicians' trust in the system and improves their understanding of how the system works.

- The hospital requires training and provides at-the-elbow support. Even for providers who have participated in workflow and order set development, training is imperative. Training must cover not only screen navigation but also workflow considerations. Once a unit goes live, daily briefings with clinical staff should identify issues and address ways to overcome them. An efficient feedback mechanism for providers themselves must be in place. The comments and suggestions received must be addressed in a timely and satisfactory manner.

- The hospital measures success. Although care must be taken on what to measure and when, simple things such as the number of physician log-ins or the number of orders placed via CPOE can be measures of success. Part of measuring success is also acknowledging the work of the teams and celebrating accomplishments in tasteful ways.

- Internal and external marketing is conducted. Educational programs, posters providing orientation to key elements of the system, countdown clocks, and other elements that demonstrate the hospital's interest not only in the technology but the anticipated impact on quality and patient safety demonstrate leadership commitment. Even community outreach that emphasizes the hospital's commitment to quality and safety through information technology can spur patient and community engagement.

- Expectations are managed. Do not over- or underestimate the potential for success with CPOE, and be aware that people's expectations of CPOE technology often exceed reality. All clinicians need to be reminded that the computer does not take care of patients. The need for professional judgment does not go away.

- Differences between inpatient and ambulatory care settings are acknowledged and addressed. As providers acquire their own EHRs, misunderstandings may arise from the differences in workflows in different care settings.

  ○ In the inpatient setting, physicians write orders for various services or tests and procedures, which are completed by other clinical staff or ancillary personnel. In fact, it is difficult to obtain a service or conduct a test or procedure without appropriate documentation in the health record. Although the physician may visit a patient only once or twice a day, the healthcare team attempts to tightly coordinate all resources and services for patient care. These arrangements are beneficial, but certain information needs may not be addressed appropriately in this scenario. For example, the needs of case managers or utilization managers may not be addressed during routine documentation, which can lead to inefficiencies in workflow.

  ○ In contrast to the location-centered focus of the inpatient record, workflow in the ambulatory environment is patient-centered, but the record is not. All members of the healthcare team attempt to expedite an outpatient visit and all associated workflow so that the patient and the healthcare team can finish their work within the constraints of the visit time. To do so, the record is often "taken apart," or compiled in separate pieces, sometimes never to come together. For example, it is common for a multispecialty clinic to have multiple chart rooms and multiple charts for each patient, depending on the specialty areas in which they are being treated. Obviously, a centralized EHR would contribute greatly to coordinated care in such a situation. This may be why EHR systems have matured and grown more in the ambulatory environment despite the greater change required in workflow.

Check Your Understanding 14.2

Indicate whether the following statements are true or false:

1. Data visualization is a form of active advice.

2. Drug lab checking is a requirement of the MU program.

3. The ability to graph laboratory test data is evidence of a results management system.

4. Integrating RIS and PACS is a form of health IT optimization.

5. In hospitals, POC documentation is largely performed by nurses.

6. An optimization strategy to increase physician use of POC documentation may be to offer differential diagnosis support.

7. Optimization efforts should be made to require all physician notes in structured format.

8. Hospitals are more likely to have issues with CPOE than physicians have with e-prescribing.

9. Workarounds are most common in results management.

10. A more advanced function of CPOE as a candidate for optimization is drug-age contraindication

Clinical Decision Support

CDS systems are interactive programs that directly assist clinicians with decision-making tasks. CDS is incorporated into many EHR components but also may be acquired as separate modules. Some of these modules are accessible to other components of the EHR, and some are standalone, including in the form of an app on a personal device. Additionally, the organization's EHR system may include analytical tools that can help create new CDS based on the experience of the hospital. Table 14.3 describes the variety of CDS options available in EHRs:

CDS generally requires three technological components, illustrated in figure 14.10, to operate:

- Dynamic **knowledge base**, which includes updated evidence from scientific research

- Inferencing mechanism, or **rules engine** (also called **inference engine**), which is the set of rules derived from scientific evidence

- **User interface**, which presents questions, checks responses for legal answers, and supplies user's responses to the inference engine

A taxonomy of functionality that the three components serve to provide has been defined (Osheroff et al. 2006; Wright et al. 2009; NQF 2010):

- *Trigger* is the event or events that cause a decision support rule to be invoked. Examples include prescribing a drug, ordering a laboratory test, or entering a new problem on a problem list.

Table 14.3.　Types of CDS in EHRs

Type	Examples
Data display	• Flow sheets • Dynamic displays • Summary creation • Data abstraction
Data retrieval	• Choices of navigational aids • Customized screens
Data visualization	• Workflow • In-baskets • Dashboards • Workgroup tools • Messaging
Data entry	• Context-sensitive templates • Infobuttons • Required field alerts • Edit checks
Decision making	• Access to knowledge bases • Drug-drug interactions • Drug-lab checking • Clinical pathways • Evidence-based guidelines • Differential diagnosis support • Patient/family preferences • Real time surveillance

Source: Summarized from National Learning Consortium 2013.

Figure 14.10.　Components of CDS

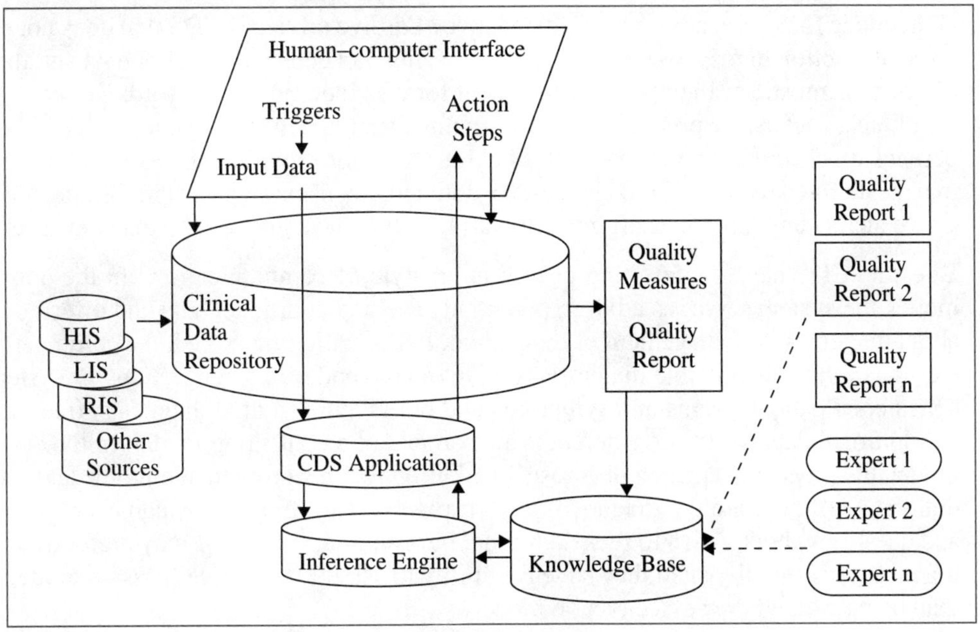

- *Input data* are the data elements used by a rule to make inferences. They do not need to be input at the time the rule is triggered; more commonly they are stored in the EHR's clinical data repository. Examples include laboratory test results; patient demographics, such as age, gender, race/ethnicity, height, weight, and vital signs; the patient's problem list, medication list, and medication allergy list; and other information, such as reason for admission, surgical history, hospital formulary, and diagnostic study inventory.

- *Interventions* are the possible actions the information system can take to deliver information. Examples include sending a message to a clinician, showing a guideline, providing defaults or pick lists, or logging that an event took place.

- *Offered choices*, sometimes called *action steps,* are the choices the recipient of the proposed intervention can take. For example, if a rule fired because a physician entered an order for a drug to which the patient is allergic, the system may allow the physician to cancel the order, choose an alternative drug, or override the alert and keep the order as written. Entering additional information, deferring a warning, adding a narrative note, or supplying a rationale for an override may be other options, depending on the context and hospital policy.

A study conducted by Wright and colleagues (2009) found that the trigger, input data element, and intervention functions were generally well covered by major EHR vendors. Offered choices, however, were not nearly as well covered and were believed to be a factor contributing to a lack of success with CDS in general and CDS in CPOE applications in particular. The following are other factors that contribute to how well CDS is accepted by clinicians; they may require optimization to improve their value:

- Does the CDS focus on reminding the clinician about what is true about the patient (for example, the patient's drug allergy), or can it offer suggestions for what to do for the patient (for example, what data to collect about a patient, what drug to order for a specific diagnosis)? Clinicians may prefer decision support that deals with what they should do, rather than with what is true about a patient—although errors occur more frequently in the latter situation.

- Is the mode for giving advice passive or active? **Passive advice** is CDS that does not require a specific action in response. For example, the clinician enters a subset of data and the CDS offers a diagnostic or therapeutic assessment for consideration. **Active advice** requires that the clinician act before proceeding. At minimum, the clinician must acknowledge the advice, perhaps by closing a pop-up window, clicking "OK," or providing a specific action, which may be directed by the offered choices. As noted in the discussion of alert fatigue, too many active alerts can blunt the usefulness of warnings that have greater clinical significance.

- Does the CDS have a consulting or critiquing style of communication? In the consulting model, the system serves as adviser, potentially seeking additional data and offering advice about diagnosis or management of the patient. In the critiquing model, the computer evaluates the clinician's possible diagnosis or plan of care and offers suggestions. A system that considers a patient's signs and symptoms and offers a differential diagnosis, fine-tuning it as additional data points are entered, is an example of a consulting model. In the critiquing model, the physician enters a diagnosis in addition to the signs and symptoms and requests that the CDS evaluate the diagnosis with responses that offer other diagnoses to consider and questions about which to seek additional information. Clinicians may prefer the critiquing model, especially when they have the ability to ask for the advice (passive mode) rather than being offered the advice (active mode).

- What is the underlying decision-making process? Early CDS systems were algorithmically based (that is, they had a structure that one can draw with a flowchart). In general, however, these kinds of systems have proven to be overly simplistic for routine use. Today, most CDS systems draw from more sophisticated processes, including Bayesian modeling, decision analysis, artificial neural networks (ANNs), and artificial intelligence. A number of CDS diagnostic programs have been developed using Bayesian modeling, which is a method of statistical inference where probabilities are determined from observations of patient-specific parameters to derive recommendations. Decision analysis adds explicit decision recommendations to the Bayesian modeling technique. CDS systems with decision analysis have been less successful, perhaps because they result in more active and consulting types of offerings. ANNs take input, classify it, and output the likelihood that a particular classi-fication explains the findings. ANN technology is widely used in statistical pattern analysis, such as speech and handwriting recognition. Because the user of ANN cannot directly see the network created to understand how the particular conclusion was reached, ANN has been less successful in CDS except for problems where it is known that a result is difficult to predict. Artificial intelligence is a process where concepts derived from experts in a field are stored in a knowledge base and then used to provide problem analysis and advice such as an expert might provide. Because decision making in healthcare requires reasoning under uncertainty, knowledge-based systems incorporating Bayesian or other probabilistic processes are most successful for CDS systems.

- Does the CDS promote successful human-computer interactions? CDS systems may pro-vide good decision support, but clinicians will not use them if logistical, mechanical, and psychological aspects of use of the system are not addressed. Van der Sijs and colleagues (2006) have done an extensive study of why clinicians override alerts and offer the follow-ing recommendations for creating useful systems. CDS systems should be:

  ○ Specific to the patient, relevant and important, accurate, with actions that can be followed.

  ○ Clear and unambiguous, with a justification that is easy to understand, is concise, enables additional information to be readily accessible if desired, and presents alternative courses of actions.

  ○ Context-sensitive and supportive of clinician workflow. Such CDS should be generated for all dangerous cases, directed to the right person (according to log in), and knowledge-specific (for example, specialists may receive fewer alerts than residents), and annoying repetition should be prevented—perhaps tied to previous performance of user (Lee et al. 2010).

  ○ Designed such that overriding fatal alerts should not be easy, reasons for noncompliance should be clear, and alerts promote action rather than stop intended action.

  ○ Reflective of characteristics of good computer usability, including system speed, screen design, and navigation.

  ○ Embedded within the larger computer system being used (such as the EHR) so that CDS use is a by-product of ordinary work processes (Musen et al. 2008).

Berner identifies two other aspects of CDS systems as important to optimizing use of CDS (2009). First, the accuracy of the underlying source data (that is, the quality of the data in the EHR) must be maintained. High rates of alert overrides may occur when source data are not up to date—for example, if the system does not indicate that a medication has been discontinued or if a new problem is not added to the problem list. Second, knowledge in the system must also be maintained. Medical knowledge is burgeoning, with new drugs and diagnoses continually being discovered. New evidence is continually being accumulated. One solution to this challenge is to use commercial knowledge bases that provide frequent updates. For example, the drug knowledge bases embedded in most CPOE and eprescribing systems may be updated as frequently as daily using the National Library of Medicine's **DailyMed** publication. The AHRQ has funded a Clinical Decision Support Consortium that is developing a web-based repository of CDS knowledge in relation to hypertension and diabetes guidelines. Local sites using the knowledge base can access the information over the Internet when changes are made.

In addition to medication management, many other aspects of healthcare can benefit from CDS systems (Versel 2011; CMS 2014). Hospital infection control has reportedly improved through real-time infection surveillance of laboratory test results and decision support recommending antimicrobial drugs (Young and Stevenson 2008); inappropriate medical imaging studies have been controlled (Curry 2011); and nurses have adhered to guidelines for head-of-bed positioning for patients receiving mechanical ventilation (Lyerla et al. 2010). CDS has been instrumental in improving fall/injury prevention through fall-risk assessment tools (Hook et al. 2012; Lytle et al. 2015). Also, as was previously noted, physicians use CDS to consider differential diagnoses. Knight (2010) and Roy et al. (2009) have found diagnosis decision support systems are beneficial in emergency department diagnosis situations.

Optimizing CDS

Just as with any other component of the EHR, it is important to ensure proper implementation and optimization of CDS systems throughout their lifecycles. Osheroff (2009) has suggested that just as there are five rights to medication administration, there are five rights to CDS—a CDS system should provide the right information, to the right people, in the right intervention formats, through the right channels, and at the right points in workflow. This framework is an excellent starting point for reviewing how an EHR's CDS components can be optimized to ensure they are used for their intended purpose. Osheroff and colleagues have published an *Implementers' Guide* (2012), which outlines a formal process that hospitals can follow to improve outcomes with CDS. All stakeholders need to be involved. Goals of the program and specific clinical objectives need to be clear. Supporting information systems need to be assessed to determine whether they can supply the necessary data for CDS. Various approaches to CDS interventions need to be identified, assessed, developed, and tested before they are put into practice. The CDS program needs to be monitored on an ongoing basis to ensure that it achieves its goals to improve clinical outcomes.

Reporting

The last component that defines the EHR is reporting. Obviously, reporting can mean any number of things, from a seemingly simple list of patients that may need follow-up after hospitalization to sophisticated data mining for quality improvement, patient risk stratification for health reform initiatives, and many other tasks. Unfortunately, EHRs are notorious for not being report-friendly. There are a number of reasons why EHRs do not effectively generate reports.

First, the EHR's clinical data repository is optimized to perform online transaction processing, not online analytical processing. As described in chapter 10, different database structures are needed to support these different functions.

Second, the amount of structured data being collected in hospitals, other than in the medication management applications and potentially some nursing documentation, is currently quite limited. Because EHRs are hugely challenging applications to implement, it may seem that more data should be available than actually are. Some key data, such as a problem list, may not be in structured format or reflect standards that make them most useful for reporting (Holmes 2011).

Third, even where data are in structured format, the hospital may not have a clinical data repository to integrate all the data, or it may have a repository but it cannot process data residing in standalone applications. For example, many hospitals have standalone emergency department systems, surgery scheduling systems, and outpatient department or clinic systems. Their laboratory and radiology information systems may not generate structured data. Some of the data in these standalone systems and reports may be the very data that, combined with EHR data, are of most interest to hospital management and basic quality improvement studies.

A final reason EHRs are not set up to perform and report a range of analytics is that many hospitals do not have personnel trained in sophisticated analytical processing and interpretation, and therefore have not demanded more capabilities in their products. Hospitals may struggle to acquire personnel who are both knowledgeable about health data and facile with query strategies and report writing software. (See figure 14.11 for a sample job description of a health informatics specialist/report writer.) Instead, they rely on their EHR vendor to construct canned report tools, or **report wizards**, that enable them to run routine reports or make small modifications to standard reports themselves. More sophisticated analytics may be used in revenue cycle management that draws primarily from claims data or may be available for use in academic research and teaching hospitals. In the case of the latter, data needed for such studies are put into a separate clinical data warehouse or other separate databases. In academic environments, the data collected for such purposes may not even derive from the EHR but from separate research processes.

As part of the MU incentives program, the Centers for Medicare and Medicaid Services (CMS) require electronic generation of clinical quality measures (eCQMs), which has increased interest in and demand for reporting functionality in EHRs. Issues with the multiplicity of measures and incompatible data definitions are discussed in chapter 4. To optimize the results of eCQMs and other measures, stakeholders in healthcare will need to collectively decide which measures are most important and align metrics across all users of those measures. AHRQ has compiled a set of continuous quality improvement (CQI) tools and factors to promote use of health IT to support quality

Figure 14.11.   Sample job description for health informatics specialist/report writer

---

Position: Health Informatics Specialist/Report Writer

Reports to: Clinical Informatics Project Director

Responsibilities
- Will be part of a team implementing a data warehouse across the integrated delivery network
- Responsible for working with administrative and clinical users to formulate query and report format solutions to their management, patient care, quality, compliance, and research needs
- Collect feedback on report performance
- Manage Crystal Enterprise report delivery, producing timely reports drawing on data in Microsoft SQL server
- Contribute to data analysis and interpretation of reports
- Propose modifications to the schema of the data warehouse to facilitate queries and optimize performance
- Employ informatics applications to design and/or implement new models to resolve any clinical issues
- Evaluate new or modified informatics solutions, data structures, and support mechanisms
- Maintain up-to-date knowledge of health informatics and related technology and software as it relates to healthcare practice

Qualifications
- Experience with electronic health records, ideally with XXX vendor products
- At least three years' experience in health informatics analysis
- At least three years of reporting experience in a healthcare environment using SQL server and Crystal Reports
- Sound knowledge of medical data and terminology
- Strong self-sufficiency and initiative to take on data projects
- Strong project management skills and attention to detail
- Excellent verbal and written communication skills
- Experience with Transactional SQL and advanced queries in an MS SQL environment

improvement (Higgins et al. 2015). Case studies from this work suggest that activities to optimize CQI include the following:

- Having a CQI committee

- Implementing a system for selecting and acting on feedback relating to the measures

- Developing an approach for identifying needs and gaps that would benefit from improvement strategies

- Using CDS to remind clinicians to address needs at the point of care

- Monitoring progress toward meeting quality goals over time

Interestingly, better data integration for reporting is also improving access to data for patient care (Narcisi 2010). One quite sophisticated example is that of **data mining at the bedside**. CHRISTUS Health deployed a real-time predictive tool to retrieve and present integrated data to help providers identify high-cost and high-risk patients so that the providers can be guided to perform and track interventions that may reduce length of stay and 30day readmissions (Goth 2010).

Another example of reporting used to improve patient care is the integration of a **real-time location system (RTLS)** with EHR data. These systems label medical devices with RFID and use global positioning systems (GPS) to track the whereabouts of the devices within the hospital. Although RTLS is largely used for inventory management, hospitals can also use it to identify what equipment may have come in contact with patients infected with Methicillin-resistant Staphylococcus aureus (MRSA) bacterium or other contagions; this report can contribute to reduced spread of infections and lower overall costs to the healthcare delivery system (Huvane 2008). In 2007, the Food and Drug Administration Amendments Act was signed into law, requiring the establishment of a **Unique Device Identification (UDI)** system. When it is fully phased in (a process expected to take several years), the UDI system will be usable locally for tracking infection exposure, facilitate device recall, be able to track allergic reactions to devices, and improve studies on medical device effectiveness (FDA 2006; FDA 2016).

The UDI system may also improve the ability to integrate medical device data with EHRs. A lack of standards for medical device interoperability and integration with EHR systems is challenging the ability to fully close the loop on electronic documentation, because nurses must transcribe data from the (monitoring) device attached to the patient to the EHR at the bedside (Day 2011; McAlpine 2009).

Examples of Other Health Information Technology in Hospitals

Although many applications of health IT have been used in hospitals for decades, some health IT applications are just now being more widely implemented or implemented as a result of EHR system capability. Following is a selection of examples.

Patient-Flow Management System

The ability to determine where a patient is at all times in a facility and to link staff requirements to patient location can be a challenge. For example, knowing when the patient has been prepared for surgery can improve the time management of an anesthesiologist. Linking patient location through a **patient-flow management system** to the BC-MAR can assist nursing in documentation of medications administered or not administered. These systems originated in the emergency department (ED), but the Joint Commission requirements for improved patient flow throughout the hospital have made them key enterprise-wide systems (Jensen 2004).

Supply Chain Management Systems

Supply chain refers to the ability to requisition, inventory, and track usage of supplies. **Supply chain management systems** linked to EHRs can help capture data for invoice matching, usage tracking, contract compliance, and rebate attainment. Such systems have helped reduce day-of-surgery delays and cancellations and enhanced safety outcomes (Pendergrass 2005). They also support device registries used to identify patients in the event of a device recall.

Smart Bed Technology

Smart bed technology combines medical device technology that is embedded in patient beds to adjust bed angle, assist in turning patients, and so on, with an interface to the EHR to support real-time monitoring and compliance. For example, if a patient's bed is required to have rails up and the patient lowers the rails, the smart bed can communicate directly to the nurse, perhaps in time to prevent a fall, or at least to prove that the rails were taken down from the bedside and not the external side.

Automated Informed Consent

An **automated informed consent system** can improve standardization of information and consistency in supplying it to the patient when seeking informed consent. With the enhancement of visualization tools, patients' comprehension can be improved. Modifications to the consent can also be controlled by the system, which can provide reminders to clinicians of allowed and disallowed changes. Additions or changes made to the consent are legible, and the patient can easily be given a copy. Hospitals have found that these systems pay for themselves in the cost of defending lawsuits where consents were not understood, a common cause of litigation (McKenzie and Karnstedt 2010).

Patient Education

Patient education has always been an important element of the care delivery process, but there are concerns that it is missing the mark as an effective tool to ensure patient safety and quality outcomes. Patients anxious to leave the hospital may not pay sufficient attention to the discharge instructions they are given. Often, these instructions are provided in a brief discussion by the nurse, who is also busy with discharge-related documentation and other processes (Jones 2010). Automated forms of education, some of which are available as components in EHR systems, can be tailored to the specific patient needs and can include pictures and diagrams in multiple languages. Paper-based educational materials can include a **quick response**, or **quick read (QR) code** (a matrix form of bar code that can be read by a smartphone app, which will take the holder of the phone to a specific web address). QR codes can direct patients to appropriate educational materials; additionally, they can be used for a variety of other purposes in the healthcare environment (Whaley 2010). Educational materials presented via a patient portal can be referenced after the patient returns home or when a caregiver needs information. Although these types of patient education materials are not a substitute for in-person education, they are important tools that enhance the experience for patients.

Today, patient education about the EHR itself may be warranted. In 2010, results of a Harris Interactive poll on consumers' perceptions about EHRs were reported (Enrado 2010). Although nearly half of the survey participants believed that EHRs would make healthcare delivery more efficient, respondents did not know how EHRs would specifically affect them as patients. To address such uncertainties and encourage patients to feel comfortable with systemic changes, physicians and other care providers need to talk to their patients about the EHR and its impact on care and offer tangible evidence of how the EHR is being used, such as for personalized patient education materials provided at discharge.

Tracking Meaningful Use

In the early days of the MU incentive program, there were concerns that hospitals could have certified EHR technology and actually be making meaningful use of the system, but would not be able to generate evidence of the use if audited. Patient education may be a good example of this. The CMS frequently asked questions (FAQs) on MU (2010) note that "education resources or materials do not have to be stored within or generated by the certified EHR. However, the provider should utilize certified EHR technology in a manner where the technology suggests patient-specific educational resources based on the information stored in the certified EHR technology. The provider can make a final decision on whether the education resource is useful and relevant to a specific patient." Whether or not hospitals produce the educational materials from the EHR, they are still left with the need for evidence that patient-specific education resources were supplied to the patient. This is an important consideration in conducting a MU assessment, with potentially many options, including ones that seem like extreme workarounds or added costs. For example, one hospital described how it anticipated asking the patient to sign a copy of the educational materials to acknowledge receipt and then scanning the document back into the EHR. Another expected to use a kiosk where the patient would log in and retrieve the educational material. Although this process would also serve to assign patients access to the hospital's portal and educate them about using the portal later, the expense of such kiosks is not trivial (although they could also be used for providing the informed consent, HIPAA notice of privacy practices, and potentially other information) (Mitchell 2011). Perhaps the QR codes will supply not only the link to educational materials but also a link to the EHR that indicates at least the QR-coded document was supplied to the patient.

Suffice it to note, however, that evidentiary documentation of MU or other incentive program, such as merit-based incentive payment system (MIPS) (see chapter 1), for up to six years after submission for funds may be a necessary part of the EHR that is overlooked when the criteria for MU do not explicitly include a requirement for how such evidence should be generated, maintained, and later produced if necessary (C3 Partners 2010).

Check Your Understanding 14.3

Match the term with its description:

    A. Active advice

    B. Alert fatigue

    C. Data mining at the bedside

    D. Drug-drug interaction

    E. Edit checks

    F. Fall/injury assessment

    G. In-basket

    H. Inference engine

    I. Knowledge base

    J. RFID

1. Requires user to address

2. Example of successful use of CDS by nurses

3. Part of reporting technology for inventory management

4. Form of CDS for use in data entry

5. Result of overuse of CDS

6. Rules engine

7. Form of CDS for use in workflow management

8. Least-liked form of CDS

9. Real-time use of predictive analytics

10. Evidence from scientific research that feeds CDS

References and Resources

American Association of Colleges of Nursing (AACN). 2014 (September). Nursing shortage (fact sheet). http://www .aacn.nche.edu/media-relations/fact-sheets/nursing-shortage.

Agarwal, R., et al. 2008 (September). Eliminating paper: Quantifying the impact of computerized clinical documentation systems (CCDS). Presentation at eHealth Initiative's 5th Annual Conference.

American Hospital Association (AHA), Health Research and Educational Trust, and the Institute for Safe Medication Practices (ISMP). 2002. *Pathways for Medication Safety: Assessing Bedside Bar-Coding Readiness*. http://www.ismp .org/selfassessments/PathwaySection3.pdf.

Agency for Healthcare Research and Quality (AHRQ). n.d. Patient safety network glossary. http://www.psnet.ahrq.gov/ glossary.aspx.

Barrameda, M. 2011 (January 24). EHR lessons for nurses: Nurse CIO of Generations+/Northern Manhattan Health Network offers tips for EHR success. Advance Healthcare Network for Nurses. http://nursing.advanceweb.com/ Columns/Nursing-Informatics/EHR-Lessons-for-Nurses.aspx.

Bates, D.W., et al. 1997. The costs of adverse drug events in hospitalized patients. *Journal of the American Medical Association.* 277(4):307–311.

Berner, E.S. 2009 (June). *Clinical Decision Support Systems: State of the Art.* AHRQ publication no. 09-0069-EF. Rockville, MD: Agency for Healthcare Research and Quality. https://healthit.ahrq.gov/sites/default/files/docs/page/ 09-0069-EF_1.pdf.

Boochever, S.S. 2004. HIS/RIS/PACS integration: Getting to the gold standard. *Radiology Management.* 26(3):16–24.

Bonsall, L. 2011 (May 27). 8 rights of medication administration. *Lippincott Nursing Center eNews.* https://www .nursingcenter.com/NCBlog/May-2011/8-rights-of-medication-administration.

Bowman, S. 2013 (October 1). Impact of electronic health record systems on information integrity: Quality and safety implications. *Perspectives in Health Information Management.* http://www.ncbi.nlm.nih.gov/pmc/articles/ PMC3797550.

Braunstein, M.L. 2014. *Contemporary Health Informatics.* Chicago, IL: AHIMA.

Briggs, B. 2004. The top 10 CPOE challenges. *Health Data Management Magazine.* 12(7):20–22, 24, 26

C3 Partners. 2010 (October 14). Meaningful use monitor requirements. Everything HITECH. http://www .everythinghitech.com.

Callen, J. A. Georgiou, J. Li, and J.I. Westbrook. 2011. The safety implications of missed test results for hospitalized patients: A systematic review. *BMJ Quality and Safety.* 20:194–199.

Cannon, J., and S. Lucci. 2010. Transcription and EHRs: Benefits of a blended approach. *Journal of AHIMA.* 81(2):36–40.

Cape Cod Health. N.d. What's new—PACS. http://www.capecodhealth.org/body.dfm?id=366.

Chapman, S. 2014 (November). Report analyzes EHR patient safety concerns. *For the Record.* 26(11):20.

Charles, D., M. Gabriel, and T. Searcy. 2015 (April). Adoption of electronic health record systems among U.S. non-federal acute care hospitals: 2008–2014. Office of the National Coordinator for Health Information Technology. ONC Data Brief no. 23. https://www.healthit.gov/sites/default/files/data-brief/2014HospitalAdoptionDataBrief.pdf.

Chavis, S. 2010 (March 29). Physician documentation slow no more. *For the Record.* 22(6):10.

Centers for Medicare and Medicaid Services (CMS). 2010 (November 7). Eligible professional meaningful use menu set measures: Measure 6 of 10. https://questions.cms.gov/faq.php?faqId=2907.

Centers for Medicare and Medicaid Services (CMS). 2014 (November). Clinical decision support: more than just "alerts" tip sheet. eHealth University. https://www.cms.gov/regulations-and-guidance/legislation/EHRincentiveprograms/downloads/clinicaldecisionsupport_tipsheet-.pdf.

Curry, H. 2011 (January 4). Clinical decision support systems help control inappropriate medical imaging, study suggests. *Journal of the American College of Radiology.*

Darcy, T. and S. Kretzschmar. 2010 (May 4). Patient safety and the electronic health record: The laboratory perspective. Presentation at Clinical Laboratory Management Association ThinkLab '10.

Davis, J. 2015 (November 30). Health IT: Driving care delivery. *Healthcare IT News.* http://www.healthcareitnews.com/news/health-it-driving-care-delivery.

Day, B. 2011. Standards for medical device interoperability and integration. *Patient Safety and Quality Healthcare.* 8(1):20–23.

Diagnostic Imaging. 2003 (August 14). PACS workstation hardware comes right off the shelf: Hospitals find it cheaper, easier to reconfigure licensing agreements and shop around for PCs. http://www.diagnosticimaging.com/display/article/113619/1178397?verify=0.

Dixon, B.E., and A. Zafar. 2009 (January). *Inpatient Computerized Provider Order Entry: Findings from the AHRQ Health IT Portfolio.* AHRQ publication no. 09-0031-EF. Rockville, MD: Agency for Healthcare Research and Quality. https://healthit.ahrq.gov/sites/default/files/docs/page/09-0031-EF_cpoe.pdf.

Douglas, P.S. 2008. ACCF/ACR/AHA/ASE/ASNC/HRS/NASCI/RSNA/SAIP/SCAI/SCCT/SCMR 2008 health policy statement on structured reporting in cardiovascular imaging. *Journal of the American College of Cardiology.* 53:76–90.

Dowding, D. 2013. Using computerized decision-support system. *Nursing Times.* 109(36): 23–25. http://www.nursingtimes.net/clinical-subjects/healthcare-it/using-computerised-decision-support-systems/5063003.fullarticle.

Embi, P.J., et al. 2004. Impacts of computerized physician documentation in a teaching hospital: Perceptions of faculty and resident physicians. *Journal of the American Medical Informatics Association.* 11(4):300–309.

Enrado, P. 2010 (June 14). Survey points to patient outreach and education on EHRs. *Health Record Review.*

Essin, D. 2011 (January 24). EHRs: Think clinical process, not automation. Physicians Practice blog. http://www.physicianspractice.com/blog/content/article/1462168/1781523.

Farrell. 2008 (February 6). Implementing wireless technology in healthcare? Learn from others' experiences. *Healthcare Informatics.*

Feldbaum, J., and K. Fuller. 2007 (June). Point of failure: Getting physicians on board with CPOE can be a battle, but is one well worth the fight. *Healthcare Informatics.* http://www.healthcare-informatics.com/article/point-failure.

Few, S. 2013. Data visualization for human perception. Chapter 35 in *The Encyclopedia of Human-Computer Interaction, 2nd ed.* Edited by Soegaard M., and R.F. Dam. Interaction Design Foundation. https://www.interaction-design.org/literature/book/the-encyclopedia-of-human-computer-interaction-2nd-ed/data-visualization-for-human-perception.

FitzHenry, F., et al. 2005. Measuring the quality of medication administration. *AMIA Annual Symposium Proceedings.* http://www.ncbi.nlm.nih.gov/pmc/articles/PMC1479849.

Food and Drug Administration (FDA). 2004 (February). FDA issues bar code regulation. http://www.fda.gov/oc/initiatives/barcode-sadr/fs-barcode.html.

Food and Drug Administration (FDA). 2006 (March 22). ERG final report: Unique identification for medical devices. http://www.fda.gov/downloads/MedicalDevices/DeviceRegulationandGuidance/UniqueDeviceIdentification/ucm054270.pdf.

Food and Drug Administration (FDA). 2016 (July 25). Unique device identification—UDID. http://www.fda.gov/MedicalDevices/DeviceRegulationandGuidance/UniqueDeviceIdentification.

Gilchrist, A. 2015 (July 19). Top 10 symptom checkers online. *Pharmacy Times.* http://www.pharmacytimes.com/news/top-10-symptom-checkers-online.

Goth, G. 2010 (April 26). From DNA to dashboards—data mining on the brink. *For the Record.* 22(8):20.

Gunningberg, L., et al. 2009. Wound care and pressure ulcers: Improved quality and comprehensiveness in nursing documentation of pressure ulcers after implementing an electronic health record in hospital care. *Journal of Clinical Nursing.* 18(11):1557–1564.

Hagland, M. 2010 (June). CPOE revelations. *Healthcare Informatics.* http://www.healthcare-informatics.com/article/cpoe-revelations.

Hale, D. 2009 (May). Documenting skin ulcers: The pressure is on. *ACP Hospitalist.* http://www.acphospitalist.org/archives/2009/05/coding.htm.

Han, Y.Y., et al. 2005. Unexpected increased mortality after implementation of a commercially sold computerized physician order entry system. *Pediatrics.* 116(6):1506–1512.

HCI Group. 2014 (April 7). EHR optimization: Planning for success. http://blog.thehcigroup.com/ehr-optimization-planning-for-success.

Health Story Project. 2009 (October). Integrating narrative notes and the EHR. http://www.healthstory.com.

Higgins, T.C., et al. 2015. *Using Health Information Technology to Support Quality Improvement in Primary Care.* AHRQ Publication No. 15-0031-EF. Rockville, MD: Agency for Healthcare Quality and Research. https://pcmh.ahrq.gov/sites/default/files/attachments/Using%20Health%20IT%20Technology%20to%20Support%20QI.pdf.

Hirschtick, R.E. 2006. Copy-and-paste. *Journal of the American Medical Association.* 295:2335–2336.

Holmes, C. 2011. The problem list beyond meaningful use: Part I: The problems with problem lists. *Journal of AHIMA.* 82(2):30–33.

Hook, M.L., et al. 2012. *Using Nursing Practices and Health IT to Reduce Fall-Related Injuries: Final Report.* AHRQ publication no. 11 (12)-0103-EF. Rockville, MD: Agency for Healthcare Quality and Research. https://healthit.ahrq.gov/sites/default/files/docs/citation/actionnursingpracticeshealthitfalls_070612comp.pdf.

Huvane, K. 2008. Follow that infection: CIOs are finding that asset tracking technologies can help keep tabs on some nasty bacteria. *Healthcare Informatics.* 25(6):94–99.

Institute of Medicine (IOM). 2000. *To Err Is Human: Building a Safer Health System.* Washington, DC: National Academies Press.

James, J.T. 2013. A new, evidence-based estimate of patient harms associated with hospital care. *Journal of Patient Safety.* 9(3):122–128.

Jensen, J. 2004. United Hospital increases capacity usage, efficiency with patient-flow management system. *Journal of Healthcare Information Management.* 18(3):26–31.

Joint Commission. 2006 (January 25). Using medication reconciliation to prevent errors. *Sentinel Event Alert.* Issue 35. Oakbrook Terrace, IL, Joint Commission.

Jones, C. 2010 (April 29). How education impacts patient care and reduces hospital costs. *CNNMoney.*

Keenan, G.M. 2008. Documentation and the nurse care planning process. Chapter 49 in *Patient Safety and Quality: An Evidence-Based Handbook for Nurses.* Edited by Hughes, R.G. Rockville, MD: Agency for Healthcare Research and Quality.

King, L.A., A. Wasdovich, and C. Young. 2004. Transforming nursing practice: Clinical systems and the nursing unit of the future. *Journal of Healthcare Information Management.* 18(3):32–36.

Knight, N.B. 2010. The impact on users of a web based diagnosis decision support system. Poster session. The 32nd Annual Meeting of the Society for Medical Decision Making. http://www.isabelhealthcare.com/pdf/Poster_42x72_2_cme_carle.pdf.

Koppel, R., et al. 2005. Role of computerized provider order entry systems in facilitating medication errors. *Journal of the American Medical Association.* 293:1197–1203.

Koppel, R., et al. 2008. Workarounds to barcode medication administration systems: Their occurrences, causes, and threats to patient safety. *Journal of the American Medical Informatics Association.* 15(4):408–423.

Koriwchak, M. 2011 (January 6). Over-automation of EMR note creation encourages missed diagnosis and incurs medical-legal risk. *Wired EMR Practice Newsletter.* http://www.wiredemrdoctor.com/2011/01.

Kuhn, T., et al. 2015. Clinical documentation in the 21st century: Executive summary of a policy position paper from the American College of Physicians. *Annals of Internal Medicine.* 162(4):301–303.

Lang, K. 2009 (April). Speech recognition supports evidence-based radiology. *Imaging Technology News.* http://www.itnonline.com/article/speech-recognition-supports-evidence-based-radiology.

Langlotz, CP. 2006. RadLex: A new method for indexing online educational materials. *RadioGraphics.* 26:1595–1597.

Langlotz, C.P. 2009 (October). Structured radiology reporting: Are we there yet? *Radiology.* 253(1). http://pubs.rsna.org/doi/full/10.1148/radiol.2531091088.

Lee, E.K., et al. 2010. Improving patient safety through medical alert management: An automated decision tool to reduce alert fatigue. *AMIA 2010 Symposium Proceedings.* http://www.ncbi.nlm.nih.gov/pmc/articles/PMC3041356.

Ligon, K.J., and A.E. de los Reyes. 2005. Nursing goes high-tech. *ADVANCE for Health Information Executives.* 9(4):33–38.

Lipsitz, C. 2010 (June 25). Top 5 physician documentation errors. *Washington & West Resources.* http://washingtonwest.com/resources/2010/06/top-5-physician-documentation-errors.

Liu, D. 2003. The use of structured radiology reporting at a community hospital: A 4year case study of more than 200,000 reports. *Applied Radiology.* 32(7):23–26.

Lum, C., and M.J. D'Amarino. 2009. Use of laboratory robots for transport and delivery of blood products. *Lab Medicine.* 40(9):517–522.

Lunney, M. 2008. Critical need to address accuracy of nurses' diagnoses. *Online Journal of Issues in Nursing.* 13(1):1–13. http://www.nursingworld.org/MainMenuCategories/ANAMarketplace/ANAPeriodicals/OJIN/TableofContents/vol132008/No1Jan08/ArticlePreviousTopic/AccuracyofNursesDiagnoses.html.

Lyerla, F., et al. 2010. A nursing clinical decision support system and potential predictors of head-of-bed position for patients receiving mechanical ventilation. *American Journal of Critical Care.* 19(1):39–47.

Lytle, K.S., et al. 2015. Clinical decision support for nurses: A fall risk and prevention example. *CIN: Computers, Informatics, Nursing.* 33(12):530–537.

Mack, M. 2005 (February). To integrate or not to integrate: That is the question! http://www.imagingeconomics.com/issues/articles/MI-2005-02_07.asp.

Massat, M. 2008 (March). Building the PACS ROI case. *Imaging Technology News.*

McAlpine, B. 2009. Biomedical device integration: The impact on clinicians at the point of care. *Patient Safety and Quality Healthcare.* 6(4):28–32.

McCann, E. 2014 (July 18). Deaths by medical mistakes hit records. *Healthcare IT News.* http://www.healthcareitnews.com/news/deaths-by-medical-mistakes-hit-records.

McKenzie, K., and P. Karnstedt. 2010. Automated informed consent: Patients and institutions benefit alike. *Patient Safety and Quality Healthcare.* 7(5):38–44.

Means, C. 2009 (December 2). Product spotlight: Picture archiving and communication systems. *Healthcare IT News.* http://www.healthcareitnews.com/news/product-spotlight-picture-archiving-and-communication-systems.

Meeks, D.W., et al. 2014. An analysis of electronic health record–related patient safety concerns. *Journal of the American Medical Informatics Association.* 21:1053–1059.

Miliard, M. 2014a (October 20). Nurses not happy with hospital EHRs. .*Healthcare IT News* http://www
.healthcareitnews.com/news/nurses-not-happy-hospital-ehrs.

Miliard, M. 2014b (March 13). RNs key to EHR improvement, says CIO. *Healthcare IT News*. http://www
.healthcareitnews.com/news/rns-key-process-improvement-says-cio.

Mills, P.D., et al. 2006 (August 1). Improving the bar-coded medication administration system at the Department of
Veterans Affairs. *American Journal of Health-System Pharmacy*. 63:1442–1447.

Mitchell, R.N. 2011 (February 23). Health systems must boost patient education on EHRs. *InformationWeek*.

Moody, L.E., et al. 2004. Electronic health records documentation in nursing: Nurses' perceptions, attitudes, and
preferences. *CIN: Computers, Informatics, Nursing*. 22(6):337–344.

Musen, M.A., et al. 2008. Clinical decision-support systems. Chapter 20 in *BioMedical Informatics*: *Computer
Applications in Health Care and Biomedicine*. Edited by Shortliffe, E.H., and J.J. Cimino. New York: Springer Science
+ Business Media.

Narcisi, G. 2010 (March 29). Clinical data repositories: Boosting patient care and research for a data-intensive future.
CMIO Magazine. http://www.clinical-innovation.com/topics/interoperability/clinical-data-repositories-boosting-patient-
care-research-data-intensive-future.

National Learning Consortium. 2013 (September 30). Strategies for optimizing an EHR system: Checklist. Developed
by Health Information Technology Research Center (HITRC) and STRATIS Health. https://www.healthit.gov/
providers-professionals/implementation-resources/strategies-optimizing-ehr-system.

National Library of Medicine. n.d. DailyMed. http://dailymed.nlm.nih.gov.

National Quality Forum (NQF). 2010. *Driving Quality and Performance Measurement—A Foundation for Clinical
Decision Support*. Washington, DC: NQF. http://www.qualityforum.org/Publications/2010/12/Driving_Quality_and_
Performance_Measurement_-_A_Foundation_for_Clinical_Decision_Support.aspx.

Neal, R. 2011 (February 18). Don't forget CPOE's dramatic impact on nursing. HealthSystem CIO.com blog. http://
healthsystemcio.com/2011/02/18/dont-forget-cpoes-dramatic-impact-on-nursing.

Oregon Patient Safety Commission. 2015 (January 30). The impact of electronic health records on patient safety. Blog
post. http://oregonpatientsafety.org/blog/blog/the-impact-of-electronic-health-records-on-patient-safety/1721.

Osheroff, J.A., ed. 2009. *Improving Medication Use and Outcomes with Clinical Decision Support*: *A Step-by-Step
Guide*. Chicago, IL: Healthcare Information and Management Systems Society.

Osheroff, J.A., et al. 2006 (June 13). A roadmap for national action on clinical decision support. American Medical
Informatics Association. https://www.amia.org/public-policy/reports-and-fact-sheets/a-roadmap-for-national-action-on-
clinical-decision-support.

Osheroff, J.A., et al. 2012. *Improving Outcomes with Clinical Decision Support: An Implementers' Guide*, 2nd ed.
Chicago, IL: Healthcare Information and Management Systems Society.

Pendergrass, A. 2005. Supply chain generates newfound savings. *ADVANCE for Health Information Executives*.
9(8):47–49.

Phansalkar, S., et al. 2013. Drug-drug interactions that should be non-interruptive in order to reduce alert fatigue in
electronic health records. *Journal of the American Medical Informatics Association*. 20(3):489–493.

Phillips, M.T., and E.S. Berner. 2004. Beating the system: Pitfalls of bar code medication administration. *Journal of
Healthcare Information Management*. 18(4):16–18.

Radiological Society of North America (RSNA). 2011. Radiology reporting initiative. http://reportingwiki.rsna.org/
index.php?title=Main_Page.

Raimey T. 2010 (August 23). A hidden quality functional requirement—the physician documentation challenge. CSC
Meaningful Use Community and C.J. McDonald. https://community.csc.com/community/meaningful_use/blog/2010/
08/23/a-hidden-quality-functional-requirement-the-physician-documentation-challenge.

Roe, K.A. 2008 (December 1). CLIA poses barrier to lab results in EHRs, states HHS revisit CLIA and its implications.
Managed Healthcare Executive. http://managedhealthcareexecutive.modernmedicine.com/managed-healthcare-
executive/content/clia-poses-barrier-lab-results-ehrs.

Rogoski, R.R. 2005. The enterprise take on patient safety. *Health Management Technology.* 9(8):12–22.

Rollins G. 2005. The prompt, the alert, and the legal record: Documenting clinical decision support systems. *Journal of AHIMA.* 76(2):25–28.

Romney, A.D., and L.R. Hayward. 2014 (April 16). Emerging EHR risks: When documentation may not be enough (or too much). Davis Wright Tremaine, LLP blog. http://www.dwt.com/Emerging-EHR-Risks-When-Documentation-May-Not-Be-Enough-or-Too-Much-04-16-2014.

Roy, P., et al. 2009. A computerized handheld decision-support system to improve pulmonary embolism diagnosis. *Annals of Internal Medicine.* 151(10):677–686.

Ruscin, J.M., and S.A. Linnebur. 2014 (June). Drug-related problems in the elderly. *The Merck Manuals.* http://www.merckmanuals.com/professional/geriatrics/drug-therapy-in-the-elderly/drug-related-problems-in-the-elderly.

Santell, J.P. 2005. Medication errors: Experience of the United States Pharmacopeia (USP). *Joint Commission Journal on Quality and Patient Safety.* 31(2):114–119, 161.

SAS. n.d. Data visualization: What it is and why it is important. http://www.sas.com/en_us/insights/big-data/data-visualization.html.

Schadow, G. 2009 (July 18). The unified code for units of measure. http://www.unitsofmeasure.org.

Shareableink.com. 2011. Shareable ink physician progress notes. http://www.shareableink.com/applications-physician-progress-notes.html.

Silow-Carroll S., J.N. Edwards, and D. Rodin. 2012 (July). *Using Electronic Health Records to Improve Quality and Efficiency: The Experiences of Leading Hospitals.* Commonwealth Fund publication no. 1608. Vol. 17. http://www.commonwealthfund.org/~/media/files/publications/issue-brief/2012/jul/1608_silowcarroll_using_ehrs_improve_quality.pdf.

Slight, S.P., et al. 2016. The vulnerabilities of computerized physician order entry systems: A qualitative study. *Journal of the American Medical Informatics Association.* 23(2):311–316.

Smaling, J., and M.A. Holt. 2005. Integration and automation transform medication administration safety. *Health Management Technology.* 26(4):16, 18, 20.

Swenson, D. 2007. Point-of-care medication error prevention: Best practices in action. *Patient Safety and Quality Healthcare.* 4(3):1–10.

Tieche M., J. Gump, M.E. Rieck, and A. Schneider. 2010. *Picture Archiving and Communication Systems: A 2000–2008 Study.* Chicago, IL: Dorenfest Institute for Health Information. http://apps.himss.org/foundation/docs/PACS_ResearchWhitePaperFinal.pdf.

Tomczak, D. 2002 (September). Demystifying RIS/PACS integration. *Axis Imaging News.* http://www.axisimagingnews.com/2002/09/demystifying-rispacs-integration.

Tyagi, M., and T.E. Hagen. 2006 (February 6). Examine PACS: Monitoring monitors. http://www.rt-image.com.

US Department of Health and Human Services (HHS). 2014 (February 6). CLIA Program and HIPAA Privacy Rule: Patients' access to test reports. *Federal Register.* 79(25):7290. https://www.federalregister.gov/articles/2014/02/06/2014-02280/clia-program-and-hipaa-privacy-rule-patients-access-to-test-reports.

Van der Sijs, H., et al. 2006. Overriding of drug safety alerts in computerized physician order entry. *Journal of the American Medical Informatics Association.* 13:138–147.

Van der Sijs, H., et al. 2008. Turning off frequently overridden drug alerts: Limited opportunities for doing it safely. *Journal of the American Medical Informatics Association.* 15(4):439–448.

Versel, N. 2011 (December 14). 10 innovative clinical decision support programs. *Information Week.* http://www.informationweek.com/healthcare/clinical-information-systems/10-innovative-clinical-decision-support-programs/d/d-id/1101834.

Webmedx. n.d. *Practical Steps for Meaningful Physician Documentation in Healthcare.* http://www.webmedx.com/corporate/about-us/CaseStudies/Webmedx_Physician_Documentation.pdf.

Weiss, D.L., and C.P. Langlotz. 2008. Structured reporting: Patient care enhancement or productivity nightmare? *Radiology.* 249(3):739–747.

Weston, M., and D.W. Roberts. 2013 (September 30). The influence of quality improvement efforts on patient outcomes and nursing work: A perspective from chief nursing officers at three large health systems. *Online Journal of Issues in Nursing.* 18(3). http://www.nursingworld.org/Quality-Improvement-on-Patient-Outcomes.html.

Whaley, M.P. 2010 (September 9). 22 ways you will use QR (Quick Response) codes in healthcare in the future (if you're smart!). Manage My Practice blog. http://managemypractice.com/22-ways-you-will-use-qr-quick-response-codes-in-healthcare-in-the-future-if-youre-smart.

Wideman, M., et al. 2005 (February). Barcode medication administration: Lessons learned from an intensive care unit implementation. In *Advances in Patient Safety: from Research to Implementation.* Vol. 3: *Implementation Issues.* Edited by Henriksen, K., et al. Rockville, MD: Agency for Healthcare Research and Quality. http://www.ncbi.nlm.nih.gov/books/NBK20569..

Wiedemann, L. 2010. Correcting lab results in an EHR. *Journal of AHIMA.* 81(5):38–39.

Wright, A., et al. 2009. Clinical decision support capabilities of commercially-available clinical information systems. *Journal of the American Medical Informatics Association.* 16(5):637–644.

Yackel, T.R., and P.J. Embi. 2010. Unintended errors with EHR-based result management: A case series. *Journal of the American Medical Informatics Association.* 17:104–107.

Young, J., and K.B. Stevenson. 2008. Real-time surveillance and decision support: Optimizing infection control and antimicrobial choices at the point of care. *American Journal of Infection Control.* 36(3):S67–S74.

Chapter 15
Optimizing the Ambulatory Care EHR

Key Terms

Active directory
Care management
Care maps
Care pathways
Care plans
Clinical messaging
Clinical research
Community offering
Controlled substances
Evaluation and Management (E&M)
E-prescribing for Controlled Substances (EPCS)
E-visits
In-basket
Legacy systems
Longitudinal study
Medication list
Patient-centered medical home (PCMH)
Patient clinical summary
Patient-provided documentation
Physician extender
Practice guidelines
Registration
Scheduling
SCRIPT
Self-administered history assessment

Learning Objectives

- Compare and contrast elements of EHRs for acute and ambulatory settings.

- Describe the functions of an EHR for use in the ambulatory setting.

- Recommend tactics for optimizing use of EHR in an ambulatory setting.

The Office of the National Coordinator for Health Information Technology (ONC) tracks adoption and use of electronic health records (EHRs) in physician offices via an online dashboard. In April 2015, it was reported that 54 percent of all office-based physicians (and 12 percent of nurse practitioners and less than 2 percent of physician assistants) had demonstrated meaningful use (MU) of certified EHR technology (CEHRT). Demonstration of MU varies somewhat by specialty, with practitioners in internal medicine, family practice, primary care, geriatrics, obstetrics and gynecology (OB/GYN), and pediatrics adopting MU at almost twice the level of other specialists. Interestingly, data from 2014 show that 83 percent of office-based physicians had adopted *some form* of EHR, although that form may not be CEHRT. It is uncertain whether the difference between those having adopted some form of EHR and those demonstrating MU (requiring CEHRT) relates solely to the certification of the product or if there are other factors. Just the same, there is clearly opportunity for optimization of CEHRT (and potentially selection of another EHR; see also chapter 7) for ambulatory care settings. As optimization strategies are planned, selection of another EHR (reselection) is almost always a possible option in a physician office (unlike for the hospital). Reselection may entail the office acquiring the hospital's EHR, disengaging from the hospital's EHR if that is the product currently in use in the office, or simply acquiring a different EHR. Therefore, understanding the similarities and differences between EHRs for hospitals and for offices can be helpful. Other optimization strategies may also differ between the two environments (ONC 2015).

Ambulatory Versus Acute Care EHR Systems

Every EHR is intended to capture data from multiple sources and be used at the point of care for clinical decision making. The MU incentive program requires exchange of data across the continuum of care, and various emerging forms of reimbursement for physicians (which ultimately may replace the MU incentive program) will compensate physicians for using technology to support quality, cost, and practice improvement (CMS 2015). The EHRs used in acute care and ambulatory care settings share similarities but are also different in several respects. It can be helpful to appreciate the differences and similarities between the ambulatory care and acute care environments because physicians are expected to use an EHR in both locations.

Existing IT Infrastructure

There are several challenges with respect to information technology (IT) infrastructure in ambulatory settings. These include systems, IT staffing, and interoperability with the hospital or hospitals with which physicians are affiliated.

Legacy Systems
One difference between an EHR in an ambulatory setting and one in an acute care setting has nothing to do with the EHR itself but concerns the applications that were used before EHR implementation, which are generally referred to as **legacy systems**. Legacy systems are older and generally have much more limited functionality than their newer counterparts. Very small physician offices may have had no other IT at all prior to implementation of an EHR, or they may have had only a billing system or practice management system (PMS). (See chapter 19 on revenue cycle management for a discussion of the differences between a billing system and a PMS.) Those physicians

with an existing billing system or PMS may have opted to retain this system when acquiring an EHR, especially as the MU program does not require CEHRT to have billing or practice management functions. Unfortunately, most standalone billing systems and PMS cannot share data with a new EHR. If the EHR is acquired from the same vendor as the billing system or PMS, the vendor may be able to create an interface to help such sharing of data between the old billing system or PMS and the new EHR, although this set-up will have less functionality than a newer PMS component that is integrates with the EHR. Many offices worry about the expense of giving up their old system. However, the incremental cost of acquiring the new PMS from most vendors is not that great, and the cost of converting from the old system to a new one is not as high as many offices fear. As requirements to verify patient eligibility for health insurance, accept electronic funds transfer from payers, and integrate financial and clinical data for health reform increase, offices will find it difficult to manage without implementing new PMSs or billing systems, either for the first time or to replace legacy systems.

In ambulatory settings where there was no or very little IT in place, application service provider (ASP) or software as a service (SaaS) models of acquiring an EHR may have advantages (refer to chapter 7 for more information on these models). Physicians initially tended to shy away from such offsite applications over concerns about security and loss of data in the event the vendor goes out of business. However, the cost of these offerings is often considerably lower than a traditional leased model, which makes them attractive to physician offices, and the companies offering these products are garnering stronger reputations surrounding their security. Just the same, it is critical that the office do due diligence and have a strong contract with the vendor. One fairly large vendor of office management software agreed to a settlement of $250,000 with the Federal Trade Commission (FTC) for falsely advertising that its product used encryption that met MU requirements (that is, NIST Advanced Encryption Standard). However, the vendor is only required to pay the settlement amount and notify its clients, who seem to be responsible for acquiring their own encryption (HCPro 2016).

Other legacy systems found in some ambulatory environments include e-prescribing, laboratory and/or radiology information systems, and registries. Prior to acquiring an EHR, an office may have used a standalone e-prescribing system to participate in the federal government's Physician Quality Reporting Initiative (PQRI), which provided incentives for use of e-prescribing before the MU program was initiated. Such standalone systems are largely being replaced by an equivalent, and often more sophisticated, component in an EHR. Integration of e-prescribing and the EHR is highly desirable for the clinical decision support (CDS) functionality. Although many of the standalone e-prescribing systems do not support data conversion well, they also did not contain much historical data. Consequently, starting records from scratch for each patient seen with the new EHR was not as troublesome as some anticipated. Many laboratory information systems (LISs) likely needed to be upgraded to be Health Level 7 (HL7)–compliant or support structured data output. Relatively few ambulatory care environments have a legacy radiology information system (RIS) or legacy picture archiving and communications system (PACS), but these also may require updating to work with the EHR.

Finally, physician offices often contribute data to registries to manage their patient follow-up (see chapter 10). Some of these registries serve as a module of an EHR and some have even become a pared-down EHR with upgraded functionality to become certified under federal MU requirements. In this case, patients were registered into the registry at the time an appointment was made, the registry generated a data collection form for the appointment, and the completed form was sent back to the registry service for scanning. The next time the patient made an appointment, another data collection form was generated, which included key information from the previous visit. Obviously, not all such registry services have become EHRs, so it is necessary to determine the volume of data and how the registry has been used to determine whether it is feasible to consider any form of data conversion from registry records into an EHR. Registries—and registry functionality that supports population health—are key to improving quality of care across the continuum (Goedert 2011) and contribute to new forms of reimbursement for health reform, such as value-based payments (VBPs), in which physicians are reimbursed for the quality of care and outcomes rather than the number and types of services provided (see also chapter 4).

IT Staffing

Another common IT infrastructure challenge in physician offices relates to IT staffing support. Very small practices generally have no IT staff and use a contractor for assistance as needed. Slightly larger practices may have one person who is dedicated part time to IT, but a full-time IT staff person is unusual in practices with fewer than 10 physicians (Amatayakul 2010a). Offices that lack IT staff support may prefer an ASP or SaaS model for the EHR. However, even these offices will have local networking and devices that need IT staff support. Some offices will use contractors for this support. Alternatively, moderately sized and larger practices may employ dedicated IT staff to perform maintenance activities and also help make workflow changes, run reports, assist with system upgrades, train new users, provide help desk functionality, serve as the information security official, and perform other IT operations tasks.

One challenge that hospitals face that physician practices may find somewhat easier to address is engagement of physicians. Physicians in ambulatory settings have a more vested interest in ensuring that the EHR is implemented correctly because they generally are the owners of the ambulatory care organization (except for hospital outpatient departments, although the physicians may then be a contracted group or a faculty practice plan that manages themselves). That is not to suggest that all ambulatory offices do a better job of implementation or that there may not still be resistance to the use of the EHR in ambulatory environments. The point is only that there are likely to be at least some physicians interested in serving in the capacity of chief medical informatics officer—even if that is not a formal title for a smaller practice.

Interoperability

Because ambulatory offices have typically few internal source systems, they tend to have fewer interoperability challenges than are seen in the acute care hospital setting. However, as noted earlier, the clinic may have interoperability issues between its existing PMS and the EHR, as well as with any ancillary source systems. Also, much the same as hospitals, ambulatory facilities can find it difficult to integrate the EHR with external source systems, such as a reference laboratory, commercial laboratory, imaging center, the hospital where its physicians admit patients, and, increasingly, other providers with whom patient data are shared.

Interfaces with Source Systems

Most EHR vendors are well aware of the need to interface EHRs with laboratory systems. To retain customers' business, at least one company has provided a laboratory system interface to physician office EHRs at no cost to the physician practices. As previously discussed, an interface does not necessarily achieve full interoperability. Ideally, a laboratory interface should enable the transmission of an order for a laboratory test to be transmitted to the laboratory (outbound interface) and for the results to be returned in structured format (inbound interface). The same general process would be used for the results of diagnostic imaging, although, of course, the diagnostic image itself would come across as a digital image.

Interfaces with Hospitals

Creating interoperability between the hospital and clinic is challenging because the workflows and processes are different in the two settings. The predominant strategy has been to provide a physician portal into the hospital's system with view and document download capabilities (Lawrence 2009). Some hospital system vendors have created templates where physician offices can enter data for scheduling an admission or surgery via the portal. However, in such cases, the office's PMS or EHR does not supply demographic data directly through an interface; it must be keyed in separately. These portals are not inexpensive—potentially costing the hospital upwards of several hundred thousand dollars. Of course, hospitals may also provide remote access directly to their EHR to members of their medical staff. Again, however, this strategy requires a separate process apart from the office's EHR. When a physician wants to write an admission order at the conclusion of a patient visit, the physician must leave the office's EHR application and log on separately to the hospital's EHR. When physicians are performing professional services in the hospital, they often use an app on a mobile device to capture their professional services billing information and then connect the devices to their office systems or arrange for wireless transmission once they are back in the office.

To address the less than satisfactory means to achieve interoperability between physician office and hospital (especially when the sites use different vendor products), many hospitals and integrated delivery networks, in conjunction with their vendors, are offering a somewhat different version of an ASP commonly called a **community offering**, which is a means to acquire licenses for the ambulatory EHR offered by the hospital's EHR vendor (Mostashari et al. 2009). A community offering provides many of the same benefits of an ASP, such as elimination of the hassles of data center maintenance and staff support. However, because it is offered by a hospital via additional licenses instead of a vendor or true ASP, there is one **active directory** (component of the Windows operating system that manages identification of data and their relationships within a system) and one repository of data. Depending on how the community offering is structured, providers may be able to view only patient records they created, or all records created by any other provider in the community offering for their patients. This provides for continuity of care across the community.

A community offering lets physicians use the same product as their hospital—so the "look and feel" is the same wherever they may be treating patients. It also gives them the ability to share data seamlessly with their hospital and is an opportunity for ambulatory offices to acquire an EHR with little overhead. However, there are some concerns surrounding the community offering. First, only access control technology separates the clinic's data from the hospital's data. Second, a hospital is typically not in the business of providing IT services so it may not effectively support the community offering. Third, customization is limited to that performed by the hospital for all providers. Finally, the license cost may be higher than what the practice might otherwise choose to pay for a standalone product.

In addition to these concerns, a community offering must comply with the Stark Law and Anti-Kickback Statute, which prohibit arrangements of economic value among providers. In 2006, the Department of Health and Human Services (HHS) made certain exceptions, called a "safe harbor" under the Stark Law (42 CFR 411) and Anti-Kickback Statute (42 CFR 1001) for e-prescribing and EHR software donations. This safe harbor was originally set to be eliminated by 2013, but it has been extended until December 31, 2021; notably, the extension eliminates the electronic prescribing requirement for EHR systems (since CEHRT require e-prescribing to be a part of the EHR) and updates the interoperability' requirements to conform with the current MU requirements.

Data Presentation and Workflows

The nature of data and workflows surrounding use of data vary between acute and ambulatory care environments. As a result, how data are presented to the user and how data are used in clinical decision making varies.

What reviewers of both acute and ambulatory care EHRs may find when they compare systems is that the ambulatory care EHR integrates functions much more closely, and consequently the EHR often has a greater impact on overall workflow in the ambulatory setting. For example, physicians are expected to use the hospital EHR for computerized provider order entry (CPOE), but they may not use it for much of anything else, preferring instead to dictate notes, history and physical exams, operative reports, discharge summaries, and so on. In contrast, physicians in their offices find that they need to document almost everything directly in their EHR. Merely recognizing workflow differences between acute and ambulatory care, however, is not the only factor in successfully addressing differences. Ambulatory care facilities have as much need (if not more) for focused workflow and process mapping and redesign. In the ambulatory environment, physicians become intimately involved in their EHR—and also need to be able to trust it. A workflow issue as simple as "did the nurse get the order for the patient to be taken for a blood draw?" represents a change in workflow that can be disconcerting to both the nurse and the physician if the associated processes and workflows are not mapped out and changes understood and agreed on by all.

As previously noted in this book, vendors typically do very little work to understand how workflows in a particular office will change and what processes need redesign. Depending on the vendor, the company may or may not offer customization in support of workflow improvements. For example, a clinic that wanted to improve its preventive screening rate studied the workflow and process surrounding how the EHR could be used for this goal. The clinic found that the EHR system displayed preventive screening reminders when a patient's record was opened, but that was not the point in the physicians' workflow that such a reminder was desired. Rather, the physicians would have liked to have seen the reminders at the point when they were documenting their assessment and plan for patients. In this particular case, the clinic physicians told the vendor about this issue, and the vendor not only made the change for them but also added some additional features that helped even more—and then enhanced their overall product for other customers. Unfortunately, not all vendors are willing to be so accommodating or able to make changes outside of their normal versioning cycle. This has had partly to do with the tremendous changes in EHRs brought about by the MU requirements. The functionality vendors have had to add to their products as a result of MU has generally been important—if potentially not always designed in a fully usable manner.

EHR Functionality

The functions that an EHR supports are somewhat different between the ambulatory and acute care environments because of their inherent differences in workflows. A hospital collects a dense and large volume of data about a patient for a relatively short period of time. Although hospitals may need to access data for a few months after the patient is discharged, hospitals have considerably less need to access these records once that period of time is over. Even for subsequent admissions, hospitals may have little need to go back to records from a previous admission. In contrast, clinics collect a small amount of information at any given time about a patient, but they typically build on that information over multiple encounters that potentially span a long period of time. The nature of the physician's specialty also makes a difference. The primary care provider will likely see the patient fairly often, potentially for many different types of conditions. For many primary care providers, it is imperative to be able to review past information to determine whether there are patterns that might suggest a new diagnosis or give insight into the management of chronic conditions. By comparison, orthopedic surgeons may maintain records more like a hospital in that they treat a patient for one broken leg and then may never see the patient again. The different data needs affect everything from whether offices assign an account number to each visit (which they generally do not) to the need for chart conversion during implementation (generally more likely in a clinic than a hospital).

Data entered into a hospital EHR must be available for all members of the care team to view, and these data must be date- and time-stamped to identify the time an entry was made and by whom. Any error that is made must be annotated properly. Because things happen quickly in a hospital, it is conceivable that an erroneous entry could be seen by another caregiver and used to inform a subsequent action, even when the error is caught as quickly as the very next time the author of the erroneous entry documents. Diligence in authenticating the author of an entry in an ambulatory EHR is required by the Health Insurance Portability and Accountability Act (HIPAA), state licensing laws, and other requirements, but the fact of the matter is that, in many small practices, it is primarily the physician who enters data into a chart. In some offices, even the medical assistant or nurse who rooms a patient, takes vital signs, and inquires about the reason for the visit does not record information into the chart. He or she may write all such information on scratch paper for the physician. As a result, some clinic EHRs do not have robust means to switch from one user to another, annotate errors, or even permit more than one user to access the EHR at a time. These are important functions to evaluate when a physician office or clinic is reviewing vendor offerings.

Many ambulatory EHRs include all functionality in a tightly integrated manner and can provide multiple data points simultaneously in a single view or set of windows, whereas hospital EHRs typically do not have similar functionality. This difference significantly affects the type of human–computer interface devices chosen for the respective environments. For example, EHR users in an ambulatory setting often use a laptop device because they move from one exam room to another, but there is adequate space in these rooms to place a laptop when not directly being used for review or documentation. In a hospital, however, nurses prefer workstations on wheels (WOWs) because there is rarely sufficient space to rest a laptop in a patient room. They also move quickly from one room to another and find a WOW outfitted with a medication drawer and other utilities helpful. Physicians in a hospital tend to prefer desktop computers, often away from the patients and flow of visitors. This set-up enables them to spend time thinking about their orders or other documentation without interruption.

Another element of data integration relates to patient identification. Clinics have largely relied on a sign-in sheet at the reception desk and verbal communication to validate that they are addressing the right patient in the exam room. With an EHR, clinics are able to take a digital picture of the patient and refer to it as another means of positive identification, along with verbal communication. On the other hand, some hospitals use bar code technology to support positive identification because the patient may not always be able to communicate verbally and his or her face may not be clearly visible at all times.

Finally, a clinic may be able to quickly achieve a "paperless" state whereas the hospital frequently must exist in a hybrid state, potentially for several years. The fact that a clinic can move more quickly to a paperless environment, however, does not always mean that the transition occurs rapidly. It is very important for a clinic to develop a chart conversion strategy and a roll-out plan to ensure that it moves to electronic format in a logical sequence.

To convert office charts, some facilities scan all previous records or at least records of its active patients. Other clinics apply a strategy of abstracting key data from active patients' records to have available as soon as the new user begins to use the system. Having some data prepopulated in this manner facilitates the immediate use of CDS, providing value back to the new user and making the learning curve more palatable. Still other clinics use a combination of chart conversion strategies, and some even decide not to undertake conversion of old charts at all but to pull old charts for a period of time. Physicians themselves may abstract pertinent information from the old charts during or immediately before or after a visit to eliminate their subsequent pulling. There are advantages and disadvantages to each strategy.

Check Your Understanding 15.1

Indicate whether the following statements are true or false. Choose the best answer:

1. Over 80 percent of office-based physicians have some form of EHR.

2. Physicians will not have to use EHRs after the MU program ends.

3. Lack of a PMS or its connectivity to an EHR will affect an office's ability to keep up with healthcare payment reform.

4. Registries are sometimes used as a "lite" form of EHR.

5. The ability to communicate between the hospital EHR and office EHR is being facilitated by small, niche vendors offering specialized interfaces.

6. EHR functionality is generally more tightly integrated in an ambulatory EHR than in a hospital EHR.

Ambulatory EHR Functions

There are several ways to categorize ambulatory EHR functions with respect to information sources and uses. Figure 15.1 displays key clinic/office processes in a sequence as they might logically occur during a visit or separate from a visit.

Another way to categorize EHR functions might be by the functions performed on the data. Figure 15.2 illustrates this approach.

As an office looks to improve the value it is deriving from its EHR, it is important to consider what functionality (beyond that required by MU or other policies or programs) is desired and conduct a vendor selection process that ensures such functionality will be present (or is being planned for as specified in the vendor contract) and is usable (see chapter 7). As the MU program draws to an end, it is important to evaluate the functionality that may become needed in light of other, new healthcare initiatives. Some providers may be tempted to "drop" consideration for having a CEHRT or the equivalent going forward. Although some MU functionality has been challenging for vendors to build and providers to use, the newer functionality is reflective of what most experts anticipate will be future needs. In other words, as an organization undertakes optimization of the EHR—whether by reselection or by adding to the existing suite of products—it is important to not repeat mistakes made when the EHR was first implemented.

Looking critically at the marketplace is essential. During stage 1 of the MU program, more than 4,000 ambulatory EHR vendors were certified. Today, only a handful of these vendors remain viable, and an even a smaller number are used in the majority of offices. ONC tracks data associated with vendor use by the number of physicians attesting to use of CEHRT. By March 2015, 62 percent of all physicians in the MU program were using 10 vendors. Another 20 vendors were used by 12 percent of physicians. The remaining 755 vendors were being used by the remaining 26 percent of physicians. Essentially, over 95 percent of the vendors in the ambulatory EHR market (755 out of 785 total) were at risk for going out of business due to insufficient market share. Furthermore, only about 20 percent of the vendors that initially entered the marketplace are still offering CEHRT products (ONC 2015). Anyone considering EHR reselection should reflect on these data. Reselection may be right for some offices; however, offices that move forward could regret the decision if they do not fully understand functionality needs, improve upon workflows, and perform vendor due-diligence. Finally, taking time to strategically plan, including anticipating what the office and

Figure 15.1.   Key clinic processes

Key Processes	EHR Goals	Baseline Metrics	Outcomes
Typical Visit-Related Processes (Clinical decision support and documentation included in all processes)			
1. Previsit registration, scheduling, insurance verification			
2. Check-in			
3. Patient intake			
4. Chart review			
5. Medical history interview			
6. Physical examination			
7. Assessment			
8. Diagnosis			
9. Care planning			
10. Health maintenance			
11. Staff tasking/back office orders			
12. Procedure			
13. Prescribing/samples			
14. Lab/radiology ordering			
15. Coding			
16. Charge capture and billing			
17. Referral management			
18. Patient instructions			
19. Visit summary			
20. Checkout			
Special Types of Visits			
21. Nurse-only visit			
22. Same-day/urgent visit			
23. Annual physical exam			
24. Occupational medicine			
25. Consultation			
26. Other: _____			
Non-visit Related Processes			
27. Results review and management			
28. No-show management			
29. Prescription refill/renewal requests			
30. Other phone calls/e-mail			
31. Patient follow-up/recall			
32. Release of information			
33. Forms completion			

(continued)

Figure 15.1.   Key clinic processes (Continued)

Key Processes	EHR Goals	Baseline Metrics	Outcomes
34. Patient document management			
35. Chronic disease management			
36. Quality improvement			
37. Required reporting			
38. Pay for performance			
39. Patient self-management/PHR			
40. Clinical trials			

Copyright © 2016, Margret\A Consulting, LLC. Reprinted with permission.

healthcare more broadly might look like in five to ten years, should help an office decide whether to switch systems or optimize use of its existing systems. If the existing system's vendor has struggled to meet stage 2 requirements for MU, the office should consider two questions: First, will that vendor survive beyond the end of MU? Second, what are the chances that desired functionality for the future can come from this vendor? It may be that the office does not necessarily want all of the functionality in stage 2 MU or what has been proposed for stage 3. But the office may want some of that functionality or seek functionality that is not a part of MU as currently designed.

Whatever the office decides about acquiring a new system or building on the existing one, it should attend to workflow and process improvements and change management. As offices identify desired functionality and seek ways to optimize current functionality, they will find it helpful to review the functionality already in place. Some offices find that their systems actually have more functionality than they thought—but their physicians and other staff do not know how to use or get value from these functions.

Scheduling, Registration/Check-In, Documentation, In-Basket, and Checkout

Scheduling, registration/patient check-in, in-basket, and checkout are related functions. Although scheduling always occurs first and checkout always occurs last, the registration/check-in and in-basket functions, along with potentially additional other functions, vary by EHR capability and preferred workflow of the clinic.

Scheduling

The **scheduling** function is used to locate and record the time the patient is to be seen. Some ambulatory EHR systems provide a patient portal that permits patients to request or possibly schedule an appointment.

Some scheduling systems prompt staff to initiate a benefits eligibility inquiry. Clinics may make inquiries for all or only a selection of patients. Clinics may use a portal made available by some payers. Some PMS/EHR products support eligibility inquiry and response using the HIPAA transaction standards (ASC X12 270/271 Eligibility Inquiry and Response).

Currently, most clinics find the portal form of inquiry to be cumbersome and not available for all benefits plans; however, it yields more complete information for a given patient than the Eligibility Inquiry and Response standard. This is changing as the Affordable Care Act of 2010 (ACA) in its health reform provisions (HHS 2015) has mandated adoption of standard operating rules for all HIPAA transactions (see chapters 13 and 19). Via these operating rules, providers receive more consistent and predictable data, regardless of health plan. For example, in the past, providers who wanted to check whether a patient has health insurance would send an eligibility transaction to

Figure 15.2.   EHR functions for ambulatory care environments

1. **Patient data capture functions**
    a. Capture and record patient demographics
    b. Capture and record patient medical history
    c. Capture and record patient medication history
    d. Capture and record patient allergy information
    e. Capture and record vital signs; perform BMI calculation
    f. Receive diagnostic studies results
    g. Record clinical documentation: visit notes, physical exams, assessments, plans
    h. Record temporary notes to self or others
    i. Capture key health data for minimum data sets
    j. Capture external clinical documents
    k. Capture images from PACS and other medical devices
    l. Capture patient-originated data
    m. Capture and display advance directives

2. **Patient data management functions**
    a. Manage problem list
    b. Manage medication list
    c. Perform medication reconciliation
    d. Manage allergy and adverse reaction list
    e. Manage patient-specific care plans, guidelines, and protocols
    f. Capture variances from standard care plans, guidelines, and protocols
    g. Trend data from multiple sources (e.g., labs, meds impact on labs)

3. **Prescription/ordering function**
    a. Manage medication formularies
    b. Write prescriptions
    c. Approval refills/renewals
    d. Receive refill notifications
    e. Drug, food, allergy, lab interaction checking
    f. Drug-condition/indications checking
    g. Patient-specific dosing and warnings
    h. Order diagnostic tests
    i. Order referrals

4. **Clinical decision support functions**
    a. Receive results notification
    b. Receive support from standard assessments
    c. Receive support from patient context-enabled assessments
    d. Receive information on most cost-effective services, referrals, devices, etc. to recommend to patient
    e. Support clinical trial recruitment
    f. Support for health maintenance, preventive care, and wellness
    g. Support automated surveillance for ADE, disease outbreaks, bioterrorism
    h. Support chronic disease management
    i. Support drug/device recall
    j. Manage rules presentation: passive, context-sensitive, mandatory, reference

(continued)

Figure 15.2.   EHR functions for ambulatory care environments (Continued)

5. **Patient support functions**
   a. Provide patient-specific instructions
   b. Generate patient reminders
   c. Provide patient-friendly summary
   d. Provide patient-specific education materials
   e. Provide electronic access to key information
   f. Provide electronic copy of patient record
   g. Support home monitoring/tracking capability

6. **Clinic workflow functions**
   a. Schedule and manage clinical tasks (work queues, personnel, rooms, equipment)
   b. Provide personalized in-basket/dashboard support
   c. Automatically generate administrative data from clinical record
   d. Enable printout of documents when necessary
   e. Enable deidentification of protected health information when necessary
   f. Enable specialized views of data
   g. Support multimedia: images, waveforms, scanned documents, pictures, sounds

7. **Administrative and reimbursement functions**
   a. Automatically generate administrative and financial data from clinical record
   b. Provide rules-driven financial and administrative coding assistance
   c. Manage external accountability reporting/outcomes measures
   d. Contract management

8. **Electronic communication and connectivity functions**
   a. Enable transfer of data to notifiable registries (reportable diseases, immunizations)
   b. Provide a current directory of provider information
   c. Manage provider identifiers
   d. Manage (external) trading partners: retail pharmacy, insurer, lab, radiology
   e. Provide secure messaging
   f. Support remote access
   g. Provide secure authentication, including two-factor authentication with digital certificate for e-prescribing of controlled substances
   h. Provide access management and audit log services
   i. Enforce patient privacy and confidentiality, including documenting notice of privacy practices, accepting requests for confidential communications and other restrictions, making amendments, and providing accounting for disclosures
   j. Ensure integrity, data retention, and availability
   k. Provide encryption for data at rest and data in motion
   l. Manage system versioning (change control)
   m. Support interoperability through compliance with data interchange standards and agreements
   n. Support data comparability through use of controlled vocabularies

9. **Quality measurement, reporting, and improvement**
   a. Calculate and submit data on clinical measures specified by CMS and others
   b. Provide feedback on quality metrics to providers and patients
   c. Be able to define goals for quality improvement and measure results
   d. Utilize quality improvement data to feedback into EHR templates, evidence-based decision support, and other uses of EHR

inquire about the patient's eligibility for services. The response often was a simple yes or no; but, under the operating rules, additional information is required to be supplied, such as whether the patient has a deductible or co-insurance amount due.

After a patient is scheduled, some clinics encourage the patient to complete an online patient **self-administered history assessment** (Wenner et al. 1994; Bachman 2003; Vogel et al. 2012; Murray et al. 2013). If the patient has access to the Internet, the assessment may be made available through a secure portal in advance of the visit. If the patient does not have access to the Internet, he or she may be asked to arrive earlier than the scheduled appointment to complete the assessment at a kiosk in the waiting room. A kiosk combines a physical enclosure and a computer that uses special software to deliver applications in a secure manner, often having touch screens with large buttons and font sizes. In addition to various health-related applications, including scheduling, bill payment, and educational resources, a kiosk may also include biometric identification, insurance card scanners, cameras, and payment transaction devices. Some clinics set up a special area where patients can use the kiosk in private but also receive assistance from staff, if necessary.

Although such an assessment process is not new, it has not yet been broadly adopted. However, more clinics are starting to realize that the self-administered history assessment is a useful way to collect a comprehensive—and consistent—set of data about the patient. The assessment is context-sensitive, so only questions related to the encounter are asked (for example, male patients would not be asked for pregnancy information, and a person with a recurring appointment for a chronic condition would not be asked for a complete history at every visit). Patients can take their time to answer all pertinent questions in the assessment, and the data are entered in structured form that is ready for use in the EHR. When the provider is ready to see the patient, the information gleaned from the assessment can be validated and any additional documentation added as necessary. The self-assessment also reduces the amount of data entry the physician must perform, freeing time for discussion with the patient.

Registration

The **registration** function generally occurs immediately prior to or at the time of check-in. At the time of check-in, all pertinent registration functions, if not previously performed, can be conducted or information updated as necessary. The patient's check-in updates the in-basket function with the patient's arrival information.

Some clinics take digital pictures of their patients to incorporate into the EHR as a means of positive patient identification. They also may have a card or document scanner in the check-in area to scan the patient's insurance card, photo identification, and potentially other documents the patient may need to sign or bring with them for incorporation into the EHR. These processes may be even more automated by using a touchscreen kiosk that enables patients to identify that they have arrived, swipe their credit card for co-pays, sign the acknowledgment of receipt of the notice of privacy practices, and perform other functions as desired by the clinic (Rhoads and Drazen 2009). Registration also starts the clock for monitoring patient wait times. Some EHR vendors have incorporated this functionality as an option; there are also niche vendors that sell such systems and interface them to the practice management side of the PMS/EHR.

Patient-Provided Documentation

The incorporation of **patient-provided documentation** into the EHR, such as from a personal health record (PHR), should be a matter addressed in the clinic's policies. Some clinics accept virtually any and every document the patient may bring from other providers. Other clinics, however, are more discriminating, accepting only documents they have specifically requested and sometimes accepting them only directly from another provider. In other cases, the physician may review documentation brought to the visit by a patient and select what will be scanned into the EHR or will summarize key factors as a note, returning the documentation to the patient (Amatayakul 2010b).

In addition to a policy about what may be incorporated into the EHR, it is a good idea to have a policy describing the communication with the patient that is appropriate to accompany incorporation or rejection of such documents. Some patients may view provision of such documents as their right under the HIPAA Privacy Rule to request an amendment to their health record, when often the content is not directly related to existing documentation and not appropriately considered an amendment. Providers are concerned about liability for accepting a voluminous set of documents that they must spend time reading and which may contain information they do not address in a particular visit. Many legal experts believe it is best to return these documents to patients, suggesting the documents are their personal records and should be kept for their own reference and used as a way to jog their memory about what they might want to discuss with their providers. As the PHR gains greater popularity, it is more often supported directly by a provider organization, and it may even serve as the consent management function (see chapter 13) of a health information exchange (HIE). (See chapter 17 for additional information on PHRs.) Providers need to keep abreast of changes in both the legal/regulatory environment and the movement under ACA's health reform initiatives to empower consumers to become more engaged in their health and healthcare (see chapter 20), often with the aid of a PHR.

In-Basket Function

The **in-basket** is a scheduling and reminder function that provides workflow information to various system users based on their individual needs. It is named for the in-basket on the desk where papers are left for the person who sits at the desk to review. In the physician office setting, the in-basket function alerts the medical assistant or nurse to the patient's arrival for an appointment, the physician when the patient is ready to be seen in the examination room, the office manager (and potentially all users) regarding how long the patient has been waiting, and so on. It also lists results to review, prescription refills to be approved, transcribed reports to be authenticated, and so on. Some in-baskets have telephone autodial features to facilitate calls to patients, and most also incorporate email. At least one vendor has linked up with a smartphone vendor and provides in-basket functionality via the smartphone (Dolan 2010). Smartphone apps also increasingly include functionality that permits physicians to record their professional services conducted in the hospital. Figure 15.3 displays an example of an in-basket screen.

Checkout

Many physician offices do not have a checkout process. Some think they are too small and do not need this function. Staff at very large clinics may believe that too many patients wander away from examination rooms without understanding where to go to be checked out. With an EHR, however, checkout can be managed better and in multiple locations, if necessary. Functions performed at checkout include having the patient schedule the next appointment, obtain instructions, and pay the bill (or co-payment if that was not collected at check-in). Just as with scheduling, all these activities can be automated and performed from any location. They generally contribute to enhanced patient satisfaction as well as improved cash flow and potentially increased revenue for the clinic.

At the time of checkout, some clinics use a nurse to provide patient education materials and offer specific instructions that either were not covered during the visit with the provider or are in addition to information provided by the provider. These educational and instructional materials should be patient-specific and can be generated by the EHR. Many EHR vendors incorporate a subscription to educational materials in their product offerings, or they can recommend vendors who supply such materials. The Institute for Clinical Systems Improvement (ICSI) offers a number of patient education resources free of charge from its website (2009). Not only do patients appreciate the specific nature of the instructions (and the clinic is able to check this function off for its MU compliance), but providing more specific information and spending more time on this function may also reduce subsequent phone calls and improve quality of care, at least on a short-term basis, although subsequent interventions may be needed for chronically ill patients (Matthews et al. 2007).

Figure 15.3. Example of an in-basket screen

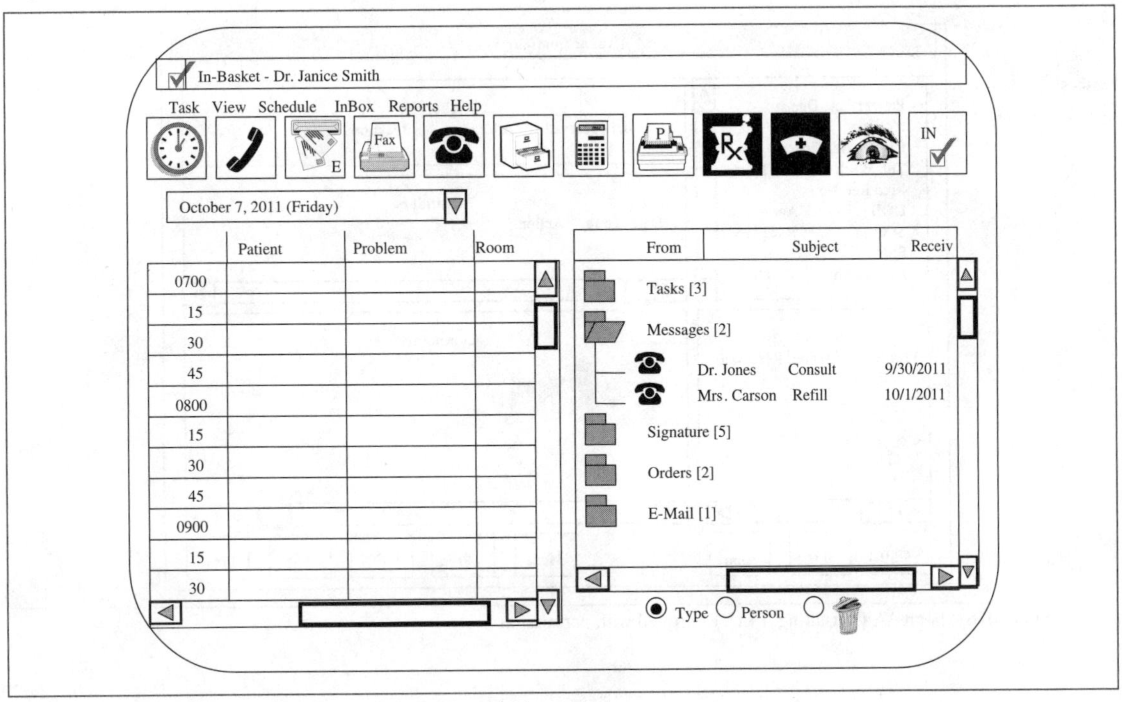

Copyright © 2016, Margret\A Consulting, LLC. Reprinted with permission.

Patient Summary

Physicians are likely to view the **patient clinical summary** as one of the most desired functions in an EHR. For the provider, the patient summary usually displays basic demographic information, a problem list, a current medication list, and a listing of recent visits and results available for review. Figure 15.4 shows an example of a patient summary screen. Providing patients with such a summary (and with timely, electronic, and direct access to their EHR) is a requirement of the MU program and has been shown to help facilitate continuity of care and improve patients' engagement in their healthcare (Patel and Siminerio 2014; ONC 2014). Sustained continuity of care improves the quality of care by decreasing hospitalizations, emergency department use, and even referrals (Maude and Tomlinson 2010). It also improves the receipt of preventive services to keep individuals healthy (Cabana and Jee 2004).

The current **medication list**, which identifies all medications the patient is currently taking, may be compiled in a number of ways. For example, physicians and nurses may enter medications directly through a prescribing function or history-taking function. In such cases, the medication list will contain all the medications the clinician believes the patient is taking, including over-the-counter (OTC) drugs.

A medication list also may be compiled through a subscription service to a **pharmacy benefits management (PBM)** consolidator, such as SureScripts. A PBM is a company that manages the variety of prescription drug programs offered by health plans. SureScripts is currently the predominant company that supplies an e-prescribing gateway, which is a standardized communication framework linking prescribers, pharmacies, PBMs, and health plans for the purpose of sharing prescription benefit information and exchanging prescriptions electronically between providers and retail drug stores or mail order drug suppliers (SureScripts 2011). A subscription to this or another similar service may provide the physician office EHR a consolidated list of all medications for which the patient has filed

Figure 15.4.   Sample patient summary screen

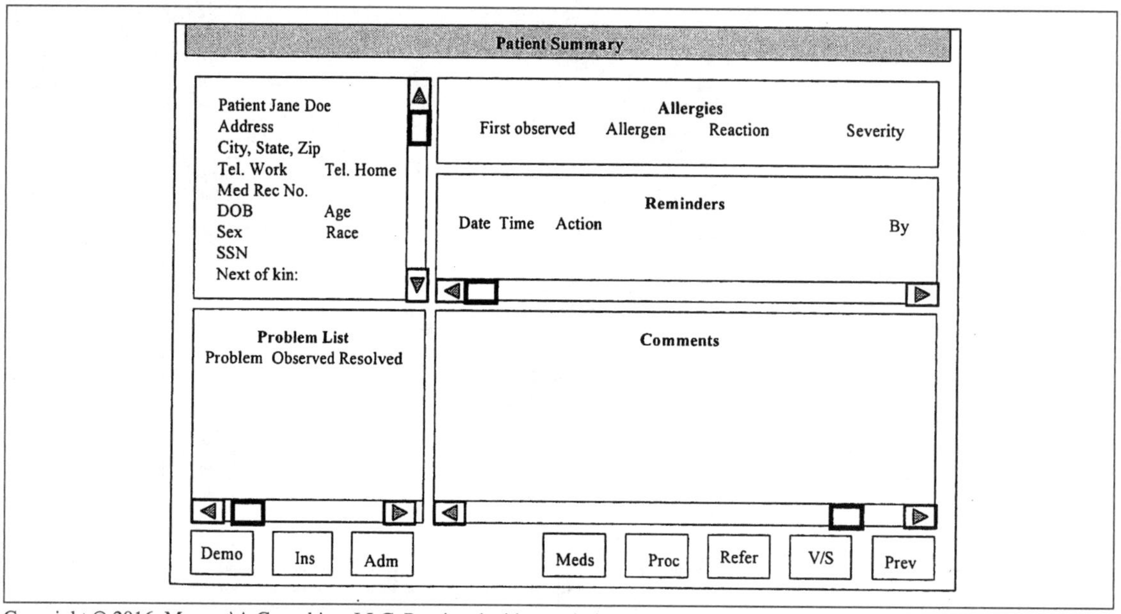

a claim. However, if the patient paid for a prescription by cash or credit card, there would be no claim and the transaction would not be included in this list. Also, OTC medications would not be included. Notably, at least one large retail pharmacy chain is attempting to capture OTC medication information through its point-of-sale merchant function, although such a list must be verified with the patient because it might include OTC medications purchased for someone else.

Documentation

Although documentation for the EHR can occur through transcribed dictation notes or scanned paper documents electronically fed into the EHR, most clinics want their EHRs to support as much structured data entry as possible, while still supporting some narrative notes. Structured data are essential for the CDS function.

Templates

To aid in entering structured data, templates are used to guide data collection. Templates are generally built around care plans, clinical guidelines, protocols, or pathways that have been created by the EHR vendor, using either publicly or commercially available sources, or through their own clinical design team or user community.

Care plans, clinical guidelines, protocols, or pathways are important clinical workflow devices. Paper versions of these devices are cumbersome to use and essentially serve only as a reference device—although using paper forms to collect structured data can be a way to ease providers into better understanding and use of structured data (Edsal 2006). An EHR can make these sorts of devices interactive and support not only information and workflow but also documentation. Some experts draw distinctions among these terms, as follows:

- **Care plans** are treatment plans created for individual patients. Although all physicians document some form of plan for treating their patients, the term *care plan* is used in the context of care coordination conducted as part of health reform initiatives to describe integrated health and social care needs. *Care plan* is also commonly used to describe the documentation that identifies nursing orders during a hospitalization as well as the formal plan of care for nursing home, hospice, and home health patients for which the Centers for Medicare and Medicaid Services (CMS) requires specific oversight by a provider.

- *Guidelines* are generally considered recommendations based on systematic statements or clinical algorithms of proven care options (see also the discussion of evidence-based medicine later in this chapter). They are often developed by professional organizations, payers, or government agencies (such as the Agency for Healthcare Research and Quality [AHRQ]) and increasingly are part of clinical quality measurement support for analyzing physician outcomes. **Practice guidelines** are widely used in physician, nursing, and multidisciplinary teams (AHRQ 2016).

- Protocols are an agreed-upon framework outlining either the care that will be provided to patients by practitioners in a designated area of practice (for example, what home health nurses are permitted to do) or in a clinical trial based on investigations done by professional societies, drug companies, or individual researchers (Ebling Library 2015).

- **Care pathways**, or **care maps**, delineate the standardized, day-to-day course of care for a group of patients with the same diagnosis or procedure to achieve consistent outcomes. Pathways are often developed by the local facility or health plan and are more commonly used by nurses than by physicians (Carpenito-Moyet 2009, 17–18).

Physicians have routinely developed care plans, although the plans may not be documented explicitly as such in the health record. In hospital records, evidence of the physician's care plan is generally found at the conclusion of the history and physical examination report as the "plan," and in the orders for care. In the inpatient setting, nurses also routinely develop care plans. In the paper environment, nursing care plans may have been recorded on temporary forms and were not incorporated into the permanent health record. As nursing documentation systems have been implemented, the care plan is being incorporated into nurses' documentation. Nurses also have begun to adopt more formalized clinical guidelines, protocols, or pathways of their own or as instituted by the organization with whom they work or the state in which they are licensed. In the ambulatory environment, physicians develop care plans that they often document in their encounter notes.

Care management, including care planning, care coordination, and population management, is a cornerstone of the **patient-center medical home (PCMH)**. PCMH is an approach to providing comprehensive primary care wherein partnerships between patients, their personal physicians, and—when appropriate—the patient's family are formed. Increasingly, PCMH is also related to new models of physician payment, such as VBP. Care is coordinated and/or integrated across all elements of the healthcare system, including subspecialty care, hospitals, home health agencies, and nursing homes and with the patient's community services. Care is facilitated by registries, IT, HIE, and other means. The purpose of PCMH is to improve quality and safety, enhance access to care, and appropriately recognize the value of care delivered through a PCMH in reimbursement. The Patient Centered Primary Care Collaborative, a partnership of the American Academy of Family Physicians (AAFP), American Academy of Pediatrics (AAP), American College of Physicians (ACP), and American Osteopathic Association (AOA), has developed joint principles of the PCMH (AAFP et al. 2007). The National Committee for Quality Assurance (NCQA) accredits practices as PCMHs. The AHRQ has reported on the roles of PCMH and accountable care organizations (ACOs) called for in the ACA with respect to care coordination. Although there are many attributes of PCMHs and ACOs that are not technology-based, they both rely on using evidence-based medicine and CDS tools to guide shared decision making with patients and their families, engaging in performance measurement and improvement, measuring and responding to patient experiences and patient satisfaction, and practicing population health management (AHRQ 2011). ACOs are one way that providers organize themselves to participate in the ACA health reform initiatives, including for Medicare, Medicaid, and a number of commercial health plans. ACOs are generally provider-led with a strong base of primary care physicians (as well as hospitals and other provider types) that collectively are accountable for quality and total per capita costs across the continuum of care for a population of patients. Medicare payments are linked to quality improvements that also reduce overall costs.

Evidence-based Medicine

The enormous variation in how physicians treat patients has come under scrutiny from parties seeking to improve care and reduce healthcare costs by identifying and instituting best practices for patient care. Much of the variation in physician practice is due to differences in physician training, changes in diagnostic and therapeutic modalities, and/or the volume of patient visits. Variations in practice are especially great among primary care physicians because they face a huge variety of diagnostic challenges and cannot possibly be expected to keep up with all the latest drugs and treatment protocols. Where the average physician may see 20 or so patients a day, some primary care physicians may see two, three, or even four times that number of patients in a day—especially during flu season or at back-to-school times.

Increasingly, physicians are turning to **evidence-based medicine (EBM)** support in their EHRs. EBM is the explicit use of clinical guidelines, protocols, or pathways that have been developed through research or other formal analysis of best practices. EBM, however, is both controversial and in need of care investigation.

According to Tonelli (2006), there can be tension between the clinical experience of the physician, evidence from research, and patient goals and values. Tonelli, who is a physician and professor, highlights a case in which best practices conflict with an unusual set of patient signs and symptoms, causing the best-practice evidence to potentially be inapplicable to this particular case. Much as EHR vendor contracts stipulate that EHRs are not substitute for professional judgment, so too must EBM become a key part, but not the totality, of the decision making in patient care. In a later article on this subject, Goldman and Shih (2011) observe that while EBM is important, "continuing to incorporate joint decision making into clinical practice . . . safeguards the importance of individual patient values" and may lessen unintended consequences of exclusive reliance on EBM.

When EBM is acquired for use in an EHR (or embedded in an EHR being selected), how it was developed and its quality should be investigated. Downing and colleagues (2009), as shown in figure 15.5, illustrate how EBM is generated and used in CDS and for clinical quality measurement (CQM). Ideally, longitudinal data are combined with research data to produce evidence. **Longitudinal data** are data collected from a sample population over different points in a long period of time (NLS n.d.). Such data collection allows for the measurement of changes over time without the bias associated with variations in the sample. For EBM, it would be ideal to collect data from health records reflecting patients' birth-to-death experiences, but that is currently an almost impossible task. As a result, longitudinal data are rarely a contributory factor in current EBM. **Clinical research** is a study carried out on a sample of patients. The quality of clinical research varies with the degree to which there are controls designed to mitigate variation. In reality, a third component is probably most prevalent in generating EBM. This third component includes case studies and expert opinions of knowledgeable persons.

Because EBM generally lacks longitudinal data, draws from research of varying types, and uses other forms of knowledge, it is important to consider the quality of evidence used in any EBM system. EHR systems have been known to embed templates and/or CDS rules with EBM from a very wide variety of sources, from literature reviews conducted by a single professor to reports from companies or organizations whose primary work product is collecting best evidence from research studies and other sources. Sometimes, the EHRs report the levels of evidence, or grades, assigned by the sources that analyze the evidence. Such grades have been developed over time to help users of EBM evaluate the quality of the data contributing to the system (Burns et al. 2011). Figure 15.6 summarizes the general schema used in levels of evidence systems (without differentiating nuances

Figure 15.5.   Generation of EBM for use in CDS and CQM

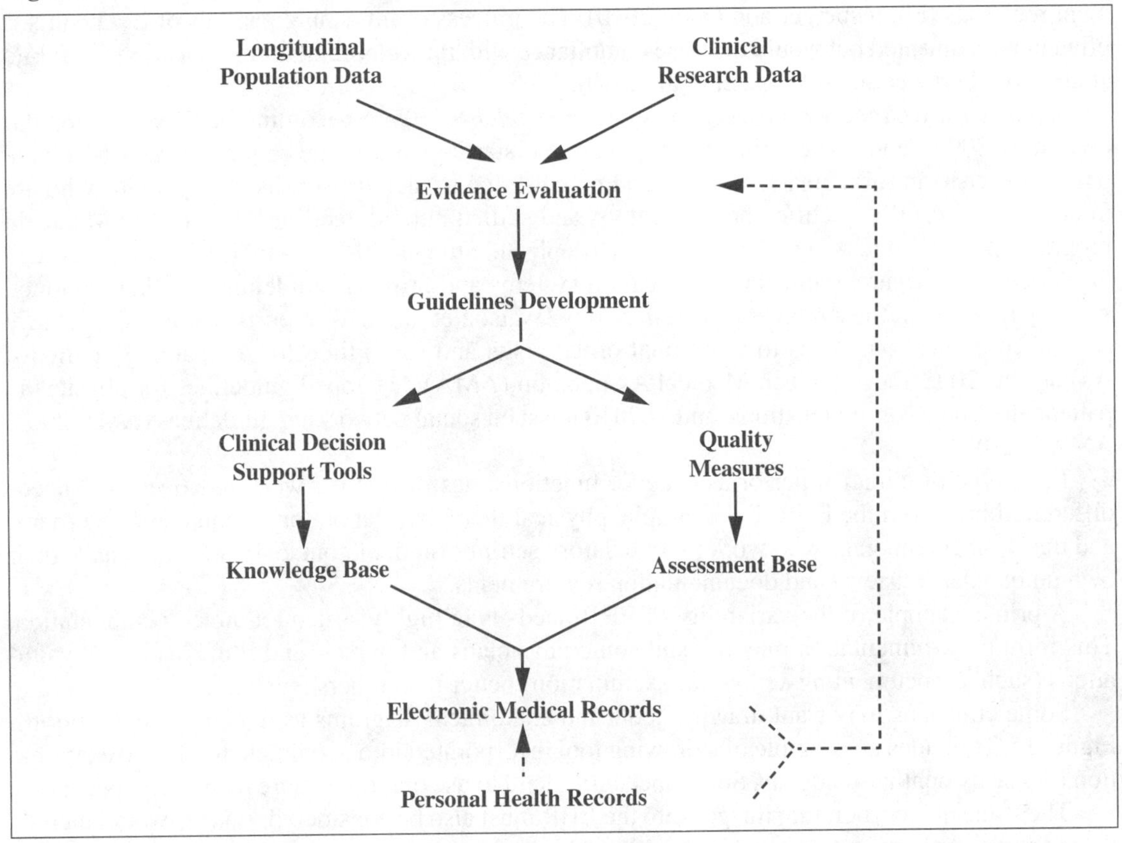

Source: Downing et al 2009

Figure 15.6.   Summary schema of levels of evidence

Level	Therapy	Prognosis	Diagnosis	Economic Decision Analysis
I	Best evidence: At least one high-quality randomized controlled study			
II	Lesser quality randomized controlled study or well-designed controlled study without randomization			
III	Controlled case studies, retrospective comparative studies, or systematic review of level III studies			
IV	Case studies			
V	Least evidence: Opinions of respected authorities based on clinical experience, descriptive studies, or reports of expert panels			

Source: Summarized from DeVries and Berlet 2010.

associated with each use). Some of the newest schemas also differentiate between evidence for use in therapy, prognosis, diagnosis, and economic decision analysis (DeVries and Berlet 2010).

Other Documentation Needs

Much of the documentation in the ambulatory EHR is performed during a patient encounter by the physician or midlevel provider, also called **physician extender** (such as physician assistant, nurse practitioner, or nurse midwife); however, it should be noted that documentation also occurs at other times and can be done by other clinicians. Documentation of telephone and e-mail encounters, refill and renewal documentation, recall management, and other documentation must be supported.

Proactive patient outreach helps patients with chronic conditions engage and better track their treatment regimens (Ehrensberger and Odell 2010). The process of informing patients of test results is often not documented but would increase compliance with this important communication (Casalino et al. 2009; Ferris et al. 2009; Elder et al. 2010).

E-visits (also called *virtual visits* or sometimes *telehealth*) are becoming increasingly popular (Williams 2009), and some commercial payers are starting to provide reimbursement Medicare pays for e-visits in rural areas and is expanding coverage to include e-visits with patients who are in hospitals, federally qualified health centers, and skilled nursing facilities. Some state Medicaid programs pay for e-visits in patients' homes (Joseph and Stuhan 2015). AAFP (2013) supports such visits over safe, secure, online communication systems and provides guidelines for their conduct. A study reported in the *Archives of Dermatology* (Watson et al. 2010) reports that e-visits achieve equivalent clinical outcomes to traditional office visits and saves time for dermatology patients. As early as 2002, the American Medical Association (AMA) developed guidelines for physician–patient electronic communications, and in 2010 it issued social networking guidelines (AMA 2002; AMA 2010).

Each type of clinician performs specific functions, has distinctive work practices, and needs different things from the EHR. For example, physical therapists, laboratory technicians, dietitians, and many other clinicians who work in ambulatory settings (and, of course, in hospitals) have their own unique data retrieval and documentation requirements.

A prime example of the variability of EHR needs is in highly structured note documentation. This form of documentation may not suit some physicians and nurses, and it may suit some situations (such as documenting a physical examination) better than others (such as a consultation).

Some clinicians may want drawing tools and anatomical diagrams as documentation options. Figure 15.7 provides an example of a drawing tool incorporated into a template for an eye examination for use by ophthalmologists. Some specialties tend to use diagrams more than other specialties.

The value of incorporating images into the EHR must also be considered. Images would include those from radiology, potential macroscopic and microscopic laboratory specimen images, waveforms from electrocardiograms and other medical devices, and pictures of a patient's rash, disfigurement, or other condition for before-and-after comparisons. All these functions and forms of data

Figure 15.7.   Example of structured data entry screen with drawing tools

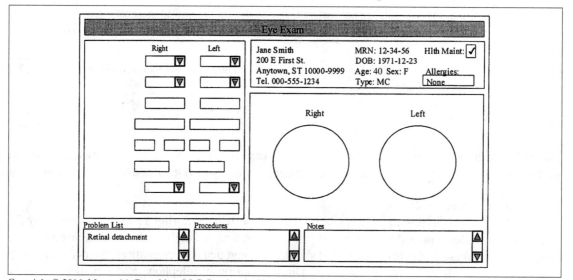

must be evaluated against the costs associated with the storage of data, retrieval time, and physician time spent working with data. Following is a case study.

> During the review of one EHR system, it was noted that no drawings were included in the documentation. A dermatologist was asked whether physicians knew that they could draw diagrams showing the locations or appearance of skin conditions. The dermatologist responded that, in the paper environment, physicians made such diagrams, and everyone was aware that such tools were available through the EHR system; however, people were not inclined to learn how to use the drawing tools. The expressed fear among dermatologists was less about the learning curve that would be required and more about the possibility that more time would be spent making "pretty pictures" than was warranted. The ophthalmologists in this practice were still drawing images on paper that were scanned into the EHR. They, too, expressed concern that drawing images in the EHR would be time-consuming. To address these concerns, plans were made to modify the software to simplify the drawing tools and incorporate some drawing macros.

An EHR should be capable of presenting various views of the same data. Again, because clinicians work in different ways and may need different views, the ability to view data in narrative, table, flowchart, or graphic form should be considered. It also may be desirable to be able to copy and paste data from one place to another. For example, when sending laboratory results to a referring physician, one may want to copy a graph into a secure email message.

The ability to create graphs and flowcharts is especially important as patients are introduced to EHR system use. Customized views, reports, and instructions may be developed for them and used during the patient encounter as well as to supply the patient with information for a PHR or instructions for care.

CPOE and E-Prescribing

CPOE and e-prescribing are specialized functions of an EHR. The CPOE functions of ordering laboratory tests, making referrals, and issuing other, nonmedication orders are relevant in the ambulatory environment. In many cases, however, such ordering in the clinic setting entails not only the documentation of what was ordered for a patient but also clinical messaging to an external party rather than to an internal, ancillary system. (Clinical messaging is described shortly.)

E-prescribing is a special case of CPOE in the ambulatory environment. It refers to the writing of a prescription to be filled by a retail, community, or mail-order pharmacy, instead of the ordering of a drug from a clinical pharmacy that is a department of a hospital. There are several important distinctions between CPOE relating to medication ordering in a hospital and e-prescribing in the ambulatory world:

- E-prescribing is used exclusively to route prescriptions to retail pharmacies. Note that e-prescribing is used for not only prescriptions written in a physician office or clinic but also those written on discharge of a patient from a hospital or emergency department and in an outpatient clinic.

- E-prescribing systems may be standalone or embedded in an EHR. Although CEHRT must include e-prescribing, it is possible that some physicians prefer a standalone product instead of an EHR or even with an EHR. When embedded in an EHR, further CDS is potentially enabled, and access is provided to additional information about the patient, such as whether he or she has recently made an appointment for a visit to the physician. The benefits of standalone products are generally in the mobility they afford the users, although this preference will likely go away soon as access to EHRs from mobile devices expands.

- Incentives for use of e-prescribing have been available to physicians since 2007, initially under the CMS Physician Quality Reporting System (PQRS) and then, not separately, rolled into the MU incentive program.

- Most benefit plans pay for almost any drugs ordered in the hospital, and the few that are not covered are well known. In contrast, in the ambulatory setting, a particular prescription drug may or may not be included in the patient's drug benefits. If the EHR or e-prescribing system can indicate that a drug is on- or off-formulary for a patient and what the patient's co-payment would be for the drug, the physician writing the prescription could consider the cost for the patient and perhaps prescribe a less-expensive medication prior to the patient going to the pharmacy. Such knowledge reduces phone calls from pharmacies back to the physician and can decrease wait time for patients. Access to a benefits formulary, then, is often not a function of CPOE, but it is an important function of e-prescribing.

- E-prescribing systems should be able to produce both a legible prescription on paper, if necessary, and an electronic transaction using the National Council for Prescription Drug Programs (NCPDP) **SCRIPT** standard protocol. The paper copy can be handed to the patient if the patient is not sure which pharmacy will fill the prescription. If the patient identifies the pharmacy of choice, the electronic transaction is sent to the pharmacy via an e-prescribing gateway. This gateway is most commonly SureScripts, although there may be other gateways and intermediary gateways that connect from the clinic to SureScripts. SureScripts provides three primary functions: It provides benefits information (as described previously in this chapter); it supplies medication history based on claims previously supplied and in support of drug-drug checking; and it routes prescriptions between providers and pharmacies. It performs these functions by credentialing users to use the system and providing a secure technical infrastructure.

E-prescribing systems are applications that support a variety of prescribing functions. Figure 15.8 illustrates these transactions.

Today, most providers who use e-prescribing primarily do so to submit a new prescription to a retail or mail order pharmacy. They may need to tap into the e-prescribing system's drug knowledge base to look for alternatives or may be presented with alternatives as part of the system's CDS. If

Figure 15.8.   E-prescribing transactions

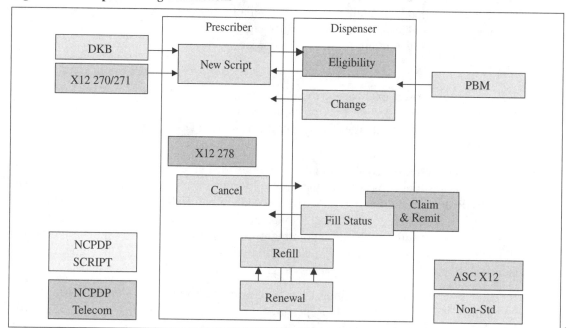

they are unable to check the formulary—perhaps the PBM is not supported by the system—they may be called by the pharmacy to consider an alternative. If the pharmacist interviews the patient and determines there is an allergy to an ingredient in the drug prescribed, the pharmacist will also call the provider. The NCPDP transaction set enables such messaging to occur electronically (that is, the "change" request transactions), but many pharmacies and providers have not yet activated this functionality. Additional functionality available to the provider is the ability to send a request to cancel a prescription—perhaps in response to the just-revealed allergy information.

Managing refill requests and renewals of prescriptions is another function that is widely used today by those with e-prescribing systems. Instead of the patient calling the physician office, or the pharmacy calling the provider to obtain approval for a refill or renewal, these requests can be achieved through the NCPDP transactions. *Refill* is typically a term used to describe the number of times a patient may have the prescription filled without the physician's explicit approval. This number should be recorded on the initial prescription for the drug and the pharmacy should be able to track that. *Renewal,* however, refers to the fact that the patient seeks more of the drug when there are no more refills available without approval. In this case, the physician may want to see the patient again, perform diagnostic studies, and so on before deciding whether to renew the same prescription, change the dose, change the drug, or discontinue it. When a renewal is needed, the pharmacy can initiate a renewal transaction to the physician who can determine what to do and respond indicating approval or disapproval. Often, the physician approves a renewal for a small amount of the drug until the patient has been seen and a new prescription issued.

Another transaction that is available from NCPDP is the fill-status notification. This tool is not widely in use, but it enables a pharmacist to send a transaction back to the physician to indicate a prescription has been filled. Recording this information in the EHR may be helpful in the patient's care management. Certainly, if the prescription is not filled, the physician may opt to remind the patient or discuss this issue on a subsequent visit. Some physicians like the idea of having this information; others believe monitoring the filling of prescriptions is too time-consuming and too closely involves the physician in supervising patient behavior. Under health reform payment strategies, however, it is likely that this function will see more use. Reaching out to a patient who has not filled a prescription can help overcome whatever obstacles there are for the patient and is worth the time in light of improved outcomes.

Originally, e-prescribing was not permitted when prescribing **controlled substances** (Schedule II–V, which include narcotics and other addictive drugs), but the Drug Enforcement Administration (DEA) issued an interim final rule in 2010 for **electronic prescriptions for controlled substances (EPCS)**, although this regulation did not preempt state law that is more stringent. The DEA requires a number of special security controls above and beyond HIPAA requirements (see chapter 12). Some e-prescribing/EHR vendors offer two types of e-prescribing products, those without and those with EPCS. The demand for EPCS varies by specialty, and some specialists may decide they do not want to incur the additional cost of setting up EPCS. The cost to send the e-prescription itself is borne by retail pharmacies or PBMs, but providers are responsible for hardware, software, and networking costs—most of which are included in the overall package of an EHR (HRSA n.d.). By mid-2015, all state boards of pharmacy had made e-prescribing of controlled substances legal in their states (Versel 2015).

Clinical Messaging Versus Portals

Clinical messaging is the secure transmission of clinical information from one entity to another, including providers to providers, patients to providers, payers to providers, and among members of a healthcare community, such as within a health information exchange organization (HIO). The e-prescribing process is a type of clinical messaging—with specific standards and a gateway that provides the security and the exchange capabilities.

A key element of clinical messaging is the security afforded by the process. Although any email system could be used to conduct clinical messaging, sending an unencrypted email containing protected health information is not advisable (and would be subject to breach notification if attacked). (See chapter 12 for more information about breach notification.)

Several companies serve as communications channels for clinical messaging. Each company providing clinical messaging does so in a slightly different manner. Some offer web portals, which are sites on the Internet that provide personalized capabilities to their visitors using a secure protocol (for example, SSL, TLS). Others are only a means to encrypt email that can be sent through any network connection used by the office. Still others are virtual private networks or other point-to-point network connections that transmit content directly into a system configured to accept it.

Whereas clinical messaging is essentially the secure exchange of email messages, which may be facilitated through a portal, portal technology is more sophisticated than simple secure messaging and may also provide greater functionality. A *portal* is literally an entranceway. It may provide entrance to an email server, or it may provide entrance directly into an application. As noted earlier in the chapter, some physicians in their offices may connect to a provider portal offered by their hospital and actually enter orders or retrieve laboratory test results, and patients may use a portal to access the office scheduling system, to obtain access to their clinical summaries, and—if offered by the office—a PHR.

Coding and CDS

Observers from Harvard Medical School (Mostaghimi et al. 2006) have suggested that the EHR "is the doctor's new black bag . . . of the 21st century physician." The most powerful, and some would say most controversial, instrument contained within an EHR is CDS. For ambulatory care, there are two primary forms of decision support: (1) that for professional service documentation and coding (using **Evaluation and Management [E&M]** in the Current Procedural Terminology) in support of reimbursement, and (2) clinical decision support.

E&M Documentation and Coding Support for Reimbursement

Although documentation in support of correct coding for reimbursement could equally well have been discussed in the section on documentation, the level of decision support provided behind the scenes to support coding qualifies this aspect of documentation as decision support. Virtually all EHRs for ambulatory care provide E&M documentation and coding guidance, but a research study conducted by the American Health Information Management Association (AHIMA) found that less than half the practices that reported using an EHR used it for coding support (Fenton and Gamm 2007). The fees attached to these E&M codes are the primary source of physician income. However, the rules about such coding are complex, and the penalties for supplying claims without supporting documentation are severe sanctions and financial penalties (Health Law Offices 2013). As a result, many providers "undercode," losing reimbursement that potentially could be theirs. The fact that EHR tools are available to monitor the completeness of documentation, prompt for specific data requirements, and recommend codes to match the level of service provided should improve the accuracy of documentation and coding, but those who fear that the system can be gamed may still be reluctant to use the tools.

As part of the due diligence in evaluating EHR products, documentation and coding support should be reviewed thoroughly so that those acquiring the products feel confident that the system supports adequate controls. Fishman (2013) offers an excellent recommendation that there should be evidence that the EHR vendor keeps up to date with coding requirements and provides system output that is comparable to coding performed by an expert. In a case study published by a software vendor, two pediatricians further recommend that the EHR should support the ability for staff to review documentation and codes prior to submission of claims to reduce risk of fraud (Aprima

Medical Software 2010). The staff review can also reduce the number of denials that require refilling of claims.

AHIMA (2007) provides guidelines for EHR documentation to prevent fraud. These guidelines highlight four areas of concerns that should be monitored in an EHR environment:

- *Authorship integrity*—that entries pertain to the given patient and are not copied and pasted from another record. In fact, in 2013 testimony to a federal committee hearing on clinical documentation on the issue of cloning/copy-paste practices, the director of research and development for AHIMA Foundation testified that, despite policies in both physician offices and hospitals, noncompliance remains an issue (AHIMA 2013). Skrocki (n.d.) has suggested that academic plagiarism detection software may be a tool compliance officers should use to automate their detection of such practices.

- *Auditing integrity*—that there is an adequate process to detect when an entry was modified or borrowed from another source. One EHR vendor encourages its clients and prospective clients to be aware of and avoid specific documentation tendencies related to E&M coding. This company urges physicians to challenge their vendors to demonstrate their coding tools and how they not only comply with published E&M coding guidelines but also support pattern analysis to suggest that certain codes may not be appropriate for the documentation or have attracted the interest of auditors (eMDs 2011).

- *Documentation integrity*—that there is clinical relevance to the data entered; that is, response to prompts for additional information should result in documentation only as applicable to the patient's condition and reflect the level of service actually provided. Some physicians believe that poorly designed EHRs exacerbate problems because it is so time-consuming to enter structured data or the output is so undesirable that they use copy and paste instead (Eramo 2013).

- *Patient identification and documentation accuracy*—that demographic and registration entries generate correct patient identification and justifiable level of care.

To ensure compliance, clinics must develop and maintain policies and procedures on E&M code selection and responding to prompts for documentation. Tech University Health Sciences Center Office of Billing Compliance has developed an Electronic Medical Record Playbook (Johnson 2010) that addresses billing compliance policies, E&M coding prompts, applicable CMS guidance, development and use of E&M documentation templates—including use of copying and pasting and macros—and other documentation issues including corrections, amendments, and audit trails. AHIMA (2009) and Nunn (2009) also provide guidance on these critical areas of documentation.

CDS

In defining the state of the art in CDS, Berner (2009) describes CDS as a system that provides "clinicians, staff, patients, and other individuals with knowledge and person-specific information, intelligently filtered and presented at appropriate times, to enhance health and health care." Berner recounts that "early CDS systems were derived from expert systems research, with developers striving to program the computer with rules that would allow it to 'think' like an expert clinician when confronted with a patient." While replacing human thought may have been a novel research agenda, the reality is that CDS systems are best used to "assist clinicians in decision making by taking over routine tasks, warning clinicians of potential problems, or providing suggestions for clinician consideration." The functions of CDS systems are illustrated in table 15.1.

The functionality of CDS can be provided in various ways. Ideally, the functionality is incorporated in the EHR. Murphy (2014) describes characteristics that make CDS more effective, and identifies integration into workflow as most important. Most EHR vendors work with specific CDS

Table 15.1.   Functions of CDS systems

Function	Example
Alerting	Highlighting a critical blood potassium level
Reminding	Annual flu vaccine
Critiquing	Rejecting duplicate diagnostic test orders
Interpreting	Diagnosing atrial fibrillation on ECG
Predicting	Predicting mortality risk from a severity-of-illness score
Diagnosing	Listing a differential diagnosis for patient with chest pain
Assisting	Modifying antibiotic choice for patient with renal failure
Suggesting	Generating suggestions for mechanical ventilator weaning

Source: Carter 2001, 182.

partners and generally will not incorporate alternative CDS applications. As such, it is important to evaluate the CDS in the same manner as the overall functionality is evaluated during a vendor selection. There are also CDS products that are available as standalone applications, generally suitable for using on an accessory device, such as a tablet or smartphone (Versel 2011).

CDS is not without its controversies or concerns. These include everything from annoyance to accuracy and whether patient outcomes in an ambulatory environment are improved (Garg et al. 2005). There are a number of white papers, technical reports, demonstration projects, and case studies that offer ways to approach the implementation and optimization of CDS (Byrne et al. 2012). The recommendations are essentially the same: To overcome issues associated with CDS, the clinician should be engaged in reviewing the CDS structures, integrate CDS into workflow, train and support users throughout the lifecycle of CDS, and routinely use the EHR at the point of care. All CDS does not have to be active, "in your face;" it may also be in a passive form that provides support when desired. Active CDS requires action. It may be a pop-up box or field that must be completed before advancing to the next field, screen, or chart completion. These are typically the forms of CDS that are considered most annoying and lead to alert fatigue. Specific active alerts should be studied thoroughly to determine their necessity. In the most customizable EHR systems, active CDS can be tailored to specific user preferences so that primary care physicians may have more alerts than specialists, or new physicians to the practice may have more alerts than established physicians. Passive CDS aids or guides a user. It is the structure of a template or an icon that appears on a screen that leads to further information. None of these forms of passive CDS require action; they are simply informational.

Sufficient structured data also must be available to ensure that the CDS has all the necessary data to operate properly. There is a life cycle associated with CDS software. It must be kept up to date and reviewed regularly for accurate and current information. Evidence from new research is continually being produced and must be incorporated into CDS. A physician who knows that a CDS alert is based on old information may not trust the CDS in the future. An assessment of the impact of CDS is also critical. When clinicians can see it helping improve patient safety and quality of care, they are more inclined to use it.

One use of CDS is to reduce medical errors. The AHRQ has commissioned a number of studies to learn about how CDS is used and to understand medical errors and find ways to reduce their occurrence (Mardon et al. 2014). The assumption here is that by collecting and assessing medical error data, potential harms to patients can be identified and steps taken to prevent or mitigate them. A number of proprietary reporting systems are currently used to collect such data—but reporting is typically voluntary and limited in scope. AHRQ believes an ontology of medical errors is one approach to solving the problem and, with the National Library of Medicine, sponsored the development of one (Mokkarala et al. 2008).

Medical errors traced to EHRs can be an issue in lawsuits, although the problem could be EHR itself, how it is implemented, or how users are trained on it. Allen (2015) reported an example of a woman who stabbed herself with a garden fork. An emergency department nurse selected "unknown/last five years" for the status of the woman's tetanus shot. While this actually was the correct choice, the physician interpreted the entry to mean the patient had been inoculated within the last five years and did not need a tetanus shot. Later, the woman died of tetanus.

As suggested in the earlier discussion of EBM, it is very important the physicians and other clinicians always apply professional judgment. A case could be made that the physician should have double-checked with the patient on the status of her tetanus vaccine, especially as that would have been the primary mode of treatment for the injury. Alternatively, some may observe that there is no point in having an EHR as a communication tool if the communication cannot be interpreted correctly—in this case, "unknown" should not have been included in the same field as "last five years." Absent the EHR, the physician may have asked the patient directly about the status of the vaccination, or conferred with the nurse, who could have validated in the conversation that the physician understood the status. In summary, CDS holds great promise and has been shown to be very useful when implemented properly. Focusing on decision support of all kinds for optimization of EHR value may be the most important step any provider can take going forward.

Data Analysis and Report Generation

Data analysis and report generations functions are typically associated with a patient visit or the conclusion/follow-up to a visit. There also are many nonvisit functions that EHR systems can support. An important element of such nonvisit functions is the ability to work with the data being collected, analyze them, and develop reports from them. This functionality is the essence of many of the new external reporting programs (for example, report cards and benchmarking), disease management functions promoted by health plans, and pay-for-performance incentive programs associated with health reform. Additionally, there are functions relevant only for internal use, such as managing workload, evaluating coding quality, recredentialing staff, or customizing patient education material. Data analysis functions may include generating letters to remind patients about upcoming appointments or the need for preventive care screenings, sending drug recall notices, requesting patient satisfaction surveys, or mailing newsletters and announcements.

Although most EHR systems acquired by physician offices have some ability to generate some reports, not all EHR systems have the ability to easily conduct sophisticated analysis (Vaughan 2009). A data analytics solution has been cited as one of the three most important "add-ons" to an EHR to boost office efficiency (Cryts 2015). As previously noted, it may be necessary to move data into a clinical data warehouse, which is a database optimized for analytical processing, in order to process a large sampling of data or even the universe of data for a given patient population. While data analytics solutions have historically been out of reach for many physician offices that do not have the staff to program such analyses or the financial resources required to support a clinical data warehouse, a number of tools are available for all sizes of organizations. Many offices contribute data to external warehouses, in the form of the Medicare claims data file, disease registries, and so on. Most of these have been uni-directional, where the office did not receive back any analysis of the data. However, registry services can provide a variety of analytics (see also chapter 20 on population health). If an office is part of an integrated delivery system, the system is very likely to support, if not require, participation in a data warehouse for the purpose of monitoring quality of care and to support health reform initiatives. For example, stratifying patients by risk and assigning more resources to higher-risk patients can improve their outcomes, hence lowering the cost to care for them and expanding the possibility of sharing savings with the health plans (AAFP 2015). Learning about the quality and cost profiles of other providers to whom the office refers patients can also create a more "narrow network" of providers to whom to refer patients, thereby lowering cost, and increasing reimbursement (Pawlak and Fadel 2014).

As a prelude to any data analysis, the data must be assessed to ensure they are appropriate for analysis. A controlled, and ideally standardized, vocabulary should be used to make valid comparisons. The system's vocabulary and metadata should be updated at least annually, or as directed by facility policy. The system's metadata may need to be reviewed to limit the scope of data included to those that will be consistent. The accuracy of data entry should be validated. If a field is optional, what is the frequency with which data are entered? If narrative documentation is permitted, how frequently are narrative notes made instead of using the discrete data field? If narrative notes can be converted to discrete data, is the conversion accurate?

Data analysis can provide powerful insights. At one provider location, data analysis was used to create new alerts, analyze physician ordering patterns to reduce cost, and reengineer laboratory specimen turnaround times. In another setting, a data analysis team studied keystrokes to redesign screens (Spencer 2010).

Analysis of data from an EHR also can be used to support clinical research. Some EHR products include the ability to manage data for clinical trials and even prompt physicians to recruit patients for clinical trials.

Check Your Understanding 15.2

Choose the best answer:

1. A critical step in optimizing the office EHR is to:

   a. Assess needed functionality

   b. Participate in a vendor community offering

   c. Plan to discontinue use of EHR

   d. Reselect a better EHR

2. Whether or not an office selects a new vendor to optimize the value it can get from an EHR, it should:

   a. Address workflow and process improvement

   b. Retrain all staff on how to use the EHR

   c. Rework its existing vendor contract

   d. Scan the marketplace for new vendors

3. A tool that can help improve physician productivity and engage patients is:

   a. In-basket

   b. Patient clinical summary

   c. Patient portal

   d. Self-administered history assessment

4. Which of the following is the best way to ensure that the medication list in the EHR includes all drugs a patient is taking?

    a. Interview the patient.

    b. Integrate retail store information into the e-prescribing functionality.

    c. Obtain PBM-generated medication information.

    d. Use a combination of all of the above.

5. An office-based physician would be most likely to use:

    a. Care map

    b. Care pathway

    c. Practice guidelines

    d. Protocol

6. An approach to providing comprehensive primary care and structure physician payment is:

    a. Care coordination

    b. Care management

    c. Patient-centered medical home

    d. Value-based payment

7. The explicit use of research or other formal analysis of best practices is:

    a. Clinical decision support

    b. Evidence-based medicine

    c. Practice guidelines

    d. Protocol

8. Which of the following is a function of e-prescribing that is not commonly used today but will likely be important under health reform?

    a. Change communication

    b. Electronic prescribing of controlled substances

    c. Fill-status notification

    d. Refill request

9. The form of clinical decision support that may prove to be most risky to use is:

    a. Differential diagnosis

    b. Drug-drug interaction

    c. E&M coding support

    d. Preventive services reminders

10. Which of the following is an example of analytics useful to targeting where more time should be spent with patients?

    a. Narrow network

    b. Patient-centered medical home

    c. Registry functionality

    d. Risk stratification

Optimizing Use of the Ambulatory EHR

The overall steps for optimizing EHR and other health IT described in chapter 14 work as well for physician offices as for hospitals. Small physician offices with few source systems may not find it necessary to plot a migration path. However, once the office starts to acquire source systems or use "add-on" applications such as those described in this chapter, plotting a migration path can ensure that there is an inventory of all application and hardware types. Some offices may find that one or more physicians have acquired and are working happily with specialized applications which others may not be aware of. Ideally, these applications should be incorporated into the overall design of the EHR for privacy and security and compliance, as well as for overall efficiency. In addition, plotting a migration path that focuses on not just the hardware and software but also the people, policy, and process aspects of a health IT *system* can highlight everywhere there is need for attention.

Once the office's strategic view of its health IT infrastructure is known, appropriate stakeholder input should be obtained, goals set, metrics identified and measurements taken, and corrective action implemented—and plans should be made for this life cycle to continue for ongoing improvement. Some of the ways that stakeholder input is obtained may be different in a physician office than in a hospital. Considering what has worked best in other major change initiatives in the office can help identify the best way to obtain such input. It is very important, however, to obtain input from all parties—physicians, nursing staff, front office staff, back office staff, managers, and patients. Reliance on "satisfaction surveys" will probably be insufficient to obtain quality input. Such surveys also have the disadvantage of being of being so commonplace that they may be ignored, and they do not support a direct feedback mechanism to the stakeholders so they know their input is being valued.

Another key difference between the hospital and physician office with respect to optimizing use of EHR and health IT may be that "simple" solutions are more prevalent in offices. One physician office observer notes that the basic process of contacting the vendor to ask questions (for example, about how to modify a template, or what shortcuts can be effective, or how to control CDS triggers) can be quite foreign to office staff. The EHR vendor—like it or not—is a partner in the success of EHR in the office. This partner has a responsibility to support the EHR but may not want to come across as constantly being in sales mode. Engaging the vendor in optimization efforts can have significant benefits for both the office and the vendor. Even if the office needs to pay for some focused help, the investment is likely to pay off in much enhanced value from the EHR (Westgate 2015).

Because physician offices do not have large IT departments, keeping the EHR up to date can be a challenge. However, relatively easy solutions, such as simply updating the EHR to a new version or applying a patch to correct an issue that other offices may have raised, may be in reach.

Similar to hospitals, physician offices must analyze workflows, determine the root cause of problems, take corrective action, and communicate what is going on and what improvements have been made and their results. Training should never end in an EHR environment. Finding ways to share lessons learned among users is invaluable.

There have been EHR "failures" in physician offices, and more are likely in the future, especially if system selection is not performed with the full due diligence necessary to ensure the right product for the organization and if implementation is performed poorly. However, it should be noted that there is no clear information on the number of failures or what constitutes an EHR failure. Renner (2009) reports that the AC Group observes that "research shows that roughly 73% of all EMR [electronic medical record] implementation fail." However, neither a specific citation for the source of the estimate nor a definition of what constitutes a failure is provided. Just the same, Renner describes the AC Group's "failure sources"—which are valid points and something organizations should consider as they approach their migration path. Failure sources identified include "software issues, slow documentation, bad vendors, not enough 'buy in,' first year pains, limited initial return on investment, procrastination or delaying the inevitable, and 'big bang' implementation."

Because there is no definition of what "failure" means with respect to EHR, it is very important that each organization identify its goals and continuously work to achieve them, as described in chapter 4. The term *failure* generally implies a significant lack of success, even to the point of being unable to use something or perform a task—even though dictionary definitions may suggest less harsh alternative meanings, such as nonperformance or subnormal quantity or quality. Describing less than desirable performance as failure is demoralizing, but well-defined goals can focus on the positive—how close the organization is to achieving the goals—and lead to corrective action—what can be done to get closer to achieving the goals.

Another key to success is to focus more on operational elements than on the hardware and software. Morton and Wiedenbeck (2009) have developed a framework for predicting EHR adoption attitudes. Eight constructs were identified that clearly focus not at all on the technology:

- Management support
- Physician involvement
- Adequate training
- Physician autonomy
- Doctor-patient relationship
- Perceived ease of use
- Perceived usefulness
- Attitude about EHR usage

These constructs can be helpful to consider when identifying the people, policy, and process elements that must be addressed to make an EHR successful. For instance, clinics need to consider whether their management team is functional. Adler (2007) has observed that, "if your practice is broken, you need to fix it before you try to bring an EHR on board. Dysfunctional organizations are likely to have dysfunctional implementations." A physician's office may wish to identify on its migration path that conducting a leadership assessment is necessary and that clear lines of authority and decision-making structures need to be made explicit. Miller et al. (2003) suggests that clinics "identify an EMR champion—or don't implement." Communicating with patients about the EHR (Merrill 2010), learning how to communicate with patients while using the EHR (O'Malley et al. 2010), and adjusting workflows and examining room layouts (Keller 2010) are operational considerations that address the doctor-patient relationship and perceived ease of use. One thing that seems very certain is that if the EHR is not used and there are negative consequences (that is, there is a perceived failure), the cost to mitigate the consequences could far exceed the value of the current incentives from MU or other programs and policies.

References and Resources

42 CFR 411. 2013 (December 27). Medicare program, physicians' referrals to health care entities with which they have financial relationships; exceptions for certain electronic prescribing and electronic health records arrangements: Extension.

42 CFR 1001. 2006 (August 8). Medicare and State Health Care Programs: Fraud and abuse; safe harbors for certain electronic prescribing and electronic health records arrangements under the Anti-Kickback Statute: Final rule.

Adler, K.G. 2007. How to successfully navigate your EHR implementation. *Family Practice Management.* 14(2):33–39. http://www.aafp.org/fpm/2007/0200/p33.html.

Agency for Healthcare Quality and Research (AHRQ). 2011. What is PCMH? AHRQ's definition of medical home. http://www.pcmh.ahrq.gov.

Agency for Healthcare Quality and Research (AHRQ). 2016 (July 15). National Guideline Clearinghouse. Inclusion criteria. https://www.guideline.gov/help-and-about/summaries/inclusion-criteria.

Allen, A. 2015 (May 4). Electronic record errors growing issue in lawsuits. *Politico.* http://www.politico.com/story/2015/05/electronic-record-errors-growing-issue-in-lawsuits-117591.

Amatayakul, M. 2010a. *Electronic Health Records: Transforming Your Medical Practice,* 2nd ed. Denver, CO: Medical Group Management Association.

Amatayakul, M. 2010b. *The No-Hassle Guide to EHR Policies,* 2nd ed. Marblehead, MA: HCPro.

American Academy of Family Physicians (AAFP). 2013. e-Visits. http://www.aafp.org/about/policies/all/e-visits.html.

American Academy of Family Physicians (AAFP). 2015 (December). Value-based payment http://www.aafp.org/about/policies/all/value-based-payment.html.

American Academy of Family Physicians (AAFP), American Academy of Pediatrics (AAP) American College of Physicians (ACP) American Osteopathic Association (AOA). 2007 (March). *Joint Principles of the Patient-Centered Medical Home.* http://www.aafp.org/dam/AAFP/documents/practice_management/pcmh/initiatives/PCMHJoint.pdf.

American Health Information Management Association (AHIMA) eHIM Work Group. 2007. Guidelines for EHR documentation to prevent fraud. *Journal of AHIMA.* 78(1):65–68.

American Health Information Management Association (AHIMA). 2009. Amendments, Corrections, and Deletions in the Electronic Health Record Toolkit. http://library.ahima.org/xpedio/groups/public/documents/ahima/bok1_044679.pdf.

American Health Information Management Association (AHIMA). 2013. Testimony of Michelle Dougherty, MA, RHIA, CHP on behalf of the American Health Information Management Association to the HIT Policy Committee Hearing on Clinical Documentation February 13, 2013. Panel 4: Role of Clinical Documentation for Legal Purposes. http://library.ahima.org/PdfView?oid=106848.

American Medical Association (AMA). 2002. Guidelines for physician-patient electronic communications. http://www.ama-assn.org.

American Medical Association (AMA). 2010. Guidelines for social networking. http://www.ama-assn.org.

Aprima Medical Software. 2010. BeittelBecker Pediatric Associates, LLC case study. https://www.aprima.com/case-study/beittel-becker-pediatric-associates.

Bachman, J.W. 2003. The patient-computer interview: A neglected tool that can aid the clinician. *Mayo Clinic Proceedings.* 78:67–78.

Berner, E.S. 2009 (June). *Clinical Decision Support Systems: State of the Art.* AHRQ publication no. 09-0069-EF. Rockville, MD: Agency for Healthcare Research and Quality. https://healthit.ahrq.gov/sites/default/files/docs/page/09-0069-EF_1.pdf.

Burns, P.B., et al. 2011. The levels of evidence and their role in evidence-based medicine. *Plastic and Reconstructive Surgery.* 128(1):305–310. http://www.ncbi.nlm.nih.gov/pmc/articles/PMC4386019.

Byrne, C. et al. 2012. Advancing clinical decision support: Key lessons in clinical decision support implementation. Westat Insight. https://www.healthit.gov/sites/default/files/acds-lessons-in-cds-implementation-deliverablev2.pdf.

Cabana, M.D., and S.H. Jee. 2004. Does continuity of care improve patient outcomes? *Journal of Family Practice.* 53(12):974–980. http://www.jfponline.com/pages.asp?aid=1830&UID=.

Carpenito-Moyet, L.J. 2009. *Nursing Care Plans and Documentation: Nursing Diagnosis and Collaborative Problems.* Philadelphia, PA: Wolters-Kluwer Health/Lippincott, Williams & Wilkins.

Casalino, L.P., et al. 2009. Frequency of failure to inform patients of clinically significant outpatient test results. *Archives of Internal Medicine.* 169(12):1123–1129.

Centers for Medicare and Medicaid Services (CMS). 2015. Medicare Access & CHIP Reauthorization Act of 2015. https://www.cms.gov/Medicare/Quality-Initiatives-Patient-Assessment-Instruments/Value-Based-Programs/MACRA-MIPS-and-APMs/MACRA-MIPS-and-APMs.html.

Cryts, A. 2015 (May 21). Three EHR "add-ons" to boost your practice's efficiency. *Physician Practice.* http://www.physicianspractice.com/ehr/three-ehr-add-ons-boost-your-practices-efficiency.

DeVries, J.G., and G.C. Berlet. 2010. Understanding levels of evidence for scientific communication. *Foot and Ankle Specialist.* 3(4):205–209. http://www.ncbi.nlm.nih.gov/pubmed/20664009

Dolan, B. 2010 (January 13). Epic Systems launches iPhone EHR app, Haiku. *Mobile Health News.* http://Mobihealthnews.com/6030/epic-systems-launches-iphone-ehr-app-haiku.

Downing, G.J., et al. 2009 (October 8). Information management to enable personalized medicine: Stakeholder roles in building clinical decision support. *BMC Medical Informatics and Decision Making.* 9:44. https://bmcmedinformdecismak.biomedcentral.com/articles/10.1186/1472-6947-9-44.

Ebling Library. 2015 (December 8). Nursing resources: Standard, guideline, protocol, policy. University of Wisconsin, Madison, Health Sciences. http://researchguides.ebling.library.wisc.edu/c.php?g=293229&p=1953402.

Edsal, R.L. 2006. The *FPM* encounter forms collection: "Paper automation" of your progress notes. *Family Practice Management.* 13(8):63–68. http://www.aafp.org/fpm/2006/0900/p63.html.

Ehrensberger, R., and J. Odell. 2010 (October 13–15). Proactive patient outreach: How providers can identify, engage, and track their chronic patients. Presentation at the Forum-10.

eMDs. 2011 (August 12). Press Release: How to avoid the potential pitfalls of automated E&M coding in EHRs. http://www.e-mds.com/news/how-avoid-potential-pitfalls-automated-em-coding-ehrs.

Elder, N.C., et al. 2010. The management of test results in primary care: Does an electronic medical record make a difference? *Family Medicine.* 42(5):327–333.

Eramo, L.A. 2013. Read between the lines: Identifying harmful copy-and-paste documentation can help curb serious coding errors. *For the Record.* 25(8):18.

Fenton, S., and L.D. Gamm. 2007. Who's coding and how in physician practices: A survey of E/M documentation and coding practices. *Journal of AHIMA.* 78(7):52–55.

Ferris, T.G., et al. 2009 (January). Electronic results management in pediatric ambulatory care: Qualitative assessment. *Pediatrics.* 123(Supplement 2):S85–S91.

Fishman, E. 2013 (August 21). Evaluation and management coding and electronic health records. *EMR Consultant.* http://www.emrconsultant.com/emr-education-center/emr-selection-and-implementation/evaluation-and-management-coding-and-electronic-health-records.

Garg, A.X., et al. 2005. Effects of computerized clinical decision support systems on practitioner performance and patient outcomes. *Journal of the American Medical Association.* 294(10):1223–1238.

Goedert, J. 2011 (February 24). Registries a key ACO component. *Health Data Management.* http://www.healthdatamanagement.com/news/registries-a-key-aco-component.

Goldman, J.J., and T.L. Shih, 2011. The limitations of evidence-based medicine—applying population-based recommendations to individual patients. *AMA Journal of Ethics Virtual Mentor.* 13(1):26–30. http://journalofethics.ama-assn.org/2011/01/jdsc1-1101.html.

Greenes, R.A. 2014. *Clinical Decision Support: The Road to Broad Adoption*, 2nd ed. New York: Elsevier.

HCPro. 2016 (January 18). FTC fines software vendor over false encryption claims. *HIM-HIPAA Insider*. http://www .hcpro.com/HIM-324560-865/FTC-fines-software-vendor-over-false-encryption-claims.html.

Health Law Offices. 2013 (June 2). Blog post: OIG report on physician compliance with e/m coding: 6 key takeaways. http://www.healthlawoffices.com/physician-compliance-em-coding.

Health Level Seven (HL7). 2007. EHR system functional model. http://www.hl7.org/ehr.

Health Resources and Services Administration (HRSA). n.d. How much does an e-prescribing system cost? http://www .hrsa.gov/healthit/toolbox/HealthITadoptiontoolbox/ElectronicPrescribing/costofepres.html.

Institute for Clinical Systems Improvement (ICSI). 2009 (August 10). Guidelines providing patient education. https:// www.icsi.org/guidelines__more/search_results_-_browsing/?catalog_search_panel_query=1#results_header.

Johnson, M.L. 2010 (December 6). Electronic medical record playbook. Tech University Health Science Center Office of Billing Compliance. http://www.ttuhsc.edu/billingcompliance/documents/EMR_Playbook_12_10.pdf.

Joseph, A., and C. Stuhan. 2015 (February 18). Practice notes: The reimbursement outlook for virtual visits. Advisory Board Company. https://www.advisory.com/research/medical-group-strategy-council/practice-notes/2015/february/ virtual-visits.

Keller, M. 2010. EHRs, workflow, and the patient experience. *For the Record*. 22(13):6.

Lawrence, D. 2009 (May). Footing the bill—patient portals, part 1. *Healthcare Informatics*. http://www.healthcare- informatics.com/article/footing-bill-patient-portals-part-i.

Mardon R., et al. 2014 (June). *Findings and Lessons from AHRQ's Clinical Decision Support Demonstration Projects*. AHRQ publication no. 14-0047-EF. Rockville, MD: Agency for Healthcare Research and Quality. https://healthit.ahrq. gov/sites/default/files/docs/page/findings-and-lessons-from-clinical-decision-support-demonstration-projects.pdf.

Matthews, J.C., et al. 2007 (December). The impact of patient-specific quality-of-care report cards on guidelines adherence in heart failure. *American Heart Journal*. 154(6):1174–1183.

Maude, J., and A. Tomlinson. 2010 (October 25). The impact of a web based diagnosis checklist system on specialist referrals from primary care: Results of a survey of general practitioners. Poster session: 32nd Annual Meeting of the Society for Medical Decision Making. http://Smdm.confex .com/smdm/2010on/webprogram/Paper5940.html.

Merrill, M. 2010 (June 9). Survey highlights need for docs to talk to patients about moving to an EHR. *Healthcare IT News*. http://www.healthcareitnews.com/news/survey-highlights-need-docs-talk-patients-about-moving-ehr

Meyers, D., et al. 2010 (December). *The Roles of Patient-Centered Medical Homes and Accountable Care Organizations in Coordinating Patient Care*. AHRQ Publication no. 11M005-EF. Rockville, MD: Agency for Healthcare Quality and Research.

Miller, R.H., et al. 2003 (October). Electronic medical records: Lessons from small physician practices. *iHealth Reports*. California Health Care Foundation. http://www.chcf.org/publications/2003/10/ electronic-medical-records-lessons-from-small-physician-practices.

Mokkarala, P. et al. 2008 (August). Development of a comprehensive medical error ontology. In *Advances in Patient Safety: New Directions and Alternative Approaches*, vol. 1: *Assessment*. Edited by Henriksen, K., et al. AHRQ publication no. 08-0034-1. Rockville, MD: Agency for Healthcare Research and Quality. http://www.ncbi.nlm.nih.gov/ books/NBK43635.

Morton, M.E., and S. Wiedenbeck. 2009 (Fall). A framework for predicting EHR adoption attitudes: A physician survey. *Perspectives in Health Information Management*. 6:1a. http://www.ncbi.nlm.nih.gov/pmc/articles/ PMC2804456.

Mostaghimi, A., et al. 2006. The doctor's new black bag: Instructional technology and the tools of the 21st century physician. Medical Education Online. http://www.med-ed-online.org/pdf/L0000012.pdf.

Mostashari, F. et al. 2009. A tale of two large community electronic health record extension projects. *Health Affairs*. 28(2):345–356.

Murphy, E.V. 2014. Clinical decision support: Effectiveness in improving quality processes and clinical outcomes and factors that may influence success. *Yale Journal of Biology and Medicine*. 87(2):187–197. http://www.ncbi.nlm.nih.gov/pmc/articles/PMC4031792.

Murray, M.F., et al. 2013. Comparing electronic health record portals to obtain patient-entered family health history in primary care. *Journal of General Internal Medicine*. 28(12):1558–1564. http://www.ncbi.nlm.nih.gov/pubmed/23588670.

National Committee for Quality Assurance (NCQA). 2011. NCQA Patient-Centered Medical Home 2011.

National Longitudinal Surveys (NLS). n.d. What are longitudinal data? US Bureau of Labor Statistics. https://www.nlsinfo.org/content/getting-started/what-are-longitudinal-data.

Nunn, S. 2009. Managing audit trails. *Journal of AHIMA*. 80(9):44–45.

Office of the National Coordinator for Health Information Technology (ONC). 2014 (September 11). Dr. Maselli leverages health IT to increase patient engagement. Health IT Success Stories. https://www.healthit.gov/providers-professionals/dr-maselli-leverages-health-it-increase-patient-engagement.

Office of the National Coordinator for Health Information Technology (ONC). 2015 (April). QuickStats Dashboard. Office-based physician electronic health record adoption: 2004–2014. Percent of REC enrolled physicians by specialty live on an EHR and demonstrating meaningful use. Health care professional EHR vendors: March 2015. http://dashboard.healthit.gov/quickstats.

O'Malley, A.S., et al. 2010 (April). Electronic medical records and communication with patients and other clinicians: Are we talking less? Center for Studying Health System Change issue brief no. 131. http://www.hschange.com/CONTENT/1125.

Patel, V., and E. Siminerio. 2014 (September 15). Consumer access and use of online health records: It takes two to tango. HealthIT Buzz. Office of the National Coordinator for Health Information Technology. http://www.healthit.gov/buzz-blog/consumer/consumer-access-online-health-records.

Patient Centered Primary Care Collaborative.. http://www.pcpcc.net.

Pawlak, V., and M. Fadel. 2014 (July 9). Narrow networks help create value in a more regulated healthcare landscape. *Becker's Hospital Review*. http://www.beckershospitalreview.com/hospital-management-administration/narrow-networks-help-create-value-in-a-more-regulated-healthcare-landscape.html.

Renner, P. 2009. Why most EMR implementations fail: How to protect your practice and enjoy successful implementation. A white paper from StreamlineMD.

Rhoads, J., and E. Drazen. 2009 (March). Touchscreen check-in: Kiosks speed hospital registration. California Health Care Foundation. http://www.chcf.org/publications/2009/03/touchscreen-checkin-kiosks-speed-hospital-registration.

Skrocki, M. n.d. Will Academic Plagiarism Detection Software be a Tool for Compliance Officers? http://www.svsu.edu/~mel/ICHITA_Skrocki.pdf.

Spencer, G. 2010 (June). Enhancing patient care through data analysis. *Journal of AHIMA*. 81(6):58–60.

SureScripts. 2011 (November 9). Press Release: SureScripts announces that majority of doctors in U.S. now use e-prescribing. http://surescripts.com/news-center/press-releases/!content/surescripts-announces-network-upgrade-for-e-prescribing-of-controlled-substances.

Tonelli, M. 2006. Commentary: Evidence-based medicine and clinical expertise. *AMA Journal of Ethics*. 8(2):71–74. http://journalofethics.ama-assn.org/2006/02/ccas1-0602.html.

US Department of Health and Human Services (HHS). 2015 (August 28). Affordable Care Act of 2010. Read the law. http://www.hhs.gov/healthcare/about-the-law/read-the-law.

Vaughan, C. 2009 (October 6). Three barriers to effectively using information stored in EHRs. *HealthLeaders Media*.

Versel, N. 2011 (December 14). 10 innovative clinical decision support programs. *Information Week*. http://www.informationweek.com/healthcare/clinical-information-systems/10-innovative-clinical-decision-support-programs/d/d-id/1101834?

Versel, N. 2015 (August 28). Vermont becomes final state to legalize e-prescribing of controlled substances. *MedCity News*. http://medcitynews.com/2015/08/vermont-e-prescribing-of-controlled-substances.

Vogel, T.J., et al. 2012. A self-administered family history questionnaire improves identification of women who warrant referral to genetic counseling for hereditary cancer risk. *Gynecologic Oncology*. 125(3): 693–698.

Watson, A.J., et al. 2010. A randomized trial to evaluate the efficacy of online follow-up visits in the management of acne. *Archives of Dermatology*. 146(4):406–411.

Wenner A.R., M. Ferrante, and D. Belser. 1994. Instant medical history. *Proceedings of the Annual Symposium on Computer Applications in Medical Care*. p. 1036. http://www.ncbi.nlm.nih.gov/pmc/articles/PMC2247777.

Westgate, A. 2015 (January 8). Ten ways to use your EHR more efficiently. *Physician Practice*. http://www.physicianspractice.com/ehr/ten-ways-use-your-ehr-more-efficiently.

Williams, D.E. 2009 (December 22). e-Visits continue their slow, steady rise. Health Business blog. https://healthbusinessblog.com/2009/12/22/evisits-continue-their-slow-steady-rise.

Chapter 16
Specialty-Specific EHRs

Learning Objectives

- Describe the overall need for EHR products that address specialty functions or special needs of certain provider types.

- Identify what efforts are being undertaken to address specialty EHR needs.

- Review functions of EHRs for nursing homes and home health agencies.

- Review functions of EHRs for behavioral health.

- Discuss the pros and cons of specialty EHRs versus general, or multispecialty, EHRs in the broader context of health IT and health information exchange.

While the focus of electronic health record (EHR) utilization has been primarily in hospitals and physician offices/clinics (especially with the meaningful use [MU] incentive program), there is growing interest in EHRs in other provider settings. Note that the term **provider** has been used in this book as defined by the Centers for Medicare and Medicaid Services (CMS) to mean any individual or organization that provides and gets paid for providing healthcare services. Providers include not only physicians—in both primary care and specialist practices—but certain other healthcare professionals whose scope of licensure includes providing medical care as billable services (that is, physicians assistants, nurse practitioners, and clinical nurse specialists), hospitals, skilled nursing facilities, home health agencies, pharmacies, laboratories outpatient physical therapy centers, comprehensive outpatient rehabilitation facilities, end-stage renal disease facilities, hospices, durable medical equipment (DME) suppliers, and others.

As coordination of care for health reform initiatives becomes increasingly important, nursing homes, home health agencies, behavioral health facilities, and public health departments want to be able to share health information electronically with hospitals and physician offices or clinics. In July 2015, CMS issued a proposed rule that would support improved opportunities for sharing data by long-term care facilities. The proposal did not require an EHR but signaled federal intention to move the long-term care industry in the direction of automation improvements (CMS 2015a).

As of early 2016, the rule has not yet been finalized. In the mental health arena, providers who are doctors of medicine (MDs), doctors of osteopathic medicine (DOs), and nurse practitioners (NPs) qualify for earning MU incentives, but other mental health providers, who represent the majority of the field's providers, are excluded. The mental health profession acknowledges challenges and barriers to use of the EHR but advocates for the expansion of the MU incentive program to other providers, a belief also held by some members of Congress who have introduced bills to extend the MU program (Getz 2013). Chiropractics, dentists, optometrists, and podiatrists were also eligible professionals (EPs) under the MU incentive program, although many of these professionals found that EHRs were either not available for their specialty or many of the MU requirements were difficult to meet, even as they use considerable technology in other aspects of their work. Physicians (MDs and DOs) may also specialize, such as in dermatology, pediatrics, or oncology, and want their EHR to be specific to their needs. Although not providers, health plans (payers) often consider their individual member records compiled from claims data and other sources to be "electronic health records" that they use for case management and contract negotiation. Public health departments may be a mix of social services and provider services and are beginning to adopt health information technology (health IT) to better exchange data with providers of all types.

Although there is an emerging interest in EHR by provider types other than hospitals and ambulatory care environments, the marketplace for many specialty-specific EHRs is challenged by the fact that many of these providers tend to be less able to afford the prices of more traditional ambulatory and hospital EHRs. As a result, vendors addressing these specialty-specific EHRs may not have the ability to put as much money into product research and development. The result of such "laws of supply and demand," then, is that certification-ready products to meet specialty needs have lagged behind EHRs for hospitals and ambulatory care settings.

New vendors are emerging to meet some of these needs. Some of them are companies that already service specialty facilities in other ways and are adding EHRs to their portfolio of products and services. New technology, such as cloud computing, is enabling some of these vendors to bring products to market more quickly and deliver them at a lower price point. Many traditional ambulatory EHR vendors advertise specialty products, but these tend to only include specialty templates for notes and tailored clinical decision support (CDS). Workflow differences are often not accommodated. Those vendors who do offer a truly specialized product are also reaching out to partner with billing software vendors, medical management system vendors, registry services, data warehouse companies, and others in an attempt to meet some of the specialty-specific needs of their customers.

Addressing Needs for Specialty-Specific EHRs

Because **specialty EHRs** are not a single, specific type of EHR but many different types that are specific to different special needs, it is difficult to generalize about them. However, they all have one thing in common: their users have specialized needs not addressed by EHRs designed for general acute care hospitals or ambulatory care in general. This may seem like an obvious statement, but vendors did not even initially recognize that one type of EHR does not fit both acute and ambulatory care settings. Only recently have companies offered complementary acute care and ambulatory care EHRs that present similar and usable user interfaces, accommodate workflow differences, and enable sharing of health data. For example, the MU program requires that EPs record smoking status for patients 13 years old or older, and an exclusion is made for those who do not see such patients. The US Surgeon General (2006) had suggested that exposure to secondhand smoke, especially in small children, would be an important smoking status type that should be included in the measure (45 CFR 170.302[g]), but this suggestion was ultimately not part of the regulation. Therefore, the exception generally makes sense (why ask a question that does not apply to the patient group?). However, a number of other specialists have indicated smoking status is not a commonly collected piece of information in their area of practice. Again, an argument could potentially be made there are many risks associated with smoking, such that it is every provider's responsibility to promote smoking cessation, and that is the reason for including the requirement to ask about smoking status in the incentive program. Still, there must be a balance that reflects the right data and the burden to collect data that may preclude use of EHR altogether.

Functionality for Specialist Providers

Some degree of tolerance for measures of limited relevance to the specialty, such as smoking status, may be acceptable to most specialist providers, but products will not be acceptable if they do not accommodate information for the specific specialty. For example, a nephrology practice may use many of the same functions in an EHR as a primary care provider, but it will also want to be able to apply the Kidney Disease Outcomes Quality Initiative (KDOQI) classification of chronic kidney disease to each of its patients. KDOQI classification is not a common measure found in general-use EHRs but has been a recommendation of the National Kidney Foundation since 2002 (MacGregor 2007) and updated periodically (Levey and Inker 2016). An EHR that is specialty-specific to nephrology should be counted on to provide such functionality. As another example, oncologists look for assistance with tumor staging in their EHRs (American Society of Clinical Oncology 2009). The list of specialty functionality is nearly endless.

In addition to information needs, different workflows must be accommodated in the functionality of EHRs for different specialty practices. Some specialists, such as surgeons, obstetricians, and others, frequently travel between the hospital and their offices. For these providers, an integrated, seamless EHR across the sites of care would be much more important than for a primary care physician who spends most of his or her time in the office or clinic setting. Some specialists conduct much of their work in special types of facilities that may be affiliated with a hospital or are freestanding, such as dialysis centers and imaging centers. These specialists may prioritize integrated access to data from each setting over a seamless interface.

Long-Term and Post-Acute Care

Long-term and post-acute care (LTPAC) has both similarities to and significant differences from hospitals and clinics. LTPAC data requirements are highly prescribed by the federal government for reimbursement purposes. Workflows are very different from those found in hospitals and clinics and also vary among types of LTPAC facilities. For example, nursing home residents stay for a fairly long time (potentially 30 days or more); clinicians employed by home health agencies provide care for clients at home; and hospice care provides special end-of-life services that may be delivered in a hospital or nursing home, or at the client's home. EHRs for nursing homes have functional requirements associated with medication administration that are very similar to those in hospitals, but the functional requirements are not the same with respect to physicians ordering medications—in nursing homes, medications are ordered through a prescription process that is even somewhat different than the usual ambulatory prescription process.

Home health workers may not only need mobile devices but also need customer relationship management software. Home health agencies may also use a global positioning system (GPS) to help clinicians locate their clients' homes and for agency management to ensure that home visits occur—the GPS functionality could be used to enter a "location stamp" in the visit note in the EHR, much as computers date- and time-stamp entries. If telehealth is integrated with home health, as some have advocated (Russell 2009), the EHR must be able to accommodate different types of data and data feeds from remote medical devices and caregivers.

Many different provider types may provide hospice services. Although the nature of the data needed may be the sameacross hospices, the EHR must support the collection and use of data in multiple settings.

Behavioral Health

Like providers working in medical ambulatory settings, behavioral health providers need health IT with the functionality to book appointments and bill for services. Unlike their medical counterparts, however, many behavioral health providers do these tasks themselves rather than have office staff perform them. Therefore, behavioral health providers may prefer that these functions be integrated directly into the EHR whereas medical clinics may use a separate practice management system (PMS) (see chapter 15).

Clinical charting in behavioral health is distinctive from medical charting because the primary diagnostic resource in behavioral health is the *Diagnostic and Statistical Manual of Mental Disorders,* Fifth Edition (DSM-5), although physicians who provide behavioral health services use ICD-10-CM codes for billing. DSM-5 functionality for diagnostic support is therefore important. Behavioral health providers may also need to document group therapy. Settings in which behavioral health is provided also vary significantly, from a traditional office setting to inpatient settings, homeless shelters, prisons, schools, and long-term care facilities (Simon 2014). Telepsychology in various forms is increasingly being used as the number of behavioral health providers is shrinking (AHA 2012). The American Psychological Association (APA) provides a guidance document to help behavioral health specialists use communications equipment for delivering services (2013). The American Telemedicine Association (ATA) also has several guidance documents on using telehealth in behavioral health, such as its Evidence-Based Practice for Telemental Health (ATA 2009).

Some behavioral health providers are concerned about using an EHR during provision of the behavioral health services—fearing that their clients may not be comfortable having information collected about them in this manner. Providers are learning that client resistance to EHR use is less of a factor than they expected, but there are still some concerns (ATA 2009; Lovett 2014) and, of course, special provisions are needed for consent management.

Other Provider Settings

There are many other provider settings that need to capture "traditional" content of a health record and exchange data across settings much like hospitals and physician practices do, but the providers in these settings also have special data and workflow needs. The following is a partial list of examples of other provider settings and their EHR needs that are not further addressed in this chapter:

- Emergency departments (EDs) in hospitals need to compile data, especially from physiological monitoring devices, in a highly concise manner. EDs also need to rapid access to protocols to support differential diagnosis. For example, a dizziness diagnostic tool for EDs can help differentiate between a viral infection and stroke in the nearly half a million people presenting in EDs with acute vestibular syndrome (Monsen 2011). Finally, EDs can benefit from systems to track patient location and status.

- Public health departments have special challenges in acquisition, analysis, and dissemination of information from specific reports—for communicable disease reporting, biosurveillance, immunization administration, and other screenings. These departments may use traditional ambulatory EHRs in public health department clinics, but they also have special needs for registry functionality and aggregating and mining data for population health management (Maddux 2015). See chapter 20 for more information on this topic. Public health departments also use electronic clinical quality measure (eCQM) reporting for public health surveillance (Heisey-Grove et al. 2015).

- Clinical research facilities have a great need to integrate clinical trials data with the EHR for both better recruitment of subjects as well as less repetitive data collection and better access to more longitudinal data. Because of the nature of clinical trial data, it may be necessary to partition research data from care delivery data amassed at the same location to ensure data are appropriate for their respective purposes (Kahn 2007; Thorman 2010).

- Human service agencies are public, quasi-public, or private organizations dedicated to providing programs for meeting basic health, welfare, and other needs of a special group. They need to document the healthcare services they provide—which are usually limited in scope and do not require the extensive clinical decision, billing, or other support of a typical EHR. However, these agencies need access to directories of other social service agencies, community services, and potentially a local pharmacy with which they may have an arrangement to supply a limited formulary to its authorized patients (Carpenter n.d.).

- Assisted living centers, when operated independently of other long-term care facilities, have an interest in being able to connect their residents with community services (for example, carpools), use healthcare alert systems to notify caregivers of emergency medical needs, perform remote monitoring for vital signs and to deliver medication prompts, and aggregate data for tracking referrals and marketing (Healthcare Scene 2011).

- DME providers may not need an EHR with full functionality, but they do need to support orders for DME equipment and supplies. One company has developed health IT for DMEs that resembles the e-prescribing model currently used between providers and retail pharmacies. The idea is to streamline processes as this market expands exponentially because hospital stays are becoming shorter and more people are receiving home health care (Stratice Healthcare 2015).

- Correctional facilities look for a distinctive mix of features and functions in an EHR. They generally want to track the status of all of their inmates' health (including preventive screening needs), manage sick calls, and ensure documentation of medication administration. The record is something of a blend of inpatient and outpatient functions. Reducing costs through better monitoring and care delivery as well as reducing grievances and litigation risk are key benefits for correctional facilities (Paris 2013). In 2013 CMS changed the requirements for the Medicaid MU incentive program to enable correctional providers to qualify for the incentives (NCCHC 2013).

- **Retail clinics** are clinics that treat uncomplicated minor illnesses and injuries and provide some preventive healthcare services under physician oversight. They are often located in pharmacies and some other retail stores, and, more recently, they have begun operating via

mobile telehealth (services using mobile technology placed in a patient's home or offered through a specially equipped vehicle [Siwicki 2016]). They are generally staffed by a nurse practitioner, who can provide services only within the scope of license. They are able to keep costs low, with many accepting health insurance, because they are small operations with no room for x-ray machines and other expensive equipment. Because retail clinics offer low-cost services and convenience, a number of employers are encouraging their use as a way to treat conditions before they become more complicated or severe (Ham 2014). The Veterans Affairs Health Care system has partnered with a retail clinic chain to address long wait times for urgent care (Kaiser Health News 2016). Quality of care is being ensured as some major healthcare facilities are connecting with some of these retail clinics in major pharmacies (Siwicki 2016). According to Bachrach and Frohlich (2016), publicly reported performance measures in Minnesota found that retail clinics ranked highly among other primary care providers in at least three measures. They note that "it is hard to fathom a better way to increase access, at low cost, in a manner that doesn't generate excess utililization . . . [especially as] primary care access is projected to get considerably worse." The EHR typically entails a point of registration that identifies whether the nurse practitioner can manage the patient's complaint or directs the patient elsewhere because the complaint is not within scope. Some retail clinics have registration kiosks that also track wait time at all of the facilities to advise patients when there might be a shorter wait at a clinic a few miles away. Routine documentation is required, and patients receive a printout of the results of their physical examination, treatment, and medications prescribed.

- Planned Parenthood organizations provide sexual and reproductive healthcare to women, men, and adolescents and have characteristics of both a primary care physician office and a human services agency, and they have the unique feature of being affiliated with a large network of other providers through the Planned Parenthood Federation of America (PPFA). Each provider operates independently with respect to its EHR purchases, generally seeking "lite" EHRs to capture health-related documentation across the continuum of care and needing access to community service directories (PPFA n.d.).

- Community health centers and federally qualified health centers are somewhat similar in their EHR needs, as they often combine primary care with behavioral health and dental services—a combination of functions generally not addressed by a single EHR vendor. These centers often rely on a practice management system, which has fewer components than an EHR, to logically link patient records. These facilities are also reimbursed by different structures and have special state reporting requirements that are more extensive than in the typical primary care provider setting.

- Pharmacies seek to add EHR functionality to their pharmacy dispensing software systems to better retain a complete and accurate medication history and associated fill status for each customer and streamline pharmacist medication therapy management documentation (Gans 2009).

- Occupational health services have unique documentation requirements. Although documentation for each individual who receives occupational health services is similar to the documentation in any physician office, records for these services generally must be kept separate from records for any other type of care provided to the individual in the same setting because the regulations surrounding privacy and ownership are different than those for health records in medical settings (Burton et al. 2013). Providers of occupational health services also have specific requirements for the reporting and billing that must go to the employer who has engaged them.

- Emergency medical services require the ability to document their communications and procedures as the ambulance or other transport is en route to an ED (Teslow et al. 2009).

- Imaging centers and radiology departments typically use radiology information systems (RIS) and picture archiving and communication systems (PACS), but use of a dedicated EHR is uncommon in these settings. However, radiologists who provide more than 10 percent of their services outside of the inpatient and/or ED setting may be able to earn MU incentives, especially if they practice in a freestanding imaging center. Some EHR vendors have modified their products—and earned certification—for this market (Roat 2011).

Efforts to Address Specialty EHR Needs

Efforts to address specialty EHR needs have largely been driven by specialty societies/associations and, in some cases, specialists or affiliates themselves who participate in other forums to promote EHR.

Specialty Societies/Associations

A number of specialty medical societies have formed workgroups or other structures within their memberships to create EHR guidance documents for their members. Some of these efforts are natural outgrowths of work on clinical practice guidelines and have focused on functionality of EHRs. The work of the American Society of Clinical Oncology (ASCO) is a good example. In 2009, ASCO convened a working group with the National Cancer Institute and related specialties to develop clinical oncology requirements for the EHR (CORE). Other specialty societies, however, have focused more on advising members about the administrative/ practice management aspect of selecting and implementing an EHR without as much regard to functionality unique to the specialty. In both cases, however, such guidance has been helpful to members but seemingly of limited value to vendors in creating product.

For example, for many years, the American College of Obstetricians and Gynecologists (ACOG), in conjunction with the American Academy of Pediatrics (AAP), has developed guidelines for perinatal care (often referred to simply as the "ACOG guidelines"). Now in their seventh edition, the guidelines outline basic, specialty, and subspecialty levels of perinatal care and provide information on maternal transport, dental care during pregnancy, human immunodeficiency virus (HIV), childbearing at 50 years or older, hyperbilirubinemia, breastfeeding, obesity, multiple gestation, newborn screening, and patient safety (AAP and ACOG 2012). These guidelines have been widely adopted, including by state Medicaid agencies. ACOG has also developed guidelines for other practices, such as for other pregnancy events, Pap smear, cancer screening, and tracking and reminder systems (ACOG 2012). Most obstetricians and gynecologists follow these guidelines, but many EHR vendors do not fully incorporate the ACOG guidelines in their products.

Although a number of providers have urged their specialty societies to endorse products for their use, few have chosen to do so over concerns for liability. Many societies offer toolkits to assist their members with EHR selection and implementation, and some include product listings on their websites. When companies pay to be listed, they very likely self-screen so that those with an affinity for a certain specialty will more likely advertise on that site.

Group purchasing organizations (GPOs) are entities created to help providers achieve deep discounts by applying economies of scale to purchasing supplies. **Management services organizations (MSOs)** are businesses that provide nonclinical services (such as practice management) for physician offices (Anderson and Grey 2013). These organizations have been helpful, especially for small and midsize providers, to select and negotiate for favorable pricing on EHR systems, although the choice is sometimes based more on price than functionality. With respect to the specialty societies and GPOs/MSOs, there can be a disconnect between physicians' clinical needs and the practice management interests.

Unlike medical specialty societies, associations representing specialty providers, such as those representing nursing homes, home health agencies, and assisted living facilities have included EHR on their radar screens and vendors exhibit at their conferences, but the associations themselves have done little to otherwise promote EHR. Many of these associations rely on other organizations, such as the Healthcare Information and Management Systems Society (HIMSS) and American Health Information Management Association (AHIMA), for information relating to the EHR. Although these are certainly appropriate resources for information about the EHR, the specific association is frequently in a better position to advocate on behalf of their members, such as for federal funding.

Standards Development Organizations

As noted, individual professionals within special provider fields are working to address specialized EHR functional requirements. Some of these efforts have been recognized by Health Level Seven (HL7), which maintains a registry of functional profiles for specialty EHRs. **Functional profiles** are statements of functions and conformance criteria deemed important for EHR systems used in a given specialty. HL7 keeps the registry because HL7 wants to ensure that EHRs for specialty providers are consistent with the two primary functional models (one for the EHR and one for the patient health record [PHR]). Hence, the registry process ensures that the specialty functional profiles draw from either the HL7 Electronic Health Record–Systems Functional Model (EHR-S-FM Release 2) or HL7 Personal Health Record–Systems Functional Model (PHR-S-FM), or both. The specialty functional profiles are developed by subject matter experts who come together voluntarily to promote a common set of functionality for their EHR or PHR needs. Registration of the functional profiles attests to their conformance with the EHR-S-FM or PHR-S-FM. The HL7 Functional Profile Registry is cosponsored by the National Institute for Standards and Technology (NIST). Some of the registered functional profiles have received federal funding support from the Department of Health and Human Services Office of the Assistance Secretary for Planning and Evaluation (HL7 2016).

Registration of a functional profile may facilitate its adoption by increasing public awareness and making it publicly available for use—ideally, for vendors to consider in product development. In addition, the HL7 registry may reduce the proliferation of profiles by making people aware of the ones that exist and thus minimize the need to create new and different profiles. The HL7 wiki (n.d.) is a forum for individuals interested in learning more and communicating broadly about functional profiles (and other communications about HL7 matters in general).

Table 16.1 lists the functional profiles that have been registered with HL7 (2016).

Table 16.1.   HL7 functional profiles for specialty EHRs and related health IT

* EHR Behavioral Health
* EHR Child Health
* EHR Clinical Research
* EHR Pharmacist/Pharmacy
* EHR System Long Term Care
* EHR System Vital Records
* EHR System Electronic Nutrition Care Process Record System
* EHR System ePrescribing
* EHR System Implementation Guide: Pharmacist/Pharmacy Provider for Community Practice
* EHR System Public Health Functional Profile
* HL7 Version 3 Specification: Data Elements for Emergency Department Systems (DEEDS)

Specialty EHR Product Certification

The Certification Commission for Health Information Technology (CCHIT) was a certifying body that created a voluntary certification program for EHRs, funded in part by AHIMA and HIMSS and with federal grants. Upon adoption of the federal MU incentive program, CCHIT also became an authorized testing body to certify EHRs for the MU incentive program. CCHIT was approached by several specialty organizations to also create specialty certifications, often used as an add-on to the MU certification. Several specialty certifications especially for those specialties that had also created HL7 functional profiles were offered. Unfortunately, as a nonprofit organization in a competitive, largely for-profit EHR certification business, CCHIT was not able to sustain itself and is no longer in existence. The MU incentive program's certification process does not address specialty certification at this time. HL7's functional profiles registry, however, is expanding. These profiles can be used as guidance documents in identifying functional requirements for EHR selection.

Check Your Understanding 16.1

Match the specialty with its most unique need:

A. Behavioral health

B. Emergency department

C. Home health

D. Corrections

E. Imaging center

F. Public health

1. Patient location tracking

2. PACS viewer

3. GPS

4. Appointment booking

5. Integrated inpatient and outpatient documentation

6. Registry

EHRs in Nursing Homes, Home Health Agencies, and Hospices

EHRs for nursing home, home health, and hospice care (referred to collectively as *long-term and post–acute care* [LTPAC]) are among the more widely adopted special EHRs. Their rates of adoption, functionality, benefits, and challenges are further explored here. Post–acute care generally includes assisted living, community-based services, rehabilitation facilities, wellness providers, and other types of services (LTPAC HIT Collaborative 2016). The expanded focus of LTPAC is important from a healthcare delivery perspective, but it may not yet reflect the same level of health IT adoption as in the more limited focus.

EHR Adoption Rates in LTPAC

Getting good data about the use of EHRs and other health IT in LTPAC is difficult. LeadingAge is an association of over 6,000 not-for-profit organizations that care for older Americans. Its Center for Aging Services Technologies (CAST) maintains an EHR portfolio with various EHR selection and implementation tools, case studies, and other useful information (LeadingAge CAST 2015). According to LeadingAge's latest survey (Magan 2014), two-thirds of all LTPAC providers do not have or are not fully using information systems technology and patient data exchanges. The survey also indicates that most (84 percent) large skilled nursing facilities (SNFs) have funding allocated for technology improvements, whereas 89 percent of single or standalone nursing homes and SNFs had no money so allocated. This 2014 study also identified that funding for health IT is made even more difficult because 21 percent of all LTPAC foresaw bankruptcy, dissolution, or closed services in 2015.

The above data, however, does not reflect the fact that most LTPAC facilities use electronic systems for reporting Minimum Data Set (MDS) and Outcome and Assessment Information Set (OASIS) data as required by Medicare (CMS 2015b; CMS 2015c; CMS 2015d). Resnick and colleagues (2009) found that 91.6 percent of LTPAC facilities used technology for billing in 2004.

The low rates of adoption of electronic systems in nursing homes reported in the 2014 LeadingAge survey are surprising given the emphasis that the Office of the National Coordinator for Health Information Technology (ONC 2013), AHIMA (2014), LeadingAge CAST (2015), and other organizations place on the use of at least health IT, if not a fully functional EHR. Also, the LTPAC Health IT Collaborative, which includes AHIMA, LeadingAge, and other professional associations, hosts an annual summit and publishes a road map to advance strategic priorities and inform provider organizations, policy makers, vendors, payers, and other stakeholders (LTPAC HIT Collaborative 2016).

LTPAC facilities operate with very low margins; however, they are under pressure to reduce medication errors, improve clinical documentation, and improve administrative efficiency and effectiveness (AHIMA 2014). A survey from Maestro Strategies (2007) reflects the difference between goals for health IT in LTPAC compared to acute and ambulatory care—in LTPAC, improving the productivity of staff is the most important goal, followed by improved reimbursement, and then reduction in errors. The Maestro Strategies survey distinguished between "electronic information systems for medical records," which were used by nearly 50 percent of the nursing home respondents and presumably more comprehensive "electronic health records/electronic medical records," which were reportedly used by 20 percent of nursing home respondents. These rates were clearly higher than those suggested by Leading Age CAST in 2015.

Several distinctive factors about LTPACs would seem to potentially facilitate adoption of health IT in this setting. First, nursing home data requirements are more highly regulated, and hence somewhat easier to accommodate in electronic systems, than the highly variable data that must be documented in an acute care hospital. Second, the acuity of the patients in nursing homes is not as high as in acute care hospitals, so the level of clinical decision support (CDS) typically needed in a nursing home system would not be as extensive or costly to program. Third, many nursing homes are part of large, national, for-profit chains that have standardized procedures—also more readily accommodated by simpler information systems—and may be more likely to see the value of automation and, of course, benefits of economies of scale in group purchasing.

Recent data on the use of EHRs by home health and hospice agencies have not been reported. The most current data are from 2007, which were reported in 2010 by Resnick and Alwan (2010). At that time, 38.6 percent of home health agencies, 49.1 percent of hospices, and 66.4 percent of home health and hospice agencies were using EHR systems The study also revealed that only 20 percent of the agencies with EHR had information sharing functionality, and only about half of those were using such functionality. Of course, the lack of sharing functionality should come as no surprise, considering that those with whom they would likely share data (hospitals and physicians) are also not far along in adopting interoperable health IT. The study also found that 20.6 percent of home health and hospice agencies were using telemedicine in 2007.

LTPAC EHR Functionality

Many functions performed by health IT in LTPAC resemble functions of health IT in hospitals, but health IT in LTPAC is considerably less focused on deep clinical functionality. Functions typically automated in LTPAC include those listed in table 16.2.

Health IT Benefits for LTPAC

Benefits from health IT in LTPAC include those for organizations and for state governments, which often foot a large percentage of the costs for long-term care services. Two studies of EHR use in SNFs (Ford 2010; Kruse et al. 2014) identified the benefits listed in table 16.3.

Table 16.2.   Information technology functions in LTC

Clinical
MDS (nursing home) or OASIS (outcome and assessment information set for home health)
Care and service plans
Resident assessment profiles
Patient records*
Electronic health records*
Activities of daily living (ADL) documentation
Vital signs documentation
Therapy management
E-prescribing
E-medication administration record (e-MAR)/e-treatment administration record (e-TAR)
Computerized pharmacy administration (CPA) (drug dispensing technology)
Pharmacy interfaces
Outcomes measurement/quality management
Physician order entry/processing
Rehabilitation
Transfer records
Advance directives (DNR)

Financial/Administrative
General ledger, accounts payable, and payroll
Admissions planning
Discharge planning
Training
Policies and procedures
Compliance surveys
Resident/customer satisfaction surveys
Marketing
Case management
Flags for LUPA or PEP (home health)
Executive dashboard

Resident Services
Resident demographics/customer relationship management
Scheduling (home health)
Resident billing
Admissions and census management
Resident identification (bar coding)
Meals processing

Facilities
Maintenance management
Project management

*"Patient records" and "electronic health records" were cited in a number of lists of LTC functionality without further clarification. Where already implemented, it appears that "patient records" often describes record tracking and completion systems and sometimes document scanning. "Electronic health records" appears to be used in a manner more consistent with the concept of EHR in acute and ambulatory care—a more integrated approach to applications and higher level of clinical decision support.

Source: CCHIT Certified Criteria for LTPAC; Long-Term Care-Nursing Homes EHR-Systems Functional Profile: Release 1; HIT Toolkit for Nursing Homes, Stratis Health; HIT Toolkit for Home Health Agencies, Stratis Health.

Table 16.3.   Benefits of EHRs in skilled nursing facilities

- Readily accessible diagnoses and demographics information on residents.
- Ability for nurses to respond more quickly to a change in a resident's condition from alerts such as weight change or out-of-range vital signs.
- Easy-to-read documentation.
- Easy-to-prepare transfer records.
- Easy-to-process physician orders because the order is written only once and automatically sent to the pharmacy and to the medication administration record or treatment administration record
- Time savings in shift documentation and searching for charts.
- Improved consistency, accuracy, and quality of documentation as nurses are guided by the EHR in necessary documentation.
- Improved documentation of events monitoring (for example, falls, fever) on computerized templates.
- Continuing education for nurses to become more adept at physical assessment and event monitoring.
- Higher resource utilization group (RUG) levels for increased reimbursement.
- Improved employee satisfaction and staff retention from an elevated perception of working in a SNF with an EHR.
- Fewer medication errors and reduced spending for Medicare or Medicaid reimbursement mediations with a computerized pharmacy administration system.
- Improved satisfaction from residents and their family members. One family saved almost $700 per month (when using private insurance) per month by changing from a name-brand to generic medication. Another resident commented on the convenience of having a printed medical record when a patient has a medical appointment outside the facility.

Source: Ford 2010; Kruse et al. 2014.

In a study sponsored by the Texas Department of Aging and Disability Services (Cherry et al. 2009), the state found that health IT in LTPAC reduced medication expenditures through waste avoidance (saving between $3,000 and $4,000 per month), reduced hospital admission due to better care in the LTPAC program, and increased quality and efficiency in care documentation. The Texas report also cited improved facility oversight, development of evidence-based practices, and the ability for improved reporting to provide compelling population-level outcome and forecast data for appropriation requests. Several other states have found that care coordination can be enabled when LTPAC facilities use directed exchange messaging from the nursing home to the hospital emergency department (see chapter 13 for more on directed exchange messaging). In Oklahoma, for instance, a transition of care document and universal transfer document are sent via Direct (ONC 2013). Remote monitoring to the home is also used by some LTPAC providers. In Maine, Tele-HomeCare services have expanded chronic disease management for diabetes, congestive heart failure, and hypertension (ONC 2013).

Home health agencies with fully functional EHR and health IT systems can create a "virtual care team" to supplement the home health nurse when at a client's home. Clients and their families can be more engaged in their own health monitoring through improved data visualization, checklists, and decision support. Workflow tools, such as customer relationship management and other coordination tools may enable home health nurses to be both more efficient and effective in their care delivery (CIOC and NEC 2013).

Challenges to EHR Use in LTPAC

The Texas study just cited also included a survey of consumers (residents and their families), administrators, supervisory nurses, direct care nurses, certified nursing assistants (CNAs), and other professionals, including health information managers, social workers, consultant pharmacists, and office managers (Cherry et al. 2009). The results highlight both benefits and challenges that nursing homes face in implementing health IT (see figure 16.1).

EHRs in Behavioral Health

EHRs are becoming more popularin behavioral health, although EHR use in this specialty still lags significantly behind use by medical providers and, by some measures, behind use in LTPAC. The American Psychiatric Association (Simon 2014) reports that in 2012 only 7 percent of behavioral health providers who are eligible to earn the MU incentive have attested (in comparison to medical specialties [excluding primary care, family medicine, and internal medicine] that at the time were

Figure 16.1.   Role-based experiences with EHR in nursing homes

Role	Positives	Negatives
Consumers	Acknowledged EHR as "wave of the future," recognized cost savings in medications, appreciated printed copies of records to take to other providers, and believed staff were less overburdened with their jobs	Less personal contact with staff, concerns about accuracy of information. Interestingly, no consumer reported concerns about privacy.
Administrators	Time savings, security and HIPAA compliance, improved access to information enabled being more responsive to inquiries from residents' families. Improved consistency, accuracy, and quality of documentation; support for higher RUG levels for increased reimbursement. Improved employee satisfaction and staff retention.	Internet outages, system downtime, and computer glitches, especially as most administrators served as the IT support for the organization
Supervisory nurses	Immediate access to records, consistent and legible documentation, streamlined method for processing physician orders, ability to monitor residents' changing conditions, ability to monitor staff performance, ability to monitor nurse aide activities	Difficulties with downtime, especially at night; desire for regular meetings with vendors for system improvements; desire for additional training
Direct care nurses	More readily available information, alerts, notes easier to read, information on resident events more readily available, easy to generate transfer records, and easier to process physician orders	Inconsistent reports concerning time it took to chart, time to complete and maintain care plans, time to process admissions, and concerns from patients and supervisors that nurses were "playing on the computer" or abusing their Internet privileges. New nurses often felt overwhelmed with the learning curve in general and typing in particular; and downtime.
CNAs	Almost exclusive use of point-of-care touch screen technology, often at kiosks for documenting ADL and intake and output were well liked by CNAs and they felt their use of computers generated higher respect	CNAs wanted more information about residents than the kiosks provided, and more explanation of the information; as with direct care nurses, half felt the system took more time and half felt the system took less time for documentation than paper
Other professionals	Easy to find information, greater efficiency, easier readmission process, accurate and detailed reports, greater oversight for improved quality of care, increased reimbursement	None identified

Source: Long-Term Care Facilities Adoption of Electronic Health Record Technology: A Qualitative Assessment of Early Adopters' Experiences, Prepared by the Cherry, B., et al for the Texas Department of Aging and Disability Services, October 1, 2009.

averaging attestation at the rate of about 45 percent). APA attributed the low rate of EHR use to multiple factors: the lack of EHRs that support the needs of psychiatrists; the fact that many psychiatrists work in solo or small practices that do not have the time or resources to implement an EHR; and expense. In addition, many psychiatrists consult at many different facilities and are often not able to meet the MU measures required by CMS. Furthermore, only 55 percent of psychiatrists participate in Medicare and only 43 percent participate in Medicaid (APA 2014).

The National Council for Behavioral (formerly National Council for Community Behavioral Healthcare) represents 2,000 community behavioral health and addiction treatment organizations. In 2012, only 2 percent of the organizations had EHR usage among psychiatrists for these psychiatrists to meet MU requirements. However, the National Council did find that the organizations were "eager" to move forward because they believed that EHRs facilitated communication with other healthcare organizations to improve care coordination, improved quality care and streamlined operations, and positioned their organizations for growth and expansion in emerging healthcare delivery systems. Barriers to adoption included the lack of skilled staff to select, implement, and maintain the EHR or manage projects. The National Council also identified 24 EHR products most used in community behavioral health organizations, with two vendors dominating.

There has been interest in incorporating behavioral health into the federal MU incentive program. In both 2010 and 2011, bills were introduced in Congress that would support inclusion in the MU incentive program. In 2011 Senator Sheldon Whitehouse (D-RI) introduced Senate bill 539, which would make incentive payments available to mental health care, behavioral health care, and substance misuse treatment professionals and facilities.

The federal agency directed by Congress to target substance abuse and mental health services to the people most in need and to translate research in these areas more effectively and rapidly into the general healthcare system is the Substance Abuse and Mental Health Services Administration (SAMHSA). Since forming in 1992, it has garnered support for and distributed grant funds to organizations to help improve the agency's work. It has identified eight strategic initiatives, among which is health IT and EHRs for behavioral health, including putting a significant level of support into incorporating behavioral health clinical data standards into the open-source EHR collaboration known as VistA, the Veterans Administration's EHR system that is made available to the public through the Freedom of Information Act (Clark 2010).

ONC has also contributed to overcoming barriers for behavioral health providers to use EHRs by conducting several consent management projects. Data segmentation for privacy (DS4P) was described in chapter 12. Another project being spearheaded by SAMHSA through the S&I Framework (2014) is **Consent2Share (C2S)**, which is an open-source tool for consent management and data segmentation designed to integrate with existing EHR and health information exchange (HIE) systems. C2S includes a front-end, patient-facing user interface that allows patients to define their privacy policy, and the tool has informed consent and access control services at the back end that provide privacy policy configuration, management, decision making, and enforcement. Aspiring to Awesome (A2A) is an ONC-funded pilot program that focuses on offering patients specific access control choices. An analysis of the pilot results will help create an understanding of patient preferences on HIE, establish an ethics framework, and contribute to the design a browser-based interface to allow patients to specify their privacy preferences (ONC 2014).

Behavioral Health Services

In considering functionality for behavioral health EHR, it is important to recognize the nature of behavioral health incorporates a variety of different types of professionals, therapies, and settings in which such services are provided. There are also a host of state laws regulating behavioral health care and even some controversy surrounding the nomenclature and categorization of types of care provided under this rubric. Although *behavioral health* is the term used in this chapter, some people prefer to use *mental health* to describe this domain of care (Sandler 2009).

A key difference between behavioral health providers and general medical providers is that behavioral health is largely provided through psychologists, social workers, and licensed professional counselors or therapists and not medical doctors and nurses (NAMI 2011). *Psychology Today* (n.d.) lists over 40 different types of credentials and licenses plus a number of different types of educational degrees that individuals may hold as they practice in the behavioral health field. Psychiatrists are the only providers with an MD or DO and are often the only providers who may prescribe medication, although depending on the setting, state, and level of education, nurses with special training in psychiatric/mental health care may also be authorized to prescribe and monitor medication. The number of psychiatrists and psychiatric nurses in any given facility is typically very small, and, in some cases, they serve a facility only on a limited contract basis. As such, any Medicare or Medicaid incentive program for MU of certified EHR technology would need to clarify the eligibility of types of behavioral healthcare providers.

Just as there are many types of behavioral health professionals, there are also many different types of behavioral health services provided. Some states have strict requirements for the separation of behavioral health/mental health records from substance abuse records, while, at the same time, others are urging their integration. In some states, regulations about the release of patient/client information extends to records on developmental disabilities and HIV (Gordon 2000).

Behavioral healthcare can include individual, group, and family sessions—all of which must be documented. Patients range in age from the very young to the elderly, so behavioral healthcare addresses pediatric, women's health, men's health, and geriatric health concerns. Behavioral health services may be provided in many settings, including schools, day treatment centers, assisted living facilities, clinics, hospitals, nursing homes, homeless shelters, residential treatment centers, correctional facilities, social service agencies, and others (Raths 2009).

Behavioral Health EHR Functionality

Obviously, with the wide variance in professionals, types of patients and therapies, and settings of care, functions that may be described for behavioral health EHRs vary depending on the needs of a specific organization. Typical functions that are unique or need to be more extensive for behavioral healthcare than in a general medical acute or ambulatory care environment are identified in figure 16.2.

Behavioral Health EHR Benefits and Challenges

In reviewing the literature on benefits of behavioral health EHRs, it is observed that this segment of the healthcare delivery system not only suffers from a paucity of implementations but is also at a level of maturity in anticipating benefits equivalent to where the medical segment was probably 10 years ago. What literature exists on benefits of behavioral health EHR is primarily focused on financial return on investment, security, accessibility, and other administrative functions (O'Connor 2013) and says little about qualitative benefits and even less on benefits for quality improvement. Behavioral health EHRs are very much perceived to be replacements for paper records without much enhanced utility. Clinical decision support is identified as a clinical function in only about half the products in the 2015 *Behavioral Healthcare* IT Vendor Survey. Interestingly, interoperability is described as a benefit in many of the more recent articles—even as interoperability is not listed in the 2015 vendor survey and is challenging for all EHRs, not just those intended for behavioral health providers (Lovett 2014).

Improvement in staff productivity is perceived as a significant benefit for EHR in behavioral health. Connors (2007) estimates that the cost of pulling charts, entering redundant data, and searching the chart is $5,200 per provider per year, or $208,000 annually for an agency with 40 providers. Connors also observes that the EHR could "mitigate the risk of required or essential data being missing or buried within progress notes."

Figure 16.2.   Behavioral health EHR functionality

- Call processing requiring incoming and outgoing caller ID management
- Referral and waiting list management; access to community service directories
- Patient registration and demographics, including special needs, guardian or conservator information, and capturing signatures of those not authorized access to the system, such as probation officer and others
- Insurance eligibility and prior authorization management
- Client scheduling, including recurring appointments, group appointments, linked appointments (e.g., medication and therapy), medical transportation requirements, administrative appointments, and cancellation management
- Provider scheduling and caseload management
- Provider desktop, schedule, and task list; integrating unique timeframe requirements for documentation tasks and flagging providers and supervisors for events outside specified parameters
- Standardized diagnostic assessments (DA), often that must meet state-specific requirements and are based on DSM IV differential diagnosis
- Standardized treatment plan, often that must meet state-specific requirements and are populated from the DA, and link client goals, treatments, and interventions to symptoms
- Prompts for additional assessments based on practice standards
- Assignment of one or more providers to specific interventions within a treatment plan
- Association of clinical notes with treatment plan
- Enable normative scaling of outcomes
- Support home monitoring, personal health records, telepsychiatry
- Billing system supporting a full range of DSM to ICD-9-CM crosswalk, CPT (including E&M coding support), claims, eligibility verification, remittance advice, coordination of benefits, and production of RVU reports

Sources: CCHIT Certified Criteria for Behavioral Health EHR; Behavioral Health Functional Profile: Release 1; Mental Health EHR – Request for Proposal, Stratis Health; Wilder Foundation RFP for EHR and Integrated PMS; Planning Your EHR System: Guidelines for Executive Management, Mental Health Corporations of America, Inc. (MHCA) and Software and Technology Vendors' Association (SATVA); 2010 Behavioral Healthcare IT Vendor Survey, Behavioral Healthcare.

In a 2008 article in *Behavioral Healthcare* titled "A Fuller Picture of ROI," Turso reported that in the Lutheran Social Service of Minnesota, bad debt expense decreased by almost 93 percent, outstanding accounts receivable of 151 days or more were reduced from 24 percent to 9 percent, and the time staff spent entering state remittances and applying payments to claims dropped from 40 hours per week to just 10 minutes with electronic processes. Turso also stated that "an EMR investment's other benefits may be less tangible and not immediately apparent, which is why an EMR often is mistaken for an expense." For example, he noted that improvements in workflow would get clients quicker access to behavioral health services, but that the value of this was difficult to express. He concluded his article by acknowledging that, in light of the organization's goals and mission, it was also a priority to have data readily available to allow staff to make informed decisions about care, a "return that is difficult to quantify or represent solely in financial terms."

There are two barriers—other than cost and MU exclusions—that are especially prevalent in behavioral health EHR adoption. These are workflow and clinician/patient relationship (McCarthy 2015).

Introducing use of a computer at the point-of-care is especially challenging in behavioral health. Many behavioral health specialists communicate with their clients without the aid of templates directing their assessments or counseling sessions, and they rarely document their findings and recommendations until at least after the client leaves, and frequently days, weeks, or even months thereafter. All documentation is typically narrative, although most specialists do tend to type their own notes, citing confidentiality as an issue for turning dictation over to others.

The second barrier concerns the potential deleterious effect that EHR use might have on the provider-patient relationship. Getz (2013) notes that behavioral health specialists have "a patient relationship that is based on paying attention and recognizing the behavior of the person in the room with you." Therefore, behavioral health providers may worry that care could suffer with the introduction of technology into the care session. However, this anticipated effect may not become a reality.

McCormack conducted a study in 2014 of patient attitudes about use of an EHR in the exam room. Because the study selected a random sample of 4,500 patients in the medical arena, its findings may not be completely relevant to behavioral healthcare. Just the same, the findings generally point to the fact that most patients do not mind electronic note-taking during exams, although their reactions varied somewhat depending on the type of device used. Desktop computers were somewhat more bothersome to patients than laptops, which were less bothersome than tablets—a finding that probably reflects the ability of the provider to interact with the patient while documenting on different types of devices. Patients expressed more concern when scribes were using during exams than when a computerized device was used, and had an equal amount of concern when audio recordings were made during the exam. In summary, 24 percent of patients preferred that their doctor used electronic systems, 18 percent somewhat preferred the use of electronic systems, and 47 percent had no preference. Only 4 percent of patients somewhat preferred the use of pen and paper, and 8 percent strongly preferred pen and paper. Lack of preference was higher in older patients, and factors other than EHR contributed more significantly to patient dissatisfaction with their visit experience. In order of frequency, 95 percent of the dissatisfaction was related to long wait times, unfriendly staff, short visit duration, and trouble scheduling an appointment, with only 5 percent of dissatisfaction related to the doctor using a computer during the exam.

A study conducted by Montague (2013) looked at the impact of nonverbal interpersonal interactions in clinical encounters and patient perceptions of empathy. The study's chief finding was that clinical environments using health IT should be designed to facilitate clinicians' ability to have positive nonverbal interactions with their patients, such as eye contact and social touch (for example, a light touch on the forearm).

In its Health Information Technology Toolkit for Behavioral Health (2014), Stratis Health offers guidance to providers on communicating with clients about EHR and HIE. Strategies for using the EHR at the point of care suggested in this toolkit include the following:

- Have a positive attitude when using the EHR in the presence of clients.

- Position oneself and the client so that eye contact can be maintained.

- At the beginning of the encounter, explain directly to the client what will be entered into the computer, how information is being secured, and how use of the EHR helps the client.

- Use the EHR to share information with the client, thus demonstrating its value to the client. For example, showing a client how assessment scores have changed over time can be a motivating factor for the client.

- Indirectly reinforce the value of the EHR to clients by asking them to look at their medication list and verify if it is current.

- Engage clients by talking through the information being entered, providing a summary, giving them access to view their records, and enabling them to enter some of their own information.

- Stop using the EHR at any point where it appears there is a client concern. Depending on the situation, asking the client about concerns with the EHR can be helpful. This discussion may initiated at the point the concern is recognized or at the conclusion of the visit. Referencing how the client also uses a computer can help the client recognize this is not an unusual activity. In fact, determining the extent to which a client conducts texting and uses social media can be insightful, as it is known that excessive use can cause depression, isolation, and other issues.

EHRs and the Integration of Data from Specialized Care

Although specialty care requires special functionality in the EHR, there is also a critical need for integrating data across care settings. For example, the following statement was made in 2009 to describe the link between oral health and overall health (Rudman et al. 2010):

> A fully integrated patient record and care model for both systemic health (medical) and oral health (dental) is needed for health information technology (HIT) standards, implementation, and interoperability to avoid discrepancies between records and to support quality of care, safety, and cost reduction initiatives.

A surprising number of patients see their dentist more frequently than their primary care provider, which makes the clinical quality measures of smoking cessation, blood pressure management, weight screening, and others very applicable to dental practice (Hoover 2011). Similarly, optometrists are in a position to identify early warning signs of hypertension and diabetes (Guttman 2009). Use of integrated EHR products in these specialties could therefore contribute to better treatment of chronic disease.

Behavioral health is one area where the integration of specialty healthcare and primary healthcare seems especially desirable and especially promising. The need for integration is great. Nardone and colleagues (2014) cite a study that shows that adults with serious mental illness die, on average, 25 years earlier than the general population. It has also been recently demonstrated that depression, anxiety, and dementia are associated with higher 30-day readmissions after hospitalization for heart failure, acute myocardial infarction, and pneumonia (Boggs 2015). One hospitalist notes, "What happens in the inpatient setting is no longer confined to just one provider and one patient" (Maguire 2014).

Steinfeld and colleagues (2006) observed that the EHR can "bring all of healthcare together." To support this claim, they cited evidence from the two-year implementation of an EHR system by Group Health Cooperative in Washington state. They found that consumers felt it was important for their primary care physicians to be aware of basic information regarding their behavioral healthcare while preserving the confidentiality of the information.

The integration of behavioral health and primary care—and their health records—is now made possible by data segmentation strategies and other automated tools (Cifuentes et al. 2015; McCarthy 2015). Use of EHRs with behavioral health components can help primary care providers recognize as early as possible when there may be a behavioral health condition in order to refer the patient to a specialist. In one study, Klein and coauthors (2006) found that EHRs contributed to improvements in overall healthcare when primary care providers incorporated results of the PHQ-9 questionnaire for depression into the EHR and used the EHR to score the results in order to provide a differential diagnosis.

Check Your Understanding 16.2

Choose the best answer:

1. All EHRs should have:

    a. Conformance with MU incentive program

    b. Full integration with other EHRs

    c. Same functionality

    d. Similar "look and feel"

2. A key difference in how EHRs are used across specialties concerns:

   a. Balance of structured data and narrative

   b. Need for evidence-based clinical decision support

   c. Types of computer devices

   d. Workflow

3. Behavioral health specialists currently document care using:

   a. Scribes

   b. Self-typed narrative notes

   c. Speech recognition

   d. Structured templates

4. The primary use of automation in many nursing homes today is:

   a. Assessment documentation

   b. E-prescribing

   c. Medication administration recording

   d. Transmission of data to CMS

5. Behavioral health specialists will have better success with EHR if they:

   a. Avoid using the EHR during a counseling session

   b. Document using speech dictation

   c. Have the patient enter all data

   d. Tell the patient what is being entered into the EHR

References and Resources

45 CFR 170b. 2010 (July 28). Health information technology: Standards, implementation specifications, and certification criteria for electronic health records technology, final rule.

American Academy of Pediatrics (AAP) and American College of Obstetricians and Gynecologists (ACOG). 2012. *Guidelines for Perinatal Care.* 7th ed. Elk Grove Village, IL: AAP, and Washington, DC: ACOG.

American College of Obstetricians and Gynecologists (ACOG) Committee on Patient Safety and Quality Improvement. 2012 (December). Committee opinion: Tracking and reminder systems. http://www.acog.org/Resources-And-Publications/Committee-Opinions/Committee-on-Patient-Safety-and-Quality-Improvement/Tracking-and-Reminder-Systems.

American Health Information Management Association (AHIMA) Longitudinal Coordination of Care Practice Council E-HIM Strategy Team. 2014. Electronic health record adoption in long term care (2014 update). *Journal of AHIMA.* 85(11): expanded web version. http://library.ahima.org/doc?oid=107519#.V73OX5grI2w.

American Hospital Association (AHA). 2012 (January). Bringing behavioral health into the care continuum: Opportunities to improve quality, costs, and outcomes. *AHA TrendWatch.* http://www.aha.org/research/reports/tw/12jan-tw-behavhealth.pdf.

American Psychological Association (APA) Joint Task Force for the Development of Telepsychology Guidelines for Psychologists. 2013. Guidelines for the practice of telepsychology. *American Psychologist.* 68(9):791–800. http://www.apa.org/practice/guidelines/telepsychology.aspx.

American Society of Clinical Oncologists (ASCO). 2009 (October 6). Clinical oncology requirements for the EHR (CORE). A Collaborative Project of the American Society of Clinical Oncology and the National Cancer Institute.https://www.asco.org/practice-guidelines/quality-guidelines/health-it-work-group/clinical-oncology-requirements-ehr-core.

American Telemedicine Association (ATA). 2009 (July). *Evidence-Based Practice for Telemental Health*. http://www.americantelemed.org/docs/default-source/standards/evidence-based-practice-for-telemental-health.pdf?sfvrsn=4.

Anderson, G.D., and E.B. Grey. 2013 (February 11). The MSO's prognosis after the ACA: A viable integration tool? Presentation at Physicians and Physician Organizations Law Institute, Phoenix, AZ. https://www.healthlawyers.org/Events/Programs/Materials/Documents/PHY13/B_anderson_grey.pdf.

Bachrach, D., and J. Frohlich. 2016 (May 20). Retail clinics drive new health care utilization and that is a good thing. *Health Affairs Blog*. http://healthaffairs.org/blog/2016/05/20/retail-clinics-drive-new-health-care-utilization-and-that-is-a-good-thing.

Behavioral Healthcare. 2015 (November). The 2015 Behavioral Healthcare IT vendor survey. www.behavioral.net/category/technology/annual-it-vendor-survey.

Behavioral Healthcare. 2010 (September). The 2010 Behavioral Healthcare IT vendor survey. *Behavioral Healthcare* 30(8):14–17.

Boggs, W. 2015. Depression and anxiety linked to higher hospital readmission rates. Psych Congress Network. http://www.psychcongress.com/article/depression-and-anxiety-linked-higher-hospital-readmission-rates-21918.

Burton, B., et al. 2013. The privacy and security of occupational health records. *Journal of AHIMA*. 84(4):52–56.

Carpenter, T. n.d. Building an effective model of EHR governance and support. Defran Systems.

Cherry, B., et al. 2009 (October 1). Long-Term Care Facilities Adoption of Electronic Health Record Technology: A Qualitative Assessment of Early Adopters' Experiences. Final report submitted to the Texas Department of Aging and Disability Services. http://www.nursinghome.org/pro/HIT/Content/HIT%20early%20adopters%20lessons%20learned_%20guide.2009.pdf.

Cifuentes, M., et al. 2015. Electronic health record challenges, workarounds, and solutions observed in practices integrating behavioral health and primary care. *Journal of the American Board of Family Medicine*. 28(supplement): S63–S72.

CIO Consortium (CIOC) and Nurse Executive Council (NEC). 2013 (June 12). Electronic health record (EHR) solutions LTPAC providers need today, version 1.0. American Health Care Association health IT resources. http://www.ahcancal.org/facility_operations/hit/Documents/2013-06-12%20CIOC-NEC_EHR_WhitePaper_FINAL.pdf.

Clark, H.W. 2010 (October 1). SAMHSA strategic initiative #6: Health information technology, electronic health records and behavioral health. https://store.samhsa.gov/shin/content/SMA11-4629/08-HealthInformationTechnology.pdf .

Centers for Medicare and Medicaid Services (CMS). 2015a (July 16). CMS reform of requirements for long-term care facilities proposed rule. *Federal Register*. 80:42167 http://federalregister.gov/a/2015-17207.

Centers for Medicare and Medicaid Services (CMS). 2015b (October 16). Home health agency billing. Chapter 10 in *Medicare Claims Processing Manual*. https://www.cms.gov/regulations-and-guidance/guidance/manuals/internet-only-manuals-ioms-items/cms018912.html.

Centers for Medicare and Medicaid Services (CMS). 2015c (December 17). *MDS 3.0 RAI Manual*. https://www.cms.gov/Medicare/Quality-Initiatives-Patient-Assessment-Instruments/NursinghomeQualityInits/MDS30RAIManual.html.

Centers for Medicare and Medicaid Services (CMS). 2015d (June 26). Home Health Quality Initiative. https://www.cms.gov/Medicare/Quality-Initiatives-Patient-Assessment-Instruments/HomeHealthQualityInits/index.html?redirect=/homehealthqualityinits.

Certification Commission for Healthcare Information Technology. 2011 (February). Certification update. Certification Commission for Health Information Technology. http://www.cchit.org.

Certification Commission for Healthcare Information Technology. 2010 (July 26). CCHIT Certified 2011 Behavioral Health EHR Certification criteria. http://www.cchit.org.

Connors, W.R. 2007. EHRs: Back to the basic benefits. *Behavioral Healthcare*. 27(9):47–49.

Ford, E. 2010 (September 10). Electronic health records hold great promise for long-term care facilities. *iHealthBeat*. http://www.ihealthbeat.org/perspectives/2010/electronic-health-records-hold-great-promise-for-longterm-care-facilities

Gans, J.A. 2009 (June 26). Letter to ONC on draft recommendations for the term "meaningful use" of electronic health records. American Pharmacists Association.

Getz, L. 2013. EHRs in behavioral health—a digital future? *Social Work Today*. 13(3):24.

Gordon, E.L. 2000 (December). Release of behavioral health, developmental disabilities, HIV, and substance abuse information: Guidelines for legal compliance. *Health Care Law Monthly*. pp. 3–17.

Guttman, C. 2009 (October 1). ODs have critical role in caring for those with hypertension, diabetes. *Optometry Times*. http://optometrytimes.modernmedicine.com/optometrytimes/Modern+Medicine+Now/ODs-have-critical-role-in-caring-for-those-with-hy/ArticleStandard/Article/detail/650406.

Ham, B. 2014 (September). Retail clinics: What's in store for health care. Center for Advancing Health. http://www.cfah.org/prepared-patient/prepared-patient-articles/retail-clinics-whats-in-store-for-health-care.

Healthcare Scene. 2011 (April 27). Verizon, HealthSense team to bring home health solutions to FiOS-equipped senior and assisted living communities. *Healthcare Scene News*. http://www.emrandhipaa.com/news/tag/assisted-living-housing.

Health Level 7 International (HL7). n.d. HL7 wiki. http://wiki.hl7.org.

Health Level 7 International (HL7). 2016. HL7 standards—EHR profiles. http://www.hl7.org/implement/standards/product_section.cfm?section=4,

Heisey-Grove, D., et al. 2015 (May 1). Using electronic clinical quality measure reporting for public health surveillance. *Morbidity and Mortality Weekly Report*. http://www.cdc.gov/mmwr/preview/mmwrhtml/mm6416a3.htm.

Hoover, T.J. 2011 (May 13). Personal conversation.

Kahn, M.G. 2007. Integrating Electronic Health Records and Clinical Trials: An Examination of Pragmatic Issues. NCRR Workshop.

Kaiser Health News. 2016 (May 25). Veterans Affairs Health Care System tries experimental partnership with CVS to cure long wait times for urgent care. *Healthcare Finance*. http://www.healthcarefinancenews.com/news/veterans-affairs-health-care-system-tries-experimental-partnership-cvs-cure-long-wait-times.

Klein, E.W., et al. 2006. Depression screening interface with an electronic health record: A feasibility study in a primary care clinic using optical mark reader technology. Primary Care Companion. *Journal of Clinical Psychiatry*. 8(6):324–328.

Kruse, C.S., et al. 2015 (January 28) Adoption factors associated with electronic health record among long-term care facilities: A systematic review. *BMJ Open*. 5(1). http://bmjopen.bmj.com/content/5/1/e006615.abstract.

LeadingAge Center for Aging Services Technology (CAST). 2015 (August 20). CAST updates EHR portfolio with enhanced selection tools and 6 case studies. http://www.leadingage.org/CAST_Updates_EHR_Portfolio_with_Enhanced_Selection_Tools_and_6_Cases_Studies.aspx.

Levey, A.S., and L.A. Inker. 2016 (July). Definition and stages of chronic kidney disease in adults. UpToDate. http://www.uptodate.com/contents/definition-and-staging-of-chronic-kidney-disease-in-adults.

Long Term and Post Acute Care Health Information Technology (LTPAC HIT) Collaborative. 2016. LTPAC HIT Collaborative wiki. https://ltpachitcollaborative.wikispaces.com.

Lovett, M. 2014 (July 14). Implementing an EHR in the behavioral health setting. *Healthcare IT News*. http://www.healthcareitnews.com/blog/implementing-ehr-behavioral-health-setting.

MacGregor, M.S. 2007. How common is early chronic kidney disease? *Nephrology Dialysis Transplantation*. 22(Suppl 9):ix8–ix18.

Maddux, D. 2015 (April 13). EHRs in the new age of population health management. Acumen Physician Solutions blog. http://acumenmd.com/blog/ehrs-in-the-new-age-of-population-health-management.

Maestro Strategies. 2007 (April). Information technology in long term care—state of the industry. Multi-facility research report. Conducted for American Health Care Association and National Center for Assisted Living. https://www.ahcancal.org/facility_operations/hit/documents/informationtechnologyinlongtermcare.pdf.

Magan, G. 2014 (February 18). Survey: What's the state of IT in post-acute settings? LeadingAge. http://www.leadingage.org/Survey_Whats_the_State_of_IT_in_Post_Acute_Settings.aspx.

Maguire, P. 2014 (August). How depression affects readmissions. *Today's Hospitalist.* http://www.todayshospitalist.com/index.php?b=articles_read&cnt=1915.

McCarthy, K. 2015 (July 16). How can behavioral health practices effectively use EHRs? NueMD News. http://www.nuemd.com/news/2015/07/16/can-behavioral-health-practices-effectively-use-ehrs.

McCormack, M. 2014 (April 25). Survey: Do patients really care if you use your EHR in the exam room? *The Profitable Practice.* http://profitable-practice.softwareadvice.com/do-patients-care-about-ehrs-0414.

Mental Health Corporations of America (MHCA) and Software and Technology Vendors' Association (SATVA). 2006. Planning Your EHR System: Guidelines for Executive Management. MHCA/STVA.

Monsen C. 2011 (May 30). Dizziness diagnostic tool. SMART Apps for Health. http://smartapps.devpost.com/submissions/3131-dizziness-diagnostic-tool.

Montague, E. 2013 (August 14). Nonverbal interpersonal interactions in clinical encounters and patient perceptions of empathy. *Journal of Participatory Medicine.* 5. http://www.jopm.org/evidence/research/2013/08/14/nonverbal-interpersonal-interactions-in-clinical-encounters-and-patient-perceptions-of-empathy.

Nardone, M., et al. 2014 (February 12). Integrating physical and behavioral health care: Promising Medicaid models. The Henry J. Kaiser Family Foundation. The Kaiser Commission on Medicaid and the Uninsured. http://kff.org/medicaid/issue-brief/integrating-physical-and-behavioral-health-care-promising-medicaid-models.

National Alliance on Mental Illness (NAMI). 2011. Mental health professionals: Who they are and how to find one. http://www.nami.org.

National Commission on Correctional Health Care (NCCHC). 2013 (March 18). Federal EHR incentive program now applicable to correctional providers. *CorrectCare.* 27(1). http://www.ncchc.org/ehr-incentive-program.

National Council for Community Behavioral Healthcare. 2012 (June). HIT adoption and readiness for meaningful use in community behavioral health: Report on the 2012 National Council survey. http://www.thenationalcouncil.org/wp-content/uploads/2012/10/HIT-Survey-Full-Report.pdf.

O'Connor, S. 2013. (February 22). 5 benefits of using EHR for behavioral health practices. Advanced Data Systems Corporation blog. http://healthcare.adsc.com/blog/bid/257238/5-Benefits-of-Using-EHR-For-Behavioral-Health-Practices.

Office of the National Coordinator for Health Information Technology (ONC). 2013 (March 15). Issue brief: Health IT in long-term and post acute care. https://www.healthit.gov/sites/default/files/pdf/HIT_LTPAC_IssueBrief031513.pdf.

Office of the National Coordinator for Health Information Technology (ONC). 2014 (September 15). Behavioral Health Consent Management. https://www.healthit.gov/policy-researchers-implementers/consent-management.

Paris, J.E. 2013. What correctional practitioners want in an electronic health record. *Journal of Correctional Health Care.* 19(3):218–228. http://jcx.sagepub.com/content/19/3/218.abstract.

Planned Parenthood Federation of America (PPFA). n.d. Impact of health information technology on Planned Parenthood's health care delivery: Two case studies. Sexual Health and Reproductive Health Promotion Training and Technical Assistance Center. http://shrpttac.jsi.com/wp-content/uploads/2016/04/Planned_Parenthood_EHR.pdf.

Psychology Today. n.d. The therapy directory. http://therapists.psychologytoday.com/rms/content/therapy_credentials.html.

Raths, D. 2009. Behavioral health IT forecast: Cloudy. *Behavioral Healthcare.* 29(8):26–27.

Resnick, H.E., et al. 2009. Use of electronic information systems in nursing homes: United States: 2004. *Journal of the American Medical Informatics Association.* 16(2):179–186.

Resnick, H.E., and M. Alwan. 2010. Use of health information technology in home health and hospice agencies: United States, 2007. *Journal of the American Medical Informatics Association.* 17:380–395.

Roat, R.J. 2011. Meaningful use planning for radiologists. *Radiology Today.* 12(11):20.

Rudman, W., et al. 2010. Integrating medical and dental records: A new frontier in health information management. *Journal of AHIMA.* 81(10):36–39.

Russell, K.G. 2009 (October). Bringing healthcare home: Technology and telehealth adoption in home care. *2009 AHIMA Convention Proceedings.* http://bok.ahima.org/doc?oid=98465#.V72x15grI2x

S&I Framework. SAMHSA 2014 Consent2Share Project. http://wiki.siframework.org/ SAMHSA+Consent2Share+Project.

Sandler, E.P. 2009 (November 17). Behavioral health vs. mental health: Battle conformity. *Psychology Today.*

Simon, L. 2014 (January 28). American Psychiatric Association behavioral health provider perspectives. APA EHR Committee. https://www.healthit.gov/archive/archive_files/FACA%20Hearings/2014/2014-01-28%20Certification%20 %26%20Adoption%20Workgroup%20Virtual%20Hearing%20on%20BH%20EHR%20Certification/012814_ONC_ BehavioralHealthProviderPerspectives.pdf.

Siwicki, B. 2016 (April 14). Cleveland Clinic inks deal with CVS, doctors to conduct telehealth visits through MinuteClinics. *Healthcare Finance News.* http://www.healthcarefinancenews.com/news/ cleveland-clinic-inks-deal-cvs-doctors-conduct-telehealth-visits-through-minute-clinics.

Steinfeld, B., et al. 2006. EMRs bring all of healthcare together. *Behavioral Healthcare.* 26(1):12–17.

Stratice Healthcare. 2015. eDMEplus. For EHRs page. http://straticehealthcare.com/healthcare_ehr .php.

Stratis Health. 2014. HIT toolkit: Behavioral health: Communicating with clients about EHR and HIE. https://www .stratishealth.org/expertise/healthit/behavioralhealth/index.html#implement.

Stratis Health. 2009a. HIT Toolkit: Nursing Homes. http://www.stratishealth.org.

Stratis Health. 2009b. HIT Toolkit: Home Health. http://www.stratishealth.org.

Stratis Health. n.d. Mental Health EHR—request for proposal (developed for Stratis Health by Margret Amatayakul).

Teslow, M., et al. 2009. Street smart: Understanding the context of emergency medical services communication and documentation. *Journal of AHIMA.* 80(3):46–49.

Thorman, C. 2010 (March 19). Electronic health records and clinical trials: An incentive to integrate. *Health IT News.* http://www.healthcareitnews.com/blog/electronic-health-records-and-clinical-trials-incentive-integrate.

Turso, C. 2008. A fuller picture of ROI. *Behavioral Healthcare.* 28(11):30–32.

US Surgeon General. *The Health Consequences of Involuntary Exposure to Tobacco Smoke: A Report of the Surgeon General.* Atlanta, GA: US Department of Health and Human Services, Centers for Disease Control and Prevention, Coordinating Center for Health Promotion, National Center for Chronic Disease Prevention and Health Promotion, Office on Smoking and Health, 2006. http://www.surgeongeneral.gov/library/reports/secondhandsmoke/fullreport.pdf.

Whitehouse, Sen. Sheldon (D-RI). 2011. S 538, The Behavioral Health Information Technology Act of 2011. (Legislation sent to the Senate Finance Committee on March 16, 2011.)

Wilder Foundation. 2010 (April 20). Request for proposals: Electronic health record and integrated practice management system. http://www.wilder.org/fileadmin/wilder/pdf/Wilder_EHR_RFP.pdf.

Chapter 17
Health IT for Consumers

Learning Objectives

- Define PHRs and identify their attributes, functionality, and supporting standards.

- Discuss the current state of PHR utilization, including PHR benefits and barriers for its adoption.

- Identify policies and practices that may aid in overcoming barriers and facilitate adoption of PHRs.

- Describe mobile health devices and other digital health technology, their appropriate use, and ways providers may encourage their safe use.

- Describe the impact of consumer empowerment on PHRs and their role in value-driven healthcare initiatives.

Health information technology (health IT) for consumers is rapidly growing. At one time, health information aids for individuals may only have been in the form of a MedicAlert bracelet worn to alert good Samaritans and others that the wearer has diabetes and may be experiencing an event related to this illness (bracelets for other conditions were later added). Many individuals have found it useful to keep track of health information—such as immunizations, medications, and responses to treatment regimens, especially for chronic illness for themselves or others. Before the advent of computers, this information would have been kept in the form of handwritten notes or paper copies of information accompanying medication prescriptions. Patients might have also asked their providers for copies of parts of their health records.

More recently, individuals began creating personal health records (PHRs) on personal computers by compiling scanned images of documents or using a spreadsheet. Next came software for PHRs supplied by vendors. These programs were often made available by a health plan or employer wellness program. Use of PHRs was spurred by the Health Insurance Portability and Accountability Act (HIPAA) Privacy Rule, which requires providers to afford individuals' rights to access their records. Now, health apps are available for downloading onto a smartphone. As providers started to adopt EHRs and provision of access to health information became encouraged, PHRs came to be integrated with electronic health records (EHRs) and offered to patients through a provider portal.

Even more recently, personal health devices, often called *digital health technology* or *mHealth,* such as in-home pregnancy tests, blood sugar (glucose) monitoring devices, automated drug dispensing, and many others, have become popular. Some of these devices, such as one of the latest screening kits for colorectal cancer, require that the individual collect a specimen and send it to a laboratory for testing, which may require a prescription for devices or laboratory testing. Personal health devices for physiological monitoring have become especially popular. Social media is also playing a role in personal health. (See section on mobile devices later in this chapter.)

The federal government has taken a keen interest in PHRs and other forms of health IT for provision of access to health information as a means to support consumer empowerment and patient engagement for its value-driven healthcare initiatives.

PHR Definitions

Definitions of the term *personal health record* abound. Here are discussed some of the most notable ones.

American Health Information Management Association (AHIMA)

Since as early as 2005, AHIMA has been at the forefront of supporting PHRs in a variety of ways. It defines the **personal health record (PHR)** as follows (AHIMA 2010):

> An electronic, universally available, lifelong resource of health information needed by individuals to make health decisions. Individuals own and manage the information in the PHR, which comes from healthcare providers and the individual. The PHR is maintained in a secure and private environment, with the individual determining rights of access. The PHR is separate from and does not replace the legal record of any provider.

Connecting for Health

Connecting for Health (2006) observed that "PHRs encompass a wide variety of applications that enable people to collect, view, manage, or share copies of their health information or transactions electronically. Although there are many variants, PHRs are based on the fundamental concept of facilitating an individual's access to and creation of personal health information in a usable computer application that the individual (or a designee) controls." Connecting for Health offers a version of five PHR dimensions that characterize PHRs. The following dimensions and their discussion were adapted from Connecting for Health (AHIMA 2006; AHIMA 2008):

- *Sponsor:* Who is supplying the PHR for the individual—provider, payer, employer, health information exchange (HIE), affinity group (for example, a professional organization or disease-related group), or commercial vendor? There may be different functions supplied by different sponsors and possibly different privacy and security concerns raised.

- *Integration:* Is the PHR **tethered** (that is, connected largely to a provider, but possibly to a payer or other sponsor) or **standalone** (that is, independent of any sponsor; also considered "commercial")? If tethered to a HIPAA-covered entity, the consumer may feel more confident of the privacy and security protections. A corollary to this question may better be—how will the data in the PHR be used? There are web-based PHRs and other products (including EHRs) that clearly state that the product is provided free of charge in return for the ability to mine the data collected for marketing and other purposes. Data mining is not necessarily bad so long as consumers are provided clear information about what data are collected and for what purposes. For example, one of the most sophisticated health social networking sites is PatientsLikeMe, which helps patients put their (usually incurable) conditions in context; organize the status of their symptoms, treatments, and side effects; and prepare themselves for a clinician encounter. Connections with similar patients are supported while, at the same time, PatientsLikeMe contributes data to a pharmaceutical companies and researchers to help find innovative treatments (Braunstein 2014). Interestingly, another similar site is much more controversial. 23andMe is a direct-to-consumer genomics company that launched in 2006 and has as its business model selling services to consumers interested in learning about their personal genetics and also aggregating those data and selling them to pharmaceutical and biotech companies. Consumers may have understood 23andMe to be just another ancestry information service; however, it was learned in 2015 that the company had forged deals with two major companies to look at Parkinson's disease (Genentech) and lupus (Pfizer). Salisbury (2015) asks, "Are 23andMe customers suckers or empowered consumers?"

- *Platform:* How is the PHR supplied from a technical standpoint? The PHR may be web-based, an app for smartphones, downloadable software to a PC, or on paper. Each platform has its own set of advantages and disadvantages for privacy, security, convenience, price, and so on.

- *Data source:* Often, the source of the data (for example, provider, payer, consumer, or other) is related to the sponsor, although sources can also be mixed. Closely related to the data source should be the ability for the consumer to exercise control over who is provided access.

- *Business model:* How is the PHR funded? Options include licensed, as any other software is; fee for use (also called *subscription*), a model frequently used to acquire a web-based product; through advertisements; and through investment by the sponsor—such as an employer seeking a healthier workforce. The value proposition is one many sponsors are considering, because value may improve process efficiency, brand loyalty, messaging, and behavioral change and outcomes improvement.

To add to their definition of PHR, Connecting for Health released in 2008 a Common Framework for increasing consumers' privacy and control of their health information on online PHRs. The Common Framework is based on a set of principles that provides the foundation for managing personal health information within consumer-accessible data streams. These principles include the following:

- Openness and transparency with respect to all uses and disclosures of health information

- Purpose specification for each use or disclosure of health information

- Collection limitation and data minimization to ensure that only minimum necessary health information is collected and maintained

- Use limitation to ensure that only minimum necessary health information is used

- Individual participation and control over their health information

- Data quality and integrity

- Security safeguards and controls

- Accountability and oversight for managing health information

- Remedies for wrongful use and disclosure of health information

Finally, the Common Framework makes a distinction between consumer access services and PHRs. Consumer access services are an emerging set of services designed to help individuals make secure connections with health data sources (for example, providers, laboratories, pharmacies, health plans, and disease management companies) in an electronic environment. These services are essentially portals that consumers can use to request and schedule an appointment, pay bills, request copies of their health records, view their laboratory test results, and perform several other functions, including accessing a tethered PHR.

Both AHIMA and Connecting for Health emphasize the importance of distinguishing between not only the PHR and the portal but also the provider's business record, in which individuals have access rights, and the PHR, which is the individual's own record. Both organizations support the fact that the PHR should provide the ability for consumers to include copies of some or all health information from one or more providers' records, add personal annotations, restrict the ability to alter any health information sourced to a provider or health plan, and enable the individual to control who may have access. Despite these premises, current portal functionality, and especially tethered PHRs, may have only a few of the functions in use or even available for use (Studeny and Coustasse 2014).

Health IT.gov

The federal government's portal for health IT defines the basics of a PHR as follows:

An electronic application used by patients to maintain and manage their health information in a private, secure, and confidential environment. PHRs:

- Are managed by patients

- Can include information from a variety of sources, including health care providers and patients themselves

- Can help patients securely and confidentially store and monitor health information, such as diet plans or data from home monitoring systems, as well as patient contact information, diagnosis lists, medication lists, allergy lists, immunization histories, and much more

- Are separate from, and do not replace, the legal record of any health care provider

- Are distinct from portals that simply allow patients to view provider information or communicate with providers

Properly designed and implemented, PHRs can help patients manage their health information and become full partners in the quest for good health. (HealthIT.gov 2013)

This statement reflects the federal government's growing interest in consumer empowerment and patient engagement.

PHR Attributes

Definitions of the PHR can be supplemented with descriptions of their attributes, which often include recommendations that urge more formal definition and standardization of PHR development and implementation. Attributes have been proposed by the National Committee on Vital and Health Statistics (NCVHS), Health Level Seven (HL7), and AHIMA.

National Committee on Vital and Health Statistics

In 2005 NCVHS stated:

PHRs are broadly considered as a means by which an individual's personal health information can be collected, stored, and used for diverse health management purposes. There is no uniform definition, and the concept continues to evolve. Lack of consensus makes collaboration, coordination, and policymaking difficult.

NCVHS concluded that "it is not possible or even desirable, to attempt a unitary definition at this time."

In 2009 recommendations to the Secretary of the Department of Health and Human Services (HHS), NCVHS urged HHS to promote fair information practices with respect to PHRs and recommended that transparency and informed consent to information uses and disclosures with respect to PHRs be incorporated in policy. It further asserted that PHR vendors should support national standards for interoperability, ensure the ability to correct information in PHRs, and provide additional privacy and security protections surrounding disclosures of information from PHRs.

Health Level 7

The standards development organization HL7 notes that its PHR System Functional Model does not attempt to define the PHR but identifies the features and functions in a system necessary to create and manage an effective PHR. HL7 also makes a clear distinction between a PHR and a PHR system: The PHR is the underlying record that the software functionality of a PHR system maintains. This distinction is consistent with HL7's EHR System Functional Model, in which it defines the attributes of an EHR system but does not explicitly define the EHR. See the PHR standards below.

AHIMA

AHIMA (2005) organizes PHR attributes into six categories:

- *Functionality,* including supporting individual health education and decision making, selected retrieval by providers, and many others.

- *Format and content,* including that the standard format is electronic but not restricted by any one format; and appropriate content is recommended to include lifelong health information but not necessarily considered a complete record. Common data elements for the PHR are recommended.

- *Privacy, access, and control,* which are strictly controlled by the individual but accessible in an emergency.

- *Maintenance and security* to provide for an audit trail, which identifies what may have been amended by the original source of the PHR data. This helps maintain record integrity as the individual decides what is incorporated in his or her PHR.

- *Interoperability,* which helps achieve easy, accurate, and consistent exchange with others (as authorized by the individual). A recent finding is that interoperability may actually be hindered by requirements of the meaningful use (MU) incentive program, because each provider now believes it is necessary to offer a PHR, which often results in patients having multiple PHRs that do not communicate with one another (Studeny and Coustasse 2014).

- *Ownership of the PHR,* which is by the individual or designee.

PHR Standards

In 2009, the HL7 standards development organization released its **HL7 PHR System Functional Model**. This model was subsequently reviewed and re-released in 2014. It is illustrated in figure 17.1. HL7 is also promoting PHR interoperability as it works on its latest V2.x message standard (V2.6) (Sujansky & Associates 2013).

Figure 17.1.   HL7 PHR functional model

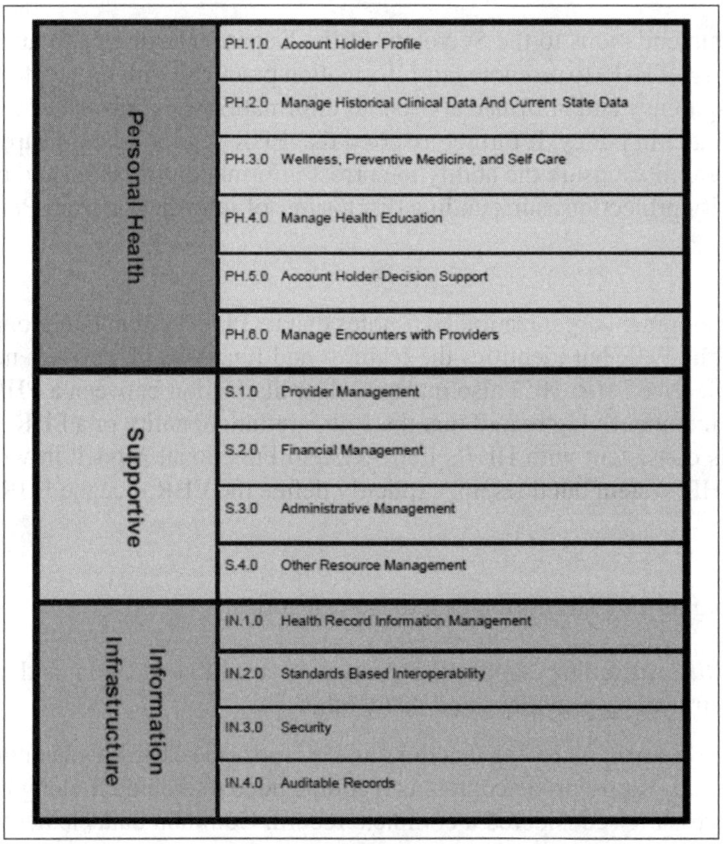

Personal Health	
PH.1.0	Account Holder Profile
PH.2.0	Manage Historical Clinical Data And Current State Data
PH.3.0	Wellness, Preventive Medicine, and Self Care
PH.4.0	Manage Health Education
PH.5.0	Account Holder Decision Support
PH.6.0	Manage Encounters with Providers

Supportive	
S.1.0	Provider Management
S.2.0	Financial Management
S.3.0	Administrative Management
S.4.0	Other Resource Management

Information Infrastructure	
IN.1.0	Health Record Information Management
IN.2.0	Standards Based Interoperability
IN.3.0	Security
IN.4.0	Auditable Records

Figure 17.2.   Standards related to HL7's Consolidated-Clinical Document Architecture (C-CDA)

ASTM CCR + HL7 CDA = CCD
+ More CDA Documents = C-CDA

Two standards that are important to recognize for their contribution to PHRs are the ASTM International's Continuity of Care Record (CCR) and HL7's Clinical Document Architecture (CDA), which together form the Continuity of Care Document (CCD).

ASTM's E31 Committee on Health Informatics, the Massachusetts Medical Society, the American Academy of Family Physicians, and the Healthcare Information and Management Systems Society (HIMSS) teamed up and recognized the need to organize a set of basic information about a patient's healthcare that can be provided to referring physicians. Developers of the CCR content specification emphasize that the specification is not an EHR. It is not a record of a patient's life-long health status and healthcare; it does not provide interactive clinical decision support; it is not universally accessible; and it does not have a universal patient identifier or record locator service. It is simply a content specification that can be used to improve the quality of information supplied to providers during the transfer of healthcare.

The HL7 CDA is a document markup standard that specifies the structure and semantics of clinical documents for the purpose of exchange. A CDA document is a defined and complete information object that can include text, images, sounds, and other multimedia content.

The result of the harmonized ASTM CCR and HL7 CDA is the CCD. As described in chapter 13, various types of document templates are being created by HL7 using the CDA. The consolidation of these additional documents in CDA format and the CCD is referred to as the Consolidated-Clinical Document Architecture (C-CDA). The relationship between these standards to yield the C-CDA is illustrated in figure 17.2.

Although the ASTM CCR may be rendered in extensible markup language (XML), it also may be rendered as a document when combined with the CDA. A key element of the CCD and other CDA documents in the C-CDA that makes them desirable for use in PHRs is not only the standard data content but also that all data may be sourced to their original author. When data are sourced, access controls on the data enable viewing but not alteration. The potential lack of data integrity in a PHR has been a major concern of providers—and this solution is frequently not well known or understood. It is also the reason that many PHRs tethered to a provider EHR are constructed so that the consumer cannot supply information. This prohibition is unfortunate because it prevents effective documentation of information related to the individual's care. For example, if the source of a prescription is a specific provider or a pharmacy benefits manager reporting a drug claim, a consumer may want to annotate that he or she is taking only half the dose, or stopped taking the medication halfway through the prescribed treatment regimen, or experienced an adverse reaction. This annotation would provide valuable information associated with the drug but would not alter records that the drug was prescribed by a certain provider and filled by a pharmacy.

Check Your Understanding 17.1

Indicate whether the following statements are true or false:

1.   A PHR is the legal health record for a provider.

2.   Most provider-sponsored PHRs are tethered.

3.   A PHR can be maintained on paper.

4.   A PHR is a portal.

5.   A consumer access service is a portal.

6.   Many tethered PHRs are not interoperable with other PHRs.

7.   Standard content for a PHR is defined by HL7.

8.   The CCD is a PHR.

9.   Many provider-sponsored PHRs do not permit patients to enter information.

10.   Documents structured using the CDA can be sourced to their origin.

Current Status of PHR Utilization

The following titles of articles identified during research to determine the current status of PHR utilization suggest a need for more definitive information on PHR usage:

What has happened to the personal health record? (Finn 2014)

Harris Poll Survey finds patients want a deeper digital connection with their doctors (Caouette 2015)

It has always been difficult to identify the current status of PHR utilization; however, in the past, there were relatively frequent and reliable surveys about PHR usage, most pointing to the fact that about 10 percent of Americans used PHRs. Today, it seems there are many fewer surveys being conducted, and those that are conducted are done either by health IT vendors, which are very likely to have some bias and hence interest in casting findings in the best possible light, or by employers whose employees have long distrusted with their health information.

The titles of the two articles noted above seem contradictory, and yet they may tell the real story: It is not clear what a personal health record is to many Americans. Is it a collection of paper copies of records obtained from a physician? Is it a portal on which one can schedule appointments or obtain test results? Is it a PHR as defined by AHIMA and others? When use of a PHR is discussed, is it hypothetical or planned? The results of the following polls make it clear that there is no clarity surrounding use of PHR:

- Data from 2011 (Archer et al.) suggest that among the 47 percent of patients who maintained health records, 87 percent said they were on paper.

- A study conducted in 2010 by the California HealthCare Foundation (CHCF) found only 7 percent of Americans using a PHR.

- The Harris Poll commissioned by eClinical Works identified in the above list of titles (Caouette 2015) revealed that 60 percent of people are "likely" to schedule appointments with their doctors via a patient portal or secure website. Furthermore, 61 percent of the physicians who actively use a patient portal to communicate with their patients would recommend telehealth visits at least sometimes to their patients. (Note that the number of such physicians was not cited.)

- An annual survey conducted by Xerox (2014) found that 64 percent of baby boomers said they "do or would" access/review "medical records/test results" online. Considering the words in quotes from just this sampling of results, it appears that the actual percentage of users is something less than the 64 percent suggested by other surveys.

- A Digital Health Consumer Adoption survey conducted by Rock Health (Dahl 2015) was reported to have found that 24 percent of respondents had "either asked for [a paper copy of] or downloaded" their personal health records. This same survey was also reported to have found that among "super adopters" (individuals who have adopted five or six forms of digital health technology), 7 percent had downloaded their records, versus 2 percent in the general population.

Another telling finding from the article titled "What has happened to the personal health record?" (Finn 2014) is a reply to posted comment on the article by a user named Michael (October 28, 2014), who states:

> I have kept a Word-based record for many years, covering data from 1969 to the present. So far, I have only found one physician who has read it. In one case, I was to have an MRI, and the provider wanted a "complete history of all radiation exposure". They gave me about 1″ of space on their intake form for this, so I just said "see attached" and attached my 2 pages' worth of data. They never even looked at their form, let alone mine—just marched me into the lab and zapped me.
>
> My principal provider locally just instituted an on-line system to great fanfare, which as far as I can tell is just an ultra-secure e-mail system, a pain in the neck to use, and riddled with incorrect data.
>
> We're doomed.

The plethora of articles about portals, personal health devices, health apps, social media, tele-health visits, and other digital health technology is very likely blurring the picture of what a PHR is in the minds of most Americans, and likely in the minds of providers as well. This observation is not to suggest that the wealth of technologies is bad, but that the principles upon which PHR is predicated by organizations like AHIMA or the federal government may be getting lost in the confusion. It would also be helpful to have accurate data about use of PHRs and each of the other technologies, in order to ensure that, as Finn notes in the article questioning what has happened to the PHR, "every patient can benefit from more efficient, cost effective, and safe medical practice."

Benefits of PHRs

The value of PHRs is of strong interest to various sponsors for many different purposes. For example, a BlueCross BlueShield of Massachusetts member-facing website, A Healthy Me (2015), notes that PHRs are "an important technology for consumer engagement and a key tool to enhance care coordination and improve patients' ability to make more informed health decisions." BlueCross BlueShield (2016) further notes that there is a need to educate consumers and providers about the value of PHRs. This payer offers a detailed brochure highlighting PHR benefits, providing testimonials, displaying screen shots, and offering a glossary of terms. A number of provider specialty societies, health affinity groups (American Cancer Society, American Heart Association, and others), and the Medical Group Management Association collaborated on the development of the brochure as well as two quick reference guides, one for consumers and one for providers.

Many physicians also view PHRs as extremely valuable to both their patients and themselves—when the PHR information from disparate sources is a structured and legible manner. The American Academy of Family Physicians (AAFP) identifies the following seven major benefits in using PHRs (Endsley et al. 2006):

- Empowerment of patients:
    - Patients can use PHRs to verify the information in their records—a study conducted by the Office of the National Coordinator for Health Information Technology (ONC) found one-third of individuals surveyed reported a gap in health information among their

providers or between themselves and their providers (Patel and Siminerio 2014). Such verification could also reduce, or at least mitigate, the impact of medical identity theft, which affected nearly 5 million individuals in 2015, and which Accenture has projected to rise to 25 million by 2019 (Miliard 2015).

○ Patients with chronic disease can also use PHRs to monitor their health data for improved care management.

• Improved patient-provider relationships, fostered through improved communications and more timely conveyance of test results.

• Increased patient safety as PHRs may provide drug alerts, missed procedure alerts, and documentation of interactions.

• Improved quality of care because of the opportunity for more continuous communication across the continuum of care through patient-mediated health information exchange.

• More efficient delivery of care as PHRs help avoid duplicative testing and unnecessary services:

○ The Center for Information Technology Leadership (CITL) estimated in 2008 that $9.4 billion per year could be saved in redundant testing if PHRs were used.

○ Overall, CITL found that the net value of interoperable PHRs could be $19 billion annually (Kaelber et al. 2008).

• Better safeguards on health information privacy because patients have control over who may access their records and how PHRs are shared.

• Bigger cost savings as a result of improved documentation with use of PHRs lowering malpractice costs.

In addition to these benefits identified by AAFP, PHRs may help reduce disparities in the level of, or access to, treatment—not only with respect to race and ethnicity differences in quality of care but also in bridging geographic isolation (IOM 2002; Garvin et al. 2009).

AAFP did note that patients are concerned about their privacy and therefore PHRs must offer strong security features. Patients entering their own information into their PHRs raised concerns among providers over data accuracy, although it was pointed out that proper development of the PHR can reduce this concern (Endsley et al. 2006).

In 2015, HHS highlighted the need to better engage and empower healthcare consumers through PHRs and other steps in order to achieve national goals for better care, smarter spending, and healthier people. However, to best utilize PHRs as one (of many) ways to improve the quality, cost, and experience of care, barriers to using PHRs—for both physicians and patients—must be found.

Barriers to PHR Use and Suggestions for Addressing Them

David Lansky, executive director of the Personal Health Technology Initiative at the Markle Foundation, is quoted as suggesting that most physicians are "not opposed to PHRs, but they anticipate challenges" (Lowes 2006). Robeznieks (2007a) quotes a chief medical informatics officer as saying that "[doctors] like me are terrified of PHRs and what patients will bring to us"—envisioning mounds of paper, some of which may be inaccurate or incomplete, and fearing liability for not being able to manage the volume of information.

Some concerns raised by physicians may reflect an incomplete understanding of how some of the PHR offerings capture, consolidate, and coordinate information. Physician willingness to use

PHRs also seems to vary by location, gender, and practice, with rural physicians, male physicians, and certain specialists (surgery, obstetrics, and psychiatry) more willing to use PHRs (Wynia et al. 2011). Witry and colleagues (2010) conducted focus groups of family physicians to gauge their perceptions of PHRs and found considerable variation in thoughts about benefits and concerns, how PHRs would actually be used, maintenance of a PHR, and what interest their patients would actually have in a PHR.

Finally, in 2015, Vydra and colleagues reported that continued lack of reimbursement for time spent in portal communication was a major barrier to providers' engagement with this technology. In 2014, Hostetter and associates similarly found that there was a lack of evidence that use of digital health technologies had any impact on cost and outcomes. This study also found that the lack of collaboration between clinicians and technologists in product development was a concern to clinicians. In summary, some of the concerns most commonly cited in the literature and suggestions for overcoming them include the following:

- Will patients faithfully and accurately maintain a "do-it-yourself" PHR or attempt to use PHRs in a fraudulent manner? It is important that any PHR a provider offers or uses be appropriately sourced, so it is clear who made each entry. Just as in a paper-based medical record or EHR, there should be access controls that do not permit deletions or alterations, but permit amendments.

- Will physicians bother reading these PHRs? Currently, there is no reimbursement for PHR review, although some physicians believe patient data entry into templates that can be moved into the EHR may increase productivity (see figure 17.3).

- If physicians do not read the content of a PHR, would they be liable for overlooking red-flag medical symptoms? To limit malpractice liability, some attorneys advise physicians to ask their patients to use their PHRs as important but personal references. They suggest that physicians be proactive in encouraging patients to maintain a record of their care for themselves and use it during an encounter as a resource to recall information, but not to supply to the physician. This advice is contrary to the intent of a patient-managed HIE architecture, but the legal stance may also change as use of patient-managed records becomes more common.

- Will patients understand the content of their health records? If they do not, will they be at greater risk because they seek explanations from uninformed or unscrupulous resources

Figure 17.3.   Patient as clinical data entry partner

One physician has created an interactive website that is used to make patients "clinical data-entry partners." Structured clinical interview forms help capture patient-supplied information in advance of an appointment. The clinical interview with the patient is then structured to follow the data entered by the patient, plus any remaining history questions the physician believes necessary. This physician has found that condition-specific, structured clinical interviews completed by the patient in advance of the appointment (or in the waiting room at a kiosk with or without staff assistance) has improved physician productivity significantly, reduced transcription costs, and heightened patient education and satisfaction. The notes resulting from this collaborative effort:

- Are clear, thorough, and legible, representing approximately 80 percent of the information needed for a specific visit

- Form a consistent baseline of information collected for each condition (and limit the amount of data collected to the essential)

- Create a searchable database of clinical attributes

- Aid in coding and reimbursement because physician activities and patient education are tied to the reason for the visit

Source: Blasingame 2003.

online? Again, education goes a long way. PHRs can be designed to hyperlink to appropriate explanatory information, and many physicians have found that a modification to their workflow to contact patients to explain results can actually save them time downstream. PHR sponsors can highlight and activate "cyberseals" of approval to validate legitimate websites.

- If patients have the ability to share health information from one provider with another provider without the author being aware of the exchange, how does that transfer of information affect these providers' liabilities and their relative positions in a competitive marketplace? Ideally, an HIE environment where appropriate agreements concerning legal matters are addressed up front would head off any problems in this regard.

- Finally, are PHRs secure? Physicians may have security concerns if they accept a flash drive or download a file from a patient. Certainly, virus protection and other measures should be the norm for any provider in any information technology environment.

There are also perhaps some deeper challenges to the use of PHRs that several individuals and organizations have identified and started working through. Three clinics, in particular, have been at the forefront of PHR use, and leaders at those organizations have raised some interesting issues that providers must address. Paul Tang, at the Palo Alto Medical Foundation, John Halamka, at Beth Israel Deaconess, and Kenneth Mandl, at Children's Hospital Boston, have different types of PHR systems but have all posed similar questions with similar responses (Halamka et al. 2008):

- Should sensitive diagnoses be shared? All indicate yes, with appropriate security measures and where state laws do not pose legal barriers.

- Should the entire medication list be shared? All indicate yes, urging provider-based and patient-maintained lists be kept side by side, showing origin of documentation and updates.

- Should all laboratory test results be shared? Variations in workflow due to state law restrictions were noted, but the main expectation of the PHR functionality was to improve the timeliness of physician review so that results could be shared.

- Should all clinical notes be shared? Access should be supplied on request.

- Should patients be authenticated to access PHR? Yes.

- Should minors have access to PHR, or should patients be able to share access via proxies? Variations in practice due to state law were noted. (For information on state laws, see Pritts et al. 2009.)

PHR Policies and Practices

Best Practices

On a blog for a corporate wellness company, Morgan reports that a 2013 study by researchers at Virginia Commonwealth University showed that patients are more likely to use a PHR if their personal physician endorsed the technology (2013). As a result of this finding, Morgan suggests that physicians should answer the following questions:

- Are you proactively inviting your patients to register in your EHR [portal] at a time that's connected to their care needs?

- Are you or a staff member proactively endorsing the portal, combined with verbal explanation (not just a handout)?

- Are you or a dedicated staff member using the portal to proactively communicate with patients once their in-office care has concluded (not just a massive distribution to all patients)? (Morgan 2013)

Morgan concludes that a "no" answer to any of the questions means the practice should reevaluate its patient engagement strategy. These three questions also reflect best practices for use of not only portals—which are potentially set up only for appointment scheduling and/or to view test results—but for PHRs as well.

West Virginia Health Information Network (2014) has also posted online its policies and procedures for PHRs. Its purpose in doing so was to explain the process by which a patient may populate his or her PHR with protected health information from the West Virginia's HIO. Individual physician offices and hospitals offering PHRs may also find such a posting to be a best practice.

PHR Policies and Procedures

To ensure that physicians and staff fully understand the PHR's purpose and how it may (and may not) be used and shared, best practices should be codified in written policies and procedures (with potentially more detailed policies and procedures for internal use only) and in training. A recent study on use of tethered PHRs in primary care (Vydra et al. 2015) found that physicians were interested in using patient portals to improve communications with patient, but they generally overestimated the time spent per week on such communications. Attention to workflow and how such communications would be best performed would help overcome both erroneous assumptions that portals are time-consuming to use and any real issues with productivity.

Another important policy that should be established is the relationship of the tethered PHR content to the organization's legal health record and its designated record set. Using AHIMA tools on the fundamentals of these constructs, dispute resolution, and other legal matters, an organization should be able to construct a content description for its PHR and policies and procedures on information management (Haugen et al. 2011; Washington et al. 2009). Access and amendment policies in place in an organization should also be reviewed in relationship to its PHR (AHIMA 2011). The PHR is not the same as the EHR, and such analysis should not be construed to suggest that the same policies apply; however, consistency in policies can be helpful for staff as they help implement and manage patient portals (Baldwin et al. 2015).

Supporting Patient Use of PHR

Offering assistance to patients in understanding and using PHRs can further encourage their use. In 2003, AHIMA launched a website (myPHR.com) as a guide to understanding and managing personal health information for the general public.

The myPHR site explains to consumers what a health record is, identifies consumers' health information rights, describes how to select and maintain a PHR, and provides additional resources on PHR products and services. This website also provides an Understanding Your Medical Record guide (AHIMA 2012). It may also be useful to consider the set of questions posed in figure 17.4 as providers start to supply PHRs and patients start to use them (AHIMA 2006; AHIMA 2010).

The myPHR site also describes the Blue Button initiative (see also chapter 13). The **Blue Button initiative** is a project to ensure access for every American to their digital health information and to help application developers use the data to build products and services that help individuals with their health. The initiative was started by the US Department of Veterans Affairs (VA) and is also used by the Department of Defense, Social Security Administration, and Medicare; it is now led ONC.

MyHealtheVet is the VA's PHR portal, with the VA Blue Button providing a simple, secure, and convenient way for veterans to access and download their available personal health information (see figure 17.5). Veterans can also self-enter demographic information, emergency contacts,

Figure 17.4.   Ten questions to ask about PHRs

1. Will this PHR enable me to record all the health information I want?
2. Will information automatically be added to my PHR from other sources?
   - What information will be added? How will it be added? Is transfer auditable?
   - Is there opportunity to delete, correct, or add information? How? Is there an audit log?
3. Does the PHR host or sponsor have any ownership rights to the information in the PHR?
4. Can the PHR host or sponsor sell the information to anyone for any reason?
   - If so, how can I ensure my privacy is protected?
   - Can I specify that my information not be sold?
5. Will my information be used for employment or insurance coverage decisions?
6. Who has access to information in my PHR?
   - Can I control who (provider, insurer, employer, caregiver, family member) has access to what information (for example, demographics/insurance, medical, behavioral) and under what circumstances (for example, specific healthcare encounter, emergency only, other)?
   - Is there an audit log of who has accessed my PHR?
7. If I no longer am employed, insured, or a patient of the host/sponsor, can I still continue to use the PHR?
8. How do I get my data if host/sponsor goes out of business? How can I transfer my PHR information to another PHR sponsor?
9. Will there be any cost for me associated with use of this PHR? Upfront, ongoing maintenance, per access, other?
10. Do you apply targeted advertisement to my PHR? If so, is there a way to use my PHR without this advertisement? How am I assured that advertisers do not get access to my health information?

Source: Adapted from AHIMA Personal Health Record Practice Council, 2006.

Figure 17.5.   VA Blue Button

Source: http://www.va.gov/bluebutton/

providers they are currently using, other health insurance, personal medical history, over-the-counter and other nonprescription drugs they are taking, adverse reactions, and much more (VA n.d.).

Other organizations are also able to use Blue Button technology, and the Departments of Education and Energy have created a Green Button for access to information on their websites–for example, utility companies can use Department of Energy information accessed via that site's Green Button. Private insurers also use Blue Buttons as a convenient way for people to access health information held by these companies (Dimick 2012).

Check Your Understanding 17.2

Indicate whether the following statements are true or false:

1. Around 75 percent of Americans currently use an automated form of PHR.

2. More timely access to laboratory test results is a common benefit of PHRs to both patients and providers.

3. PHR use by providers can reduce healthcare costs.

4. Physician concerns about patient-entered data accuracy can be overcome by using the CDA.

5. Physicians are being reimbursed for review of PHRs in e-visits.

6. It is generally agreed that physicians should not share sensitive diagnoses with patients.

7. A PHR best practice for a provider setting is to encourage its patients to use a health insurer–sponsored PHR.

8. A provider should study workflow to determine the most appropriate way to engage with PHR.

9. Patients should not be permitted to change data they enter into a PHR.

10. The VA permits veterans to enter personal medical history into their PHR.

Mobile Health Devices and Other Digital Health Technology

As previously discussed, many healthcare consumers today are tech-savvy. According to Dahl (2015), the Digital Health Consumer Adoption Survey found no significant differences across the demographics of age, gender, income, education, and geography with respect to use of, or at least interest in, digital health technology.

Many consumers want to be able to go online and e-mail their physician, schedule an appointment, see physician reviews, view their medical records, and document their own healthcare experiences in the quickest and easiest way. A number of large integrated delivery networks are enrolling their physicians to use Directed exchange (see chapter 13) for heightened e-mail security with their patients.

Patients also seek easy ways to manage their health through wearable fitness devices, personal testing tools, health apps, and other digital health technology. PwC, an international network of professional services companies, identifies that 43.6 percent of patients needing electrocardiogram monitoring and 42.6 percent of patients with a pacemaker or defibrillator who need their devices checked can have this occur wirelessly through the device attached to their phone (2016). Rhodes (2014) summarizes a number of such trends and raises awareness that use of such devices leave "digital footprints." Providers and consumers must be concerned about the privacy of such information, including addressing data ownership, informed consent, data sharing and access, and data quality. AHIMA urges information governance in this growth industry and is committed to working with HL7 and the Institute of Electronics and Electrical Engineers (IEEE) as they create standards for real-time plug-and-play interoperability for medical, healthcare, and wellness devices. The IEEE 11073 Health Informatics–Medical/Health Device Communication Standards are a suite of standards that address semantic interoperability for device data, general application services, networking and gateway standards including HL7 and DICOM interfaces, and technical interoperability transports, such as cable-connected or wireless. The Food and Drug Administration (FDA) has recognized IEEE 11073 for medical device interoperability (Kelly 2013).

Reliable and easy-to-understand information about health conditions is important for consumers. While there are many websites devoted to supplying information about health, they vary in their quality. Many consumers may not be aware that they should be concerned about the accuracy of such information. Several organizations have emerged to filter and qualify the information available to consumers on the Internet. The most widely recognized organization is the Health on the Net Foundation. (See figure 17.6.)

Patients are also building communities to help them deal with their health conditions through use of social media. Many consumers, especially younger ones, use social media to research to make health decisions. Belbey (2015) describes such users as members of a tribe who tend to trust others on social media more than other sources. Thus, social media is the contemporary equivalent of a coffee klatch or quilting club, where people once sought referrals, comfort, and sage advice from their trusted friends. In 2013, Honigman, a blogger on the social media site ReferralMD, posted 24 statistics from various sources that describe how social media has affected the healthcare industry. He reported that 40 percent of consumers say that information found via social media affects that the way they deal with their health. Honigman also indicated that 31 percent of healthcare organizations have specific social media guidelines in writing—this statistic should cause providers to take note and address this important aspect of the consumer empowerment movement (Braunstein 2014). Honigman also noted that 31 percent of healthcare professionals use social media for professional networking, two-thirds of physicians use social media for professional research—preferring the open forum as opposed to a physician-only online community, and 60 percent of physicians say social media improves the quality of care delivered to patients—largely due to its transparency. YouTube traffic to hospital sites has increased 119% year-over-year (Honigman 2013), and even the HHS Office for Civil Rights (OCR) is on YouTube and Twitter—with significantly more hits than its traditional website has garnered (Seeger 2015).

Privacy and security of health information remain important issues, although in ways that may need continuing education of consumers to address. For example, Snell (2015) reported that 89 percent of individuals in a recent survey conducted by Wakefield Research did not include medical records in their top-three selections for personal data they would be most concerned to lose in a data breach (the top three were Social Security numbers, credit card data, and financial account information). Few of those surveyed seemed to realize that loss of their medical data is potentially much more dangerous than a loss of financial data. This same survey also found that individuals may not know enough about the benefits of data encryption; with 91 percent of respondents saying they would still feel vulnerable if an encrypted file containing their data were lost. Concerns for privacy and security also have been found to be different than willingness to share data. In the Digital Health Consumer Adoption survey, nearly 80 percent of participants reported a willingness to share health data from digital health technology with their physicians, 59 percent would share their data with medical researchers, and 52 percent would share with health insurers for a discount; furthermore, 39 percent would exchange their data for money (Heath 2015). Consumers want control and governance over their data, but they are not unwilling to share data. A finding from another survey, which was conducted by a company that consults on software purchases, also highlights the need for consumer education with respect to HIE. It reports that 73 percent of patients did not know whether their state operates an HIE; however, of those patients knowing about an HIE, 73 percent

Figure 17.6.   Health on the Net

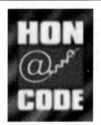

	This symbol has become recognized internationally as a symbol that the health information website agrees to the HON Code of Conduct for medical and health websites and addressed the principles of:
	Authority Justifiability
	Complementarity Transparency
	Privacy Financial disclosure
	Attribution Advertising policy

Source: Health on the Net Foundation (2016) Reprinted with permission. The HON Code is a formal and proper certification.

were very or moderately comfortable with data shared over an HIE (Loria 2016). In this survey, those individuals who were not comfortable with data sharing via HIE cited potential privacy violations (for example, a nurse who is not involved in a patient's care viewing that patient's record) and data breaches (for example, cyberattacks) as concerns.

Individuals are empowering themselves in many new and different ways—often without the aid of their personal physicians. However, a good physician-patient interface is nevertheless necessary, much as EHRs need good human-computer interfaces. One physician has even suggested that the United States needs to define "provider" more broadly to include the patient for there to truly be clinical and financial improvement (Edelstein 2016). Certainly, patients are already using alternative providers, such as a retail clinic or pharmacy, to have stitches removed or some wounds and illnesses treated. As Edelstein also points out, even patients with chronic conditions spend only a few hours annually in the care of a physician, nurse, or other clinician. A significant amount of the ownership for an individual's health rests with the individual. As such, mobile health devices and other digital health technology enable individuals to take on those responsibilities. Many parties—and especially the federal government—believe consumer empowerment will result in better clinical outcomes and lower the costs of care. Consumers need to not only become empowered, but tech-empowered (Salisbury 2014).

Consumer Empowerment and Patient Engagement

Consumer empowerment and patient engagement are concepts that are still evolving. **Consumer empowerment** in general is the investment of power or authority in those who purchase goods and services (Rollyson and Associates 2007). With the advent of social networking technologies, such as blogs, wikis, and podcasts, and intermediaries, such as Facebook, Twitter, LinkedIn and others, people are connecting and collaborating in far greater numbers worldwide. Such technology is moving us from the Information Age to the Connected Age (Zelenka 2007) and creating an entire new "Generation V" (for *virtual*) whose members are not defined by age, gender, social demographics, or geography but by a preference for conversation (rather than communication) using digital media channels for collaboration ("we" is more powerful than "me") in global communities (Prentice and Sarner 2008). As a result, a new market force is being created, which digitizes what has always been the most powerful determinant of customer relationships—word of mouth.

A movement as far-reaching as consumer empowerment enhanced through digital and web technologies has also reached healthcare. Healthcare consumerism is a natural progression from general consumerism. The idea is that patients need to be at the center of healthcare priorities and operations, including making them more financially responsible and accountable for their own healthcare.

Patient engagement has been defined by the Center for Advancing Health as "the actions individuals take to obtain the greatest benefit from the healthcare services available to them" (CFAH 2010). In 2010, CFAH proposed an Engagement Behavior Framework, summarized in table 17.1, which creates a solid physician-patient interface.

The National eHealth Collaborative (NeHC) is a public-private partnership with a close relationship to ONC. NeHC cites Cryer in describing that "properly done, patient engagement looks like shared responsibility between patients (and their families if applicable), health care providers, and healthcare administrators to co-develop pathways to optimal individual, community, and population health" (NeHC 2012). In 2012 NeHC introduced its Patient Engagement Framework & Consumer eHealth Readiness Tool, outlining five phases of patient engagement:

- *Inform me* helps inform and attract patients to appropriate services.

- *Engage me* helps providers retain and interact with patients.

Table 17.1.   Summary of health engagement behavior framework

Engaged patients:
- Find safe, decent care
- Communicate with healthcare professionals
- Organize their healthcare
- Pay (and select appropriate coverage) for their healthcare
- Make good treatment decisions
- Participate in treatment
- Promote their health
- Get preventive healthcare
- Plan for the end of life
- Seek health knowledge

- *Empower me* provides quality reports, virtual coaching, integrated EHR and PHR, and HIE to partner efficiently with patients.

- *Partner with me* creates synergy and extends reach to patients to ensure their healthcare is appropriately managed.

- *Support my e-community* delivers appropriate tools to coordinate care.

In 2013 *HealthAffairs* published A Multidimensional Framework for Patient and Family Engagement in Health and Health Care (Carman et al. 2013). According to this framework, patient engagement involves patients' beliefs about their roles, health literacy, and education; organizational policies, practices, and culture; and societal norms, regulations, and policy. Furthermore, providers need to encourage patient activation and broader patient engagement.

Currently, provider support for patient engagement is often more about providing educational material and online resources, or at best providing tools and resources to manage health information (that is, PHRs), than it is about sharing responsibility. The federal government, however, aims to get patients involved in self-management and shared decision-making. To achieve this goal, patients need access to their health records and need to be able to manage their health information—often using PHR as the vehicle. There have been a number of initiatives to promote patient empowerment.

Federal Government Initiatives

In its **Value-Driven Healthcare** initiative, HHS (n.d.) observed that:

> Consumers deserve to know the quality and cost of their healthcare. Healthcare **transparency** provides consumers with the information necessary, and the incentive, to choose healthcare providers based on value.
>
>   Providing reliable cost and quality information empowers consumer choice. Consumer choice creates incentives at all levels, and motivates the entire system to provide better care for less money. Improvements will come as providers can see how their practice compares to others.

HHS (n.d.) also identified the following steps to transparency:

- The federal government, individual private employers, and health plans commit to sharing information on price and quality in health care. Together, the government and major employers provide health care coverage for some 70 percent of Americans.

- The federal government and individual private employers commit to quality and price standards developed with the medical community. This will help guarantee a fair and accurate view of the quality of care delivered by individual providers, as well as providing consistent measures for quality.

- The federal government and individual private employers commit to standards for health information technology (IT). Health IT will be important for gathering and using the best information for consumers. These standards are also crucial to the goal of achieving EHRs for all Americans.

- The federal government and individual private employers commit to offering plans that reward consumers who exercise choice based on high quality of care and competitive price for healthcare services.

Health Plan Initiatives

Health plans have been strong advocates for consumer empowerment and PHRs. Several BlueCross BlueShield plans offer PHRs, and Aetna has also launched a PHR.

Payers and payer-affiliated disease management organizations have access to vast amounts of patient data, clinical analysis tools, best practice and best process protocols based on specialty society norms, and their own experience. They can use all of these assets to cost-effectively communicate routinely with patients and their caregivers to encourage compliance and behavior modifications when necessary (St. Clair 2005).

The recent movement by payers to reimburse providers for e-visits, often referred to as *telehealth,* is a form of consumer empowerment. Physicians had thought allowing telehealth would result in a deluge of e-mails and become one more uncompensated drain on their time, but they actually find that patients are articulate in e-mail, and the provider therefore gets much better information than when the patient and physician play "telephone tag" with nurses as intermediaries (Clark 2009). Many patients are even willing to pay for the e-visit themselves if it means they do not have to take time off from work or pay a babysitter. Many providers are coupling the e-mail with a telephone call that they arrange with the patient. As noted in chapter 15, which further discusses evisits, several medical societies, malpractice carriers, and PHR vendors who also support evisit functionality have developed guidelines for appropriate parameters for evisits (Texas Medical Association 2001; Medem 2007; Colwell 2004). It must be noted, however, that one of the first studies conducted on the impact of e-visits found accuracy in diagnoses but overprescribing of antibiotics (Zellner 2012).

Employer Initiatives

Employers were among the first parties to engage in promoting healthcare consumerism and PHRs. At the end of 2006, a group of companies announced a "plan to create a massive data warehouse that could eventually give all their employees online access to their personal health records" (Hoover 2006). They called this "Dossia." A soundbite from this announcement was, "Fed up with rising health care costs, Intel, WalMart, and others think giving employees digital records will help." The goal was to let employees compare costs, availability of services, and, to some extent, performance across care providers, thereby putting more power into consumer hands. Hoover (2006) also observed that separately, a few other major companies, such as Microsoft, had their own initiatives under way. In 2013, Nosta reported that several employers were offering Dossia to their employees, and according to the Dossia website (n.d.), Dossia Personal Health Manager is up and running in 2016. There are reports of positive experiences by employees with such PHRs and reassurances that employees (not employers) control the personal data they enter (King 2010).

However, there are also unique concerns with the employer initiatives (Burkard et al. 2010). So far, it seems that patients have been wary of employer- and health plan-sponsored PHRs (Robeznieks 2007b), believing that they could be used for employment discrimination. Employees also worry that insurance premiums could rise or even be canceled as a result of information a person may put in a health plan–sponsored PHR. Furthermore, from the employer side, there are potential legal and policy issues to investigate related to the promotion of PHRs to their employees (Goldman 2007).

Vendor Initiatives

There are numerous commercial companies on the myPHR.com website that offer PHRs either free or for a fee, and via the web or in the form of downloadable software.

In general, PHR vendors are unregulated with respect to what standards they adopt and what protections they afford consumers. The marketplace and watchdog groups have been the primary instruments to ensure solid practices. So far, it seems that their efforts have been relatively effective. The Center for Democracy and Technology (CDT) is one such watchdog group and offers recommendations for building a strong privacy and security policy framework for PHRs (CDT 2010). On December 2, 2009, the Patient Privacy Rights (n.d.) organization provides PHR privacy report cards based on information from PHR company websites. The Electronic Privacy Information Center (EPIC) is another group that tracks privacy issues in all sectors of society. For example, EPIC petitioned the Federal Trade Commission (FTC) to open an investigation into Google's cloud computing services (Albanesius 2009). Although the investigation has ended and Google is no longer offering a PHR, EPIC continues to serve as a privacy watchdog. These are just a sampling of groups and may represent only one side of the privacy debate, but they certainly serve to draw attention to important issues that the nation must grapple with as it promotes health IT that can present both opportunities and risks.

Watchdog groups are not the only organizations helping to ensure PHR privacy. In August 2009, the FTC issued the Health Breach Notification Rule that requires commercial PHR vendors to notify individuals whose information was breached and to file a report with the FTC (16 CFR 318). The FTC Report on Internet of Things "urges companies to adopt best practices to address consumer privacy and security risk" (FTC 2015).

In addition to the Health Breach Notification Rule, ONC initiated a multiphase project to create a model PHR Privacy Notice in 2008. A model notice is available online and can be used to generate a form with a company's logo on it (ONC 2016).

Check Your Understanding 17.3

Match the terms with the appropriate description:

A. Directed exchange

B. E-visit

C. Federal Trade Commission

D. HON

E. IEEE 11073

F. Physician-patient interface

G. PHR vendors

H. Physiological monitoring devices

I.   Tech-empowered patients

J.   Social media

1.   Source for physician referrals

2.   Secure e-mail

3.   Blood sugar checking

4.   Transmitting pacemaker data via telephone

5.   Reliability of health data on the Internet

6.   Consumer empowerment

7.   Tele-health

8.   PHR breach

9.   PHR Privacy Notice

10. Patient engagement

References and Resources

16 CFR 318. 2009 (August 25). Federal Trade Commission: Health Breach Notification Rule; final rule.

Aetna. n.d. Personal health record (PHR) FAQs. https://www.aetna.com/faqs-health-insurance/personal-health-record faqs.html.

Albanesius, C. 2009 (March 18). FTC asked to investigate Google's privacy breaches. *PCMag.com*. http://www.pcmag .com/article2/0,2817,2343346,00.asp.

American Health Information Management Association (AHIMA) eHIM Personal Health Record Work Group. 2005. Defining the personal health record. *Journal of AHIMA*. 76(6):24–25.

American Health Information Management Association (AHIMA) Personal Health Record Practice Council. 2006. Helping consumers select PHRs: Questions and considerations for navigating an emerging market. *Journal of AHIMA*. 77(10):50–56.

American Health Information Management Association (AHIMA). 2008. Defining the personal health information management role. *Journal of AHIMA*. 79(6):59–63.

American Health Information Management Association (AHIMA). 2010 (November). The role of the personal health record in the EHR (2010 update). http://library.ahima.org/doc?oid=103209#.V74WBJgrI2w.

American Health Information Management Association (AHIMA). 2011 (January). Patient access and amendment to health records (2011 update). http://library.ahima.org/doc?oid=103501#.V771UpgrI2w.

American Health Information Management Association (AHIMA). 2012. Understanding your medical record. MyPHR. com. http://www.myphr.com/HealthLiteracy/understanding.aspx.

Archer, N., et al. 2011. Personal health records: A scoping review. *Journal of the American Medical Informatics Association*. 18(4): 515–522.

Baldwin, K., et al. 2015. the implementation and management of patient portals. *Journal of AHIMA*. 86(4):50–55. http://bok.ahima.org/doc?oid=107601#.V772B5grI2w.

Belbey, J. 2015 (January 21). How healthcare can use social media effectively and compliantly. *Forbes*. http://www .forbes.com/sites/joannabelbey/2015/01/21/how-healthcare-can-use-social-media-effectively-and-compliantly/ #1d1b1d473bc8.

BlueCross BlueShield. 2016. Personal health records. http://www.bcbs.com/healthcare-partners/personal-health-records.

BlueCross BlueShield of Massachusetts. 2015 (February 3). Maintaining your personal health record. A Healthy Me website. http://www.ahealthyme.com/library/wellness/todaysmedicine/1,2716.

Braunstein, M.L. 2014. *Contemporary Health Informatics.* Chicago, IL: AHIMA.

Burkard, R.J., et al. 2010. Information systems and healthcare XXXVII: When your employer provides your personal health record—exploring employee perceptions of an employer-sponsored PHR system. *Communications of the Association for Information Systems.* 27(1).

California HealthCare Foundation (CHCF). 2010 (April). Consumers and health information technology: A national survey. http://www.chcf.org/publications/2010/04/consumers-and-health-information-technology-a-national-survey.

Caouette, H. 2015 (April 6). Press Release: Harris Poll Survey Finds patients want a deeper digital connection with their doctors. eClinicalWorks. https://www.eclinicalworks.com/pr-harris-poll-patient-engagement-survey.

Carman, K.L.; P. Dardess; M.Maurer; S. Sofaer; K. Adams; C. Bechtel; J. Sweeney. 2013. Patient and family engagement: a framework for understanding the elements and developing interventions and policies. *HealthAffairs* 32(2) 2223–2231.

Center for Advancing Health (CFAH). 2010. A new definition of patient engagement: What is engagement and why is it important? http://www.cfah.org/pdfs/CFAH_Engagement_Behavior_Framework_current.pdf.

Center for Democracy and Technology (CDT). 2010 (July 21). Building a strong privacy and security policy framework for personal health records. https://cdt.org/insight/building-a-strong-privacy-and-security-policy-framework-for-personal-health-records/.

Clark, C. 2009 (May 13). Physician-patient email can save both time and cost. *Health Leaders Media.* http://www.healthleadersmedia.com/community-rural/physician-patient-e-mail-can-save-both-time-and-cost.

Colwell, J. 2004 (December). How two practices are taking patient visits online—and getting paid for them. American College of Physicians. *ACP Observer.* http://www.acponline.org/journals/news/dec04/evisit.htm.

Connecting for Health. Markle Foundation. 2006 (December 7). Connecting Americans to their health care: A common framework for networked personal health information. http://www.markle.org/health/connecting-health/.

Connecting for Health. Markle Foundation. 2008 (June). Connecting for Health common framework for networked personal health information. http://www.markle.org/health/markle-common-framework/connecting-consumers.

Dahl, K. 2015 (December 7). Why consumers want their health records. Rock Health. https://rockhealth.com/why-consumers-want-their-health-records.

Dimick, C. 2012 (July 20). Blue Button program expands into private sector. *Journal of AHIMA* website. http://journal.ahima.org/2012/07/20/blue-button-program-expands-into-private-sector.

Dolan, M., and J. Wolter. 2009 (October). Using social media to promote the use of a personal health record (PHR) and the management of personal health information to consumers. *2009 AHIMA Convention Proceedings.*

Dossia. n.d. Home page. http://dossia.com.

Edelstein, P. 2016. Correcting critical misperceptions about patient engagement. *Health Management Technology.* 37(1):10–11.

Electronic Privacy Information Center (EPIC). n.d. EPIC consumer privacy project. https://www.epic.org/privacy/consumer.

Endsley, S., et al 2006 (May). An introduction to personal health records. *Family Practice Management.* 13(5):57–62.

Finn, N.B. 2014 (October 27). What has happened to the personal health record? Society for Participatory Medicine. http://e-patients.net/archives/2014/10/what-has-happened-to-the-personal-health-record.html.

Federal Trade Commission (FTC). 2015 (January 27). Press Release: FTC Report on Internet of Things urges companies to adopt best practices to address consumer privacy and security risks. https://www.ftc.gov/news-events/press-releases/2015/01/ftc-report-internet-things-urges-companies-adopt-best-practices.

Garvin, J., et al. 2009 (June). Healthcare disparities and the role of personal health records. American Health Information Management Association (AHIMA). http://library.ahima.org/doc?oid=91677#.V74sRJgrI2w.

Goldman, J. 2007 (January) Issue brief. Personal health records: Employers proceed with caution. California HealthCare Foundation. http://www.chcf.org/publications/2007/01/personal-health-records-employers-proceed-with-caution.

Halamka J.D., K.D. Mandl, and P.C. Tang. 2008. Early experiences with personal health records. *Journal of the American Medical Informatics Association.* 15(1).

Haugen M.B., A. Tegen, D. Warner; American Health Information Management Association. 2011. Fundamentals of the legal health record and designated record set. *Journal of AHIMA.* 82(2): expanded online version. http://library.ahima.org/doc?oid=104008#.V770T5grI2w.

HealthIT.gov. 2013 (May 2). Frequently asked questions: What is a personal health record? https://www.healthit.gov/providers-professionals/faqs/what-personal-health-record.

Health Level Seven International (HL7). 2014 (May 16). PHR System Functional Model, release 1-2014. http://www.hl7.org/implement/standards/product_brief.cfm?product_id=88.

Health on the Net Foundation. 2013 (September 13). The HON code of conduct for medical and health web sites. https://www.healthonnet.org/HONcode/Conduct.html.

Heath, S. 2015 (October 21). Health data privacy not a concern for health tech consumers. *Health IT Security.* http://healthitsecurity.com/news/health-data-privacy-not-a-concern-for-health-tech-consumers.

Honigman, B. 2013. 24 outstanding statistics & figures on how social media has impacted the health care industry. ReferralMD blog. https://getreferralmd.com/2013/09/healthcare-social-media-statistics.

Hoover, J.N. 2006 (December 4). Get well soon. *Information Week.* pp. 26–30.

Hostetter, M., et al. 2014 (October). Taking health to the next level: Promoting technologies that empower consumers and drive health system transformation. The Commonwealth Fund publication no. 1777. http://www.commonwealthfund.org/~/media/files/publications/fund-report/2014/oct/1777_hostetter_taking_digital_hlt_next_level_v2.pdf?la=en.Institute of Medicine. 2002. *Unequal Treatment: Confronting Racial and Ethnic Disparities in Health Care.* Edited by Brian D. Smedley, Adrienne Y. Stith, and Alan R. Nelson. Washington, DC: National Academy Press.

Kaelber, D.C., et al. 2008. The value of personal health records. Center for Information Technology Leadership (CITL). http://www.partners.org/cird/pdfs/CITL_PHR_Report.pdf.

Kelly, V. 2013 (November 12). Press Release: U.S. federal government recognizes IEEE 11073™ standards for medical-device communication. IEEE Standards Association. http://standards.ieee.org/news/2013/ieee_11073_medical-device_communication.html.

King, R. 2010 (May 3). Crafting employees' personal online health records. *Bloomberg Businessweek.* http://www.bloomberg.com/news/articles/2010-05-03/crafting-employees-personal-online-health-recordsbusinessweek-business-news-stock-market-and-financial-advice.

Loria, G. 2016. Are patients ready for EHR interoperability? Software Advice. http://www.softwareadvice.com/resources/address-ehr-interoperability-concerns.

Lowes, R. 2006. Personal health records: What's the status now? *Medical Economics.* 83(4):TCP13–TCP14, TCP16.

Medem. 2007 (January). eRisk Working Group for Healthcare's Guidelines for Online Communication. http://www.medem.com/phy/phy_eriskguidelines.cfm.

Miliard, M. 2015 (October 19). Cyberattacks could cost providers $305B. *Healthcare IT News.* http://www.healthcareitnews.com/news/cyberattacks-could-cost-providers-305b.

Morgan, D. 2015 (April 10). How does your practice rate when it comes to patient engagement? HealthWell Corporate Solutions blog. http://www.healthwellcs.com/#!How-does-your-practice-rate-when-it-comes-to-Patient-Engagement/chzy/552806860cf215f35a55b442.

National Committee on Vital and Health Statistics (NCVHS). 2005 (October). Personal health records and personal health record systems: A report and recommendations from the National Committee on Vital and Health Statistics. http://www.ncvhs.hhs.gov/wp-content/uploads/2014/05/0602nhiirpt.pdf.

National Committee on Vital and Health Statistics (NCVHS). 2009 (September 28). Protection of the privacy and security of individual health information in personal health records (letter to Kathleen Sebelius, Secretary, Department of Health and Human Services). http://www.ncvhs.hhs.gov/wp-content/uploads/2014/05/090928lt.pdf.

National eHealth Collaborative (NeHC). 2012 (November 21). Patient engagement framework & consumer ehealth readiness tool. https://www.khareach.org/sites/default/files/Patient-Engagement-Framework.pdf.

Nosta, J. 2013 (November 27). For Dossia, digital health isn't just personal anymore. *Forbes.* http://www.forbes.com/sites/johnnosta/2013/11/27/for-dossia-digital-health-isnt-just-personal-anymore/#43b7d3ea5589.

Office of the National Coordinator for Health Information Technology (ONC). 2016 (May 23). Personal health record (PHR) model privacy notice. http://www.healthit.gov/policy-researchers-implementers/personal-health-record-phr-model-privacy-notice.

Patel, V., and E. Siminerio. 2014 (September 15). Consumer access and use of online health records: It takes two to tango. *HealthIT.gov Buzz.* http://www.healthit.gov/buzz-blog/consumer/consumer-access-online-health-records.

Patient Privacy Rights. n.d. Detailed PHR privacy report cards. https://patientprivacyrights.org/detailed-phr-privacy-report-cards.

Prentice, S., and A. Sarner. 2008 (January 3). Defining Generation V: The virtual generation. Gartner. Research ID no. G00154114. https://www.gartner.com/doc/575707/defining-generation-v-virtual-generation.

Pritts, J., et al. 2009 (August). Privacy and security solutions for interoperable health information exchange. Releasing clinical laboratory test results: Report on survey of state laws. Agency for Healthcare Research and Quality (AHRQ) / Office of the National Coordinator for Health Information Technology (ONC). https://www.healthit.gov/sites/default/files/290-05-0015-state-law-access-report-1.pdf.

PwC. 2016. The empowered consumer. http://www.pwc.com/gx/en/industries/healthcare/emerging-trends-pwc-healthcare/new-entrants-healthcare-provision.html.

Rhodes, H. 2014. Accessing and using data from wearable fitness devices. *Journal of AHIMA.* 85(9):48–50.

Robeznieks, A. 2007a (June). PHR liability, data overload making docs a little queasy. *Modern Physician.* http://www.modernhealthcare.com/article/20070604/MODERNPHYSICIAN/306040004.

Robeznieks, A. 2007b (June). Patients wary of employer- and plan-sponsored personal health records. *Workforce Management.* http://www.workforce.com/2007/06/14/patients-wary-of-employer-and-plan-sponsored-personal-health-records.

Rollyson, C.S., and Associates. 2007 (June 1). Market advisory. Consumer empowerment—A rare innovation opportunity. http://rollyson.net/download/Soc_Nwkg_Mkt_advisory.pdf.

Salisbury, M. 2014 (November 21). How many heartbeats today? Are patients ready to become tech-empowered healthcare consumers? Techonomy. http://techonomy.com/2014/11/many-heartbeats-today-patients-ready-become-tech-empowered-healthcare-consumers.

Salisbury, M. 2015 (January 28). Are 23andMe customers suckers or empowered consumers? Techonomy. http://techonomy.com/2015/01/23andme-customers-suckers-empowered-consumers.

Seeger, R. 2015 (November 19). Testimony to the National Committee on Vital and Health Statistics. http://www.ncvhs.hhs.gov/transcripts-minutes/transcript-of-the-november-19-2015-ncvhs-full-committee-meeting.

Snell, E. 2015 (November 2). Healthcare data breaches not top consumer concern. *Health IT Security.* http://healthitsecurity.com/news/healthcare-data-breaches-not-top-consumer-concern.

St. Clair, D. 2005. Collaborative disease management: Leveraging MCO data to improve patient outcomes. *Health Management Technology.* 26(7):28–30.

Texas Medical Association Council on Communication. 2001. Patient-physician electronic communication. http:www.texmed.org/templateprint.aspx?id=2480

Studeny, J., and A. Coustasse. 2014 (Summer). Personal health records: Is rapid adoption hindering interoperability? *Perspectives in Health Information Management.* pp. 1–19.

Sujanksy and Associates. 2013. A standards-based model for the sharing f patient generated health information with electronic health records. Project HealthDesign. http://www.projecthealthdesign.org/media/file/Standard-Model-For-Collecting-And-Reporting-PGHI_Sujansky_Assoc_2013-07-18.pdf

US Department of Health and Human Services (HHS). n.d. Value-driven health care (archived content). http://archive.hhs.gov/valuedriven.

US Department of Health and Human Services (HHS). 2015 (September 29). Better care, smarter spending, healthier people: improving our health care delivery system with an engaged and empowered consumer at the center. http://www.hhs.gov/healthcare/facts-and-features/fact-sheets/better-care-smarter-spending-healthier-people.html.

US Department of Veterans Affairs (VA). n.d. MyHealth*e*Vet website. https://www.myhealth.va.gov.

Vydra, T.P., et al. 2015 (Spring). Diffusion and use of tethered personal health records in primary care. *Perspectives in Health Information Management*. pp. 1–16.

Washington, L., et al. 2009. Dispute resolution: Planning for disputed information in EHRs and PHRs. *Journal of AHIMA*. 80(11):25–30.

West Virginia Health Information Network. 2014 (January 30). Policies and procedures: Personal health records. http://www.wvhin.org/App_Media/assets/doc/wvhin/policies/Personal_Health_Record_Policy_-_Approved_013014.pdf.

Witry, M.J., et al. 2010 (Winter). Family physician perceptions of personal health records. *Perspectives in Health Information Management*.

Wynia, M.K., et al. 2011 (February). Many physicians are willing to use patients' electronic personal health records, but doctors differ by location, gender, and practice. *Health Affairs*. 30(2):266–273.

Xerox. 2014 (December 16). Press Release: Annual Xerox EHR survey: Americans open to viewing test results, handling healthcare online. http://news.xerox.com/news/Xerox-EHR-survey-finds-Americans-open-to-online-records.

Zelenka, A. 2007 (October 6). From the information age to the connected age. Gigaom. http://gigaom.com/2007/10/06/from-the-information-age-to-the-connected-age.

Zellner, W. 2012 (December 3). Patient e-visits seem to offer accurate diagnoses but may spur overprescribing of antibiotics. *Pitt Chronicle*. http://www.chronicle.pitt.edu/story/patient-e-visits-seem-offer-accurate-diagnoses-may-spur-overprescribing-antibiotics-mehrotra-l.

Chapter 18

Enterprise Content and Record Management as an EHR Bridge Technology

Key Terms

Adaptive case management (ACM)

Clinical messaging

Code 39 bar code standard

Code 128 bar code standard

Document imaging system

Document imaging and management system (DIMS)

Electronic document management (EDM) system

Electronic signature authentication

Enterprise content, collaboration, and communication management (EC3M) system

Enterprise content management (ECM) system

Enterprise master person index (EMPI)

File formats

Front-end speech (FES) recognition

Groupware

Hybrid record

Information as a service

Intelligent character recognition

Intelligent word recognition

Knowledge management system

Optical character recognition

Optical mark recognition

POISED

Positive patient identification

QR codes

Radio frequency identification (RFID)

Real-time location system (RTLS)

Scan on demand

Speech recognition

Two-dimensional bar code

Vendor neutral archive (VNA)

Workflow engine

Workflow management

Workflow management system

Workflow technology

Learning Objectives

- Describe sources and uses of content that benefit from ECM services.

- Define types of ECM technologies, including how they fit into the overall strategic health IT migration path.

- Summarize the key steps in acquiring and implementing ECM systems.

- Describe key technology components of ECM and special considerations for adopting these technologies.

For many years, electronic document management (EDM) systems were considered "bridge technology" for electronic health records (EHRs). An organization could scan and feed paper-based health record documents into a document repository so that they would be accessible throughout the organization and across the enterprise as authorized. This approach was a convenient way to improve access to health record documents without yet having all of the clinical components of an EHR. Although this technology is still important to fill gaps where an enterprise is phasing in its EHR components, it is increasingly used as a workflow tool and as a means to manage "stray" documents and integrate other content from other sources. Advancements in this technology and knowledge learned from implementing EHR components have led to EDM systems and related types of health information technology (IT) being used as integral tools that complement the EHR components.

As is discussed in this chapter, many terms are associated with technologies for managing documents and other content. To simplify reference to these technologies collectively, this chapter calls them *enterprise content management (ECM) tools*. The term *enterprise* is used to recognize that all the tools are electronic, with a focus on their being available for use across an enterprise—whether that refers to departments within a hospital, facilities within an integrated delivery network, or the organizations formally participating in a health information exchange organization (HIO). The term *content* reflects the full scope of what is being managed with this technology—from patient information that remains on paper or other nondigital form outside of the EHR, to integration of such information with clinical images from the picture archiving and communications system (PACS). Content also includes information from other information-gathering media, such as voice files and, potentially, web and social media content. Generally, the content managed by an ECM system is considered unstructured information. However, content can sometimes be managed as structured data. For example, it was described in previous chapters that speech dictation systems coupled with natural language processing (NLP) can create limited structured data entries in an EHR by using discrete reportable transcription (DRT). As discussed later in this chapter, there are a variety of new tools for character and word recognition, and Health Level 7 (HL7) Consolidated-Clinical Document Architecture (C-CDA) documents also are able to identify data types for location purposes. Finally, *management* is broader than just taking the necessary steps to accurately scan and appropriately store documents. Data modeling, forms management, storage management, security, interfaces of all types, workflow, and other services are all elements of ECM services. In summary, ECM focuses on managing unstructured information in ways to lend structure, improve interoperability, and gain intelligence from that information.

Sources of Content

Despite the fact that EHRs are now widely used, it has been estimated that, for many healthcare organizations, as much as 25 percent of patient information exists outside of the EHR (Hyland 2014). Such patient information may include clinical images including x-rays, wave forms, and other such content stored in PACS. Additionally, patient information is collected in many other forms:

- Photographs (for example, taken during an emergency department encounter or to document "before and after" for certain types of procedures)

- Voice files (for example, provider dictation, speech dictation, and DRT, as well as, potentially, recorded telephone messages to and from patients)

- Video (for example, recordings of a telehealth consultation)

- E-mail (for example, messages from an e-visit encounter, transmitted through a patient portal, or exchanged between providers)

- Digital pen and paper

- Fax

- Electronic forms that include optical mark, character, or word recognition or intelligent character recognition (for example, patient-documented health history)

- Scanned images (for example, insurance cards, photo identification)

- Paper documents patients supply from other providers

- Web content (for example, download or visual capture of content collected during research by a provider on a new drug)

- Information posted to social media

- Information transmitted via health apps

Not all of these forms of patient information may be collected by all providers, but many of them are—and more are likely to be collected in the future.

In addition to patient information that is generally managed by the health information management (HIM) department and the "shadow" health records that still exist either on paper or in personal databases, patient information on paper, fax, or rendered in HL7 Clinical Document Architecture (CDA) may be collected by and stored in the business office. Screenshots from payer portals regarding eligibility for services, claim status, or remittance advice may be stored by the business office. Some of what the business office keeps in separate files duplicates what exists in the patient's EHR, such as some patient admission data or discharge summaries, operative reports, and other information that needs to be sent to health plans as attachments to claims or for prior authorization of referrals or certain services. Sometimes, these data are retrieved from an EHR, printed, and scanned into a separate document imaging system.

The business office is not the only place that separate files of duplicate information may be retained. Radiology, pharmacy, laboratory, emergency department, respiratory therapy, dietary, and other departments all have need for patient information, which may be retrieved from the EHR and scanned into separate systems, potentially coupled with other department-specific information.

Finally, there are other departments in hospitals and large clinics that keep or scan paper records into separate systems that do not contain patient information, but may contain sensitive information. Human resource departments typically maintain separate files for employees, procurement departments retain invoices and contracts, maintenance departments keep records, foundations keep records for managing donations, research departments maintain separate files of research data, and others similarly maintain separate record systems. Many providers have started posting policies and procedures, internal newsletters, and other information to an intranet.

None of these sources of information outside of the EHR are unknown to provider organizations, since **hybrid records** (part paper and part electronic) have existed for some time (AHIMA 2003a). However, the full scope of content that needs to be managed has typically not been centrally managed. And, while there may be good reasons to not manage all of this information centrally, organizations may find that centralized management of at least some of such information management is cost-effective, reduces potential errors due to redundancy, and ensures better security.

Uses of Content

There are a number of uses for content that it is typically output to paper or requires significant level of workflow management. **Workflow management** in the context of ECM refers to the categorization, routing, monitoring performance, and reporting of work associated with patient information. Grzybowski (2014) describes several of the following uses:

- Coding, at a minimum, includes review of the entire health record as well as reference to the code system. The entire health record may be represented in hybrid state—some in digital form and some in paper form, even if the paper is scanned and accessible through the EHR. Still, there is often the need to view two separate sources simultaneously, or in multiple windows on a screen. Many coders use dual monitors to display the code system content alongside of the health record. Coders also need reference materials, which may be in paper or accessible through an intranet and/or the Internet and, in some circumstances, need to manage documents, digital records, and supporting materials while formulating a message to the physician concerning clinical documentation. Beyond the needs of each individual coder, coding workflow needs to be managed for the coding team. Such workflows entail routing of work based on a number of factors, such as how complete the record is, patient type, financial class or payer, facility, or need for additional reviewers. The code system software may contribute to workflow management—for example, sophisticated computer-assisted coding systems can help manage the routing functions.

- Chart analysis and deficiency completion can be aided by access to the hybrid record that is integrated through ECM. Grzybowski notes that "ensuring coders do not code records until the process of deficiency analysis and completion of the record occurs has become a frequently ignored work routing practice with the adoption of the EHR" (2014). As a result, a large percentage of health records require additional documentation. To help address deficiencies in documentation, ECM systems could, for example, include a rule requiring documentation of a pathology report be in the record before the claim is coded. This type of rule improves productivity and supports accurate coding.

- Data abstracting, especially for clinical quality measurement but also for abstraction into a registry or other uses, also requires review of the entire health record, tools for posting and submittal of the abstracted data, a set of rules associated with the measures, and, potentially, rules for routing work assignments based on the expertise of the staff doing the abstracting.

- Transcription is generally considered a source of information; however, in the process of transcribing information, the transcriber may need to access the EHR and other content to verify potential discrepancies or check on dictation content that may be somewhat garbled. This review of content is a part of clinical documentation improvement from the perspective of complete and accurate output.

- Release of information can directly generate paper from both the EHR and any scanned content. First, there must be a process to match the request to the patient, ensure that the release is authorized, and monitor other forms of consent associated with sensitive information or patient preferences. Data segmentation for privacy was described in previous chapters; not all EHRs have the capability to assign the metadata necessary to automate this function. If the tasks are not automated, staff must review records manually. Workflow tools vary depending on which staff may release which kinds of records, the nature of the request for release, and other factors. In addition, documentation associated with the release must be retained and, ideally, associated with the EHR.

- Responding to requests for access, amendment, and accounting for disclosures may also entail the location of content from multiple sources. This process involves many of the same tasks as described for release of information. In addition, however, responding to some of these requests may require access to the metadata associated with data in the EHR and in the ECM system.

- ECM can help with tracking any paper records, including paper records that are still currently being used, paper documents that are warehoused but location information is automated, and archived paper records that have been fully scanned prior to the first use of EHR. Eventually, ECM may also be needed to locate archived EHRs that may be stored separately from current EHRs. Such "chart management" functions are certainly not the same as managing a file room, but the purposes remain the same.

Workflow functionality in ECM also generates output for various uses. ECM tools, for example, can include their own form of decision support, where "rules" are established for how long it should take to perform certain functions or for what steps, in what sequence, must be taken to perform a certain function (as illustrated by the previous example of requiring a pathology report before coding). Using such tools, a supervisor can spot a potential backlog and redirect work, or identify a potential problem before work is completed in order to take corrective action. These tools can be especially useful when work is outsourced and turnaround times and accuracy need to be monitored.

Figure 18.1 illustrates how sources of unstructured data, which are excellent for presentation of content, relate to the representation of data in the structured environment of an EHR that provides for clinical decision support, analytics, and other processes to be performed on data.

Hospital Versus Physician Office Sources and Uses of Content

As described in chapter 15, physician office EHR products tend to be more inclusive than hospital EHR systems and therefore can typically produce a better representation of the legal health record. Just the same, physicians are not always enamored with data input or output strategies offered in EHR products for physician offices.

Figure 18.1.   Nature and use of information content

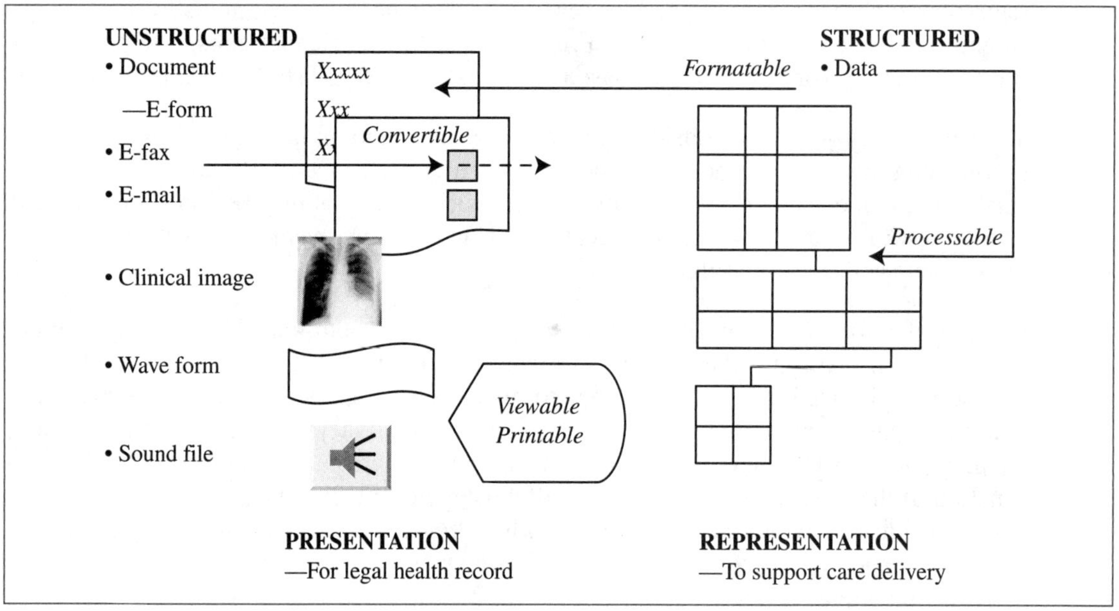

Physicians complain that "too much clicking" is required to input data (McCann 2015). They also may believe that they are less interactive with patients as they focus on data entry. The Regenstrief Institute has created a tool it calls POISED to help clinicians engage with patients during interactions while attending to patient safety. **POISED** stands for *preparing* to see patients by reviewing the record in advance; *orienting* the patient to the physician's use of the computer; gathering *information* while the patient is talking; *sharing* information with the patient by turning the computer screen to them; *educating* patients using graphical representations of information from the system; and *debriefing* with the patient to ensure understanding (Hirsch 2015a).

Physicians do not like the "choppiness" of information generated when the EHR automatically shapes structured data into phases or sentences; they believe it is too difficult to extract the patient story from such documentation (Varpio et al. 2015). Copy-and-paste functionality often produces inaccurate, outdated, and redundant information in the EHR, which can lead to sentinel events or fraudulent billing and the potential for the EHR records to be deemed too inauthentic in court (Hirsch 2015b; Hirsch 2014).

Virtually all aspects of clinical information flow and documentation within an office can be addressed by the EHR. However, some physicians will likely continue to use paper for some aspects of their documentation—for example, longer notes, certain referral letters, and complicated procedures may be dictated and transcribed. Also, various forms that patients need may have to be completed manually (for example, clearance forms for going back to work after illness or injury, camp attendance, school attendance, or sports participation), although at least some of these forms can be integrated into the EHR with ECM tools.

While physician offices may not have as many gaps in documentation in the EHR as hospitals, gaps occur in physician offices in two main areas: clinical messaging and chart conversion. **Clinical messaging**, in the electronic sense, is a service that provides a secure, electronic infrastructure to automate the delivery of health data to any site where clinical patient care decisions are made (HealthIT.gov 2014). Such messaging systems are usually considered in the context of e-mail-like systems, which are often not linked directly to the EHR or to an ECM. Additionally, orders and other information not captured in e-mail may need to be documented The use of verbal orders is becoming less common, but information from phone conversations may sometimes be recorded by the physician or patient (there is increasing evidence that patients are recording verbal conversations on their smartphones), and physicians also are audio recording at least some patient encounters (with notice to the patient) (Elwyn and Buckman 2015; Klugman 2015). Whether these are communications are transcribed or left as voice files—they still must be stored and made accessible. Furthermore, some offices may still fax admission paperwork, especially if the physician is an infrequent admitter to a particular hospital. ECM systems can be used to manage these faxes.

With respect to chart conversion in a physician office, most physicians find they need a patient's problem list, medication list, record of immunizations, recent laboratory test results, and some additional information based on the type of patient for each visit, at least across an episode of care for continuity of care purposes, if not for longitudinal reference for chronic care patients. When an EHR is acquired, this information needs to be brought forward to the EHR. This process of chart conversion may be accomplished in several ways, including abstraction, scanning of documents, or simply pulling previous records for a period of time. Although offices are frequently advised to avoid back-scanning and focus on current paper-record scanning (AAFP 2016), determining what documents to scan and what data to abstract in the transition to EHR should include a review of technology that not only scans the documents but supports workflow and content management (AHIMA 2010). The office should also consider how likely it is that a significant portion of the current record will be needed for subsequent care. Some physician offices will want to scan all past records to free up space or reduce storage costs. Others may prefer to warehouse their old records until they can be destroyed, based on the statute of limitations in their state. When there is a mix of paper and electronic records, or scanned paper and electronic records, physician offices can suffer from a hybrid record situation, which is more likely to produce errors, especially in medication reconciliation, just as much as hospitals (Perez 2013; Hirsch 2013).

Access to past charts is typically less of a priority in the hospital setting. When a patient is readmitted to a hospital, the admission may or may not be related to the reason for a previous admission. Also, a significant period of time may pass between one admission and another, and, in those cases, immediate access to previous admission information is not usually needed (Stiell et al. 2003). Still, hospital staff may need to be access to some parts of or all of a patient's previous admission(s) and some information from that review or from other providers may need to be placed into the EHR for easy access during a hospitalization. Scanning these via ECM is easiest way to afford such access. Many hospitals scan historical records as a means to free space.

Check Your Understanding 18.1

Choose the best answer:

1. In the typical provider setting, how much patient information exists outside of the EHR?

    a. Less than 10 percent

    b. About 25 percent

    c. About 50 percent

    d. More than 75 percent

2. Hybrid records are those including:

    a. Clinical and nonclinical information

    b. Paper and electronic content

    c. Paper and unstructured electronic information

    d. Structured and unstructured electronic information

3. An example of a use of workflow management is:

    a. Exchanging patient information in a health information exchange environment

    b. Quality-checking scanned documents

    c. Routing charts to various staff members for coding

    d. Scanning paper records for archiving

4. Unlike paper or scanned documents, when structured information affords:

    a. Creation of the legal health record

    b. Presentation of information for viewing

    c. Representation of information that support electronic decision making

    d. Viewing of documents formerly on paper

5. In a physician office, ECM is an important means to:

    a. Archive old records of deceased patients

    b. Create a hybrid record that eases physicians toward the EHR

    c. Overcome fear of computers

    d. Support continuity of care by making previous information available

Strategically Planning for ECM Technologies

At a Healthcare Information and Management Systems Society (HIMSS) conference in 2011, an industry observer suggested the need to "stop talking about document management and start talking about content management." The observer further noted that "if you're convinced that many EHRs remain incomplete without a document management solution, one that efficiently handles 'loose items' left out of the system . . . you're still missing half the story" (HIMSS 2011). These observations were echoed by HIMSS, as cited in a white paper from *Healthcare IT News* (2015), when it was observed that success with automation in one area of an organization, such as the clinical side with EHR, leads to benefits in other areas, such as billing and human resources. In a scanning solution, images of documents are made for retrieval or archival purposes. With an ECM solution, there are workflow functionalities and other tools that have the ability to manage documents in a logical manner. Beyond managing the documents, managing source system content in the EHR (Nunn 2008) and the actual intellectual substance of a document take ECM to an entirely different level. Strategic planning for tools that help manage documents and other content that may complement the EHR or simply improve organizational performance should encompass consideration for the variety of ECM tools available.

When considering ECM, strategic planners should be aware that various types of systems—with varying degrees of functionality—may be referred to as *document imaging systems* or *content management systems*. The following are three levels of patient information management tools:

-   **Level 1 document imaging systems** include computer systems that capture, store, and reprint images of documents. Documents are typically scanned in sequential order, and the person scanning them inserts a separator sheet to indicate where each record begins and ends. Level 1 systems have minimal workflow support, some limitations on the actual scanning capabilities (to improve image quality), and very little interoperability with the EHR. Typically, such scanned documents are accessed by an icon on the computer screen that takes the user out of the EHR to a separate system. Sometimes, there is no icon in the EHR, but it is instead on the log-on screen, so the user may have to guess whether there are scanned documents associated with the patient whose current record is displayed.

- **Level 2 document imaging and management systems (DIMS)** add enhancements to better manage, control, locate, and retrieve documents and other information in digital form. In an EDM system, bar code technology or another type of identification technology is used to identify documents within a record and potentially even parts of a document. This technology significantly aids in retrieval and may also be used to support workflow management. EDMs have more sophisticated image processing technologies than level 1 systems to ensure better quality presentation. DIMS also allow users to edit documents, including with electronic signatures, and they typically interface with storage management systems (sometimes referred to as *computer output to laser disk [COLD] systems,* even though few vendors are using laser disks any more). Level 2 DIMS may also have some limited workflow tools.

- **Level 3 electronic document management (EDM)** systems include advanced management tools that provide workflow and infrastructure support for managing the content, movement, and maintenance of the complete health record. These systems enable output from other electronic systems to be captured and stored in the same repository as scanned documents. Such output may include digital dictation files, speech dictation files, transcription (directly from a word processing system), and print files (often generated from laboratory and other ancillary information systems) (Grzybowski 2014).

Even level 3 systems do not manage additional content that may be included in a designated record set, such as PACS images, photographs, voice or video recordings, information for billing decisions, and hybrid records. **Enterprise content management (ECM) systems** are successors to level 3 EDM systems. AIIM (formerly known as Association for Information and Image Management) describes ECM as the ability to manage content through its lifecycle of content collection, processing, use, and archiving (n.d.[a]). As applied to the healthcare environment, this would include:

- Content, which includes collection of:
  - Documents
  - Forms with marks and/or handwriting
  - Speech to be recognized
  - Photos, images, video
  - E-mail and web content
- Processing, which includes:
  - Scanning, imaging, forms processing, and/or recognition
  - Categorizing and indexing
  - Workflow, integration, and repository functionality
  - Secure storage, backup and recovery, business continuity for active content
- Use, such as:
  - Search and retrieval
  - Syndication (reuse of data for other purposes, such as placing it into an analytics warehouse)

- ○ Publication (that is, the process where content gets where and to whom it needs to go through a number of tools, including not only presentation tools but also security features of authorization, authentication, and audit logging)

- Long-term archiving

In sum, because an ECM system has workflow functionalities and other tools to manage documents in a logical manner, it goes beyond a scanning solution that only makes images of documents for retrieval and/or archival purposes. ECM solutions that also manage source system content in the EHR and the actual intellectual substance of a document rise an entirely different level (Nunn 2008). ECM may begin to approach what some call **knowledge management (KM) systems** (Frost 2015; Lobach et al. 2012), where the content within the documents or other digital records are indexed such that individual components of the documents or records can be intelligently searched and where interpretation of the data within context can be added (Dirking 2010; Craciun 2014). In healthcare, ECM systems can be used to generate the continuity of care document (CCD) and other documents in the C-CDA. In this case, the ECM system must be compatible with the HHL7 Clinical Document Architecture (CDA) standard that enables a document to contain various types of information that can be processed by computers using a structure and labels (AIIM 2010). ECM may also be used to describe the management of information stored in extensible markup language (XML), which can be tagged and used to generate, for instance, the continuity of care record (Chavis 2010). Additional information about the C-CDA is described later in this chapter.

In addition to managing content (rather than just documents), new forms of ECM can provide an integrated platform on which multiple different EDM and ECM systems can exchange content. This type of integrated platform is referred to as a **vendor neutral archive (VNA)** (Rouse 2014). VNA technology was initially used to exchange PACS images across different platforms—for example, when new systems are acquired but old images remain, when different providers within an integrated delivery network work on different platforms, or when providers across the continuum of care require access to PACS images. VNA is also used in reimbursement when a payer requires that documentation for a claim or prior authorization request include radiology reports and other documents, such as invoices for special equipment, as well as PACS images.

In general, VNA separates the imaging function from the archiving function in ECM systems so it is easier to share document images across platforms (Cook 2014), which means VNA can be used to integrate documents from disparate ECM systems. Interfaces that have VNA functionality are both DICOM- and HL7-enabled and also use application program interfaces (APIs) to exchange other types of electronic documents rendered in a variety structures for which information can be stored (called **file formats**). File formats may include those used in word-processing software (e.g., .DOC or .DOCX), as PDF files (.PDF), as .JPG or other image structures, and other formats.

Enterprise Content, Collaboration, and Communications (EC3M) systems add the dimensions of collaboration and communication to ECM systems. Collaboration software, which is often called **groupware**, manages analog and digital documents according to the needs of teams or projects. For example, it enables simultaneous document editing, screen sharing, and file synchronization and sharing. It also supports discussion databases or "communities," bulletin boards, electronic schedulers, sophisticated search capabilities, instant messaging (IM, SMS, MMS, and chat), voice over Internet Protocol (VOIP), and the capture of insights, such as those generated through mind mapping, that would support knowledge management (Zinick 2010; Hinchcliffe 2014). When these functions are part of a cloud-based offering of EC3M, they are often referred to as **information as a service** (Estes et al. 2013). The communications component takes advantage of social media of many forms, including blogs, social networking sites, podcasts, and wikis and other forms of crowdsourcing (the ability to solicit information from a large group of people, especially online). The HIMSS Clinical Decision Support Wiki is a good example of a community that brought together best practices and experience to accumulate collective knowledge in one site. In addition, communications such as teleconferencing, anonymous interchanges, and structured interactions can be managed through EC3M (EMC 2015; Finances Online 2016).

Webster (2010) describes the use of EC3M for a pediatric practice where groupware and workflow management systems were combined with **adaptive case management (ACM)** in the EHR to help manage exception processing, such as appointment no-shows, abnormal laboratory test values, and capturing history of present illness. Also called dynamic case management, case management is defined by AIIM (n.d.[b]) as the process to address "any project, transaction, service, or response that is 'opened' and 'closed' over a period of time to achieve resolution of a problem, claim, request, proposal, development, or other complex activity. It is likely to involve multiple persons inside and outside of the organization, with varying relationships to each other, as well as multiple documents and messages." Swenson (2010) observes that ACM systems are able to manage the case process workflow in a flexible way that helps knowledge workers perform work. Increasingly, ACM is also the foundation for greater interoperability (Hawes 2014).

While the prospects for EC3M are appealing, it is not easy to achieve a true form of EC3M because few vendors offer a truly all-in-one enterprise collaboration platform. Furthermore, internal technology landscapes in healthcare are becoming increasingly costly to change. However, healthcare organizations are starting to deploy some of the functionality of EC3M, especially for managing organizational performance. The tools afford the ability for people from disparate locations within an integrated delivery network or who participate in HIE to communicate effectively and efficiently. As accountable care organizations form, with potentially even more disparate organizations coming together to afford care coordination across the continuum of care (and putting themselves at financial risk to be successful), EC3M tools are likely to become even more important in healthcare. Figure 18.2 illustrates the convergence of the types of ECM technology with the EHR and other health IT systems within provider settings.

Figure 18.2.   Convergence of ECRM technology

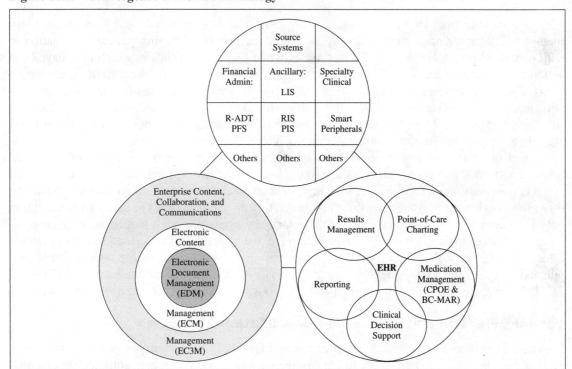

Check Your Understanding 18.2

Match the terms with the appropriate descriptions:

A. Document imaging system

B. Document imaging and management system

C. Electronic document management system

D. Enterprise content management system

E. Enterprise content, collaboration, and communication system

1. Level 3 sophistication for scanning and supporting workflow for patient information

2. Enables teams to work together from remote locations

3. Simplest system with which to transform paper records into electronic information

4. May integrate paper from multiple healthcare organization departments

5. Affords some workflow tools to help ensure the quality of scanning

6. Embeds rules that supports a full life cycle for documents

7. Often includes tools such a groupware

8. Can support integration of clinical information and images across multiple platforms

EDM/ECM Systems Acquisition, Implementation, and Use

Although various types of ECM technology are available, most hospitals and larger clinics still focus on EDM systems as their mainstay to reduce the burden of having patient information in both paper and electronic systems. In fact, the move to ECM in healthcare, which may have been anticipated with the advent of EHRs, has not been as rapid as expected. Many EHR vendors have focused on fully automating the clinical components necessary for earning MU incentives and creating new records, and have not developed systems for managing paper and other content that may still remain. Most EHR vendors have partnered with EDM or ECM vendors, but the EDM/ECM and EHR components are not always fully interoperable (Miliard 2015).

When organizations are involved in mergers and acquisitions or become part of integrated delivery networks, there are challenges in gaining interoperability between the various EDM/ECM systems used at different facilities. As such organizations seek solutions for their EDM/ECM needs, they must consider the pros and cons of truly integrating disparate systems or using a VNA solution only for access purposes—which may not necessarily be available for all platforms. When considering a full integration, organizations must recognize that each entity has defined its own workflow rules within the technology, has different policies and procedures for managing both input and output, and may be using different technology for forms identification, and other elements of EDM and ECM. All of these issues must be studied and decisions made about what and how to standardize.

Vendor Selection and EDM/ECM Consolidation Strategies

In general, the steps in vendor selection for a new EDM or ECM system are generally similar to those for any health IT system where full due diligence and strong contract negotiation are essential (see chapter 7). However, organizations reshaped by mergers and acquisitions and or by joining integrated delivery networks may not want to acquire an entirely new system, as many of the hospitals and physician offices that are part of the organization will already have some form of EDM or ECM. In these organizations, vendor selection involves deciding first whether all entities should use the same EDM/ECM (herein called an *EDM/ECM consolidation*). Then, if EDM/ECM consolidation will be performed, the next decision is to select the EDM or ECM that will become the single technology. Many organizations assume that the acquiring organization will have the platform of choice, but this assumption should not be made without due diligence.

Some considerations for organizations considering EDM/ECM consolidation include the following:

- Does the acquiring organization use a VNA for its radiology/PACS integration? If so, does the vendor have experience with integrating EDM/ECM?

- How disparate are the organizations being consolidated? Do they have many patients in common? If there are not many common patients today, is an accountable care organization (ACO) being formed that requires more integration of clinical and financial data instead of just provision of access to documents for viewing?

- Has the acquiring organization conducted an EDM/ECM consolidation in the past, and how successful was it? Did this include EDM/ECM and EHR integration?

- Has the acquiring organization conducted an EHR consolidation in the past, or is it integrating data through a centralized repository and/or warehouse to which disparate EHRs contribute?

- Which organization has the most sophisticated EDM/ECM technology? Should all organizations implement this level of technology, or is the organization with the more sophisticated technology not really using all the functionality?

- Have volumes and workflow policies and processes been analyzed to determine the scope of differences between needs, some of which may be new with the consolidation, and between comparably sophisticated technologies?

- Is a single, entirely new EDM/ECM system a better choice than cobbling together multiple systems, especially if the dominant EDM/ECM is not tightly coupled with the dominant EHR?

- Is there significant other content that would warrant acquisition of the next level of EDM/ECM for the entire integrated delivery system?

- Are there ways to reduce the volume of documents to be scanned that will affect this decision? There are many providers who embarked on an archival scanning project at the time their EHR was acquired, only to be afraid to get rid of paper, which somehow manages to continue to be used on a routine basis. There are also many provider settings that have comprehensive, enterprise-wide EHRs but still permit clinicians to handwrite orders, notes, and other documents (Chapman 2012). Many organizations have not adopted health IT to manage documents requiring patient signatures, such as acknowledging receipt of the notice of privacy practices, various consents, and other documents. However, there are best practices for use of interactive, informed-consent kiosks and other similar technologies that demonstrate enhanced patient understanding of these consents with their use (Aldoory et al. 2014).

If the decision is made to make an acquisition, it is advisable that each different entity within the organization be involved in the selection process—with the understanding that there will need to be compromises. A new system will be new to all, hence leveling the "playing field" somewhat, but the experience of each different entity can contribute value to the overall process. Much as an EHR selection committee requires stakeholders from all disciplines who will be using the EHR, so too should the EDM/ECM selection committee be diverse.

Just as the EHR is not strictly an IT system, EDM/ECM is more than information technology. With the move toward more ECM or even EC3M, the new system is also not exclusively an HIM system or a system for any other single domain. It is also important to recognize that a consolidated EDM/ECM does not necessarily mean centralized processing. Some organizations find it more effective to centralize processing, but not all do. In fact, as the amount of patient information entered into an EDM/ECM decreases and the amount of other types of information increases, some organizations may decide to move from a previously centralized processing structure to a decentralized, or distributed, one. There are many permutations of how decentralization might work. For example, some organizations may choose to have input scanned locally, documents made accessible to all as required, coding performed locally, and release of information performed centrally. Other organizations may use a **scan-on-demand** vendor service (which is much like the software as a service [SaaS] acquisition strategy for EHR, or on-demand software commonly used in other industries), which enables the customer to pay for services as they are used and not a flat monthly or annual fee (Hyland 2014). Such an organization may then push all other functions to the local organization—or decide to centralize some functions (Stryker 2013).

Services such as scan on demand and information as a service are most commonly (although not necessarily) provided through the cloud. Even when such services are not sought, decisions about storage management must be made. Although many healthcare providers have not fully embraced cloud computing due to security concerns, they seem most willing to use cloud-based applications for administrative functions, including cloud storage (HIMSS 2014). Certainly, security is a major factor, but some experts suggest that cybersecurity is less of a threat in a cloud environment than in a local environment where security is only one many functions performed by the organization's IT department (Guccione 2015). The National Institute of Standards and Technology (NIST) offers several special publications on cloud computing, including a Cloud Computing Standards Roadmap (2013) that addresses healthcare uses of cloud computing in particular. HIMSS (2014) has noted that there are over 1,000 vendors selling cloud services to the healthcare industry, so performing due diligence can be a significant challenge.

Organizations that aim to consolidate EDM/ECM must decide who will provide governance over the consolidation. If there is an enterprise-wide HIM department, it may be the natural source of such governance. On the other hand, a business office manager or radiology department director in one location may have by far more experience with the nature of the EDM/ECM being acquired and would be more appropriate. Such a decision needs to be based on qualifications and whether the focus for EDM/ECM remains patient information or is more expansive (Coots et al. 2008).

Implementation

Implementation considerations include those relating to standards for technology and processes. Critical parts of implementing EDM/ECM involve how patients are identified, how documents are indexed, the design of forms, version control and authentication, access controls and audit logs, categorization of records, and workflow designs.

Person Identification

It is virtually impossible to consolidate EDM/ECM systems without an **enterprise-wide master person index (EMPI)**. The EMPI can be created by integrating master person indexes (MPIs) from entities in the consolidating organization. This process will very likely require a MPI cleanup.

At this time, there may be additional factors relating to person identification that should be considered. These may include how patients are identified—that is, the set of data and algorithms to appropriately match patients must be determined. For example, an organization may decide to require **positive patient identification** in the form of government-issued photo identification, and processes related to this policy might be implemented at the same time that the EDM/ECM is consolidated. Enhancements to some other patient registration and admission procedures may also be considered, especially in light of new opportunities for revenue cycle management improvements (deCathelineau 2013). (See chapter 19.)

Document Indexing

To enhance retrieval of scanned documents, indexing organizes the documents. Various entities involved in a consolidation may use different indexing techniques, so these indexes must be consolidated. Ideally, each form that is scanned or otherwise created should have an automatic identification technology associated with it (Kohn 2009). Bar coding is frequently used for this purpose.

There are at least two primary types of bar code standards commonly used in EDM/ECM systems. Most EDM/ECM systems support the **code 39 bar code standard**, also called the **linear bar code**. This is an alphanumeric, self-checking, variable-length code that has been standardized by the Health Industry Bar Code Council (HIBCC). It also is the standard that the Food and Drug Administration (FDA) requires for use on drug products and biologicals. The **code 128 bar code standard**, also called a **two-dimensional bar code**, can encode more complex information. It is produced by the Uniform Code Council (UCC). Hospitals may use either or both bar codes on patient wristbands. The FDA has indicated that, although the linear bar code must be used to encode the National Drug Code (NDC) of the drug or biological, it is acceptable to add information via the two-dimensional bar code or other means, such as **radio frequency identification (RFID)**. Both linear and two-dimensional forms of bar codes are mechanically scanned via a light beam that interprets the pattern of light reflected off the white gaps between the lines of the code.

Two-dimensional bar codes also come in what is called **QR codes**. These are square, can contain even more information than the traditional two-dimensional bar code, and can be digitally scanned using the camera on a smartphone that has an appropriate app installed. The QR code can link the smartphone's app to a website to access additional information or functionality. QR codes have become quite popular in marketing and, in an EC3M environment, have the potential to link a patient to a provider's website. That being said, there are numerous issues with QR codes, including that the apps are free and open source and hence not fully interoperable, there may be unintended privacy issues when a phone has a global positioning system (GPS) that can be used to track location, and they can be used to transmit malicious code (Schottmuller 2011).

RFID, as mentioned above, is yet another form of content identification. RFID does not require direct line of sight for reading a bar code, can be read faster than bar codes, can be implanted into a product, and can afford both read and write capability. RFID is significantly more expensive to use than bar codes, but it is being used in healthcare for managing "critical inventory" (Vecchione 2015). In addition to cost concerns, another challenge with RFID is that it can read too much because of its proximity property of being able to read up to 300 feet away. For example, a nurse could use RFID to scan a sleeping patient's wristband through a sheet but could inadvertently read a second patient's wristband in a bed or chair nearby. This has been dubbed "RFID collision." Finally, different manufacturers are using different RFID standards so that these systems are not necessarily interoperable (Technovelgy n.d.).

A final identifying technology that is seeing some traction in certain healthcare environments is the **real-time location system (RTLS)**. RTLS includes a wireless (radiofrequency, infrared, or ultrasound) tag that emits signals enabling content or people wearing the tag to be tracked. Miliard (2013) describes some RTLS applications in healthcare, such as tracking patients with Alzheimer's disease, locating family members of patients, locating staff, and assessing hand-hygiene compliance and other behaviors. Although there are a variety of standards—some newer than others—a study by Van der Togt and colleagues (2008) found potentially hazardous incidents in medical devices from RTLS interference.

Although QR codes, RFID, RTLS, and other such identification systems are generally used for identification of objects and people, not documents, their use in healthcare could result in some relationship to ECM or EC3M. For example, documentation of identification actions could be transmitted to an EHR.

Forms Identification and Design

In addition to bar codes on health record documents, forms recognition systems may be available to enhance the accuracy of indexing features on forms. Instead of having to create bar code labels for such forms, optical mark recognition (OMR), optical character recognition (OCR), optical word recognition (OWR), or intelligent character recognition (ICR) systems may be used.

- **OMR** is the oldest form of optical recognition and requires pre-printed forms to contain locations for marking specific, limited information that is then read by a scanning system and content incorporated into an EDM, ECM, or any other system capable of receiving such information. The strength of OMR is ease of use, while its weakness is lack of flexibility. In healthcare, OMR has been used in collection of patient histories, and for various questionnaires such as patient satisfaction surveys and others.

- **OCR** has also been available for some time. This is the mechanical or electronic translation, usually by scanning, of printed or typewritten text in structured locations on forms into machine-editable text. Depending on the quality of the translation system, often in association with the quality of the printing or typing, the quality of OCR "readability" can be variable. Early in the adoption of EHRs, OCR was considered a significant adjunct to data entry, although the necessity to print in block letters and use of standardized forms was a significant drawback (HealthInformatics 2008; Rasmussen et al. 2012).

- **ICR** is an advanced form of OCR in which the system "learns" (through various forms of artificial intelligence, such as artificial neural networks) to recognize a specific person's handwriting and, over time, increases its accuracy (Vasudeva et al. 2012; Templeton 2015). Although higher accuracy rates are achieved with ICR use on structured forms, the system at best can reach about 97 percent accuracy. A key difference between handwriting recognition and **speech recognition**, which deploys comparable type of technology, is in their application. Most speech recognition systems are used in a transcription environment, where transcribers can listen and correct inaccuracies (AHIMA 2003b), or in uses that rely on limited vocabularies and away from a point of care, often referred to as **front-end speech (FES)**. The limited vocabulary and ability for immediate correction not only makes speech recognition useful in this environment but also contributes to improved learning by the system. Just the same, as many as half of providers polled in a study conducted in 2014 were skeptical of using FES (Miliard 2014a).

- **IWR** is an even newer technology than ICR. This is the recognition of unconstrained handwritten words. Thus, instead of reading character-by-character, IWR is able to recognize entire words or phrases. It matches these words or phrases to a user-defined dictionary to reduce character-based system errors (CMS Software 2016).

The various forms of recognition systems probably are not as reliable as bar codes for identifying records or forms for purposes related to ensuring that all content about a given patient is captured together in an EDM/ECM system. However, there may be value in using such recognition systems to categorize records (see below), and potentially to capture content that can be contributed to an EHR system.

Healthcare organizations that are just approaching adoption of EDM/ECM systems should plan ahead to incorporate bar codes on their forms or be faced with using an interim solution for indexing, such as bar coded separator sheets, to distinguish between different records of different patients and different types of documents within a given patient's health record. Those looking at enhanced EDM/ECM with sophisticated workflow components (discussed later in this chapter) should evaluate OCR or ICR as options that may improve accuracy of such management.

Version Control and Authentication

Version control is a particularly critical component when scanned documents must be included in the EHR (as opposed to scanning as a means to archive inactive charts). Depending on when documents are scanned or electronically fed into the EDM/ECM system, it is possible that some documents will not have been completed and authenticated and will need to be printed out, completed/signed, and rescanned—or an alternative form of electronic authentication applied (AHIMA 2009). Two sources of guidance on **electronic signature authentication (ESA)** are:

- *ASTM E1762–95* (2013), which is a Standard Guide for Electronic Authentication of Health Care Information. It provides a process for applying an electronic signature and guidelines for handling multiple signatures and signature attributes (for example, time stamp, signature purpose—such as addendum, modification, or administrative correction), and signer's role—especially for use when there are multiple, dual, co-, or countersignature requirements.

- *HL7 EHR-System Records Management and Evidentiary Support Functional Profile* (2010), which identifies functionality related to authentication, attestation, pending records, amendments, and version management.

Amendments, corrections, and deletions may also be made to documents (Hall et al. 2009). The organization must consider how and when and by whom such changes may be made. Additionally, what is done with a former version of a document is an important matter of healthcare organization policy. All of these considerations should be determined in conjunction with the clinicians who will use the record as well as with legal counsel. In general, displaying multiple copies of a document is not advisable because it represents a patient safety risk; however, changes to a document over time need to be tracked for legal purposes. Usually, organizations make only the most current version accessible for viewing. However, if an amendment, correction, or deletion is the cause of a new version, there must be a way for the viewer to understand that it is a newer version and be able to retrieve a former version if it is needed. In other words, the provenance of a form with multiple versions must be transparent.

Access Controls and Audit Logs

Just as with any electronic application, an EDM/ECM system requires access privileges to be authorized, established, and enforced; and a record of accesses must be kept as a means to audit. Document management technology should provide for such access controls and audit logs (see chapter 12).

Record Categorization

In addition to associating each record with a person and each document in the record with the person, and identifying each document by type of form (for example, history and physical exam, operative report, pathology report), organizations may wish to categorize the nature of the record. With respect to an EDM/ECM that is exclusively maintained for patient information, records may be categorized by type for purposes of workflow. For example, records may be categorized by payer type, potential complexity for coding, nursing unit in a hospital from which the patient was discharged, and/or other categories of information. This categorization may be done to direct certain records to certain coders who specialize (for example, coders for Medicare versus those who work with commercial payers), or to separate highly complex cases from simpler ones, such as normal mother and child records. Some organizations may wish to associate a group of coders with a nursing unit, and the physicians and nurses who work on that unit, in order to assist with clinical documentation improvement.

If EDM/ECM is going to integrate clinical and billing information, there may be a hierarchy of record categorization, such as first relating to whether the content is clinical or billing, then perhaps the type of payer, and then, finally, the nature of the case or the location of patient for the clinical records.

Workflow

Many EDM systems add a workflow component to their functionality; and workflow is a key characteristic of ECM systems. This component enables documents to be proactively directed to where work needs to be performed. For example, some logic may indicate that as soon as key documents have been scanned, the record is ready to populate a queue for coding, and the system would then send an alert to a workstation in the HIM department (or wherever such work may be performed, including to a remote coder). Cross-department communication can also be aided with workflow tools. For example, a business office that requires clinical documentation to be attached to a claim or request for prior authorization can direct such requests to the HIM department automatically.

A number of terms are associated with workflow and its management. *Workflow* refers to the sequence of tasks that need to be performed within a process. *Workflow management* is the planning, organizing, directing, and controlling of the workflow. **Workflow management systems** store workflow definitions as a collection of tasks, resources, and conditional logic. These systems retrieve workflow information from the database to guide work as transactions pass through the organization (Amatayakul 2012).

Workflow technology helps organize, automate, and improve processes by dividing them into component tasks, specifying who performs each task, identifying the business rules for performing the tasks, describing the potential outputs, and indicating who performs the next step in the process (Dooling 2011). Based on these factors, workflow technology:

- Assembles the information needed to perform each task

- Provides guidance for performing each task according to the correct and consistent business rules

- Routes the task, along with the information needed to perform it, to the appropriate person

- Potentially speeds up a process by dividing it into tasks or parts, coordinating the work of multiple people on the various parts, and reassembling the parts to complete the original process

HL7 has addressed workflow management functions in its EHR-System Functional Model and its message standards. HL7 has a Medical Document Management (MDM) message type that helps manage the transmission of new or updated documents by also transmitting important status information about the record (Corepoint Health n.d.[a]). A survey of EDM vendors reported by Andrew and Bruegel in 2005 revealed that some 60 percent to 80 percent of respondents indicated that they had workflow functionality, although just under 50 percent indicated they had a workflow engine. Andrew and Bruegel defined a **workflow engine** as a system that takes care of the management of workflow, including task assignment generation, resource allocation, activity performance, case preparation and modification, launching of applications, and the recording of logistical information. In much more recent article, Miliard (2014b) observes that, despite benefits of helping to measure and improve efficiency and minimize errors, there are relatively few fully functional workflow engines in health IT.

Use of ECM Systems

A final step in implementing an ECM system is to ensure that best-practice policies and procedures for use are established, staff are trained, and ongoing maintenance of the system and monitoring of output are performed. The American Health Information Management Association (AHIMA) provides a Document Management and Imaging Toolkit that address best practices (AHIMA 2012).

Preparation for Use

Communications with staff need to be carefully planned and initiated long before implementation of the hardware and software. Whether the organization is acquiring ECM for the first time, consolidating systems, or even just updating one, the staff performing related functions will have questions and potentially concerns for their jobs. Clinicians who will be expected to use ECM to access records will also have questions—albeit different from those of administrative staff. Clinicians may be concerned about the readability, ability to print from the systems, whether and how to authenticate their use, and interoperability with an EHR. Each such question and concern should be anticipated. Most of the responses to issues raised should be codified in policies and procedures, but, as described earlier in this book, formal and informal communications that support change management with respect to such systems are essential.

Decisions need to made, and policies and procedures written, for every aspect of scanning of documents, from ensuring that the patient's name is on both sides of a two-sided form and both sides of a form will always be scanned to addressing special needs for colored forms, large forms, and other form-related issues. As the EHR significantly reduces the need for forms which the organization has control over, the more likely there will be unusual form issues.

Training processes and procedures ensure that everyone who scans documents is equipped not only to perform the typical scanning operations but has instruction on what to do in unusual circumstances or with unusual forms. Staff to be trained on ECM in an EHR environment, especially one that is decentralized, may include nurses and others who typically have not had to perform such work.

Physical Environment

The physical environment must also be prepared for implementation. In a first-time archiving process, there is often the need for space to stage records for scanning, perform the scanning, and stage records for destruction or removal to a remote warehouse. Once such a major process is performed, usage for the space that held paper records should also be planned. Space considerations change when the initial archiving process is finished and consolidation of ad hoc scanning of loose forms and potentially other content is being done.

Space considerations largely depend on whether ECM will be performed centrally or not. If it is centrally performed, there still must be a secure, though generally smaller, staging area. ECM usually is performed using dual monitors, so the space that staff needs to actually perform the scanning may need to be enlarged. If scanning is decentralized, carefully planning for scanner location, training of those using the scanner, and space considerations are also needed. In some cases, such as on a nursing unit, a combination scanner and printer can replace an existing printer. Unless the document being scanned will be returned to the patient (such as an insurance card), temporary and secure space must be accommodated for the scanned documents or a shedder or secured shred box is needed. The space requirements depend on what is being scanned and the policies and procedures of the organizations—as well as, in some cases, state laws, which may require that documents scanned into an EHR be retained for some period of time, such as 3 to 6 months, after which they may be destroyed.

Monitoring Work Performed

As work is performed, it must be monitored to ensure that all documents that must be scanned are scanned and that the quality of scanning is acceptable. The organization must determine in advance how it will ensure that all work requiring scanning has been scanned. This process may require some form of reconciliation of scanned documents against records of patients discharged. It may also be necessary to build such monitoring into the workflow components of the ECM. As EHR use increases and there is need only for scanning of the occasional ad hoc document, tracking that all documents have been scanned becomes more difficult, especially in a decentralized environment. In fact, there may be a point in time that only the work performed using ECM/EHR (such as, coding discharges or fulfilling release of information requests) is tracked and not the actual scanning of loose documents. An exception may be if there are certain areas in a hospital or clinic that do not have health IT support and will always, or at least predictably, have documents to be scanned, which can then be tracked. Surgical areas, therapy departments, and other similar areas are often among the last to use the EHR or other health IT system (Dunn 2007).

Ensuring that the scanning performed meets organizational criteria for acceptability is an ongoing process. The level of monitoring will vary with the tenure of the staff member doing the work—those in training usually need more monitoring than those who are more experienced. However, when there are changes in either the hardware or software of the ECM system, or in the nature of forms required to be scanned, there may be periods of time when more intense monitoring is needed of all staff involved in scanning.

Productivity monitoring is also an important aspect of work associated with ECM. Some ECM systems are able to produce productivity reports. If one is acquired that does not offer this functionality, a system needs to be put into place to track productivity.

HL7 Consolidated-Clinical Document Architecture

The HL7 CDA and its C-CDA set of document templates have been referenced throughout this book. These are tools that are required for certified EHR technology (CEHRT) under the MU incentive program for EHRs. Coupled with the MU requirement to provide patient summaries, the CDA will very likely decrease the volume of release-of-information requests. The CDA should also lower costs of processing release-of-information requests as documents can be transmitted electronically using the C-CDA. Some believe that the C-CDA will increase physician adoption of EHRs because their narrative tells the patient story while still affording structured data for clinical decision support (Bonney 2015). There is also an expectation that the C-CDA will be adopted by the federal government by 2017 or 2018 as a means to provide attachments to the Health Insurance Portability and Accountability Act (HIPAA) claim and potentially other HIPAA transactions, such as eligibility, prior authorization, and postpaid claim audits (NCVHS 2016). The purpose and functionality of the C-CDA is described here.

The CDA is an XML-based electronic standard used for clinical document exchange that was developed by the standards development organization HL7. Its origins and relationship to the ASTM Continuity of Care Document were explained in chapter 17.

The CDA is a flexible document markup standard where a mandatory free-form portion enables human reading and an optional XML-structured part enables electronic processing. Text, images, and multimedia, including signatures, can be included in a CDA document. In addition, the CDA does not specify a transport mechanism. It can be supplied as an attachment via the HL7 V2.x standards or embedded in an HL7 V3 message (as shown in figure 13.4 in chapter 13). The Integrating the Healthcare Enterprise (IHE) Cross-Enterprise Document Sharing (XDS) Profile further enables specificity for using HL7 messages. The CDA can also be transported via a DICOM message (often when a document accompanies a radiological image or another type of clinical image). Not specific to healthcare, but the CDA can also be transported as a MIME-encoded attachment (that is, e-mail), hypertext transfer protocol (HTTP) for communications over the World Wide Web, or file transfer protocol (FTP) for transmission through any client/server network (Corepoint Health n.d.[b]).

The Office of the National Coordinator for Health Information Technology (ONC) offers an excellent primer on the structure of the CDA (ONC 2013). The CDA structure enables content to become increasingly structured. Figure 18.3 illustrates the fact that each CDA has a header and a

Figure 18.3.   CDA document structure

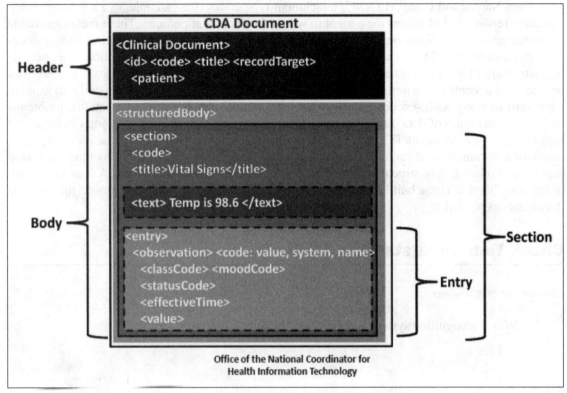

Source: ONC

Figure 18.4.   CDA building blocks

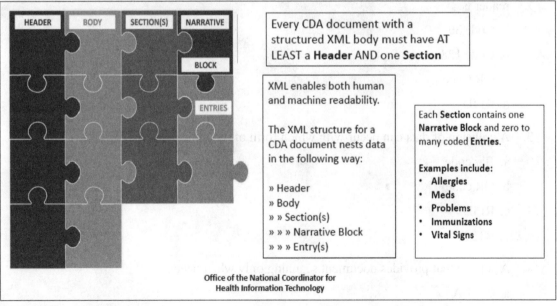

Source: ONC

body. The information in the header identifies the type of document, using Logical Observation Identifiers Names and Codes (LOINC) attachment type codes (for example, discharge summary, operative report), and identifies the patient to whom the document pertains. These metadata enable exchange across and within organizations and facilitate document management, including document placement in an EHR. The body of the CDA contains the clinical information. This may be in unstructured form or structured (XML) content organized into one or more sections. Sections are required to contain one narrative block that is the human readable component and may contain from zero to many XML-encoded entries. Entries may include allergies, medications, problems, and many other types of data. Entries provide additional markup that enables the entry to be placed into an EHR (or other health IT system) as structured data. Hence, the CDA can be used only as an image of a document, or it can include structured data content that can be used in clinical decision support and other uses of structured data. Figure 18.4 also illustrates that the CDA is actually a set of building blocks. These building blocks can be sets of related data that are moved into various documents as needed.

Check Your Understanding 18.3

Choose the best answer:

1. Which recognition system is able to recognize handwriting?

   a. FES

   b. ICR

   c. OCR

   d. QR codes

2. A two-dimensional code that enables comprehensive information to be read by a bar code reader is:

   a. Code 39

   b. Code 128

   c. QR Code

   d. RFID

3. A collision of data can occur with which form of recognition technology?

   a. Bar code

   b. QR code

   c. RFID

   d. RTLS

4. A service that provides document scanning only when needed is:

   a. C-CDA

   b. Information as a service

   c. Scan on demand

   d. Vendor neutral archive

5. Which of the following is an example of positive patient identification?

   a. Enterprise master person index

   b. Real-time location tracking

   c. Unique patient ID

   d. Verification of patient ID

6. When an organization pushes the scanning function out to the end user, what type of system is it?

   a. Centralized

   b. Consolidated

   c. Distributed

   d. Enterprise-wide

7. Which of the following is a required element in the CDA?

   a. Header in human readable form

   b. One narrative section in human readable form

   c. Structured data according to HL7 V3

   d. XML content

8. The C-CDA is required for use in:

   a. All EHRs

   b. CEHRT

   c. HIPAA transactions

   d. Release-of-information requests

References and Resources

AIIM. n.d.(a). What is enterprise content management (ECM)? http://www.aiim.org/What-is-ECM-Enterprise-Content-Management.

AIIM. n.d.(b). What is case management? http://www.aiim.org/What-is-Case-Management.

AIIM. 2010 (June 1). PDF healthcare supporting the clinical document architecture: A white paper. AIIM BP-03-2010. http://wiki.siframework.org/file/view/AIIM_PDF_CDA_Whitepaper.pdf.

Aldoory, L., et al. 2014 (July). Best Practices and New Models of Health Literacy for Informed Consent: Review of the Impact of Informed Consent Regulations on Health Literate Communications. Commissioned paper for the Institute of Medicine. http://www.nationalacademies.org/hmd/~/media/Files/Activity%20Files/PublicHealth/HealthLiteracy/Commissioned-Papers/Informed_Consent_HealthLit.pdf.

Amatayakul, M. 2012. *Process Improvement with Electronic Health Records: A Stepwise Approach to Workflow and Process Management*. Boca Raton, FL: CRC Press.

American Academy of Family Physicians (AAFP). 2016. Tips on migrating old paper records to your EHR. http://www.aafp.org/practice-management/health-it/product/old-records.html.

American Health Information Management Association (AHIMA). 2003a (October). Practice brief: The complete medical record in a hybrid EHR environment. *Journal of AHIMA*. http://library.ahima.org/xpedio/groups/public/documents/ahima/bok1_022142.hcsp?dDocName=bok1_022142.

American Health Information Management Association (AHIMA). 2003b (October). Practice brief: Speech recognition in the electronic health record. *Journal of AHIMA*. http://library.ahima.org/doc?oid=62526#.V79jZ5grI2w.

American Health Information Management Association (AHIMA). 2009. Electronic signature, attestation, and authorship (updated). *Journal of AHIMA*. 80(11): expanded online edition. Appendix A: HL7 EHR-System Records Management and Evidentiary Support (RM-ES) Functional Profile Standard excerpt. http://library.ahima.org/doc?oid= 103212#.V79lr5grI2w.

American Health Information Management Association (AHIMA). 2010 (June). Managing existing patient records in the transition to EHRs in physician practices. *Journal of AHIMA*. Web extra. http://library.ahima.org/doc?oid=101080# .V79l3ZgrI2w.

American Health Information Management Association (AHIMA).2012. *Document Management and Imaging Toolkit*. Chicago: AHIMA.

Andrew, W.F., and R.B. Bruegel. 2005. EHR workflow management review and survey results. *ADVANCE for Health Information Executives*. 9(2):34–50.

ASTM E1762–95 (2013). 2013. *Standard Guide for Electronic Authentication of Health Care Information*. Conshohocken, PA: ASTM International. https://www.astm.org/Standards/E1762.htm.

Bonney, S. 2015. 4 applications of C-CDA to consider. The case for why C-CDA is needed to advance shared savings and interoperability. *Journal of AHIMA*. (86)11: 32–35.

Chapman, S. 2012. Document management challenges. *For the Record*. 24(22):18. http://www.fortherecordmag.com/ archives/120312p18.shtml.

Chavis, S. 2010 (December 6). The CCD standard: Building blocks for better data exchange. *For the Record* 22(22):10.

CMS Software. 2016. Form processing. http://www.cmssoft.co.uk/pages/form_processing.html.

Cook, R. 2014 (April 24). Is VNA the future of image delivery? *Healthcare IT News*. http://www.healthcareitnews.com/ news/should-you-use-vna-whats-vna.

Coots, C. et al. 2008. Enterprise content and record management for healthcare. *Journal of AHIMA*. 79(10):91–98.

Corepoint Health. n.d.(a). HL7 MDM message—Medical Document Management. http://corepointhealth.com/resource-center/hl7-resources/hl7-mdm-message.

Corepoint Health. n.d.(b). HL7 CDA—Clinical Document Architecture. http://corepointhealth.com/resource-center/hl7-resources/hl7-cda.

Craciun, E. 2014 (October 29). Benefits of a knowledge management system within an organization. LinkedIn Pulse. https://www.linkedin.com/pulse/20141029121125-2108052-benefits-of-a-knowledge-management-system-within-an-organization.

Dirking, B. 2010 (December). Content in context. *KMWorld Magazine*. S13. http://www.kmworld.com.

Dooling, J. 2011. Managing records between the EDMS and EHR: Monitoring, evaluating, and redesigning workflows. *Journal of AHIMA*. 82(2):38–39.

Dunn, R. 2007. Benchmarking imaging: Making every image count in scanning programs. *Journal of AHIMA*. 78(6): 42–46.

Elwyn, G., and L. Buckman. 2015 (January 8). Should doctors encourage patients to record consultations? *BMJ*. http:// www.bmj.com/content/350/bmj.g7645.

EMC Enterprise Content Division. 2015 (April). Using interoperability to transform clinical content management & collaboration. Presentation at HIMSS15 Annual Conference & Exhibition, Chicago, IL. http://www.slideshare.net/ EMC_IIG/using-interoperability-to-transform-clinical-content-management-collaboration.

Estes, M., et al. 2013. Open Data Center Alliance Master Usage Model: Information as a Service Rev. 1.0. Open Data Center Alliance. http://www.opendatacenteralliance.org/docs/Information_as_a_Service_Master_Usage_Model_ Rev1.0.pdf.

Finances Online. 2016. Types of collaboration software: 5 groups you should know about. https://collaboration-software.financesonline.com/types-of-collaboration-software-5-groups-you-should-know-about.

Frost, A. 2015. KM Tools. http://www.knowledge-management-tools.net/knowledge-management-systems.html.

Grzybowski, D. 2014. *Strategies for Electronic Document and Health Record Management*. Chicago, IL: American Health Information Management Association (AHIMA).

Guccione, D. 2015 (July 20). Is the cloud safe for healthcare? *Healthcare Informatics*. http://www.healthcare-informatics.com/article/cloud-safe-healthcare.

Hall, T., et al. 2009. Amendments, corrections, and deletions in the electronic health record: An American Health Information Management Association toolkit. American Health Information Management Association. http://library.ahima.org/doc?oid=93657#.V79myZgrI2w.

Hawes, L. 2014 (June 26). Adaptive case management could be the foundation for networked business. *Forbes*. http://www.forbes.com/sites/larryhawes/2014/06/26/adaptive-case-management-could-be-the-foundation-for-networked-business/#34539da45d12.

Healthcare Information and Management Systems Society (HIMMS). n.d. HIMSS Clinical Decision Support Wiki. http://himssclinicaldecisionsupportwiki.pbworks.com.

Healthcare Information and Management Systems Society (HIMSS). 2011. Stop talking about document management and start talking about content management. HIMSS11 Annual Conference & Exhibition. http://www.hyland.com/industry-solutions/healthcare/document-management-integration.aspx.

Healthcare Information and Management Systems Society (HIMSS). 2014 (June 16). HIMSS Analytics cloud survey. http://www.himss.org/ResourceLibrary/genResourceDetailPDF.aspx?ItemNumber=41958.

Healthcare IT News. 2015. The value of document imaging in a digital era. http://pages.healthcareitnews.com/The-Value-of-Document-Imaging-in-a-Digital-Era.html?topic=clinicl%26ehr.

HealthInformatics. 2008 (October 16). Optical character recognition. https://healthinformatics.wikispaces.com/Optical+Character+Recognition.

HealthIT.gov. 2014 (February 24). How to implement EHRs: Step 5: Achieve meaningful use stage 2 use secure electronic messaging. https://www.healthit.gov/providers-professionals/achieve-meaningful-use/core-measures 2/use-secure-electronic-messaging.

Hinchcliffe, D. 2014 (October 23). How to deliver on a modern enterprise collaboration strategy. Adjuvi. http://adjuvi.com/how-to-deliver-on-a-modern-enterprise-collaboration-strategy.

Hirsch, M.D. 2013 (June 4). "Hybrid" medical record systems boost likelihood of errors. *FierceEMR*. http://www.fiercehealthcare.com/ehr/hybrid-medical-record-systems-boost-likelihood-errors.

Hirsch, M.D. 2014 (September 23). EHRs too inauthentic to be relied on in court. *FierceEMR*. http://www.fiercehealthcare.com/ehr/ehrs-too-inauthentic-to-be-relied-court.

Hirsch, M.D. 2015a (December 1). Docs must follow "POISED" best practices when using EHRs in the exam room. *FierceEMR*. http://www.fiercehealthcare.com/ehr/docs-must-follow-poised-best-practices-when-using-ehrs-exam-room.

Hirsch, M.D. 2015b (March 23). 4 ways providers can avoid copy-and-paste errors. *FierceEMR*. http://www.fiercehealthcare.com/ehr/4-ways-providers-can-avoid-ehr-copy-and-paste-errors

Health Level 7 International (HL7). 2010 (August 16). HL7 EHR Records Management and Evidentiary Support (RM-ES) Functional Model, release 1. . http://www.hl7.org/implement/standards/product_brief.cfm?product_id=86.

Hyland. 2014. 5 places in your hospital where enterprise content management can help. http://www.aha-solutions.org/resources/pdf-files/hyland-2014-1004-ar-5places.pdf.

Klugman, C. 2015 (April 29). Why doctors should audio record patient encounters. Bioethics.net blog. http://www.bioethics.net/2015/04/why-doctors-should-audio-record-patient-encounters.

Kohn, D. 2009. How information technology supports virtual HIM departments. *Journal of AHIMA*. 80(3):38–42.

Lobach, D., et al. 2012 (April). *Enabling Health Care Decisionmaking Through Clinical Decision Support and Knowledge Management*. Rockville, MD: Agency for Healthcare Research and Quality. AHRQ publication no. 12-E001-EF. http://effectivehealthcare.ahrq.gov/index.cfm/search-for-guides-reviews-and-reports/?pageaction=displayproduct&productid=919.

McCann, E. 2015 (September). How satisfied are you with your EHR? 2015 Satisfaction Survey results. *Healthcare IT News*. http://www.healthcareitnews.com/news/2015-ehr-satisfaction-survey.

Miliard, M. 2013 (September 11). RFID and RTLS getting "dominated" by MU. *Healthcare IT News*. http://www.healthcareitnews.com/news/rfid-rtls-getting-dominated-mu.

Miliard, M. 2014a (June 20). Speech recognition proving its worth. *Healthcare IT News*. http://www.healthcareitnews.com/news/speech-recognition-proving-its-worth.

Miliard, M. 2014b (December 3). Making workflow engines work for you. *Healthcare IT News*. http://www.healthcareitnews.com/news/making-workflow-engines-work-you.

Miliard, M. 2015 (September 18). 2015 survey results: Speaking out about EHRs. *Healthcare IT News*. http://www.healthcareitnews.com/news/survey-results-speaking-out-about-ehrs.

National Institute of Standards and Technology (NIST). 2013 (July). *NIST Cloud Computing Standards Roadmap*. NIST special publication 500-291, version 2. http://www.nist.gov/itl/cloud/upload/NIST_SP-500-291_Version-2_2013_June18_FINAL.pdf.

Nunn, S. 2008 (March). Managing source system content in the EHR. *Journal of AHIMA* 79(3):60–61.

Office of the National Coordinator for Health Information Technology (ONC). 2013 (April 5). Implementing Consolidated-Clinical Document Architecture (C-CDA) for meaningful use stage 2. https://www.healthit.gov/sites/default/files/c-cda_and_meaningfulusecertification.pdf.

Perez, M.A. 2013 (July 18). The challenges of the hybrid medical records . . . its impact on clinical, coding, and fiscal outcomes. Healthcare Financial Management Association, Oregon Chapter. http://www.oregonhfma.org/files/70864305.pdf.

Rasmussen, L.V., et al. 2012 (June). Development of an optical character recognition pipeline for handwritten form fields from an electronic health record. *Journal of the American Medical Informatics Association*. 19(e1): e90–e95.

Rouse, M. 2014 (September). Vendor neutral archive. TechTarget Search Health IT. http://searchhealthit.techtarget.com/definition/Vendor-neutral-archive-VNA.

Schottmuller, A. 2011 (December 30). Top 14 things marketers need to know about QR codes. Search Engine Watch. https://searchenginewatch.com/sew/how-to/2066777/top-14-things-marketers-need-know-about-qr-codes.

Stiell, A., et al. 2003. Prevalence of information gaps in the emergency department and the effect on patient outcomes. *Canadian Medical Association Journal*. 169(10):1023–1028.

Stryker, C. 2013 (July 17). Avoid the pitfalls of centralized document scanning for EHRs. Physicians Practice blog. http://www.physicianspractice.com/blog/avoid-pitfalls-centralized-document-scanning-ehrs.

Swenson, K.D. 2010. Case management. In *Mastering the Unpredictable: How Adaptive Case Management Will Revolutionize the Way That Knowledge Workers Get Things Done*. Tampa, FL: Meghan-Kiffer Press.

Technovelgy. n.d. Problems with RFID. http://www.technovelgy.com/ct/Technology-Article.asp?ArtNum=20.

Templeton, G. 2015 (October 12). Artificial neural networks are changing the world. What are they? ExtremeTech. http://www.extremetech.com/extreme/215170-artificial-neural-networks-are-changing-the-world-what-are-they.

Van der Togt, R., et al. 2008. Electromagnetic interference from radio frequency identification inducing potentially hazardous incidents in critical care medical equipment. *Journal of the American Medical Association*. 299(24):2884–2890.

Varpio, L., et al. 2015. The EHR and building the patient's story: A qualitative investigation of how EHR use obstructs a vital clinical activity. *International Journal of Medical Informatics*. 84(12):1019–1028.

Vasudeva, N., et al. 2012. Offline character recognition system using artificial neural network. *International Journal of Machine Learning and Computing*. 2(4):449–452.

Vecchione, A. 2015 (June 30). Patient safety driving increased RFID use in hospitals. *Healthcare IT News*. http://www.healthcareitnews.com/news/patient-safety-driving-increased-rfid-use-hospitals.

Webster, C. 2010 (April 23). Adaptive case management, clinical groupware, and routine vs. non-routine workflow in pediatric practice. Healthcare Business Process Management Blog. http://chuckwebster.com/2010/04/ehr-workflow/adaptive-case-management-clinical-groupware-and-routine-vs-non-routine-workflow-in-pediatric-practice.

Zinick, B.M. 2010 (June 2). What is SharePoint 2010? Vision and reality. *CMS Wire*. http://www.cmswire.com/cms/enterprise-20/what-is-sharepoint-2010-vision-and-reality-007513.php.

Chapter 19
Revenue Cycle Management

Key Terms

30-day readmission
Accountable care organization (ACO)
Accounts receivable (A/R)
Actuarial models
Administrative simplification
Appeals
Bad debt
Balance after insurance
Bundled payment
Care coordination
Capitation
Case management
Case mix
Charge capture
Charge description master
Chargemaster
Charity care
Claim attachment
Claim status inquiry and response
Claim submission
Claim scrubbing
Clinical documentation improvement (CDI)
Clinically integrated network (CIN)
Co-insurance
Companion guide

Consumer-driven care

Coordination of benefits

Cost accounting

Deductible

Discharge planning

Drug utilization review

Electronic data interchange

Electronic remittance advice (ERA)

Eligibility inquiry and response

Healthcare clearinghouse

Healthcare EFT and Remittance Advice Standard

Health maintenance organization (HMO)

Health plan

Health plan ID (HPID)

Implementation guide

Managed care

MAP Keys

Medically necessity

NACHA

Patient-centered medical home

Payer

PayerID

Pay for performance

Payment and remittance advice

Point-of-service payment

Point-to-point transmission

Pre-certification

Preferred provider organization (PPO)

Reassociation trace number

Request for information

Revenue cycle management

Shared risk

Shared savings

Shifting financial risk

Situational

Solicited attachment

Specialty review

Unsolicited attachment

Utilization review

Value-based payment models

Virtual cards

Learning Objectives

- Describe the current state of revenue cycle management challenges.

- Discuss enhancements to improve usage of the HIPAA financial and administrative transactions as part of an overall health IT strategy to support revenue cycle management.

- Describe the scope of revenue cycle management for which there are health IT opportunities for improvement.

- Define the current state-of-the-art in value-based payment models and structures through which they are being organized and used, and identify revenue cycle management improvements needed to support such payment models.

Healthcare has notoriously been comprised of many silos, especially with respect to clinical and financial functions. This situation has contributed to both wasted dollars and less than desirable outcomes. Revenue cycle management should no longer be considered the "other side of the house" from the clinical side; instead, it is best understood as truly an integral part of overall healthcare and a critical element of quality healthcare. Increasingly, clinical and financial data need to be integrated, especially as health reform focuses on value—the cost and quality of care. New forms of technology will be needed, and new skills for healthcare workers will be needed.

Financial and administrative transactions were actually responsible for leading the way to more automation in healthcare with the Health Insurance Portability and Accountability Act (HIPAA) of 1996. HIPAA's Subtitle F—Administrative Simplification had the stated purpose:

> To improve the Medicare program . . . the Medicaid program . . . and the efficiency and effectiveness of the healthcare system by encouraging the development of a health information system through the establishment of standards and requirements for the electronic transmission of certain health information.

Nine standards were required to effect **administrative simplification** (that is, to streamline and reduce the cost of financial and administrative operations in healthcare), primarily revolving around transactions for healthcare claims or equivalent encounter information, health claims attachments, enrollment and disenrollment in a health plan, eligibility for a health plan, healthcare payment and remittance advice, health plan premium payments, first report of injury, health claim status, and referral certification and authorization (often referred to as *prior authorization*). In addition, HIPAA also required medical and nonmedical code sets associated with the transactions; unique provider, health plan, employer, and individual identifiers; privacy; security; and recommendations for the electronic exchange of patient medical record information.

Twenty years later, revenue cycle management has become more automated, but much work remains. Only seven of the nine financial transactions required by HIPAA have been adopted by regulation, and only the claim has strong (93 percent) usage. The transactions related to eligibility, claim status, and payment and remittance advice have moderate usage (68 percent, 55 percent, and 50 percent, respectively), and the prior authorization transaction has just 10 percent usage (CAQH 2016). A health claims attachments standard (likely to be a set of standards) has yet to be adopted by regulation, although, as noted in chapter 18, it appears possible for 2017 or 2018. A first report of injury standard is likely not to be adopted as there is virtually no interest in it. Finally, standards for the enrollment and disenrollment in a health plan and health plan premium payments are those that would be used by employers to send information to health plans. They have been adopted by regulation, but they are rarely used because employers are not covered entities and therefore not required to use them under HIPAA.

As illustrated by these data, it is important to recognize that, while it has been challenging to gain full usage of the electronic health record (EHR), health information technology (health IT) for revenue cycle management has its own unique set of challenges. When considering the advent of health reform and new payment models that are to improve quality, cost, and experience of care (the Triple Aim; see chapter 4) by requiring integration of clinical and financial/administrative data, the challenge to improve revenue cycle management is now part of the broader health IT strategy to address the Triple Aim (Commins 2016).

Current Challenges in Revenue Cycle Management

Revenue cycle management is one of the top topics on the minds of both hospital and practice executives at this time. Not only are there concerns about administrative processes as described above, but there are also significant, looming challenges that are unlike those seen in the past. Examining the basics of the healthcare revenue cycle and taking innovative action is a critical activity for hospitals and physicians moving toward health reform. The following challenges are described by Bayley and colleagues (2013) and the Healthcare Information and Management Systems Society (HIMSS 2015):

- Impact of the health insurance exchange (HIX)

- More complex payment methodologies growing out of health reform goals

- Market dynamics shifting to consumer-driven health

- Limited access to capital needed for improvements in legacy systems

- Outdated business processes and revenue cycle silos

Impact of the Health Insurance Exchange

The Affordable Care Act (ACA) of 2010 created the health insurance exchange (HIX), which is an online marketplace where individuals can shop for insurance coverage and thereby avoid the shared responsibility payment requirement under ACA that is paid via the federal income tax return (Healthcare.gov 2016). Small employers may also shop for health insurance for their employees on the HIX.

While some may view the fact that approximately 30 million people who were previously uninsured (which accounted for more than two-thirds of hospital bad debt) are now insured via the HIX as positive, the changes can be a challenge to providers because it can be expected that reducing bad debt will require significantly more emphasis on collection—both at the front end of the revenue cycle with respect to co-pays and financial counseling for patients and at the back end in collecting balances due. This phenomenon affects both hospitals and physician offices. The American Medical Association (AMA) notes that the average amount due from patients at the time of visit is $110 and identifies that 25 percent of the average practice's revenue comes from direct patient payments (AMA n.d.). The AMA offers a point-of-care pricing toolkit that includes scripts for staff to talk with patients about their financial responsibilities and sample language to interact with health plans before collecting at the point of care. Levine and colleagues (2013) also note that expanded insurance coverage will probably not have a large impact on healthcare utilization, but those who can capture a disproportionate share of the increase can gain competitive advantage.

More Complex Payment Methodologies Growing Out of Health Reform Goals

As reimbursement moves from fee-for-service (FFS) to value-based payment (VBP; see chapter 4), another challenge faced by providers is that a much more complete understanding of the actual cost of care is needed. An understanding of how to attribute quality improvements to specific providers is necessary in order to allocate payments among providers (for example, among hospitals in an integrated delivery system, or among physicians in an office) in a VBP environment. To acquire this greater understanding, organizations must make capital investments in new technology that can integrate clinical and financial data, and hire persons with skills in data warehousing, actuarial, predictive modeling, and data visualization, which are typically not among the skills most hospitals or physician offices have.

Market Dynamics Shifting to Consumer-Driven Health

In the past, providers largely managed a "wholesale"-model of revenue cycle management with little emphasis on collecting from individuals. **Consumer-driven health**—where consumers must manage their health savings accounts, high-deductible health plans, debit card payments, and/or direct account payments—is shifting providers to a "retail" model that focuses on directly collecting from individuals (TripleTree 2006). Much as in the HIX movement, there are both positive and negative aspects to this shift. Consumers likely understand better the need to address payment upfront before a service is delivered. In the past, consumers paid more than twice as slowly as commercial payers, but they are more likely to pay more quickly as they assume greater responsibility (Bayley et al. 2013).

However, as consumers become more knowledgeable, so too must the provider. Providers must know in advance of services what the patients' share of payment is in order to manage collections. But even more so, providers must know what the total service is expected to cost. Consumers are more likely to shop around and will want to know the value (that is, clinical outcomes) of their expenditure. Consumers are also becoming savvy spenders. In fact, in some cases it is more cost-effective for patients to pay for a service than to have a claim go to an insurer. In a shared decision-making process, they may also be likely to weigh the cost and benefits of conservative versus aggressive treatment regimens. They will want to know what they can do to improve and preserve their health. The result is (hopefully) not only a more informed healthcare consumer, but a healthier consumer. To achieve this aim, providers must shift to a VBP system that reimburses for keeping people healthy rather than paying for ever more procedures. The ability to calculate the cost of services and patient responsibilities, however, can be even more challenging in a VBP system.

Limited Access to Capital Needed for Improvements in Legacy Systems

To effectively and efficiently manage their finances in the future, healthcare organizations likely need to invest in improvements to their existing (legacy) revenue cycle management systems. In addition, they will need new strategies to integrate clinical data from EHRs with financial data for population health. These significant needs are coming on the heels of significant health IT investments in moving to the HIPAA electronic transaction standard ASC X12 V 5010 in 2012, acquiring an EHR for the meaningful use (MU) incentive program that started in 2011, mandated adoption of operating rules in 2013 and beyond, the ICD-9-CM to ICD-10-CM/PCS transition in 2015, and an estimated 209,000 physicians being hit with 2 percent cuts in Medicare payments in 2016 for failing to meet MU requirements in 2014 (Pittman and Tahir 2016). While interest rates were relatively low in 2016, many organizations remained cautious with respect to making many new investments (HealthLeaders Media 2016). In addition to the capital investments already made for regulatory compliance and the recent frenzy of mergers and acquisitions, inpatient volume is decreasing, costs of care and payments under VBP models are not fully understood, not all states have addressed Medicaid expansion, and sizable bad debt are concerns (Ellison 2015).

Outdated Business Processes and Revenue Cycle Silos

Although new technology is needed to improve management of the revenue cycle, it cannot succeed without the institution of new business processes and changes in organizational structures and culture. Outdated business processes and revenue cycle silos are consistently identified in discussions of improvements needed in healthcare revenue cycle management. Bayley and colleagues (2013) characterize these issues as siloed functions, limited usefulness of current benchmark data, lack of standardized data definitions, and performance measurement time lags.

Those who manage the revenue cycle need a deep understanding of the revenue cycle and must ensure that all components are invested in and work together. HIMSS (2015) has brought together a revenue cycle improvement task force that represents a cross-section of the industry to create a vision for the next generation of revenue cycle management business processes and tools. Many organizations are looking at centralizing the revenue cycle processes, determining whether and how much to outsource, and instituting new performance measurement systems with clear metrics and timely reporting. The Healthcare Financial Management Association (HFMA) has developed a comprehensive revenue cycle strategy that it calls MAP (*measure* performance, *apply* evidence-based improvement strategies, and *perform* to the highest standards). HFMA's key performance indicators, called **MAP Keys**, have become the industry standard for measuring revenue cycle performance, with MAP awards being given for high-performing hospitals and physician practices (HFMA 2016). A list of the MAP Keys, their purpose, value, and equation for their calculation are supplied on the HFMA website.

Health IT Enhancements for HIPAA Financial and Administrative Transactions

In 2011, the Institute of Medicine (IOM; now Health and Medical Division [HMD] of the National Academies of Science, Engineering, and Medicine) conducted a roundtable on value- and science-driven healthcare. The topic was "The Healthcare Imperative: Lowering Costs and Improving Outcomes." In addition to Organisation for Economic Cooperation and Development (OECD) data cited in chapter 13 of this book, the IOM identified some stunning data, such as the following (Yong et al. 2011):

- Between 2000 and 2006, Medicare spending on imaging services more than doubled, with an over 25 percent increase in use of advanced imaging modalities despite the increased risks associated with such advanced imaging services.

- In several assessments of institutional and regional cost and volume of treatments variation, treatments that were 60 percent more expensive were found to have no quality advantage.

- Medicare spending per capita by hospital referral region varied more than threefold—from $5,000 to $16,000—and yet there appeared to be an inverse relationship between healthcare spending and quality scores.

As a result of these and many similar findings, the IOM explored the nature of excess health costs and the effectiveness of approaches to their control and set a goal to reduce healthcare costs by 10 percent within 10 years (by 2021) without compromising patient safety, health outcomes, or valued innovation. As the roundtable discussions were conducted, the IOM identified several prominent drivers for patterns of unnecessary costs. These included scientific uncertainty, perverse economic and practice incentives, system fragmentation, opacity as to cost and quality outcomes, changes in the population's health status, lack of patient engagement in decisions, and under-investment in population health. The IOM also identified the following key levers to address these drivers (Yong et al. 2011):

- Streamlined and harmonized health insurance regulation—which ultimately led to the ACA regulations to require health insurance for more people who were not covered by their employers, a government program, or another sponsor

- Administrative simplification and consistency—which, also under ACA, contributed to adopting operating rules for the HIPAA transactions that would "reduce the clerical burden on patients, health care providers, and health plans" (ACA 2010, section 1104)

- Payment redesign to focus incentives on results and value—which Medicare is aggressively pursuing and commercial health plans are rapidly implementing

- Quality and consistency in treatment, with a focus on the medically complex—which is associated with population health and stratifying patients at risk and improving their coordination of care

- Evidence that is timely, independent, and understandable—which is focusing on integrating financial and clinical data, improving data analytics, and utilizing data visualization tools at the point of care

HIPAA Transactions

While there are a number of tasks associated with each of the HIPAA financial and administrative transactions conducted between providers and health plans (for example, enrollment/disenrollment in a health plan, premium payment by an employer, eligibility verification, prior authorization, claims, claims attachments, claim status, remittance advice, and electronic funds transfer), the transactions and their standards and operating rules form the basic building blocks for revenue cycle management within a provider setting.

It is important to note that the terms *health plan* and *payer* are sometimes used interchangeably, but they can have very different meanings. The Public Health Service Act [(42 USC 300gg-91(a) (2)] provides the formal definition of **health plan** as adopted under HIPAA, which is an individual or group plan that provides, or pays the cost of, medical care. HIPAA regulations (45 CFR 160.103) provide a list of such types of individuals or group plans. Implicit is that a health plan establishes the policies for what services will be covered by the plan and what providers will be paid. **Payer** is a business that is engaged by a health plan to process payments on claims submitted by providers. This distinction is important because the HIPAA transaction standards accommodate a **Payer ID** that is not the same as the **health plan ID (HPID)** that has been required under HIPAA and is still undergoing regulatory development. Since health plans may be payers or hire others to perform this function, the following discussion uses the term *health plan,* which is consistent with such usage in HIPAA, to associate ultimate responsibility for compliance with the HIPAA transactions standards and operating rules to the health plan.

Transaction Standards

Standards for the financial and administrative transactions are adopted by federal regulation, based on recommendations by the National Committee on Vital and Health Statistics (NCVHS), which—among other responsibilities—has statutory oversight for HIPAA. As identified in chapter 13, the standards adopted for the financial and administrative transactions are primarily those from X12 Incorporated (formerly Accredited Standards Committee [ASC] X12). X12 develops and maintains standards for **electronic data interchange (EDI)** in business globally (X12 Incorporated 2016). EDI is the **point-to-point transmission** of business information in a standard electronic format between business partners (EDI Basics 2015), such as a provider and a health plan. The ASC X12 EDI standards adopted for healthcare transactions have been modified for use in healthcare business transactions. The name of each ASC X12 standard includes a number and a full name. For example, the ASC X12 standard for enrollment in a health plan is named ASC X12 834 Benefit Enrollment and Maintenance. Each standard also includes an **implementation guide** that explains intended usage and technicalities for the standard. The standards are updated on a regular basis, with the most current standard being V7030. However, for healthcare, each new version of the standard must be adopted by regulation. Originally, V4010 was adopted; as of January 1, 2012, the healthcare industry is now required to use V5010. It is not anticipated that a new version for health-care will be adopted until 2017 or 2018 (NCVHS 2015).

There is one current exception to the standards development organization used for the financial and administrative transactions. As required by ACA, a payment standard was adopted and required for use by January 1, 2014, for electronic funds transfer (EFT), which is produced by NACHA. **NACHA** (previously National Automated Clearing House Association) is a not-for-profit member-ship organization that comprises most of the nation's financial institutions. It is the administrator of the ACH (Automated Clearing House) Network, which is an electronic network for processing financial transactions. As the network administrator, it has developed standard processes for EFT, which have been modified for use in healthcare.

A second exception to the use of X12 standards is anticipated to be the use of a combination of the ASC X12 277 Health Care Claim Request for Information and the ASC X12 275 Addi-tional Information to Support a Health Care Claim or Encounter plus the Health Level 7 (HL7) CDA Rel. 2 and/or HL7 CDP1 (Clinical Documents for Payers Set 1), which is a repackaging of Consolidated-Clinical Document Architecture (C-CDA) sections with enhancements for claims attachments (NCVHS 2016).

Flow of Financial and Administrative Transactions

Figure 19.1 illustrates the flow of the financial and administrative transactions from the point an individual is enrolled in a health plan and premiums are paid by a sponsor to the point where pay-ment is deposited into a provider's bank account. The following sections describe this process and highlight issues associated with the current state of affairs.

Enrollment and Premium Payment

The flow of transactions begins when an employer or other sponsor contracts with a health plan to provide health insurance benefits for its employees (that is, insurance beneficiaries). The employer may then use the ASC X12 834 Enrollment transaction to enroll its employees in real time—although most employers have long been accustomed to using other means to enroll their employ-ees, including mailing health plan–provided forms in batches or supplying enrollment information

Figure 19.1.   Flow of financial and administrative transactions

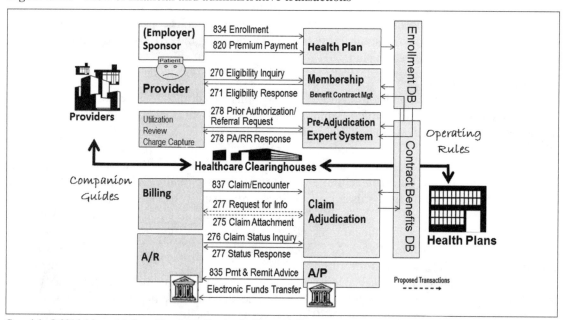

on a spreadsheet. This same transaction can also be used for **disenrollment** of an individual when that person is no longer employed or other circumstances preclude the individual from receiving health insurance benefits from the employer/sponsor. The employer/sponsor may make premium payments using the ASC X12 820 Premium Payment transaction, although, once again, premium payment using alternative manual/paper means has been and continues to be a well-established process that was also used prior to the HIPAA regulations.

While employers and payers are generally satisfied with the current manual processes, providers are increasingly concerned that health plans do not have current information about the status of individuals' health plan benefits. A chain reaction occurs when an employee leaves an employment setting and then seeks treatment from a provider a short time later. If the batch of disenrollment information does not reach the health plan for some time after the individual leaves and therefore the health plan cannot update its enrollment database system on a timely basis, the provider performing eligibility verification obtains inaccurate information from the health plan as to the individual's insurance benefits, treats the patient, files a claim, and is denied reimbursement. While some steps are being taken to require health plans to accept a claim within a defined window of time, the burden is often on the provider to negotiate for this. One recent development offers renewed hope this set of transactions may come to see greater traction. The Centers for Medicare and Medicaid Services (CMS) are requiring use of a form of these transactions by the HIX (ASC X12 2016).

Eligibility Inquiry and Response

Eligibility inquiry and response are also referred to as the *eligibility verification process*. Under this process, whenever a patient presents with insurance, the provider should use the ASC X12 270 Eligibility Inquiry in order to receive an ASC X12 271 Eligibility Response back to verify that the patient has insurance benefits as claimed.

Although providers are increasingly using the eligibility inquiry transaction in real time, the issue remains that the eligibility response transaction does not always provide sufficient information for the provider to work with the patient on making financial arrangements to make **point-of-service payments** for their **balance after insurance**—which may include the co-pay, any **deductible** amount that has not yet been fulfilled, and/or a **co-insurance** if the patient has a health insurance plan in which the patient owes a portion of the total bill, not just a co-pay and deductible (Matjucha and Giuliano 2011). For example, the provider may learn through the eligibility response that the patient has insurance but may not learn about the amount of the deductible the patient has yet to fulfill. If the patient has catastrophic coverage with a very large deductible that has not yet been fulfilled, the patient may not be able to pay out-of-pocket for treatment anticipated. High-deductible plans are increasing, with one survey finding that 25 percent of patients have a deductible of at least $1,000; and patients gaining insurance through the HIX have average deductibles from $2,567 and $4,343 (Gabriel 2014). Even for smaller amounts, such as might be charged for a prescription, a large co-pay or deductible—and increasingly co-insurance—significantly affects whether the patient will fill the prescription, or possibly cut the dose in half to reduce the cost.

Many providers are starting to conduct eligibility verification as soon as the patient makes an appointment or has an elective hospitalization scheduled. However, given the enrollment/disenrollment issue, providers also re-verify eligibility on the day the patient presents for service. Lack of reimbursement and poor outcomes for the patient are leading providers to also do a third verification at the time a claim is being readied for sending.

Many health plans have created web portals and/or call centers for providers to check eligibility. These portals often have more information than the eligibility response transaction provides. While providers are using these tools (often in conjunction with the eligibility inquiry—duplicating effort), there are also issues with both portals and call centers. Each portal requires a different log-in and has different navigational requirements that must be learned by the provider's staff. Call centers often limit the number of patients whose eligibility can be verified at one time. As a result of these issues, many physician offices—large and small—often do not verify eligibility for every patient seen every time, putting them and their patients at risk.

Prior Authorization Request and Response

The ASC X12 278 serves both as a request and a response. Prior to a claim being filed, some services—such as an expensive drug or procedure, or a referral to a special type of provider—require that additional information be sent to the health plan before it will authorize reimbursement. This process is often a part of the utilization review management called **precertification** in a managed care health plan environment (utilization review management is discussed in greater detail later in this chapter).

Managed care is a type of health insurance in which providers contract with health plans to provide care for members at reduced costs. Collectively, these providers make up the health plan's network. There are two main types of managed care plans as well as some hybrid versions. One major type is the **health maintenance organization (HMO)**, which usually pays only for care when patients stay within the network they have chosen. The other major type is the **preferred provider organization (PPO)**, which pays more if patients get care within their network but pays for a smaller part of the cost if patients go outside of their network. Managed care plans generally cost patients less than plans where there are no restrictions. For providers, the benefit of a managed care plan is the source of patients it supplies.

While providers could use the ASC X12 278 to request an authorization, the request usually entails supplying additional information. Until recently with the MU incentives for adopting an EHR, this additional information was available only on paper, so most providers would simply send a request on paper, or supply scanned images of paper through a portal, in an e-mail attachment, or by other transmission means. Today, providers typically have to print the required information from their EHRs to send the health plan because the health plan often does not have a system compatible with accepting an electronic document in the form sent by the provider. Most health plans respond in writing to such requests, and the response is then stored in the business office or scanned into a business office document imaging system. When a Claim Attachment standard is federally adopted, it is likely that the Claim Attachment transaction will be used to process more prior authorization requests electronically from start to finish using the Claim Attachment transaction for this purpose, in addition to its primary purpose of supplying additional information for claim adjudication.

Claim

The ASC X12 834 Claim (which is available for institutions, providers, and dentists) is the most widely used of the transaction standards because Medicare, under the Administrative Simplification Compliance Act of 2000, started requiring the use of the transaction by all Medicare providers in 2002 (with an extension to October 1, 2003). It should be noted here that HIPAA considers only those providers who perform any of the transactions electronically to be covered providers under HIPAA. Although covered providers do not have to perform the transactions electronically, they must use the regulated standards if they do. However, all health plans must use the electronic transaction standards for any types of transactions they perform. Requiring all Medicare providers to use the electronic claim—and hence the ASC X12 834—caused the vast majority of providers who were previously noncovered providers to become covered providers. However, providers are not required to use any of the other transactions in electronic form. Many small providers do not do so still to this day.

At this time, there are some issues with the claims transaction, although not as many as with the other transactions. One issue is that many Medicaid programs are far behind in adopting the ASC X12 standards. As of this writing, some still use the ASC V4010 standard, even though it does not accommodate ICD-10-CM codes. Another issue relates to when **coordination of benefits** must be conducted between health plans, most often between a primary health plan (usually a commercial payer) and a secondary health plan, such as Medicaid. Although the

ASC X12 Claim supports information for coordination of benefits, most providers find it easier to send this information on paper because of issues with providing proof of which health plan is primary. Coordination of benefits issues account for the large majority of the 10 percent of claims filed on paper.

CAQH, which is described in the discussion of operating rules later in this chapter, has developed a tool, called COB Smart, that is a registry of up-to-date and complete coverage information that can quickly and accurately direct coordination of benefits processes. This tool has been field-tested successfully by Blue Cross and Blue Shield of North Carolina and Kaiser Permanente (CAQH 2015).

Another issue that has not affected transactions usage, but is a growing concern among providers, is that many providers do not accept or process more than a limited number of ICD-10-CM/PCS codes, even though the V5010 claim can accommodate many more codes than the V4010. As VBP models become increasingly popular, it will be essential for providers to have a full understanding of a patient's condition and treatments. It has also been suggested that health plan use of the full set of diagnoses and procedures codes could reduce the volume of claims attachment requests (Rode 2015).

Request for Information and Claim Attachment

The **request for information** and **claim attachment** set of transactions is intended to be used when a health plan finds it cannot adjudicate a claim without additional information. The health plan would send an ASC X12 277 Request for Information, and the provider would supply the additional information via the ASC X12 275 Claim Attachment.

At this time, however, these two transactions have not been officially adopted for use by the federal government. Instead, these transactions are largely processed manually. Some providers may be able to anticipate the need for additional information and send the information with the claim (this is called an **unsolicited attachment**). There is a field in the ASC X12 Claim that allows a provider to indicate that there is an "attachment." However, because there is no currently adopted standard to associate or send an electronic attachment with the claim and to avoid filing a duplicate claim, which is fraudulent, the ASC X12 Claim requiring an attachment is often removed from the batch before transmission, printed, and mailed with the additional information. Health plans have observed that in many cases they do not need these unsolicited attachments, and receiving them disrupts their workflow. They would prefer to initiate the request for an attachment only when needed.

However, if the provider does not submit additional information with the claim and the health plan determines additional information is necessary to adjudicate the claim, the plan will deny the claim and send the provider a request for additional information (that is, a **solicited attachment**). This latter situation not only delays payment but also puts payment at risk if the health plan denies the service given the additional information. These concerns are why many providers try to anticipate what additional information may be needed.

In addition to delays and reimbursement risk, the attachment process is cumbersome and costly for both health plans and providers. An unpublished survey conducted for CAQH CORE found that 70 percent of attachments were mailed to health plans on paper and another 20 percent were transmitted to health plans via a portal as a scanned image. The remaining 10 percent were transmitted using some form of industry-neutral or proprietary transmission mode, such as FTP, or a compact disk (often when a copy of an entire health record is sent), or as an e-mail attachment (Amatayakul and Lazarus 2014). Many times, when paper is received by the health plan, it is scanned into a document imaging system.

Clearly, there is a need for an attachment standard that enables electronic transmission to be associated with the claim, the request for additional information, or the prior authorization request. Ideally, there should also be transparency in claims adjudication processes that would enable claims attachments to truly be attached to the claim rather than requiring a request sent later. This ideal situation, however, does not have any bearing on what transactions standards are used, and it is not something the federal government can regulate. There are some provider organizations that have reached agreements with their health plans about what claims require attachments to somewhat better manage this process.

A final concern with respect to claims attachments relates to the HIPAA Privacy Rule: because health plans may not be specific about their needs or the provider is uncertain about the health plans' needs for additional information, there is the risk that more than the minimum necessary information is sent. (See chapter 12 for more information on the Privacy Rule.)

Claim Status Inquiry and Response

The **claims status inquiry and response** set of transactions is the third most popular set of transactions used—essentially because of the issues with claims previously described, as well as the fact that, while ASC X12 offers two forms of Acknowledgement standards, they were not anticipated by Congress when HIPAA was enacted and have not been adopted by regulation—even though Medicare and come commercial health plans use acknowledgements broadly. The ASC X12 999 Acknowledgement for Healthcare Insurance Transaction is used to notify a provider that any functional group of *any* transaction set is accepted, accepted with errors, or rejected (that is, the ASC X12 999 is an acknowledgement for not only claims but also the end of any set of transactions). The ASC X12 277CA Claim Acknowledgement set is used to acknowledge *each claim* received in a Functional Group only when the transaction set (of claims) is not rejected (Jackson 2010). Providers are often concerned as to whether claims have been received by the health plan, or what is causing a delay in payment. The claim numbers received in the ASC X12 277CA may be used to make future claim status inquiries about those claims.

Similar to the eligibility verification process, however, the ASC X12 claim status transaction generally does not supply as much information as a portal or call center; hence, the issues in using this set of transactions are the same as for the eligibility transactions. Many believe, however, that this set of transactions may not be necessary at all if the previously described transactions were fully and properly utilized and Acknowledgement standards were in place.

Payment and Remittance Advice

Originally, **payment and remittance advice** was one transaction, the ASC X12 835 Payment and Remittance Advice, which supplied information about what payment was made on which claims. The intent was for a provider's billing system or practice management system (PMS) to receive this advice, reconcile the amounts with the provider's accounts receivables, and post payments—which should then reconcile with the provider's statement of deposits from a bank or other financial institution. Unfortunately, there is not a one-to-one correlation between a batch of claims the provider sends and the payments documented on a given remittance advice from the health plan. Some claims out of a batch sent by a provider may be held pending receipt of additional information. As a result, the reconciliation process was often cumbersome and difficult to manage electronically. As noted earlier, ACA recognized this issue and therefore mandated the adoption of an EFT standard for healthcare payments, which went into effect on January 1, 2014. The **Healthcare Electronic Funds Transfer-Remittance Advice** standard includes a requirement for a **reassociation trace number** to be used on the EFT and the **electronic remittance advice (ERA)** so it is be easier to reconcile payments. The EFT also enables funds to flow more rapidly to the provider's bank.

Unfortunately, there have been issues with the new standard from both the EFT and the ERA perspective. A number of providers became concerned about giving health plans their bank's routing number, believing that potentially the health plan would be able not only to put money into the account, but take out overpayments. Banks have reassured providers that only those who are authorized to withdraw funds are able to do so.

Another issue is that a number of health plans interpreted EFT to include not only the direct transmission of funds from a health plan's bank to a provider's bank but also the use of **virtual cards,** also called *payment cards*. The title of a blog post on the topic—"Virtual card payments to healthcare providers: Villainous or valuable?" (Haug 2015)—suggests the controversy surrounding such use. A number of provider associations have complained that providers were not given a choice, or sufficient information about the choices, for accepting virtual cards. NACHA (2014a) has supported providers in their concerns, citing excessive costs for use of the virtual card, higher risk for card number theft, manual entry requirements necessitated by the cards, the lack of the reassociation trace number in the card process, and slower time for the funds to reach the provider's bank.

Others describe benefits of these cards, such as associated rebates for use of the cards and no requirement for providers to enroll with individual health plans for EFT processing that they do not frequently use—although CAQH now offers a resource for providers to use for supplying EFT enrollment information one time, called EnrollHub (see under operating rules, later in the chapter). Those who describe the benefits of virtual cards, however, also acknowledge cost considerations for using the cards and the longer processing time between the provider's merchant account and bank. It is important for any provider to weigh the benefits and risks of each type of payment. Health plans must provide EFT payments if requested by the provider, and, by law, providers cannot be charged an interchange fee for receiving an EFT transaction from a health plan (Grosze 2015).

A final issue associated with the new remittance advice standard is that some billing system and PMS vendors have not yet updated their systems to accommodate the enhanced features that improve claim-payment reconciliation.

Companion Guides and Healthcare Clearinghouses

To complete an understanding of the flow of financial and administrative transactions, it is important to note two factors in their use relating to companion guides and healthcare clearinghouses that also contribute to administrative cost in healthcare.

Much as the HL7 V2 standards include optionality in their use (see figure 13.4 in chapter 13), the ASC X12 standards include situational data content. While *optionality* means fully discretionary, *situational* means reliance on context to determine whether or not situational data are required. For example, use of a middle initial for a patient may be optional in HL7 (that is, the middle initial is not required for use, whether or not it is known), but situational in ASC X12 (that is, if the middle initial is known, it must be used). However, determining what is situational can be open to interpretation. Such interpretation is often codified by a health plan in documents called companion guides. **Companion guides** provide the technical information and instructions for how providers must compile and transmit transactions to the specific health plan. Some of this information is critical and understandable—such as the Internet Protocol (IP) address to use to submit a batch of claims, or who is the primary contact person at the claims processing site in the event of needing live technical support. However, these instructions have also addressed format and content changes that many believe thwart the interoperability of the standards (Krager and Krager 2008).

Because any given provider must comply not only with the standard and its implementation guide but also with multiple different health plan companion guides, and transmit transactions in a point-to-point manner to many different locations, **healthcare clearinghouses** emerged a number of years ago to manage these transmissions. When the HIPAA transaction standards were first mandated, the healthcare clearinghouses also helped ease the transition from the old Uniform Bill (UB) and HCFA/CMS 1500 standard forms to the ASC X12 electronic standards by converting nonstandard transactions sent from a provider into standard transactions to be sent to the health plan in compliance with HIPAA. (In some cases, healthcare clearinghouses would also convert the standard transactions from the provider back to a nonstandard transaction format required by health plans that had not yet updated their systems.) HIPAA included the healthcare clearinghouse in its designation of covered entities because of the processing performed by such entities and to ensure their Privacy Rule and Security Rule compliance. While the costs of such conversions may seem to be unnecessary, these costs must be compared with the cost to completely upgrade information systems. Clearinghouses also offer a number of value-added services that aid other aspects of the revenue cycle. Ensuring that the claim is in conformance with health plan companion guide requirements, for instance, is part of claims reviews and edits; clearinghouse connectivity to thousands of health plans can manage large-batch eligibility verification or just-in-time eligibility verification.

Figure 19.2 illustrates use of healthcare clearinghouses. While the vast majority of providers use a healthcare clearinghouse, a few may transmit certain transactions directly to a health plan, or to a health plan's clearinghouse (denoted by the dashed lines in figure 19.2). Most health plans also use a clearinghouse (denoted by the dotted lines in figure 19.2), but some transactions will be transmitted directly to a health plan via the provider's healthcare clearinghouse (denoted by double lines in figure 19.2).

HIPAA Operating Rules

Although savings have accrued from use of the financial and administrative transactions where it is more feasible for providers to exchange electronic transactions directly, it is still estimated that the US healthcare delivery system spends 15 percent to 32 percent of each healthcare dollar on administrative costs (with variance in estimates due to variations in what is included in the definition of administrative costs). The current costs are split evenly between providers and health plans, and not all are associated directly with the financial and administrative transactions; however, it is estimated that savings of as much as $8 billion annually could be achieved with full implementation of the electronic transactions, with $7.2 billion of the savings accruing to providers (CAQH CORE and AHA 2013).

These potential savings have been demonstrated in part by voluntary adoption of operating rules developed by the CAQH CORE (AHA 2016). Originally called the Council on Affordable Quality Healthcare, CAQH was formed by a number of major health plans, representing 40 percent of all commercially insured lives in the United States, to address improvements that could be achieved by health plan standardization of certain processes. In 2005, the CAQH created the Committee on Operating Rules for Information Exchange (CORE) with a board that has equal representation between

Figure 19.2.   Healthcare clearinghouse usage by providers and health plans

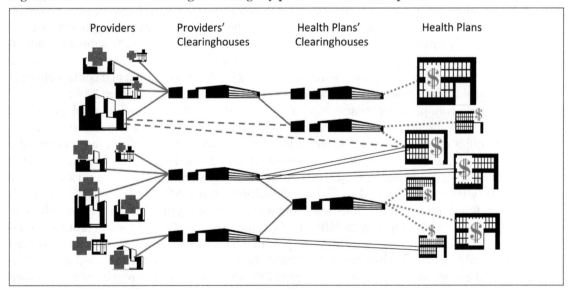

providers and health plans and also includes representatives of healthcare clearinghouses and vendors. CAQH CORE initially was focused on creating and maintaining operating rules relating to the HIPAA transactions used in the FFS environment. It first created operating rules for eligibility and claim status transactions. It next created operating rules for EFT and ERA transactions. These were voluntarily adopted through a formal certification process offered by CAQH CORE that proved highly successful. Under ACA, use of the rules for EFT and ERA transactions was mandated, and regulations required their adoption in 2013 and 2014, respectively, for all health plans and providers that used the specific electronic transactions. A final set of operating rules for the claim, prior authorization, enrollment, and premium payment were created in 2015 and are being proposed to the NCVHS for federal regulatory adoption (NCVHS 2016). CAQH CORE is now also focusing on administrative simplification for the VBP environment.

Operating rules provide the business rules that help drive consistency in connectivity, security of transmissions, response time for batch and real time transmissions, system availability, exception processing and error resolution (including rules for use of the Acknowledgement standards), roles and responsibilities for all business partners, and guidelines for companion guides (collectively referred to as *infrastructure operating rules*). They also provide support for uniform use of structured content specified in the standards and their (medical and nonmedical) code sets. Operating rules for the HIPAA transactions do not change or alter the HIPAA transaction standards, but the rules afford consistency in how the standards are used. Operating rules also do not entirely supplant the need for companion guides with respect to certain aspects of transmission instructions, but the rules do significantly reduce variation.

Check Your Understanding 19.1

Match the terms with their description of impact:

    A. Acknowledgement

    B. Claim status inquiry

    C. Companion guide

    D. Consumer-driven care

    E. Coordination of benefits

    F. Eligibility and benefits verification

    G. Enrollment and premium payment

    H. Healthcare clearinghouse

    I. Health insurance exchange

    J. Implementation guide

    K. Key performance indicators

    L. Operating rules

    M. Payer

    N. Prior authorization request

1. Patients are paying larger share of healthcare costs

2. Driving bad debt down

3. Drives evidence-based improvement in revenue cycle management

4. Business associate that manages payment distribution

5. Key to accurate eligibility information

6. Used for utilization review

7. Enables point-of-service payment

8. Explains intended usage and provides instructions for use of a transaction standard

9. Main cause of filing claims on paper

10. Not a required standard transaction under HIPAA

11. Provides instructions specific to conducting transactions with a health plan

12. Aids transmission of electronic data interchange standards

13. Supports furtherance of administrative simplification use of transaction standards

14. Transaction largely necessitated by lack of acknowledgements

Revenue Cycle Management and Opportunities for Enhancement with Health IT

Although the HIPAA transactions form the basic building blocks for revenue cycle management, there is more to revenue cycle management than the transactions. With health reform and other challenges facing the industry, it is imperative to take a solid look at the basics of financial accounting and the steps that can be taken to improve revenue cycle management with better information and other technical and nontechnical solutions.

Basics of Financial Accounting

To fully understand the revenue cycle, it is helpful to have a basic understanding of financial accounting. Figure 19.3 summarizes the sources of revenue for a provider, which today are heavily driven by the volume of patients and types of services provided; the nature of the health plan reimbursement structures for which the provider contracts; and the types of plans patients have in the community in which the provider operates. A provider organization must keep an income statement that clearly demonstrates its revenue and expenses, and it must record its assets and liabilities/equity on a balance sheet. There are many nuances to recording financial information on such financial statements, including—for example—when and how bad debt and charity care are recorded (HFMA 2012). These two basic financial statements help identify opportunities for improvement, and their use is often supplemented by the use of additional financial processes and presentations. Two very important tools for this purpose are cost accounting and accounts receivable (A/R) management.

   Cost accounting identifies the costs of products and services so those costs can be accurately reported on financial statements and used to evaluate an organization's possible courses of action. Many providers do not conduct cost accounting because of the variable nature of the services they provide; however, cost accounting is not just a way to document costs. It is also a process

Figure 19.3.   Basics of provider financial accounting

	Employer/Sponsor Individual	Provider
Health plan(s)	-Enrolls in a desired type of plan based on cost/benefit analysis -Pays premiums	Enrolls in and contracts with plans based on reimbursement rates offered and potential volume of patients
Provider	Pays providers: -Co-pays -Deductibles -Co-insurance -Self-pay	Earns revenue from: -Fee for service payments -Managed care payments -Value-based payments -Patient collections

Provider Financial Statements	
Income Statement	Balance Sheet

Gross revenue
  -Professional fees less patient & insurance refunds
  -Product sales less cost of goods sold
Net revenue
	Assets
	  -Cash -by age
	  -Accounts receivable: -by plan
	  -Inventory -by patient
	  -Property, plant, equipment

Expenses
  -Staff payroll & benefits
  -Provider compensation
  -Rent/lease, utilities, supplies
  -Office/IT expenses
Net income
	Liabilities & Equity
	  -Payroll
	  -Accounts payable
	  -Loans
	  -Retirement contributions
	Owner's equity

improvement technique. Providers moving toward VBPs must understand their costs to be able to reduce them. For example, Michelson (2014) cites a study that found that only 20 percent of orthopedic surgeons can accurately estimate the cost of common implantables within 20 percent of the actual cost, but 80 percent of those surveyed would incorporate cost information into their decisions if they had it. Michelson also describes a survey published by the American Medical Association that concluded that when physicians are presented with costs information for laboratory tests, they drove down laboratory costs by 25 percent.

Thus, cost accounting helps generate the income statement. Income is the net result of revenue minus expenses. It is the amount a practice has to compensate providers, contribute to retirement funds, and invest in new services and products. Knowing costs associated with insurance refunds, such as discounts offered providers for enrolling in a plan as well as the costs borne by patients that may not be able to be collected, can reduce expenses and improve the likelihood of more professional fees revenue being retained as income. Similarly, understanding costs associated with "product sales" (for example, implantables, laboratory tests, and others) also improves income.

Accounts receivable is the amount of money owed to a provider for services and supplies provided. Obviously, a provider should understand what services and supplies cost to provide in order to seek an appropriate level of reimbursement. At a minimum, A/R information should be presented by age (that is, time since costs were billed—for example, 30, 60, and 90 days), type of plan (Medicare, Medicaid, Blues, commercial FFS, commercial managed care, and many others), and the **case mix** (that is, the distribution of patients into categories reflecting differences in severity of illness or resource consumption). Once the domain of health plans only, providers are now applying **actuarial models** (statistical techniques for predicting financial risk) to their case mix to assess and plan for the financial impact of various types of risk (for example, tighter reimbursement rates offered by health plans, age of population in the community, impact of a major employer going out of business, and savings that may be accrued by entering into a VBP model).

Revenue Cycle Management Components

Revenue cycle management reflects the systems development life cycle (SDLC) not only with respect to the series of steps taken when a patient presents for service through collecting payment but also encompassing the feedback mechanism supplied by data that come from these tasks feeding into contract negotiation that initiates a relationship with a health plan for payment. Figure 19.4 illustrates the components of revenue cycle management.

Revenue cycle management components are often categorized as *front end* (those conducted prior to a claim being submitted) or *back end* (those conducted after a claim has been submitted). However, these distinctions are being eliminated as front-end staff members need to appreciate that their work directly affects the results of what can be accomplished in back-end processes. Similarly, some of the back-end processes must be available to and performed by those engaged in what has been traditionally considered front-end processing. The following is a brief summary of the various components of the revenue cycle, with an emphasis on health IT tool requirements.

Contract Negotiation

Contract negotiation is the process taken to establish reimbursement levels and other provisions, such as prior authorization requirements and payment terms, in order to forecast financial results

Figure 19.4. Revenue cycle management components

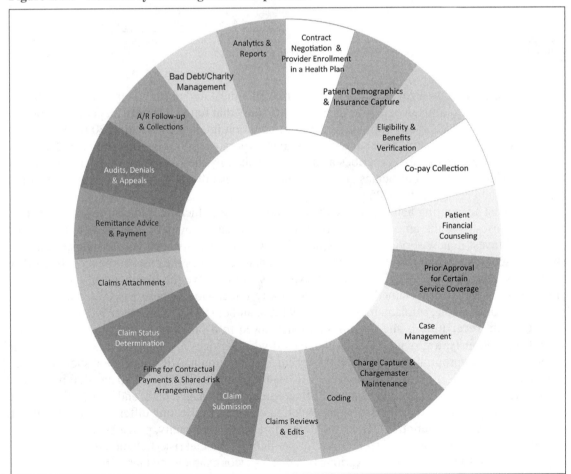

from a given health plan. In general, most providers have contracts with a variety of payers in order to optimize their potential patient pool and improve their revenue stream.

Negotiating a contract up front (usually annually, although increasingly under health reform on a five-year cycle) can be time-consuming, labor-intensive, and outright unpleasant, but the process is easier than managing payment terms on a case-by-case basis for out-of-plan patients (Davis 2011). When entering contract negotiation with a health plan, providers should prepare thoroughly, encourage collaboration, and be willing to compromise—but in a win-win mode (Vega n.d.).

An extremely important aspect of contract negotiation is the collection and analysis of information that enables the provider to demonstrate value (that is, cost and quality) and an understanding of the market that differentiates the provider from others. For example, a provider who can point to the fact that a certain health plan has historically attracted individuals who are less likely to pay their balance after insurance should be able to negotiate for increased reimbursement rates. Under health reform, these negotiations will become even more complex, with providers needing comprehensive information and predictive models to help them determine the level of risk they can assume for a bigger share of the savings. Hospitals are typically accustomed to such negotiations, whereas physicians have been generally more timid but are learning the importance of negotiating (Jones and Mills 2006).

Part of the contract negotiation process is physician enrollment in health plans—which is essentially a credentialing process for physicians. Physician enrollment is often a lengthy process, potentially taking months to perform. It is also a very repetitive process, with much of the information required for each health plan being the same, but potentially in a different format. Streamlining this function would also enable providers to keep the information up to date. To address this issue, CAQH developed CAQH ProView, a database where providers enter and maintain their credentialing information and authorize health plans to retrieve the data they need. CAQH also offers SanctionsTrack, a database that tracks healthcare provider licensure disciplinary actions.

Patient Demographics and Insurance Capture

Patient demographics and insurance capture begin the revenue cycle management process at the provider site. This step is often referred to as *patient registration* or *admissions* and has been the traditional starting point of "front-end" processing. Staff involved in registration and admission must be alert to red flags that could signal potential medical identity theft. Therefore, registration or admission includes verifying the patient's identification (for example, by checking or making a copy of the patient's government-issued photo identification and, often, taking a photo of the patient to be retained in the EHR) and confirming insurance coverage. These tasks can also be aided by health IT that provides a checklist for staff, a process for retention of patient photographs, and decision support that provides red-flags support. (For more information on red flags, see chapter 12.)

Patient registration or admission is also the time when staff should begin collection of patient co-pays and discuss with patients how they will meet any further financial obligations—which must be coordinated with eligibility and benefits verification. Of course, if a patient presents without insurance, the patient should be referred directly to financial counseling. (Eligibility and benefits verification and financial counseling are covered later in this chapter.)

Several of the responsibilities described here are new for registration/admission staff, and so retraining is necessary. Retraining needs to be done in a way that staff will retain their helpful and caring attitudes, but be firm in their obligations as part of the revenue cycle team. For example, many people who work in admissions in hospitals know that the Emergency Medical Treatment and Labor Act (EMTALA) requires emergency departments to stabilize a patient regardless of insurance or ability to pay, but they do not understand how this law might apply to admission of patients without insurance in nonemergency situations. Health IT can help provide a script for staff to use in working through these issues.

Many physician offices find that revenue cycle management actually starts at scheduling, when patients can be advised of their need to bring positive patient identification and their insurance information and be prepared to pay their co-pay. If a patient does not have insurance, the provider must have a policy on whether the patient will be referred elsewhere or required to pay a significant portion of their financial obligation up front. It is also important to determine whether and how staff may record reasons for visit in the EHR, as this entry initiates a "paper trail" that could cause problems in billing at the back end if it does not accurately reflect the visit.

For returning patients, scheduling is also the time to provide reminders about some of their preventive service needs and to ensure, when applicable, that they get their laboratory work done in advance of the visit. These processes can improve the health of patients and may contribute to revenue generation. To perform these processes, however, the EHR must feed or be integrated with the scheduling system or the scheduling component in a PMS. Decisions must also be made about what preventive services reminders will be offered by the scheduling staff. If scheduling is done electronically through a patient portal, these reminders need to be provided directly to the patient at the time of appointment scheduling.

Eligibility and Benefits Verification

Eligibility and benefits verification was introduced in the previous discussion of the transactions standards. If eligibility and benefits verification is performed in physician offices, it is often done in batch mode the day before patients are scheduled to be seen. Hospitals may do eligibility and benefits verification earlier, at the time an elective admission is scheduled. However, typically, 50 percent of patients are admitted through the emergency department (Merrill 2013), and coverage for these patients must be verified in real time. To start the payment collection process, information gathered during the eligibility and benefits verification process must be accessible to staff who will actually register or admit the patient. Issues in eligibility and benefits verifications for both hospitals and physician offices have been found to contribute to as much as 30 percent to 40 percent of claims denials (Bayley et al. 2013).

Co-pay Collection

The practice of collecting co-pays upfront is not new, but, historically, collection was more often done at the back end. When a provider attempts to collect co-pays after the patient is discharged or leaves an office, it is less likely that the fees will be collected, and collection costs increase (Matjucha and Giuliano 2011). To have effective point of service (POS) collections, eligibility and benefits verification information must be accurate. Provider policies must be very clear about what staff should say and do in the event the patient does not want to or cannot pay upfront, questions the amount, wants more information than is available, or has another issue regarding the co-pay. Scripts embedded in PMSs for talking to patients are extremely helpful to staff handling these issues.

Patient Financial Counseling

Patient financial counseling should be available to patients who are unable to make their co-pay and/or who seem to be at risk for not paying their balance after insurance. The counseling may be as simple as offering a payment plan, while still attempting to collect some portion of what is due up front. Offering small discounts for early payment, especially when payments are in the form of cash, can be a good strategy because it costs the provider less to give a discount than it would to collect payment on the back end (Owens 2013).

Patient financial counseling may also require engaging social services in arranging for public assistance and other types of financial support. Again, it is the patient registration/admission staff member who must be prepared to have the initial conversation with the patient or family and know when to refer patients to others for more in-depth support.

Prior Authorization (Precertification)

Prior authorization for coverage of specific services, now more commonly referred to as *precertification*, was described in the discussion of the standard transactions and is required in many contractual requirements with commercial health plans (or, if there is no contract, to credential the provider and authorize payment for an out-of-plan patient). Requirements for when a service must be authorized in advance will vary with the nature of the service. It may occur prior to a patient being admitted to a hospital (admission review) or when a patient is referred to a specialist physician office (specialty care review). In other cases, precertification occurs after an examination of the patient reveals the necessity for the service.

Case Management

Case management refers to a collection of services including utilization management, discharge planning, and care coordination performed by a case manager. It is required by many commercial health plans in their managed care contracts as well as by Medicare and Medicaid.

The purpose of case management is to ensure that care being delivered is medically necessary, appropriate, and aligned with clinical best practices. Such steps should reduce denial of payment. The insurance company Cigna (2016) offers a comprehensive definition of medical necessity that is similar to the definition used by many other insurers:

> Healthcare services that a physician, exercising prudent clinical judgment, would provide to a patient for the purpose of evaluating, diagnosing or treating an illness, injury, disease or its symptoms, and that are:
>
> - In accordance with the generally accepted standards of medical practice (i.e., based on credible scientific evidence, physician specialty society recommendations, view of physicians practicing in the relevant clinical areas, and any other relevant factors)
> - Clinically appropriate, in terms of type, frequency, extent, site and duration, and considered effective for the patient's illness, injury or disease, and
> - Not primarily for the convenience of the patient or physician, or other physician, and not more costly than an alternative service or sequence of services as likely to produce equivalent therapeutic or diagnostic results

Case managers are frequently nurses and are often supported by a committee of physicians, nurses, and others. They are responsible for ensuring that the provider documents in the EHR substantial information about the medical necessity for a patient's admission and continued stay, as well as the comprehensive discharge plan.

Forms of health IT that can facilitate case management include various data discovery tools, access to evidence-based guidance, predictive modeling tools that can look back at experiential information to predict areas on which to focus, and even customer relationship management tools—where the customers include patients/family members and contacts for transition-of-care services, such as long term and post-acute care (LTPAC) providers, social services, pharmacies, transportation services, and others (Miodonski 2012).

Utilization Review

Utilization review is the component of case management that requires health plans to receive clinical reviews of inpatient care that provide sufficient information for the health plan to make a determination of medical necessity. Such a determination may require that the patient's physician confer with the health plan's medical director. Some hospitals also have case management committees where the case manager can bring cases where there is disagreement about medical necessity for reconciliation prior to conferring with the health plan's medical director. Medical necessity determination is part of admission review, and it also includes classifying patients as observation or inpatient status, early discharge planning, and concurrent review.

Utilization review is also performed for readmissions. In 2013, hospitals were penalized 1 percent of their Medicare reimbursement when patients with myocardial infarction, congestive heart failure, or pneumonia were readmitted within 30-days of discharge. Penalties for 30-day readmissions increased to 2 percent in 2014 and 3 percent in 2015. Beginning in 2016, Medicare added chronic obstructive pulmonary disease and total hip or knee replacements to the list of diagnoses to which 30-day readmission penalties apply. In 2017, 30-day readmissions penalties will also apply to sepsis or respiratory failure with a secondary diagnosis of pneumonia. In fiscal 2015, 78 percent of hospitals eligible for such a penalty (2,665 of 3,400) were penalized (Rice 2015).

Discharge Planning

Discharge planning, as noted previously, should begin upon admission in order to avoid unnecessary extension of the length of stay, which usually results in denials of care and lengthy and often unsuccessful appeals processes. Execution of a discharge plan and provision for transition of care to other levels of service according to medical necessity are essential elements of discharge planning.

Care Coordination

Care coordination is process by which the patient's physician, hospital care team, and health plan case manager work together to ensure that a patient's hospital stay is not extended unnecessarily. Care coordination is most intense for high-risk patients and then also includes discharge follow-up to ensure that services such as home healthcare and medical supplies are delivered, prescriptions are filled and being taken, and other services to reduce readmission and improve chances for a healthy recovery or health improvement are made available as needed.

Drug Utilization Review

Drug utilization review is designed to promote patient safety. Health plans, such as Medicaid, conduct prospective screening of prescription drug claims to identify therapeutic duplication, drug-disease contraindications, incorrect dosage or duration of treatment, drug allergy, and clinical misuse or abuse. Plans also use retrospective reviews to identify patterns of fraud, abuse, gross overuse, or medically unnecessary care (CMS 2015a).

Charge Capture

Charge capture is the entry of items charged into an accounting system as well as clinical documentation in the health record to substantiate the claim. Entering items into an accounting system requires cataloging the supplies and services and their charges available from the organization, appropriately charging for and documenting usage of the supplies and services, and reconciling all services provided to patients (Wexler and Bucci 2016).

A **charge description master**, also called a **chargemaster**, is the cataloging in a database of all the supplies and services provided to patients and the corresponding charges for those items. It must be accurately maintained on a timely basis in order to enable a facility to capture and record patient charges as they are incurred. It also supports budgeting by providing statistics on use and affords an understanding of profitability by comparing charges to costs (Davis 2011).

Clinical Documentation Improvement and Coding

Clinical documentation improvement (CDI) is the function of improving the quality of clinical documentation. One particular aim of CDI is to ensure the complete and accurate reporting of diagnoses and procedures, especially to meet revenue cycle goals such as submission of clean claims and reduction in days in A/R (Haas 2013; Arrowood et al. 2015). A CDI program is often multidisciplinary, including health information management (HIM) professionals, physicians, and nurses. A CDI program undertakes concurrent and retrospective reviews of the health record and includes activities both to improve documentation globally for all patients and to ensure complete and compliant documentation for medical necessity and coding of each individual patient's health record. The latter function is aided by nonleading queries to physicians to address present indicators of an undocumented condition, request further specificity or degree of severity of a document condition, clarify a potential cause-and-effect relationship, and address hospital-acquired conditions (HAC)–present on admission (POA) issues (Bryant et al. 2010). AHIMA Guidance for Clinical Documentation Program (Bryant et al. 2010) notes that CDI can reduce compliance risks, minimize a healthcare facility's vulnerability during external audits, and provide insight into legal quality of care issues.

The "back-end" revenue cycle processes start with coding, and sometimes CDI when performed only retrospectively. Coding is "the process of assigning numeric or alphanumeric representations to clinical documentation" (AHIMA 2014). Examples of these representations would be ICD-10-CM/PCS or Current Procedural Terminology (CPT).

The fragmentary nature of coding can be difficult to manage. Accurate and complete coding may be aided by various types of encoder and computer-assisted coding software, clinical messaging systems, and access to educational and regulatory requirements. Easterling (2015) describes the importance of delving deeper into understanding different payment structures in order to move forward in a quality/risk-adjusted environment. This process should begin with coordinating coding and CDI with quality measure abstraction. It can be helpful to coders if they fully understand what measures are being required, and to abstractors to understand the coding process.

Use of ICD-10-CM codes contributes to successful documentation practices for CMS quality reporting, accuracy of coding for the HAC-POA program (Snow et al. 2012; Diop 2015), pay-for-performance, VBP, data used for decision making in healthcare reform, and other national reporting initiatives (Leventhal 2014). The transition to ICD-10-CM in coding has been considered a "non-event," with the Cooperative Exchange noting that sufficient planning, education, testing, and industry collaboration helped significantly (Spivey 2015).

Coding is often outsourced. Murphy (2015) found that 50 percent of healthcare systems worked with one or two coding vendors and 45 percent worked with seven or more vendors.

Claims Reviews and Edits

The process of checking claims against each health plan's specific rules and making changes to produce "clean claims" and reduce the likelihood that claims are denied due to errors is known as **claims reviews and edits**, or **claims scrubbing**. The claims-scrubbing process not only looks at coding but also checks data entry and other potential types of issues with a claim (Greene 2015). For example, it will look for a CMS POA indicator on a claim, which is necessary to group diagnoses into their proper diagnosis-related group (DRG) (CMS 2015b). DRGs are used by CMS in its acute care hospital Inpatient Prospective Payment System (IPPS) (CMS 2016), and by hospitals to benchmark and manage reimbursement (Bielby 2010).

Claims-scrubbing tasks are often performed by specialized third parties, including healthcare clearinghouses. These companies are in the business of capturing and developing software that supports claims scrubbing. Increasingly, however, providers are performing claims reviews internally. Software to automatically scrub claims and notify staff members of discrepancies based on continually updated health plan rules can be performed prior to claim submission (Optum 2016).

Claim Submission

As noted previously in the section on transaction standards, **claim submission** is the transmission of the standard claim transaction to the health plan. Most revenue cycle managers set specific goals for the number of days in total that claims are discharged not final billed (DNFB), the percentage of clean claims submitted, the number of days that claims are in A/R, and other indicators. With respect to claims submission, DNFB directly affects cash flow (Nicastro 2013). In 2015 HFMA identified the median DNFB to be 3.9 days, with those in the 90 percentile and above having a median DNFB of 1.75 days. Yarsinksy (2015) cites HIMSS data showing hospital clean claims rates of between 75 percent and 85 percent. NextGen Healthcare (2015) suggests that a top benchmark for physician practices for clean claims is 90 percent. HFMA (2015) found the median net days in A/R for hospitals to be 37.45 days and for physician practices 29.4 days.

Filing for Contractual Payments and Shared Risk Arrangements

Filing for contractual payments and shared risk arrangements may entail significantly different types of reporting than those used when filing the traditional claim. Contractual payments and shared risk arrangements may be in the form of a lump-sum payment based on contract terms, often needing to be adjusted at the end of a given period of time (such as quarterly or annually). However, at this time, experience with such arrangements is limited. Health plans that offer them often combine VBP with FFS reimbursement and therefore request that providers submit traditional claims. (See additional information on such payment arrangements under VBP.)

Claim Status Determination

As was previously described in the discussion of transactions standards, claims status determination is essential in the absence of acknowledgements for claims submission but should also be performed if an acknowledged receipt of claim does not yield a response from the health plan on a timely basis. Tracking A/R in the hospital billing system or physician PMS and close monitoring of claims are necessary to ensure that claims do not "fall through the cracks." Ideally, systems should support alerts set to timing desired by the organization to notify staff when a claim's status needs to be determined.

Claims Attachments

Claims attachments were also described in the previous discussion of transactions standards. In the absence of a transaction standard for this purpose, providers should try to clarify with health plans what types of claims will require attachments. In fact, the requirements could be part of a contractual obligation requested of the health plan. In anticipation of the claim attachment standard being the HL7 C-CDA, providers may wish to request via contract that claim attachments be accepted in this format. Even if the health plan does not yet accept such a format and denies inclusion in the contract, going on record with the request puts health plans on notice that they will need to be able to manage this. Of course, the provider must be able to generate this format from its EHR, an accommodation that is required under the MU incentive program. In addition to minimum necessary concerns, the cost of copying or printing out an entire health record should not be considered the norm.

Remittance Advice and Payment

Remittance advice and payment, which also has been addressed in the discussion of transaction standards, may be one area where physician PMS vendors need to improve functionality. The operating rules for ERA (described previously) include a significantly more uniform process for use of the Claim Adjustment Reason Codes (CARCs) and Remittance Advice Remark Codes (RARCs). Application of these rules should make it easier to understand what adjustments are made and how to address them in the A/R system. These codes permit providers to bill patients for their balance after insurance. It should be noted here that health plans send their members an explanation of benefits (EOB) when a claim has been filed by a provider. The purpose of the EOB is to notify the patient that a claim has been received and that there is an approved balance after payment for which the provider can require payment. Some providers use the term ERA and EOB as synonyms, but they are two entirely different documents.

Denials

Denials are increasing as health plans tighten their requirements for medical necessity and conduct more reviews for this purpose. Denials may include both denial of a current claim as well as a takeback of money from claims already paid where a review reveals issues. This is particularly true for the CMS recovery audit contractor (RAC) reviews wherein RACs are increasingly targeting providers with high claims denial rates (Crump 2015). Appeals, however, are important. Murphy (2015) found that hospitals appealed 47 percent of all RAC claim denials in a recent quarter of activity, and that about 60 percent of the claims reviewed by RAC appeals judges were found *not* to have an overpayment. Appeals are an expensive undertaking not only in their processing but also with regard to their impact on availability of capital resources.

Steps to manage denials include tracking their financial impact, benchmarking performance using CARCs and RARCs, targeting the root causes of denials to determine solutions (for example, are most of the denials the result of registration errors, invalid coding, fail claim edits, or another reason?), and eliminating inconsistencies in denial processing (Sanderson et al. 2015). Once a provider has a good understanding of its denials and can apply solutions, there must be feedback to the health plan at the time of contract negotiation. Bayley (2013) describes a recent health plan–provider collaboration that anticipates a 10 percent to 20 percent savings as the parties work together to improve coding; decrease eligibility errors by improving access to information (by health plan); reduce late charges by reconciling the provider's guidelines on timing for documentation and coding submission with the health plan's claims submission timelines; and consolidate audit costs by developing a recovery rate to apply to audits based on historical performance.

A/R Follow-Up and Collections

Bad debt and charity care are two forms of nonpayment for services. **Bad debt** is a payment that is not collected from a party who was obligated to pay. **Charity care** is the provision of services at no cost to people who do not have the means to pay. Bad debt and charity care expenses are both rising, as is the cost to collect balances after insurance. In addition to aggressive collection up front, aggressive follow up on relatively young A/R is necessary to limit collection costs and avoid bad debt. The strategy of offering a discount to those who pay up front was discussed previously. Similarly, a discount can be an effective means to reduce A/R and bad debt. Scoring A/R by reviewing patient credit scores can identify patients at high risk of not paying for billed services, and more effort can be focused on high-risk cases both up front and before A/R reaches 30 days. Such risk scoring can also identify those patients at low risk who may not have service waived if they are unable to pay up front—especially in clinical situations warranting such arrangements.

Providers may outsource collection of late payments to collection agencies, although many providers, especially small physician offices, do not like using a collection agency for fear of gaining a bad reputation and losing patients. Another option for postservice collection is to sell eligible A/R (as defined by the provider) at a discount from face value to a vendor that keeps any payments it collects. The sale of A/R provides cash and reduces collection costs for providers, and it does not negatively affect the balance sheet because it is not a loan. Just the same, vendors are unlikely to purchase the A/R that does not seem to be collectible. Providers will still have to write off the oldest, least collectible A/R as bad debt (Matjucha and Giuliano 2011).

Analytics and Reports

Many providers lack a strategy to address the movement toward consumer-driven care. They are somewhat optimistic about VBP but still are concerned that they are not even close to being prepared, especially from the perspective of having sufficient data and understanding of the data to assume the right level of risk. Analytics and reports are therefore essential as a means to monitor the revenue cycle and make effective decisions regarding solutions that can improve revenue cycle management.

Check Your Understanding 19.2

Chose the best answer:

1. Analytics that describe a provider's unique characteristics in a local market aids:

    a. Contract negotiation

    b. Individual enrollment in a health plan

    c. Physician enrollment in a health plan

    d. Reduction in bad debt

2. A service that can increase revenue may be obtained through:

    a. Online bill paying

    b. Point of service payment

    c. Preventive service reminders

    d. Positive patient identification

3. Failure for a provider to conduct which of the following transactions will result in a large number of claims denials?

    a. Claims attachments

    b. Claims status

    c. Eligibility verification

    d. Premium payment

4. A successful strategy to improve collection of a patient's balance after insurance is:

    a. Discount for early payment

    b. Investment counseling

    c. Late payment penalties

    d. Pre-certification

5. Services required by health plans to ensure medical necessity include:

    a. Accurate coding

    b. Co-pay collection

    c. Deductible management

    d. Utilization review

6. A form of case management addressing care after patients leave a provider setting is:

    a. Care coordination

    b. Claims audits

    c. Drug utilization review

    d. Medical necessity checks

7. A charge description master:

    a. Catalogs supplies and services

    b. Creates accounts receivables

    c. Reconciles A/R with payments

    d. Supports correct coding

8. Which of the following may no longer be necessary in a future value-based payment environment?

    a. Claims submission

    b. Coding

    c. Eligibility verification

    d. Prior authorization

9. A document sent by the health plan to patients to identify the portion of payment that is their responsibility is:

    a. Claim

    b. Electronic remittance advice

    c. Explanation of benefits

    d. Invoice

10. Information that helps providers understand the amount being reimbursed by a health plan is:

    a. Claims adjustment reason codes

    b. Electronic remittance advice

    c. Explanation of benefits

    d. ICD-10-CM/PCS or CPT codes

Value-based Payment

Although VBP has existed for a while in the form of report cards (early 2000s) and as pay-for-performance (P4P) systems linking provider reimbursement to quality (Rosenthal et al. 2005), it was not until the passage of ACA in 2010 that VBP became a national priority.

VBP Terminology

There are many terms and concepts associated with VBP. Some key terms are defined here.

Value
Value may be defined as outcomes relative to costs. Porter (2010) observes that "value—neither an abstract ideal nor a code word for cost reduction—should define the framework for performance improvement in healthcare." However, Porter also observes that "value in healthcare remains largely unmeasured and misunderstood." To that end, "value should always be defined around the customer, and in a well-functioning healthcare system, the creation of value for patients should determine the rewards for all other actors in the system. Since value depends on results, not inputs . . . value is a central challenge."

Value-Based Payment
VBP is used to describe paying for the value (cost and quality) of services, as opposed to paying for the volume of services. Damberg and colleagues (2014) defines the term VBP as "a demand-side strategy to measure, report, and reward excellence in healthcare delivery within a framework of standardized performance measurement, transparency and public reporting, payment innovation,

and informed consumer choice." Similar terms include *value-based purchasing, value-based reimbursement,* and *value-based contracting.*

Value-Based Payment Models
Value-based payment models are being used to carry out VBPs. They also vary in what they are called, with no single taxonomy able to account for the nuances that exist in every different contract. The following (as illustrated in figure 19.5) are the most common types of payment models that are value-driven. These are found in both government and private sector VBP programs.

Pay-for-Performance
Pay-for-performance (P4P) is described by Damberg and colleagues (2014) as "a payment arrangement in which providers are rewarded (bonuses) or penalized (reductions in payment) based on meeting pre-established targets or benchmarks for measures of quality and/or efficiency." Incentives are typically paid on top of FFS payments.

Patient-Centered Medical Home
Patient-centered medical home (PCMH) is both a new payment model as well as a patient care delivery model and has been defined by Mourar (2012) as "a physician practice and patient partnership that provides accessible, interactive, family focused, coordinated and comprehensive care." Reimbursement for PCMHs varies, but it generally is FFS plus care coordination fees (per member per month [PMPM]) and, sometimes, P4P bonuses for quality and/or individual services. A few health plans provide an episode-of-care payment (that is, bundled payment) or full risk capitation (Schilz 2010).

Shifting Financial Risk
Shifting financial risk, in general, refers to a program in which providers keep part of the savings realized by the health plan for specific services or the total cost of care per beneficiary or population. Within any given risk-sharing structure, there are a number of ways that financial risk is shared. It is also important to note that since shifting financial risk is very new, many providers engage in one or more of the following types of shifting risk and often retain some level of FFS or P4P as carve-outs for types of patients or types of procedures.

Catalyst for Payment Reform (2013) describes the following types of value-based, risk shifting payment models:

- **Shared savings** (also known as *one-sided risk* or *gainsharing*) is an arrangement in which all providers are reimbursed based on FFS and are then eligible to receive shared savings payments (incentive) after they meet quality performance and risk-adjusted standards. Shared savings may be applied to some or all of the services that are expected to be used by a patient population and may vary based on provider performance.

- **Bundled payment** *(episode-of-care payment)* is a method in which payments to providers are based on the expected costs for a clinically defined episode or bundle of related healthcare services, including cost associated with preventable complications.

Figure 19.5.   Value-based payment models

Fee-for-Service	Pay-For-Performance	Patient-centered Medical Home	Shifting Financial Risk (w/wo ACO, CIN, PCMH)				Provider-Sponsored Health Plan
			One-Sided (Shared Savings)	Bundled (Episode) Payments	Two-Sided (Shared Risk)	Full Risk (Capitation)	
	Incentive Payment			Transfer Risk			→

- **Shared risk** *(two-sided risk)* adds the dimension of the provider being at risk for the same portion of spending over the target as the health plan. Shared-risk programs can be based on a FFS payment system or include capitation for all (global) or some (partial) conditions or services.

- **Capitation** *(full risk)* refers to a fixed payment amount given to providers for the care that patients may receive in a given time period, such as a month or year. Full risk may be implemented globally for all services provided, or partially where the fixed payment is provided for specific services only (that is, there are FFS payments for carve-outs for high-cost items such as specific drugs or medical devices). Full capitation may also be offered with or without payment adjustments based on measured performance and/or patient acuity or level of risk.

Value-Based Delivery Models

Value-based delivery models refer to organizational structures that have been developed to support VBP models. CMS has been a leader in using the accountable care organization (ACO) structure, and some commercial health plans have encouraged creation of ACOs to share accountability and rewards. However, while CMS has required a separate ACO organization to be formed, many commercial health plans' value-based *payment* models do not result in a new *delivery* model to be formed. The following are the current types of value-based delivery models forming.

- **Accountable care organization (ACO)** is a group of providers, including physicians, hospitals, LTPAC providers, and others, who are collectively responsible for the care outcomes of a patient population. ACOs provide contracts with such providers for improving the quality and lowering total costs for the patients in the population over time. The following strategies contribute to ACO success (O'Hara 2014; Butts and Gursahaney 2014):

  - Aligned physician network, typically employed in an integrated delivery network

  - Information technology (IT) infrastructure that facilitates exchange of patient information and identification of care improvement opportunities

  - Optimal capacity strategy including a streamlined acute care enterprise and comprehensive ambulatory network

  - Transformed clinical operations using evidence-based guidelines with emphasis on primary care, transitions of care, and patient engagement

  - Partnerships with health plans willing to reward all participants for better population management (see chapter 20)

- **Clinically integrated network (CIN)** is a group of otherwise independent physicians who commit to improving quality and lowering cost by negotiating collectively (under a "safe harbor" provision in antitrust law) for commercial health plan contracts. The belief is that such contracting is necessary to support investment in performance improvement and ensure cross-referrals among like-minded physicians. Necessary strategies for success include the following (O'Hara 2014; Butts and Gursahaney 2014) include the following:

  - Key clinical and administrative metrics defined by the CIN's performance improvement goals

  - Selective membership in the CIN by only those physicians who are able to advance the goals

  - System to monitor physician performance against the goals

  - Physician-led governance structure to oversee the program, supported by staff

  - IT infrastructure to identify opportunities for improvement and facilitate exchange of patient information

- ○ VBP incentives

- ○ Joint contracting with commercial health plans/employers for physician services

- **Patient-centered medical home (PCMH)**, as previously described in the section on VBP models, is both a payment and delivery model. As a value-based delivery model, it addresses the following fundamental elements (NCQA 2014), all of which are supported by health IT such as EHRs and disease registries:

  - ○ Patient-centered appointment access

  - ○ Team-based care including primary care physicians and others who meet the cultural and linguistic needs of patients

  - ○ Population health management

  - ○ Care management and support, using evidence-based guidelines for preventive, acute, and chronic care management

  - ○ Care coordination and care transitions, including the ability to track and coordinated diagnostic studies, referrals, and care transitions across the continuum

  - ○ Performance measurement and quality improvement

Trends in VBP

There are several overarching trends in VBP, irrespective of the VBP structure. Some of the key trends include the following.

- *Rapid adoption of VBP:* Studies consistently find that the growth trend in VBP is strong and continuing. For example, McKesson Health Solutions (2014) observes that "the reimbursement landscape is changing faster than many had anticipated." Health plans and providers are also aligned on embracing payment with value measures. McKesson Health Solutions reports that 90% of health plans and 81% of providers are already using some mix of VBP combined with FFS. This white paper also indicates that providers expected to see FFS decrease from about 56% in 2014 to 34% in five years; also, providers are more aligned with VBP in regions where there are only one or two health plans. Where there is no clear market leader in a region, FFS still dominates. Large providers with a range of VBP experiences are also more likely to be further along the continuum toward VBP.

- *Growth in VBP is strong and continuing.* Medicare's VBP is gaining momentum. CMS identified that in 2015, 42% of payments were linked to value, 33% were made through P4P, and 14% through shared-risk and shared-savings programs. Medicare's goals are to increase VBP (which CMS has started referring to as *alternative payment models*) in 2016 and 2018, as illustrated in figure 19.6. Physicians identify claims under CMS's VBP through use of a value-based payment modifier (CMS 2015c).

- *Private health plan interest in VBP is following Medicare's lead.* Much less is known about VBP in the private sector, but some examples are emerging. Very early in the VBP initiative, WellPoint reported it is replacing its traditional rate increases with a mandatory program tying increases to performance on outcome, safety, and satisfaction measures, thereby reducing their cost growth by 3 to 5 percentage points (Advisory Board Company 2011). UnitedHealthcare in Illinois started providing increases in physicians' contracted rate for all services in 2013 (Milburn and Maurar 2013).

- *Provider trends are demonstrating movement toward VBP.* Trinity Health suggests that almost all of their hospitals participate in some type of VBP, with about 20% of all hospital

Figure 19.6.   Medicare Goals for VBP

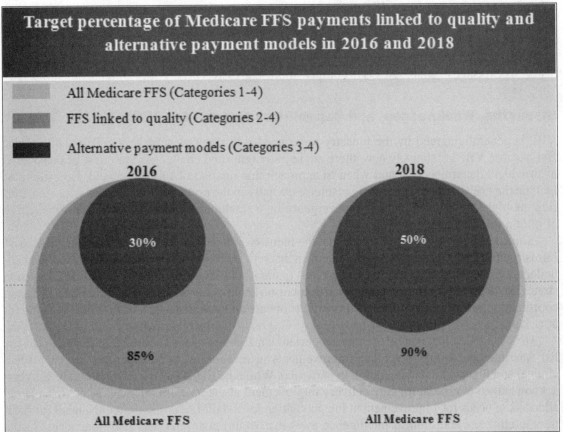

Source: CMS.gov 2015 (January 26). Better Care. Smarter Spending. Healthier People: Paying Providers for Value, Not Volume.

payments having some risk component, and 10% to 15% of primary care providers having some risk component (Evans and Herman 2015).

- *ACO growth may be slowing.* While the ACO delivery model is not the only way to shift financial risk, it has been one of the most widely recognized of the models, most likely because of its adoption by Medicare. Ghandi (2015) provides some interesting data: The total number of ACOs in the United States in 2015 was 585, up 12% from 522 in 2014, and up 127% from 258 ACOs in 2013. The number of Medicare versus non-Medicare ACOs is also shifting. In 2013, the numbers of Medicare ACOs and non-Medicare ACOs were roughly equal (134 and 124, respectively); however, by 2015, the 159 Medicare ACOs accounted for only 27% of all ACOs in the United States. Most ACOs in CMS programs also serve non-Medicare patients, estimated to be at about 35 million, up 6% from 33 million in 2014 and 120% from 15 million in 2013.

- *Outcomes of ACOs are improving.* ACOs with the best outcomes are reported to be delivering care at 20 percent to 40 percent below the typical cost of care with excellent quality and patient satisfaction, but most have not progressed that far (Advisory Board Company 2015). In fact, there is significant discrepancy in outcomes data, with some suggesting quite positive results and others demonstrating very modest or almost no significant results. For example, in a study conducted in August 2015 by the eHealth Initiative, cost savings were reportedly improved by 68 percent, quality measures improved by 54 percent, readmissions reduced by 52 percent, preventive healthcare delivery improved by 52 percent, emergency department visits reduced by 48 percent, and chronic disease management improved by 45 percent. CMS has institute a Next Generation ACO (NGACO), which holds more promise for both shared-savings payments and outcomes. It has been suggested that CMS's rules have made it difficult for some of the best ACOs to earn shared-savings payments. The NGACO model is expected to enable ACOs to compete more aggressively (Advisory Board Company 2015).

Strengths, Weaknesses, and Capabilities Needed for VBP

VBP is generally agreed by the industry to be needed in order to achieve the Triple Aim goals. But because VBP is relatively new, there are key strengths and challenges that must be considered as providers determine how and when to approach this method of reimbursement. Key strengths include the growth trends; promising results, especially in the population of patients who are incurring the highest costs; and industry convergence on a small number of VBP models after a period of pilot implementations.

Some key VBP-related challenges that the industry at large needs to address include lack of IT infrastructure, attention to process improvement that reflects best practices, the establishment of well-understood and aligned performance measures, (patient) risk stratification and (provider) attribution strategies, skills for contract negotiation that focus on benefits for all parties, and care management/coordination competencies to ensure transitions of care and maintenance of a healthier lifestyle for at-risk patients.

HFMA (2015) has identified some important capabilities needed for VBPs. At the top of the list was interoperability to achieve improvements in revenue cycle management in general and clinical and financial data integration in particular. While the EHR MU incentive program has been acknowledged as critical for care delivery improvement at the patient level, it does not adequately address the needs for improvement at the population level. HFMA has also cited the need for business intelligence and clinical intelligence tools that would give providers real-time access at the point of care to information that is based in business intelligence to make value-based decisions. Some of the tools cited by HFMA as well as additional tools are illustrated in figure 19.7.

Figure 19.7.   Business and clinical intelligence tools for VBP

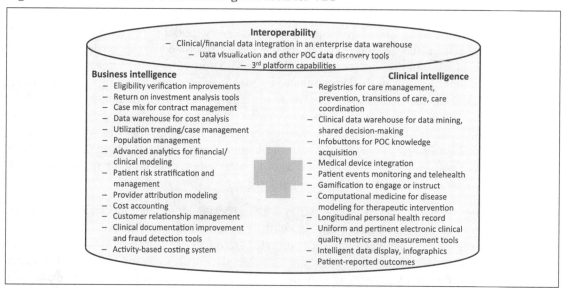

Check Your Understanding 19.3

Choose the best answer:

1. Which of the following is a new value-based *payment* model?

    a. Accountable care organization

    b. Bundled payments

    c. Clinically integrated network

    d. Health insurance exchange

2. A patient-centered medical home is a new form of:

    a. LTPAC delivery system

    b. Payment model and delivery model

    c. Primary care specialty

    d. Strategy for cost reduction

3. Pay for performance is a payment model that:

    a. Offers incentives for quality

    b. Pays for an episode of care

    c. Requires ACO formation

    d. Shifts financial risk

4. A key strength of VBP that distinguishes it from other measures to lower cost and improve care in the past is:

    a. Care coordination competencies

    b. Consensus exists among provider and health plans for its need

    c. Existence of well-aligned performance measures

    d. Information integration brought about by EHRs

5. Which of the following value-based *delivery* models includes hospitals?

    a. Accountable care organization

    b. Clinically integrated network

    c. Health insurance exchange

    d. Patient-centered medical home

References and Resources

Advisory Board Company. 2011. Accountable care economics. https://www.advisory.com/sitecore%20modules/web/research/financial-leadership-council/studies/2011/economics-of-accountable-care/a-growing-quality-premium/value-based-purchasing.

Advisory Board Company. 2015 (April 27). Daily briefing: What ACOs need to know about CMS' next generation model. https://www.advisory.com/_apps/dailybriefingprint?i={AF5F997B-5C15-47B6-BF77-7524FC24C4DA}.

Affordable Care Act of 2010 (ACA). 2010 (March 23). http://www.hhs.gov/healthcare/about-the-law/read-the-law.

Amatayakul, M., and S.S. Lazarus. 2014 (August). Market assessment of HIPAA attachments. Unpublished work for CAQH CORE.

American Hospital Association. 2016 (January). Administrative simplification strategies offer opportunities to improve patient experience and reduce costs. *TrendWatch*. http://www.aha.org/research/reports/tw/16jan-tw-adminsimp.pdf.

American Medical Association (AMA). n.d. Managing patient payments. http://www.ama-assn.org/ama/pub/advocacy/topics/administrative-simplification-initiatives/managing-patient-payments
.page?

Arrowood, D., et al; AHIMA Workgroup. 2015 (July). Best practices in the art and science of clinical documentation improvement. *Journal of AHIMA*. 86(7):46–50. http://bok.ahima.org/doc?oid=107704#.V8C0XpgrI2w.

Bayley, M., et al. 2013 (May). Hospital revenue cycle operations: Opportunities created by the ACA. McKinsey & Co. http://healthcare.mckinsey.com/hospital-revenue-cycle-operations-opportunities-created-aca.

Bielby, J.A., et al. 2010 (April). Evolution of DRGs (updated). *Journal of AHIMA*. Web exclusive. http://library.ahima.org/doc?oid=106590#.V8C8h5grI2w.

Butts, D., and V. Gursahaney. 2014 (October 3). Turning skeptics into believers: Why ACOs/CINs are still a good idea. *Becker's Hospital Review*. http://www.beckershospitalreview.com/accountable-care-organizations/turning-skeptics-into-believers-why-acos-cins-are-still-a-good-idea.html.

Bryant, G., et al. 2010. Guidance for clinical documentation improvement programs. *Journal of AHIMA*. 81(5): expanded web version. http://library.ahima.org/doc?oid=103352#.V8C1UZgrI2w.

CAQH CORE and AHA: Learn How Operating Rules Are Reducing Hospital Receivables and Expediting Healthcare Payments, Webinar, September 25, 2013.

CAQH. 2015. CAQH Solutions webinar brief: COB SMART® health plan strategies on coordination of benefits: Saving money through efficiency and collaboration. http://www.caqh.org/sites/default/files/solutions/cob-smart/cob-webinar-sept-2015-exec-summary_0_0.pdf?token=GGZ0kpvj.

CAQH. 2016. HIPAA standardized electronic transaction adoption rates for commercial health plans. In *2015 CAQH Index: Electronic Administrative Transaction Adoption and Savings Calendar Year 2014*. http://www.caqh.org/explorations/caqh-index.

Catalyst for Payment Reform. 2013. Definitions of payment model terms. http://compendium.catalyzepaymentreform.org/compendium-search/definitions-pmt.

Cigna. 2016. Cigna Healthcare definition of medical necessity for physicians. http://www.cigna.com/healthcare-professionals/resources-for-health-care-professionals/clinical-payment-and-reimbursement-policies/medical-necessity-definitions.

Centers for Medicare and Medicaid Services (CMS). 2015a (March 31). Drug utilization review. Medicaid.gov. https://www.medicaid.gov/Medicaid-CHIP-Program-Information/By-Topics/Benefits/Prescription-Drugs/Drug-Utilization-Review.html.

Centers for Medicare and Medicaid Services (CMS). 2015b (August 20). Hospital-Acquired Conditions (Present on Admission Indicator): Coding . https://www.cms.gov/medicare/medicare-fee-for-service-payment/hospitalacqcond/coding.html.

Centers for Medicare and Medicaid Services (CMS) 2015c (December 17). Fact Sheet for the 2016 value-based payment modifier. https://www.cms.gov/medicare/medicare-fee-for-service-payment/physicianfeedbackprogram/valuebasedpaymentmodifier.html.

Centers for Medicare and Medicaid Services (CMS). 2016 (February). Acute care hospital Inpatient Prospective Payment System. https://www.cms.gov/Outreach-and-Education/Medicare-Learning-Network-MLN/MLNProducts/downloads/AcutePaymtSysfctsht.pdf.

Commins, J. 2016 (February 2). HIT enters "post-EHR era." *HealthLeaders Media.* http://healthleadersmedia.com/content/TEC-325053/Healthcare-HIT-Enters-PostEHR-Era.html##.

Crump, D. 2015 (September 17). Insight: The case for revisiting denial rates. *Healthcare Finance News.* http://www.healthcarefinancenews.com/blog/insight-case-revisiting-denial-rates.

Damberg, C.L., et al. (2014). *Measuring Success in Health Care Value-Based Purchasing Programs.* Washington, DC: RAND Corporation. http://www.rand.org/pubs/research_reports/RR306z1.html.

Davis, N.A. 2011. *Revenue Cycle Management Best Practices.* Chicago, IL: American Health Information Management Association.

Diop, K. 2015. ICD-10 moves healthcare one step closer to improved documentation. *Journal of AHIMA.* 86(11):62–63.

Easterling, S. 2015 (September). Documentation and coding in a risk-based environment: Obstacles to be aware of. *CodeWrite.* http://bok.ahima.org/doc?oid=301140#.V8C4T5grI2x.

EDI Basics. 2015. What is EDI (electronic data interchange)? http://www.edibasics.com/what-is-edi.

eHealth Initiative. 2015 (September 8). 2015 ACO Survey Results Webinar. https://www.ehidc.org/resources/418-2015-aco-survey-results-webinar .

Ellison, A. 2015 (June 15). The community hospital survival guide: Strategies to keep the doors open. *Becker's Hospital Review.* http://www.beckershospitalreview.com/finance/the-community-hospital-survival-guide-strategies-to-keep-the-doors-open.html

Evans, M., and B. Herman. 2015 (January 28). Where healthcare is now on march to value-based pay. *Modern Healthcare.* http://www.modernhealthcare.com/article/20150128/NEWS/301289952.

Gabriel, S. 2014 (February 3). POS collections are up—but is it enough? Advisory Board Company. https://www.advisory.com/research/financial-leadership-council/at-the-margins/2014/02/rev-cycle-benchmarks-pos.

Ghandi, N. 2015 (April). ACO update: A slower pace of growth. Oliver Wyman. http://www.oliverwyman.com/content/dam/oliver-wyman/global/en/files/insights/health-life-sciences/2015/ACO-Update-2015-v2.pdf.

Greene, D. 2015 (December 29). What does it mean to scrub an insurance claim? *Codapedia.* http://codapedia.com/articlePrint.cfm?id=168.

Grosze, P. 2015. Healthcare virtual card payments—Just the facts! PNC Healthcare. https://www.pnc.com/content/dam/pnc-com/pdf/corporateandinstitutional/Treasury%20Management/Healthcare/Spring2015/HC-Virtual-Card-Article_188633_FINAL.pdf.

Haas, D.L. 2013 (February 12). Clinical documentation improvement: What executives need to know and the financial impact of neglect. *Becker's Hospital CFO.* http://www.beckershospital review.com/finance/clinical-documentation-improvement-what-executives-need-to-know-and-the-financial-impact-of-neglect.html.

Haug, T. 2015 (April 8). Virtual card payments to healthcare providers: Villainous or valuable? AOC Solutions blog. http://www.aocsolutions.com/blog/virtual-card-payments-to-healthcare-providers-villainous-or-valuable.

Healthcare Financial Management Association (HFMA). 2012 (December). Principles and Practices Board statement: Valuation and financial statement presentation of charity care and bad debts by institutional healthcare providers. http://www.hfma.org/Content.aspx?id=1069.

Healthcare Financial Management Association (HFMA). 2015 (May). HFMA's executive survey: Value-based payment readiness. http://www.hfma.org/value-basedpaymentreadinesssurvey.

Healthcare Financial Management Association (HFMA). 2016. About MAP. https://www.hfma.org/MAP/AboutMap.

Healthcare.gov. 2016. If you don't have health insurance: How much you'll pay. https://www.healthcare.gov/fees/fee-for-not-being-covered.

Healthcare Information and Management Systems Society (HIMSS). 2015 (April 8). Rethinking revenue cycle management. HIMSS Revenue Cycle Improvement Task Force. http://www.himss.org/library/health-business-solutions/rethinking-revenue-cycle-management.

Health Insurance Portability and Accountability Act of 1996 (HIPAA). 1996 (August 21). Public Law 104-191, Subtitle F—Administrative Simplification. Section 261: Purpose.

HealthLeaders Media. 2016. Opportunities in hospital capital access. http://healthleadersmedia.com/content/RND-90250/Opportunities-in-Hospital-Capital-Access

Jackson, J. 2010 (September 29). HIPAA version 5010: Tenth national provider call—acknowledgement transactions. Centers for Medicare and Medicaid Services. https://www.cms.gov/Regulations-and-Guidance/Administrative-Simplification/Versions5010andD0/Downloads/Acknowledgements_National_Presentation_9-29-10_final.pdf.

Jones, C.L., and T.L. Mills 2006. Negotiating a contract with a health plan. *Family Practice Management.* 13(10):49–55.

Krager, D., and C. Krager. 2008. *HIPAA for Healthcare Professionals.* Clifton Park: NY: Delmar Cengage Learning.

Leventhal, R. 2014 (May 20). Recognizing the value of clinical documentation improvement. *Healthcare Informatics.* http://www.healthcare-informatics.com/article/recognizing-value-clinical-documentation-improvement.

Levine, E. et al. 2013 (May) The impact of coverage shifts on hospital utilization. McKinsey & Co. http://healthcare.mckinsey.com/sites/default/files/793546_Coverage_Shifts_on_Hospital_Utilization.pdf.

Matjucha, K., and C. Giuliano. 2011 (December). Improving your bottom line through bad debt management. Deloitte Consulting, LLP. http://www.njhfmainstitute.org/pdf/Oct13/Improving%20Your%20Bottom%20Line%20Through%20Effective%20Bad%20Debt%20Management.pdf.

McKesson Health Solutions (2014). White paper: The state of value-based reimbursement and the transition from volume to value in 2014. http://mhsinfo.mckesson.com/rs/mckessonhealthsolutions/images/MHS-2014-Signature-Research-White-Paper.pdf.

Merrill, K. 2013 (March). Rehabbing the hospital revenue cycle. American Society for Quality (ASQ) healthcare update. http://rube.asq.org/health/2013/04/change-management/rehabbing-the-revenue-cycle.pdf.

Michelson, D. 2014 (October 21) The new cool in healthcare: "Cost accounting is sexy?!" *Healthcare IT News.* http://www.healthcareitnews.com/blog/new-cool-healthcare-cost-accounting-sexy.

Milburn, J.B., and M. Maurar 2013. New reimbursement systems and value-based compensation incentives. Chapter 4 in *Strategies for Value-based Physician Compensation.* Englewood Cliffs, CO: Medical Group Management Association.

Miodonski, K. 2012 (June 18). Aligning case management processes with revenue cycle. *Becker's Hospital CFO.* http://www.beckershospitalreview.com/finance/aligning-case-management-processes-with-the-revenue-cycle.html.

Mourar, M. (2012). *Experts Answer 95 New Practice Management Questions.* Englewood Cliffs, CO: Medical Group Management Association.

Murphy, B. 2015 (December 22). 25 things to know in revenue cycle management. *Becker's Hospital CFO.* http://www.beckershospitalreview.com/finance/25-things-to-know-in-revenue-cycle-management.html.

NACHA. 2014a. Healthcare EFT payment options: Why choose ACH? https://healthcare.nacha.org/WhyACH.

National Committee for Quality Assurance (NCQA). 2014. NCQA recognized patient-centered medical home. https://www.ncqa.org/Portals/0/PCMH%20brochure-web.pdf.

National Committee on Vital and Health Statistics (NCVHS). 2015 (June 16–17). Meeting minutes: National Committee on Vital and Health Statistics Subcommittee on Standards Review Committee hearing on adopted transaction standards, operating rules, code sets & identifiers. http://www.ncvhs.hhs.gov/transcripts-minutes/summary-of-the-june-16-17-2015-ncvhs-subcommittee-on-standards-review-committee.

National Committee on Vital and Health Statistics (NCVHS). 2016 (February 16). National Committee on Vital and Health Statistics Subcommittee on Standards hearing on HIPAA and ACA administrative simplification—Phase

IV operating rules and attachment standard: Tentative agenda. http://www.ncvhs.hhs.gov/meeting-calendar/agenda-of-the-february-16-2016-ncvhs-subcommittee-on-standards-hearing.

NextGen Healthcare. 2015 (February 18). RCM survey report: What's happening behind the billing office door. https://bridge.nextgen.com/media/3082/nextgen_healthcare_ebook_rcm_survey_report_spc1.pdf.

Nicastro, D. 2013 (January 23). Don't let DNFB cripple hospital cash flow. *HealthLeaders Media.* http://www.healthleadersmedia.com/finance/dont-let-dnfb-cripple-hospital-cash-flow.

O'Hara, S. 2014 (September 24). The care transformation alphabet: What's the difference between CI, ACO, and PCMH? Advisory Board Company Care Transformation Center blog. https://www.advisory.com/research/care-transformation-center/care-transformation-center-blog/2014/09/deciphering-the-reform-alphabet.

Optum. 2016. Healthcare business insights white paper: Infusing the revenue cycle with clinical intelligence to drive success. https://www.optum.com/landing/hfn-0213-landing-page.html.

Owens, S. 2013 (September 23). Give your front office staff the tools they need to increase POS collections. Advisory Board Company. https://www.advisory.com/research/financial-leadership-council/at-the-margins/2013/09/maximize-pos-collections.

Pittman, D., and D. Tahir. 2016 (January 12). 209,000 doctors hit with meaningful use penalty this year. *Politico Morning eHeatlh.* http://www.politico.com/tipsheets/morning-ehealth/2016/01/politicos-morning-ehealth-209-000-doctors-hit-with-meaningful-use-penalty-this-year-212129.

Porter, M.E. 2010. Perspective: What is value in health care? *New England Journal of Medicine.* 363(26): 2477–2481. http://www.nejm.org/doi/full/10.1056/NEJMp1011024.

Rice, S. 2015 (August 3). Most hospitals face 30-day readmissions penalty in fiscal 2016. *Modern Healthcare.* http://www.modernhealthcare.com/article/20150803/NEWS/150809981.

Rode, D. 2015. Public Comment. NCVHS. 2015 (June 16-17). National Committee on Vital and Health Statistics Subcommittee on Standards Review Committee Hearing. http://www.ncvhs.hhs.gov/transcripts-minutes/summary-ot-the-june-16-17-2015-ncvhs-subcommittee-on-standards-review-committee/

Rosenthal, M.B., et al. 2005. Early experience with pay-for-performance: From concept to practice. *Journal of the American Medical Association.* 294(14):1788–1793. http://jama.ama-assn.org/cgi/content/abstract/294/14/1788 abstract.

Sanderson, B., et al. 2015 (August 11). Don't be in denial: Your final denial rate is not the answer. *Becker's Hospital CFO.* http://www.beckershospitalreview.com/finance/don-t-be-in-denial-your-final-denial-rate-is-not-the-answer.html.

Schilz, J. 2010 (September). Healthcare industry/managed care story of the week: Medical home pilot uses a three-tiered reimbursement methodology. Healthcare Intelligence Network. http://www.hin.com/sw/Hindustry_MC110810_patient_centered_medical_home_reimbursement_payment_structure_quality_care_coordination.html.

Snow, C.L., et al. 2012 (June 30). Accuracy of coding in the hospital-acquired-conditions/present-on-admission program. Final report prepared by RTI International for Centers for Medicare and Medicaid Services Rapid Cycle Evaluation Group. https://www.cms.gov/medicare/medicare-fee-for-service-payment/hospitalacqcond/downloads/accuracy-of-coding-final-report.pdf.

Spivey, M. 2015 (December 17). Cooperative Exchange declares ICD-10 implementation "non-event." *ICD10monitor.* http://www.icd10monitor.com/enews/item/1555-cooperative-exchange-declares-icd-10-implementation-non-event.

TripleTree. 2006 (April). Healthcare revenue cycle management: A TripleTree industry analysis. http://www.triple-tree.com/research/healthcare-revenue-cycle-management.

Vega, K.B. n.d. Successfully negotiating managed care contracts. Healthcare Financial Management Association (HFMA). http://www.hfma.org/Content.aspx?id=16658.

Wexler J., and K. Bucci. 2016. White paper: The business of hospital charge capture. ERIS Medical Technologies. http://www.erismed.com/2010/08/white-paper-the-business-of-charge-capture.

X12 Incorporated. n.d. Health insurance exchange enrollment and health insurance exchange related payments. http://store.x12.org/store/health-insurance-exchanges.

X12 Incorporated. 2016. About X12. http://x12.org/x12org/about/asc-x12-about.cfm.

Yarsinsky, J. 2015 (January 30). Clean claims: The key to efficient healthcare revenue cycle management. Linkedin Pulse. https://www.linkedin.com/pulse/clean-claims-key-efficient-healthcare-revenue-cycle-jim-yarsinsky.

Yong, P.L., R.S. Saunders, and L. Olsen. 2011. *The Healthcare Imperative: Lowering Costs and Improving Outcomes.* Institute of Medicine Workshop Series Summary. Washington, DC: National Academies Press. http://www.nap.edu/catalog/12750/the-healthcare-imperative-lowering-costs-and-improving-outcomes-workshop-series.

Chapter 20
Population Health

Patient attribution

Population

Population health

Population health management

Provider attribution

Risk stratification

Single sign on

Uncompensated use

Validity

Value stream maps

Variety

Velocity

Veracity

Volatility

Volume

Workflow modeling

Learning Objectives

- Define population health and its scope.

- Describe the general nature of health IT needed for population health management.

- Identify specific health IT tools to support quality measurements for improved health outcomes.

- Discuss the importance and use of big data and healthcare analytics to measure quality of care, cost, and experience of care and provide intelligence for continuous improvement.

Much has been made in this book about the need to focus the use of the electronic health record (EHR) and health information technology (health IT) on achieving the Triple Aim—the national goals for improving the quality, cost, and experience of care in the United States. In 2010, the Affordable Care Act (ACA) reiterated the importance of these goals and mandated certain changes in health insurance coverage for the uninsured, tools for further administrative simplification, and a focus on value-based payment (VBP). Also in 2010, the US Department of Health and Human Services (HHS) launched the **Healthy People 2020** campaign with four overarching goals (NCHS 2015):

- Attain high-quality, longer lives free of preventable disease, disability, injury, and premature death.

- Achieve health equity, eliminate disparities, and improve the health of all groups.

- Create social and physical environments that promote good health for all.

- Promote quality of life, healthy development, and healthy behaviors across all life stages.

Health IT is not the only factor that contributes to meeting these goals, but it has played, and will continue to play, a major role. EHRs are rapidly replacing paper health records and have demonstrated value in many areas, even if they can be challenging to use. There is no doubt that EHRs will continue to be refined and their use fine-tuned to produce ever-greater value. Within provider settings, the focus for health IT is shifting to optimizing use of the EHR and achieving interoperability among EHRs. Such improvements are needed for a healthier populace because individual patients experience care throughout their lifetime in many different locations, including in their homes and workplaces.

There are multiple **health determinants** (factors that contribute to health). These include availability of health system services, physical environmental factors, lifestyle, and social and economic conditions (Woolf et al. 2013), as well as individuals' genomic makeup. As these multiple determinants come into clearer focus, efforts to address them are converging. Instead of solely building up separate fields of community medicine, public health, preventive medicine/health promotion, social epidemiology, precision medicine/genomics, and so forth, population health focuses on "the health outcomes of a group of individuals" by considering the "health determinants and policies and interventions that link these two." (Kindig and Stoddart 2003). Much as the health IT systems development life cycle (SDLC) is comprised of hardware, software, people, policy, and process with a feedback mechanism for continuous improvement and growth, population health management seeks to create an ecosystem that focuses on "care for the nation as a whole and redesigns the care delivery system around integrated, accountable, and patient-centric care processes" (Esterhay et al. 2014). (See chapter 2 for discussion of SDLC.)

Key Concepts in Population Health

Population health and population health management are relatively new concepts. As such, ways to define these terms are evolving. To gain further understanding of population health management, it can be helpful to dissect the meaning of each of the associated terms (*population, population health,* and *population management*). Therefore, the following sections review each of these terms as they are understood in the work of the **Institute for Healthcare Improvement (IHI)**, which is the source of the concept of the Triple Aim (Lewis 2014), and selected other sources relevant to this chapter.

Population

Population in the context of population health management, and as discussed in this chapter, refers to those who will receive healthcare that is accountable to the goals of the Triple Aim. Community leaders, health plans, and providers may view the question of who is accountable differently, and, frequently, the determination of who is accountable depends on how the accountability functions (that is, population health management) will be carried out. Providers typically choose from one of the following in defining the population on which they will focus (Lewis 2014):

- *Discrete/defined populations,* which are enterprise-level populations that make business sense. The population may be all individuals receiving care within a health system, or those whose care is financed through a specific health plan or entity, such as an accountable care organization (ACO).

- *Regional/community populations,* which are defined geographically (for example, within the area in which a provider offers services, within a given town, or within other geographic boundaries). Such populations may also be segmented by a common set of needs or issues, such as all low-birth weight babies within so many square miles, or all elderly patients with complex needs in a defined community.

In general, providers find it easier to identify a discrete/defined population than a regional/community population. However, community leaders and, in some cases, health plans often focus on regional/community populations. When Medicare first started its Medicare Shared Savings Program (MSSP) program, it defined the population to be served by the ACO with respect to its geographical characteristics—irrespective of where care had previously been provided or would ultimately be provided. This **patient attribution** method, which is the process used to determine which provider group is responsible for a patient's care and costs (HCP-LAN 2016a), meant that potentially some patients could be attributed to a specific ACO even after they moved away, and the expectation would be that the ACO provider would continue to coordinate their care. This aspect of the ACO program was not well liked, as providers in one community were unable to coordinate care in a totally different community. The Medicare approach to determining the responsible provider group has subsequently been changed, and the current method considers not only patient attribution that is intentionally performed but also **patient attestation**, in which patients self-report, declare, or confirm which provider is their primary care provider. If a health plan wishes to ensure that all patients in a given population area or segment are attributed to a primary care provider but patients have not intentionally done so, algorithms based on Current Procedural Terminology (CPT) evaluation and management (E&M) codes from claims within a two-year look-back period are used, or, as a last resort, claims from specialists will be considered in the same manner (HCP-LAN 2016a).

Population Health

Definitions of **population health** vary. For this chapter, relevant definitions are those of Jacobson and Teutsch (2012), Kindig and Stoddart (2003), and IHI (Lewis 2014).

Jacobson and Teutsch (2012) define population health as follows:

> A cohesive, integrated, and comprehensive approach to health considering the distribution of health outcomes in a population, the health determinants that influence the distribution of care, and the policies and interventions that impact and are impacted by the determinants.

Note that this definition includes outcomes, determinants, and policies and interventions. The Health and Medical Division (HMD) of the National Academies of Science, Engineering, and Medicine (formerly Institute of Medicine [IOM]) adopted that definition in its Roundtable on Population Health Improvement (HMD 2016).

Kindig and Stoddart were the first to define population health. Their definition is "the health outcomes of a group of individuals, including the distribution of such outcomes within the group" (Kindig and Stoddart 2003).

IHI has adopted the Kindig and Stoddart definition, which focuses solely and broadly on outcomes. However, IHI aims to make the concept of population health more specific and operational by focusing on the measures it uses for the Triple Aim, which include the following:

> Life expectancy, mortality rates, health and functional status, disease burden (i.e., the incidence and/or prevalence of chronic disease), and behavioral and physiological factors such as smoking, physical activity, diet, blood pressure, BMI [body mass index], and cholesterol. (Lewis 2014)

Although this definition is important for policy makers, Kindig (2015) has suggested that the definition from Jacobson and Teutsch is more appropriate for current usage within the provider community.

Population Health Management

Population health management has been defined by the provider-sponsored health plan Partners HealthCare (n.d.) to mean the "collection of activities, not reimbursable in the fee-for-service model, but important in the care we deliver our patients," including "primary care, specialty care, non-hospital care, patient engagement, and analytics and technology." IHI distinguishes *population health,* which "focuses on the broader determinants of health," from *population medicine,* which is defined by IHI as the "design, delivery, coordination, and payment of high-quality healthcare services to manage the Triple Aim for a population using the best resources available" (Lewis 2014). IHI further observes that effective population medicine

> Will require new partnerships among providers and payers, integrated data support, redesigned IT [information technology] structures, a focus on non-traditional healthcare workforce, new care management models, and a shift from fee-for-service delivery to bearing financial risk for the population served.

In a survey of 37 chief executive officers and other health leaders (Pizzi 2015), one respondent observed that "population health signifies the movement from a silo-focused delivery of medicine to a communal effort with the purpose of improving the overall health outcomes of a population."

The Robert Wood Johnson Foundation conducted a discussion group on defining population health in which discussants contrasted population health with public health, suggesting population health was more oriented around patients in a population whereas public health was oriented around geographic communities (Chokshi and Stine 2013). Like IHI, these discussants used the term *population medicine,* which they understood to be "evidence-based interventions and disease management to triage and allocate healthcare resources in a cost-effective manner."

Scope of Population Health Management

A curriculum framework for population health management (Harris et al. 2016) suggests that population health management includes the following:

- Clinical case reports and studies on managing major public health conditions
- Compliance programs
- Health economics
- Outcomes assessment
- Provider incentives
- Health care reform
- Resource management
- Return on investment
- Healthcare quality
- Care coordination

A strategy for successful population health management typically involves recognizing the paradigm shift from acute care to a multitude of care venues across the continuum of care, and including formal financial agreements to share accountability for results. Successful population health management means providers need to "implement technical and service components that help improvement initiatives be repeatable and scalable across the enterprise," including the following (Burton 2013):

- Systematically integrating data and measurement
- Systematically applying evidence and standardization
- Systematically changing processes and behavior

Population health management requires **financial benchmarking**, which is the process that establishes spending levels used to determine the VBP rates for providers (HCP-LAN 2016b). Providers, in turn, use VBP rates to manage resources, plan investments in delivery support infrastructure, and identify inefficiencies. Financial benchmarks for public health plans are imposed on providers through a notice-and-comment rulemaking process; while financial benchmarks for commercial health plans are negotiated between the plans and the providers and for which providers must have solid cost of care data by case mix. Within a provider organization, **provider attribution** methods are also necessary to determine how to distribute payments, which may include a share of the cost savings or losses from over spending. (See further discussion of these concepts in chapter 19.) The Health Care Payment Learning and Planning Network (HCP-LAN) also identifies two additional priority needs for population health management: data sharing and performance measurement (discussed later in this chapter).

Health IT in Population Health Management

Health IT plays a major role in population health management. In order to link health determinants with policies and interventions to improve outcomes, health IT integrates data from EHRs with other information. EHRs have the potential both to supply evidence (patient data) to inform best clinical practices and policy choices for population health and to receive and apply information on population health from external sources. However, this sort of integration of data and information will require tools and technologies that do not currently reside in EHRs.

Sources of Data for Population Health Management

Many different types of data are required for population health management. Some of these are very commonplace as they are typically captured by and residing in EHRs and other forms of health IT that exist in most provider settings, such as administrative, financial, and clinical data. Other data are collected outside of the provider setting and tend to be data that are less standardized and used for more specific types of uses, such as research data and public health data. Still other types of data are important for population health management and currently may not be collected at all or only in a limited, ad hoc manner, such as some types of patient outcomes data. Some types of relevant data may not even seem to be health-related—such as data about a person's lifestyle, socio-economic status, and physical environment—but are determinants of health.

Interoperability Challenges

Three characteristics of today's EHRs restrict their capacity to support population health management at this time. First, they are generally not interoperable, especially across disparate provider settings. While a health information exchange (HIE) process or HIE organization (HIO) may be able to support some exchange of data from disparate EHR systems, it is well recognized that there are challenges in such data sharing. Just because data are listed as being available in an EHR does not necessarily mean they are available in the EHR at the provider setting where a patient is receiving care at any one point in time. A second characteristic that hinders use of EHRs in population health management is that their data are grounded in transactional databases that support point-of-care capture and use of data but do not support advanced analytics (Leventhal 2014). The third hindering characteristic is that EHRs are predominantly built on platforms that do not support advanced search functionality. They do not have a web interface that is suitable for retrieving data from multiple patients' records at one time. Even structured search functionality in an EHR system is limited (Regard and Hedges 2015).

Privacy Concerns

Responsible use of data for population health, irrespective of their source, must respect the privacy of patients. Esterhay and coauthors (2014) identify two types of privacy concerns with respect to population health management. The first is the "traditional" issue of inappropriate access to or wrongful disclosure of protected health information and other personal health information. The second relates to the **uncompensated use of aggregate data**—that is, data that are collected from multiple sources and/or on multiple measures, variables, or individuals and compiled into summary reports, typically for the purposes of public reporting or statistical analysis. Such aggregate data may have been de-identified and hence no longer protected under the Health Insurance Portability and Accountability Act (HIPAA); however, the use of data about patients or other consumers without asking their permission or offering them compensation may be viewed as a privacy violation, even if the data are used to benefit the individuals or society as a whole. The Federal Trade Commission (FTC) has categorized some uncompensated uses of aggregate data as "unfair and deceptive" trade practices.

Addressing this second type of privacy issue may involve compensation for data use, transparency about data use, or both. For instance, there is a website that offers, for a nominal fee, genomic testing not only for ancestral information but also to supply information to individuals about their risk for certain diseases. This website has come under investigation by the Food and Drug Administration (FDA) relative to offering an "unapproved medical device"; however, most of its critics are more concerned that the company sells de-identified data to pharmaceutical manufacturers and other medical researchers, and uses the data to recruit people who suffer from the diseases being researched to add to the data pool (Seife 2013).

The FTC recently recognized the need to address consumer-generated and controlled health data in the age of the Internet of Things (that is, the burgeoning phenomenon of commonplace consumer products and services that connect to the Internet) (Han 2015). After a settlement in 2014 with PaymentsMD, a medical billing provider that misled consumers about collection of personal health data, the FTC has developed a brochure entitled *Careful Connections: Building Security in the Internet of Things* (2015). This brochure advises companies to think through the health data being collected and how they are used, to ensure that data are appropriately de-identified, to consider obtaining consent to collect health information, to build security into their products from the beginning, and to give customers the "straight story"—that is, do not use legalese, bury uses in a multiscreen privacy policy or terms of service, or use deception to get consent.

Although the concept of patient consent is not new, it is generally carried out in a limited fashion and typically through an all-or-nothing, one-on-one approach with a provider, health information exchange service, researcher, or other. Lack of a well-thought-out consent approach can result in harm if researchers do not have permission to use data that could potentially be useful or if patients do not disclose data because they fear the data will be used in ways they cannot anticipate. Fine-tuning of patient control over health data must be addressed, including how patients can become educated consumers of such control (Esterhay et al. 2014).

Dispersion of Data Needed for Population Health

To illustrate the many types of data needed for population health management, table 20.1 identifies categories of data, each with a few specific examples, that are required for population health management. The data types are categorized by whether such data are *typically* available in a given provider's EHR or must be obtained from other sources. Data included in an EHR can vary significantly according to whether the EHR is used in a hospital, primary care provider, or specialty provider. Furthermore, different EHR vendors and different providers make choices regarding whether to capture certain data or not. In some cases, data may not be retained in an EHR because they

Table 20.1.   Sources of data for population health

Type of data	Data typically included in an EHR	Data typically not included in an EHR	(Potential) source(s) for data not in an EHR
Administrative	Patient identification, location of care, healthcare professionals participating in care delivery, length of stay	Bed management data, nurse and other staff scheduling data, serial number of an implantable device, provider business hours	• Standalone systems • Credentialing system • Human resource system • Data warehouse • Enterprise master person index • Practice management system
Financial	Diagnosis and procedure codes, health plan identification	Medical necessity determination data, co-pay amounts, charges, reasons for claims denial, reimbursement rates	• Provider billing system • Practice management system • Document imaging system • Health plan systems
Clinical	Reason for admission/visit, diagnoses and their codes, laboratory test results, discharge instructions	Health plan case-management findings, data from other providers, use of evidence-based guidelines, genomic data, infection surveillance processes	• Health plan systems • HIE/HIO • Other providers' EHRs • Metadata in a clinical decision support system • Genomic data warehouse
Research		Clinical drug trials data, cancer study data	• Research databases • Disease registries • Pharmaceutical manufacturers

Type of data	Data typically included in an EHR	Data typically not included in an EHR	(Potential) source(s) for data not in an EHR
Personal reported, lifestyle, behavioral	Symptoms, diet, tobacco use, contraindication to a drug	Compliance with a treatment regimen, satisfaction survey data, outcomes of treatment regimens, sensor data, data that patients do not wish to share with a given provider or any provider	• Care coordination systems • Other providers' EHRs • Retail pharmacy point-of-sale system • Bank/credit card data • Quality data warehouse • Personal trainer • Personal physiological monitoring devices/telemetry systems • Personal health record • Health-risk appraisals
Socioeconomic	Next of kin, travel to an at-risk location	Income, education, employment, family and social support network	• Public health department • Census data • Social media
Physical environmental	Exposure to lead	Air and water quality, transportation availability, housing availability	• Public health department • Community services
Outcomes		Length of life and quality of life	• Vital records • Clinical quality outcomes measures in data warehouses

are too large (for example, genomic data) (DuBravec 2015). In other cases, data are deemed too sensitive for a variety of reasons (for example, psychotherapy notes, genomic data, research data) to document in an EHR. Other data are retained elsewhere for convenience or are not accommodated in the typical EHR. For example, one data element that may be needed for population health management (and for one-on-one patient care) is the serial numbers of implantable devices. Only a few EHRs include these data, which may more commonly reside in a surgery information, central supply, or other system. As noted, certain research data are also generally not included in an EHR, or they are not identifiable as research data per se. This may be done by intent so that bias is not introduced into the research.

The discussion here should not imply that all data need to be integrated within an EHR, that EHRs may never evolve to support population health management, or that the data types identified here are the only data needed for population health management. Instead, the discussion points to the fact that a significant amount of data is unavailable to providers today for population health management, and much more needs to be understood about population health management and health determinants to know the nature of the data actually needed.

Uses of Information for Population Health Management

Data collection obviously feeds creation of information. Healthcare is just beginning to use information for population health management. Some efforts to mine claims data have been undertaken, mostly by health plans, but many providers questioned the results (Wolfe 2015). Data used to generate information for use in population health must be captured accurately, provisioned in a manner that does not create error, and analyzed in a way that is meaningful and can accurately be interpreted (Wiedemann 2014). Data analysts may require education and tools that support ease of use (Inglesby 2015).

The list of information that may be used in population health management will very likely change and expand dramatically as more becomes understood about the nature of what information is needed and as more providers engage in population health management. For example, risk information is currently information vital to VBP. Providers and health plans want to understand both the financial risks of VBP contracts as well as the clinical risks involved in focusing care coordination on patients most in need of attention. There is also a new concept of **emergent risk**, which focuses on a tier of patients whose risk level is just below that of those patients who are at the highest level of risk for costly services. Such an emergent-risk population includes patients who are at high risk of developing a chronic disease and those who have early-stage chronic conditions, for whom better management could result in significant future value (Andrews 2015).

Business intelligence information and **clinical intelligence information**—which Henchey (2013) refers to as **clinical business intelligence**—are terms relating to technologies for gaining a deeper understanding of a variety of business and clinical information, respectively, often through integration of financial and clinical information presented to applicable users. Methods to derive such intelligence is further discussed in the section on big data analytics. Such a categorization appears useful today, but a longitudinal study over time must confirm its usefulness. Table 20.2 identifies some of the types of information used in population health management today.

Tools and Technologies Needed for Population Health Management

Tools and technologies needed for population health management include a continuum of health IT from source systems and ancillary systems that feed or complement EHRs to sophisticated data warehouse structures and software to analyze big data, present information to the user, and help exchange data across the continuum of care. Table 20.3 identifies the types of tools and technologies needed to process data into information for population health management. With one exception,

Table 20.2.   Use of information in population health management

Types of Business Information	Types of Clinical Information
Activity-based cost information	Aggregated patient-reported outcomes
Case mix information	Quality of care information
Financial risk information	Patient risk information
Financial benchmarks	Emergent risk information
Business intelligence information	Clinical intelligence information
Workforce productivity	Evidence-based guidelines
Enterprise resource information	Real-time best practices information
Performance benchmarks	Score cards and peer benchmarks
Cash flow management	On-demand comparative effectiveness information
Call center solutions	Outcomes information
Reporting compliance	Biosurveillance information

the table distinguishes between business and clinical tools merely as a matter of convenience and representation of where the industry is today with respect to these functions. The exception is the concept of big data analytics, which is a topic further discussed later in this chapter.

The tools and technologies identified in table 20.3 are generally on the cutting edge, or at least are those that are not necessarily adopted by most providers. For example, bed management systems have been available to hospitals for many years, but newer systems track more data and have more extensive management tools. Miliard (2015) reports on findings from HIMSS Analytics' hospital database that indicate that 50 percent of hospitals do not have bed management systems and perhaps rely on a basic tool, like a spreadsheet for this purpose. The HIMSS Analytics' hospital database showed that 40 percent of health systems do not have an enterprise master person index, an absolute necessity to begin the process of sharing data across an enterprise. Not surprising are findings that 65 percent of providers do not have **enterprise resource planning** (a suite of integrated tools that collect and interpret data from business activities for the purpose of planning improvements in operations, such as supply chain management, inventory management, patient relationship management, human resources, financing, and billing). Similarly, 40 percent of providers do not have a data warehouse or data warehouse service with which to manage the collection of massive amounts of data from myriad sources and upon which analytics are performed for population health management and many other uses.

Other tools listed in table 20.3 may seem simple, but they are still not widely deployed and can be tremendous workflow aids that increase efficiency and leave more time for direct patient care. An example is updated **clinical communication systems** where strong security components and pertinent apps to provide reminders and alerts are used on smartphones (Parker 2015).

Alternatively, some of the more sophisticated tools, such as predictive modeling, are equally important but may be challenging to implement. **Predictive modeling** tools apply rule-based logic to data to find statistical relationships between current patterns and future outcomes. These tools can aid providers (as well as health plans and policy makers) prospectively to predict the intended and unintended consequences of a policy intervention; they can also be used retrospectively to analyze how well various interventions have worked and how to replicate or scale such interventions; and they can be helpful by focusing on the root cause of issues to create new interventions that will be effective (Dickey 2012; Alper and Geller 2016). **Workflow modeling** is another form of modeling that also helps identify efficiencies. Sophisticated workflow modeling may target processes associated with diagnostics (for example, laboratory tests, radiology) substance therapeutics (for

Table 20.3.   Tools and technologies needed for population health management

Business Tools and Technologies	Clinical Tools and Technologies
Unit costing of services and supplies	**Laboratory outreach services** for care coordination with patients who have not had recent necessary laboratory tests performed, physician checkups, and monitoring treatment regimens (Miliard 2015)
Executive information system/dashboard	**Single-sign on** system that supports access to a mix of vendors' systems within an enterprise that has not consolidated on a single vendor (Miliard 2015)
Financial modeling	Predictive modeling
Enterprise master person index	**Infection surveillance system** that can aggregate information from multiple sources and notify an infection control nurse of a possible infection in real time
Bed management	**Molecular diagnostics** that can analyze biological markers in human genes for precision/personalized medicine (De Sa et al. 2013)
Nurse scheduling	Clinical communication systems
Staff scheduling	**Data visualization** (a process that creates a more agile information architecture by creating real-time data access, in a manner that presents information in a more user-friendly and interpretable manner, from the existing EHR and other types of health IT without changing or moving the original source code) (Caban and Gotz 2015)
Nurse communication systems that can notify a nurse in transit of a patient need (Miliard 2015)	**Risk stratification** tools that periodically and systematically review a population of patients served by a provider to categorize them according to risk factors (Stratis Health 2014)
Smart beds to notify a nurse of a patient at risk for a fall	Workflow modeling
Enterprise resource planning	Advanced clinical decision support, such as diagnostic algorithms, criteria for triage to treatment venues, indications for referrals, indications for interventions, and standard order sets and protocols
Medical-necessity checking system	**Patient activation plans** (care plans developed in conjunction with patients who are willing and able to take independent actions to manage their health and care) (Hibbard and Greene 2013)
Narrow network (insurance plans that limit subscribers to certain hospitals and physicians they believe offer the highest value) information resource (Blumenthal 2014)	**Value stream maps** for clinical service delivery and patient safety processes (lean enterprise tools used to document, analyze and improve the flow of information or services required to produce a product or service effectively and efficiently) (Barry 2013)
Big data analytics for uncovering hidden patterns, unknown correlations, and other useful information that can be used to make better decisions (SAS Institute n.d.)	

example, pharmaceuticals, nutrition), ambulatory care, emergency care, and invasive diagnostics and therapeutics. **Clinical support modeling** can also focus on things such as identification of patients who should be screened for fall risk, tracking systems to monitor compliance with treatment regimens, and modeling new processes needed for population health management, such as obtaining patient outcome information or integrating the EHRs of acute care, primary care, and LTPAC providers (Burton 2013; Mitchell 2013).

Infrastructure Needs to Support Population Health Management Tools

The tools and technologies described in table 20.3 are specific to population health management. However, these tools and technologies must be supported by an infrastructure that goes beyond what is needed by EHRs and other types of health IT used today. The following list of objectives for the infrastructure components necessary for successful and sustainable population health management is drawn from the 2014 "JASON" report commissioned by the Agency for Healthcare Quality and Research (AHRQ) and other sources. (JASON is a group of scientists, housed within the Mitre Corporation, which advises the US government on science and technology.)

- Security systems must be standardized to encrypt data at rest and in transit, separate key management from data management, and be enhanced to reduce the risk of cyber and other threats.

- Backup and recovery systems, especially for big data stored in the cloud, must ensure business continuity without cost to replace such data.

- Cloud computing—whether in public, private, or hybrid deployments—must be secure and it must provide 100 percent uptime connectivity mechanisms.

- Broadband must be universally available.

- Application performance, including EHR and other mission-critical applications, must be enhanced, and application use must be optimized.

- Data repository and data warehouse technologies must seamlessly integrate.

- Analytics as an infrastructure must become ubiquitous and not just for the few. Analytics must also support search and data discovery techniques.

- Mobile devices must be enhanced, secured, and adaptable to a variety of apps.

- Informed patient privacy controls must be in place.

- Data must be represented as atomic data with associated metadata, and the metadata, context, and provenance information must flow with data during any transmission.

- Health information exchange software must be agnostic as to the type, scale, platform, and storage location of the data and use public application program interfaces (APIs) and open standards, interfaces, and protocols.

- Interoperability must be achieved from both technology and policy perspectives.

Five Rights of Population Health Management

Groves and colleagues (2013), in describing what they call "the 'big data' revolution in healthcare," identify five value pathways that are being derived from analysis of big data. This set of five rights of population health management is based on the concept that value is derived from the balance of cost and outcomes and that the scale of big data analytics should contribute to an equally large scale, system-wide improvement. The following summary of these five "rights" describe the important aspects of population health management:

- *Right living* means patients are engaged in their health and make appropriate lifestyle choices.

- *Right care* ensures that patients get the most timely and appropriate treatment.

- The *right provider* is the one who achieves the best outcomes and has the skill set to produce the outcomes according to the complexity of the task.

- *Right value* is the result of population health management driving achievement of the Triple Aim.

- *Right innovation* addresses the feedback mechanism by which new therapies and approaches to care will be developed through the cycle of continuous population health management improvement.

Check Your Understanding 20.1

For each of the following types of data, identify if it typically is Included (I) or Not Included (N) in an EHR:

1. Provider business hours

2. Health plan identification

3. Patient satisfaction data

4. Availability of transportation

5. Family support network

For each of the above types of data, briefly describe why the data are important for population health management (drawing from chapter 19 as well):

1. Provider business hours

2. Health plan identification

3. Patient satisfaction data

4. Availability of transportation,

5. Family support network

Quality Measurement for Improved Health Outcomes

As has been previously stated, value is about quality and cost. VBP should pay for value where quality is improved and cost is lowered or the growth of cost does not escalate. Very frequently, however, the quality component is lost in discussions of population health management, or it is addressed only in the context of whether payment should establish minimum performance standards, make payment adjustments for improved performance, or make warrantied payments—which puts the responsibility for correction of quality issues solely on the shoulders of providers (Miller 2015). In another example, a white paper titled "Quality Improvement in the Advent of Population Health Management" (Caradigm 2014) identifies that "your population health strategy will drive your quality initiatives." Sadly, it seems the physicians who complain that EHRs are only a fraud prevention tool in a fee-for-service world (Halamka 2015) could be right if quality initiatives do not drive population health rather than the other way around.

Quality Metrics, Measures, and Reporting

For quality improvement to be a focal point in population health management, quality metrics, measurement, reporting, and improvement techniques must all be improved. Chapter 4 distinguishes between *metrics* and *measures* (even as the terms are frequently used synonymously) and describes the basics of quality measurement and reporting. Also identified in chapter 4 is the fact that there are a very large number of quality metrics/measures, many of which are similar but not aligned, and that there is a need to reduce the number to include only those that are most important and align any differences between programs that require their reporting.

With respect to population health management, quality metrics need to be clearer than they are today. Any ambiguity, lack of definition, or variation in metrics will produce invalid results because of data integrity issues. An example of a data integrity problem is a metric that requires measurement of a patient's arrival time in the emergency department. Suppose it is assumed that the patient's arrival time is the time when the patient is registered. There will be a significant variance in data because, in most emergency departments, some patients will be registered then triaged and others will be triaged and then registered. A solution would be to standardize another way to determine arrival time, and then figure out how such data could be collected. Unfortunately, that will not be an easy task in an emergency department. Missing data can also result from disparate systems and lack of interoperability, or simply other causes. An example is a patient who receives a urinary catheter in the emergency department and acquires an infection after being admitted to the hospital. If the EHR in the hospital does not have access to the emergency department system, the date/time of insertion of the catheter will be missing. Possible solutions for this issue would be an integrated data repository or data warehouse, or alternatively manual abstraction (Dietzel 2014).

Too many measures and misaligned measures can have unintended consequences for population health management. *The 2015 National Impact Assessment of the Centers for Medicare & Medicaid Services (CMS) Quality Measures Report* identifies that CMS quality measures reach a wide range of patients with high-impact (costly) conditions. However, CMS also notes that these measures are not evenly distributed across CMS reporting programs. Furthermore, although not stated in the report, the analysis cannot account for regional variation, which has been demonstrated numerous times to exist (for example, Spurlock and Shannon 2015). In addition, focusing measures only on such high-impact conditions could have a long term effect if more is not understood about conditions that may be emergent (see earlier discussion of emergent risk stratification).

CMS also identified that less than half of the quality measures studied by CMS are aligned with other state and federal programs. Very likely, the CMS measures are also not aligned with commercial health plan measures, which are also not aligned across plans. The result could be such a degree of variation that all measures will end up being suspect. In both scenarios of too many measures and not aligned measures, CMS proposes to create additional measures.

Another consideration with respect to CMS measures is that CMS suggests that its measures reach many more patients than the Medicare population. Forty percent of its measures include Medicaid patients and 30 percent include individuals whose care is supported by other health plan sources (in other words, the Medicare Advantage programs, in which commercial health plans assume management of payments for Medicare-eligible patients). The results of CMS measures, then, still focus primarily on Americans older than 65 years old and those who are disadvantaged. Using CMS data, then, to benchmark against commercial health plan data for a younger or more diverse population would be very misleading.

Quality Improvement

Using reports of quality measurement for quality improvement, as suggested by the previous discussion, seems to be risky. In fact, the is the risk for error increases as more measurements are required by a greater variety of types of programs—from Medicare, Medicaid, each commercial health plan with which a provider contracts, and then broken down by each type of payment model (for example, Medicare fee-for-service as compared to a Medicare alternative payment model)—if for no other reason than the quality reporting burden is made more complex by similar yet slightly different measures.

Electronic clinical quality measures (eCQM) offered by CMS are intended to reduce the reporting burden by allowing one-time reporting across all CMS programs. EHRs that support eCQM were required for stage 2 meaningful use (MU) incentives. However, in a September 2015 report, the American Hospital Association (AHA) noted that more than 60 percent of hospitals and about 90 percent of physicians had yet to attest to stage 2. Many factors, not just the ability to generate eCQMs, explain why more organizations did not reach stage 2, but the fact remains that recouping at least part of the investment in EHR through the anticipated MU incentives is delayed and potentially at risk. Many providers use outsourced services to manage quality measurement reporting, but these services must still extract the data from EHRs or data repositories to manage the variety of reporting requirements they are hired to address.

Lack of reliable information derived from quality measurement reporting has an unknown impact on the ability of providers to make improvements, although there may be a "report effect" that alone could trigger some improvement. One finding from the CMS 2015 report on quality measures is that 35 percent of the 119 measures were classified as high performing, meaning that performance rates exceeding 90 percent were achieved in each of the most recent 3 years for which data were available. One assumption that could be made is that quality improves when providers know it is being monitored. That is not a completely faulty assumption, and yet one could wonder what improvement strategies were actually used to achieve such success. Were improvement strategies intentionally created in response to the quality measures, or was improvement achieved simply because providers knew all along what would be better but, for some reason, had not implemented those better performance activities? Are whatever strategies deployed sustainable without measurement? Should, and would, CMS risk the discontinuance of the reporting requirements for high-performing measurements, assuming that lasting changes have been made?

CMS and other health plans include both process and outcomes measures in their reporting requirements. Process measures can lead to change that yields outcomes improvement. For example, CMS inpatient-hospital heart failure process measurement improvements resulted in 7,000 to 10,000 lives saved between 2006 and 2012. Still, outcomes metrics/measures need significant fine-tuning so that outcomes can reflect more than just whether a person lived or died, especially as Healthy People 2020 focuses on two outcomes: length of life and quality of life (NCHS 2015).

Population health management that focuses on payment may drive change in measurement reporting and improvement strategies. However, it remains to be seen whether such improvements can be accomplished quickly enough to encourage spread, scale, and sustainability in population health (Wizemann et al. 2015).

Healthcare Big Data Analytics

Big data is defined as "a massive amount of data available to study, but which is so big and often in unstructured format that traditional databases and methods of analysis are difficult to use" (Zikopoulos et al. 2012). Big data alone are often inconsequential unless they can be harnessed to provide useful information and intelligence (Rossi 2015). Chapter 2 describes the data-information-knowledge-wisdom (DIKW). The difference between the DIKW and intelligence is distinguished here. Data are processed into information, and experience may be added to information to generate knowledge, which, when codified into best practices, offers wisdom. *Intelligence,* however, is the ability to apply knowledge. Knowledge is an inherent feature of creating intelligence—in fact, if a person lacks knowledge in a certain area, he or she may still use intelligence to solve a problem (Colangelo 2014). Such intelligence also carries a requirement that people can trust the data and their results and that they will be open to identifying opportunities for innovation and have the will to make cultural and business changes from intelligent insights (Bean 2016).

Big Data Characteristics

Big data are indeed big and are frequently described by at least the first three of the following characteristics (Normandeau 2013):

- *Volume:* Vast amounts of data characterize big data. The amount of data accumulated between 2012 and 2013 is measured as a zettabyte (a measure of storage capacity that is equal to 10^{21} bytes of information), which dwarfs the prior record of human civilization (Shaw 2014). The ability to harness such data makes big data more accessible to use in analytics. For example, the ability to tap social media to gain insights into healthcare outcomes could prove very valuable where such data about patient opinions have been elusive to providers in the past. However, it is also observed that in many cases, data analytics can find results by examining only a representative sample of the data that are available in big data systems. Sampling must be done properly and the selection methodology must be tested to ensure accurate results (Stedman n.d.).

- *Velocity:* Velocity is the real-time, or near-real-time, speed with which data are collected. When big data are analyzed, the results also have the capability of being delivered in real or near real time. In healthcare, for example, a physician could literally tap into big data generated by all of the EHRs in an enterprise to gain insights into the efficacy of a certain drug as it relates to a wide variety of patient attributes—all of this analysis can be done at the point of care and delivered to the patient, using data visualization tools, to help in shared decision making.

- *Variety:* Big data are not limited to structured data but may also include much unstructured data, such as narrative, audio, sound, wave forms, photos, scans, videos, and other types. In healthcare, data from physiological monitoring devices can be integrated with photos, sound, and/or wave forms to help provide critical alerts for patients with congestive heart failure patients or atrial fibrillation, for instance.

- *Value:* The value of big data is drawn from their volume, velocity, and variety (Rossi 2015). In the past, structured data were essentially required for analysis, but big data analytics techniques enable data in a variety of forms to be tapped for use in creation of information or intelligence. The speed with which intelligence can be delivered to a user makes the big data valuable. For healthcare, most of the uses of information for population health require, or at least are significantly improved by the value of, big data.

- *Veracity* and *validity:* The volume, velocity, and variety of big data may provide value, but they also pose challenges. Noise, biases, and other abnormalities are characteristic of big data, which would ordinarily cause the data to not be trusted and would invalidate its use. Big data that are ungoverned and not standardized and monitored for quality can affect the empirical evidence, trustworthiness, and transparency of the intelligence derived from them. Cleansing big data is becoming a task associated with big data analytics.

- *Volatility:* Volatility refers to how long data and the information derived from data will remain useful. There is volatility in all data, but volatility may be more observable in big data because of the ability to continuously conduct analytics in real or near real time; this type of analytics highlights even subtle changes.

Big Data Analytics

Analytics identifies meaningful patterns and knowledge in data through the use of statistical, mathematical, and machine-learning techniques as well as predictive modeling. In contrast to **data**

mining, which discovers previously unknown patterns and knowledge, machine learning uses algorithms to reproduce known patterns and knowledge and apply that to other data and to decision support. Analytics is different than analysis in that analytics tends to use data to look forward and model the future or predict a result. Analysis tends to look backward over time, separating a whole into component parts that may lend insights into past experiences (Hill 2011).

It is suggested that there have been three eras of analytics, with Analytics 1.0 being the era of business intelligence that started with new techniques to conduct analysis—especially surrounding the need to prepare data for analysis (that is, recording data in a structured format, aggregating them, and applying statistical processes to understand them). Analytics 2.0 is described as the era of big data with the emergence of analytics that could build models that were forward-looking. Analytics 3.0—the era of data-enriched offerings—brings analytics into the mainstream. The near future of analytics includes customer-facing tools, such as better search algorithms and social media that puts experiential data at the fingertips of lay persons. Analytics 3.0 fully supports combining multiple types of data, offers new data management technologies (see below), provides faster technologies and processing methods, and embeds analytics in other software, such as clinical decision support (Davenport 2013).

Data discovery is also a part of the new analytics. **Data discovery** is the ability of end users to apply artificial intelligence tools to explore data for discovering trends. Data discovery is more refined than a typical Internet search, but it is easier for a nontechnical person to perform than data mining (All 2014). It supports ad hoc creation of data sets rather than using data sets that have been painstakingly created with data that may no longer be current or current, and absent data that were not previously anticipated and therefore not collected.

While Analytics 3.0 is "user-friendly," it is also cross-disciplinary with respect to sophisticated programming of the analytics techniques. A new role, the data scientist, is emerging. A **data scientist** can combine mathematics, statistics, and software engineering, and has the domain expertise that IBM calls "part analyst and part artist." A data scientist "does not simply collect and report on data, but also looks at it from many angles, determines what it means, then recommends way to apply the data" (IBM n.d.).

Technical Platform for Big Data Analytics

Some of the technology needed for big data analytics is described in the earlier discussion of health IT for population health management. At the risk of oversimplifying the technology needed to conduct big data analytics, healthcare organizations (including providers, health plans, and their service providers) need the following five types of technology to utilize big data for effective population health management:

- *Cloud services:* As previously noted, healthcare organizations have been somewhat reluctant to adopt cloud services, but no organization has the capacity to store and process big data in one place. Genomic data alone need enormous data warehouses. In fact, some big data applications are using multiple cloud service providers. IBM was one of the companies that spearheaded big data analytics with its Watson supercomputer platform that uses natural language processing and machine learning to reveal insights from large amounts of unstructured data. Even Watson, however, is now offered as a cloud service through the Watson Health unit for performing big data analytics (Wicklund 2015).

- *HIPAA-level encryption:* It is unlikely that every piece of data collected as part of big data will be de-identified according to the HIPAA safe-harbor or expert determination guidance issued by the HHS Office of Civil Rights (OCR) in 2012. Therefore, whether big data are stored in the cloud or not, it is essential that data at rest be encrypted following the National Institute of Standards and Technology (NIST) special publication 800-111, *Guide to Storage Encryption Technologies for End User Devices* (Scarfone et al. 2007), and data in transit be encrypted following the Federal Information Processing Standards (FIPS) 140-2, Annex A, which is also required under the EHR MU incentive program (CFR 170.210). It is also important to get assurances from data management vendors regarding their compliance and their key management strategies. Certification and/or audit conducted by third parties may be necessary.

- *Big data technical platform:* Two types of technical platforms may be used to manage big data. When a data set (even one with a very large volume) is slowly evolving and includes data that have predetermined schemas, parallel processing architectures, such as a data warehouse, can be used. According to Miliard (2015), up to 60 percent of healthcare providers have acquired such a platform, at least in its most basic form. For data that are not structured and change rapidly, a faster solution for analytics processing is a distributed processing solution where data reside in multiple, disperse file and database storage systems and can be processed via **in-memory computing** (using a type of middleware software that processes data stored in memory across a cluster of computers) (Ivanov 2014). Such a "virtual" environment of processing is an extended version of server virtualization. Figure 20.1 compares the two solutions.

- *Big data processing framework:* Big data are typically processed on a framework for storing data and running applications on clusters of affordable, easy-to-obtain hardware. The framework operates much like a general contractor, providing massive storage literally wherever it might be available at the lowest possible cost and processing limitless concurrent tasks or jobs virtually (wherever there is space and appropriate data analysis and analytics tools are available for such processing). The open-source software that is currently most popular and serves as a basis for other software development is Apache's Hadoop, initially developed by Java programmers at Yahoo. MapReduce is the framework for problem distribution, and the Hadoop Distributed File System (HDFS) provides the ability to integrate unstructured data into resultant computational processes. Newer versions of Hadoop and Hadoop alternatives are becoming available, each with different advantages and disadvantages (Mitchell 2014; Webster 2014).

Figure 20.1.   Technical platforms for big data analytics

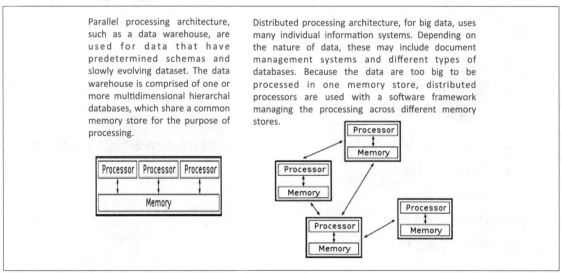

- *Data analysis and analytics tools:* As noted previously, specific data analysis and analytics tools are used to process big data in various ways, such as to offer predictive modeling, perform data discovery and conduct searches, provide data visualization, and even to clean data for more refined data warehousing applications (Jones 2014). Some of these tools are native to Hadoop, others are specifically designed to run on Hadoop, and still others work alongside Hadoop and often run with Hadoop alternatives as well. Many of the analysis and analytics tools utilize SQL or NoSQL (not only SQL) as their programming language (Henschen 2014).

Check Your Understanding 20.2

Choose the best answer:

1. Which of the following may have an unintended consequence for patients with emergent risk?

    a. Misaligned quality measures

    b. Narrow networks

    c. Provider attribution

    d. Quality improvement report effect

2. Which of the following could negatively affect a provider's ability to demonstrate value in private health plan contract negotiation?

    a. CMS reimbursement rates

    b. Lack of transparency in reimbursement rates

    c. Invalid risk stratification

    d. Misaligned quality measures

3. Which term describes the ability to apply information without necessarily having experience?

    a. Big data

    b. Intelligence

    c. Knowledge

    d. Population health

4. A key reason that a single, large database will not suffice for processing big data is the :

    a. Value of big data

    b. Variety of big data

    c. Velocity of big data

    d. Volume of big data

5. Which of the following types of tools is necessary to ensure interpretation of data from analytics?

   a. Data cleaning

   b. Data discovery

   c. Data mining

   d. Data visualization

References and Resources

Affordable Care Act of 2010 (ACA). 2010 (March 23). http://www.hhs.gov/healthcare/about-the-law/read-the-law.

All, A. 2014 (September 18). Data discovery is changing business intelligence. *Enterprise Apps Today*. http://www.enterpriseappstoday.com/business-intelligence/data-discovery-is-changing-business-intelligence.html.

Alper, J., and A. Geller. 2016. *How Modeling Can Inform Strategies to Improve Population Health: Workshop Summary*. Washington, DC: National Academies Press. http://www.nap.edu/catalog/21807/how-modeling-can-inform-strategies-to-improve-population-health-workshop.

American Hospital Association (AHA). 2015 (September 9). Fact sheet: Getting meaningful use right. http://www.aha.org/content/14/fs-meaningfuluse.pdf.

Andrews, J. 2015 (July). Analytics empower health industry. *Healthcare IT News*. http://www.healthcareitnews.com/issue/July%202015.

Barry, C. 2013 (February 27). How to use value stream maps in healthcare. Minitab blog. http://blog.minitab.com/blog/real-world-quality-improvement/how-to-use-value-stream-maps-in-healthcare.

Bean, R. 2016 (February 9). Just using big data isn't enough anymore. *Harvard Business Review*. https://hbr.org/2016/02/just-using-big-data-isnt-enough-anymore.

Blumenthal, D. 2014 (February 24). Reflecting on health reform—narrow networks: Boon or bane? *To the Point* (Commonwealth Fund blog). http://www.commonwealthfund.org/publications/blog/2014/feb/narrows-networks-boon-or-bane.

Burton, D.A. 2013. White paper: Population health management: Implementing a strategy for success. Health Catalyst. https://www.healthcatalyst.com/WhitePaper_PopulationHealthManagement.html.

Caban, J.J., and D. Gotz. 2015 (March). Visual analytics in healthcare—opportunities and research challenges. *Journal of the American Medical Informatics Association*. 22:260–262.

Caradigm. 2014 (November 20). White paper: Quality improvement in the advent of population health management. Health IT Outcomes. http://www.healthitoutcomes.com/doc/quality-improvement-in-the-advent-of-population-health-management-0001.

Centers for Medicare and Medicaid Services (CMS), Center for Clinical Standards and Quality. 2015. *2015 National Impact Assessment of the Centers for Medicare & Medicaid Services (CMS) Quality Measures Report*. https://www.cms.gov/Medicare/Quality-Initiatives-Patient-Assessment-Instruments/QualityMeasures/Downloads/2015-National-Impact-Assessment-Report.pdf.

Chokshi, D., and N. Stine. 2013 (January 23). Defining population health. Robert Wood Johnson Culture of Health blog. http://www.rwjf.org/en/culture-of-health/2013/01/defining_population.html.

Colangelo, A. 2014 (November 14). Knowledge vs. intelligence. A List Apart blog. http://alistapart.com/blog/post/knowledge-vs-intelligence.

Davenport, T.H. 2013 (December). Analytics 3.0. *Harvard Business Review*. https://hbr.org/2013/12/analytics-30.

De Sa, J., et al. 2013. Growth of molecular diagnostics and genetic testing in the USA, 2008–2011. *Personalized Medicine*. 10(8):785–792.

Dickey, D.A. 2012. Introduction to predictive modeling with examples. *Proceedings of SAS Global Forum 2012*. Statistics and data analysis section. http://support.sas.com/resources/papers/proceedings12/337-2012.pdf.

Dietzel, L. 2014 (July 29). The unintended consequences of electronic clinical quality measures. HealthCatalyst. https://www.healthcatalyst.com/electronic-clinical-quality-measures-impact-data-quality.

DuBravec, D. 2015. Can EHRs handle genomic data? *Journal of AHIMA*. 86(11):28–31.

Esterhay, R.J., et al. 2014. *Population Health: Management, Policy, and Technology*. Virginia Beach, VA: Convurgent Publishing; 2014

Federal Trade Commission (FTC). 2015. *Careful Connections: Building Security in the Internet of Things*. https://www.ftc.gov/tips-advice/business-center/guidance/careful-connections-building-security-internet-things.

Groves, P., et al. 2013 (January). White paper: The "big data" revolution in healthcare: Accelerating value and innovation. McKinsey & Company. http://www.mckinsey.com/industries/healthcare-systems-and-services/our-insights/the-big-data-revolution-in-us-health-care.

Halamka, J.D. 2015 (December 23). My 2016 predictions for HIT. Life as a Healthcare CIO blog. http://geekdoctor.blogspot.com/2015/12/my-2016-predictions-for-hit.html.

Han, C. 2015 (April 28). Using consumer health data: Some considerations for companies. Federal Trade Commission business blog. https://www.ftc.gov/news-events/blogs/business-blog/2015/04/using-consumer-health-data-some-considerations-companies.

Harris, D., et al. 2016. Population health: Curriculum framework for an emerging discipline. *Population Health Management*. 19(1): 9–45. http://online.liebertpub.com/doi/abs/10.1089/pop.2015.0129.

Health and Medical Division (HMD) of the National Academies of Science, Engineering, and Medicine. 2016 (April 22). Vision, mission, and definition of the Roundtable on Population Health. http://www.nationalacademies.org/hmd/Activities/PublicHealth/PopulationHealthImprovementRT/VisionMission.

Health Care Payment Learning and Action Network (HCP-LAN). 2016a (June). White paper: Accelerating and aligning population-based payment models: Patient attribution. Mitre Corporation. https://www.mitre.org/publications/technical-papers/accelerating-and-aligning-population-based-payment-models-patient.

Health Care Payment Learning and Action Network (HCP-LAN). 2016b. White paper: Accelerating and aligning population-based payment models: Financial benchmarking. Mitre Corporation. http://hcp-lan.org/workproducts/fb-whitepaper-final.pdf.

Henchey, P. 2013 (April 1). What is clinical business intelligence? Module 1 in *Healthcare Information and Management Systems Society (HIMSS) Clinical & Business Intelligence Primer*. http://www.himss.org/library/clinical-business-intelligence/clinical-business-intelligence-primer/what-is-clinical-business-intelligence?navItemNumber=18235.

Henschen, D. 2016 (January 28). Big data analytics: Time for new tools. *Information Week*. http://www.informationweek.com/big-data/big-data-analytics/big-data-analytics-time-for-new-tools/a/d-id/1318106.

Hibbard, J.H., and J. Greene. 2013. What the evidence shows about patient activation: Better health outcomes and care experiences. *Health Affairs*. 32(2):207–214.

Hill, C. 2011 (June 2). Analysis vs. analytics: What's the difference? 1to1Media. http://www.1to1media.com/view.aspx?docid=32968.

IBM. n.d. What is a data scientist? http://www-01.ibm.com/software/data/infosphere/data-scientist.

Inglesby, T. 2015 (April 3). Special advertising section: Healthcare analytics: Putting data to good use. *Patient Safety and Quality Healthcare*. http://psqh.com/march-april-2015/healthcare-analytics-putting-data-to-good-use.

Ivanov, N. 2014 (March 17). In-memory computing: In plain English. GridGain In-Memory Computing Performance blog. http://www.gridgain.com/resources/blog/in-memory-computing-in-plain-english.

Jacobson, D.M., and S. Teutsch. 2012. An environmental scan of integrated approaches for defining and measuring total population health by the clinical care system, the government public health system, and stakeholder organizations. Public Health Institute and County of Los Angeles Public Health Department. http://www.improvingpopulationhealth.org/PopHealthPhaseIICommissionedPaper.pdf.

JASON. 2014 (April). *A Robust Health Data Infrastructure*. Rockville, MD: Agency for Healthcare Research and Quality. AHRQ publication no. 14-0041-EF. https://www.healthit.gov/sites/default/files/ptp13-700hhs_white.pdf.

Jones, A. 2014 (June 12). Top 10 data analysis tools for business. LinkedIn Pulse. https://www.linkedin.com/pulse/20140612032806-111366377-top-10-data-analysis-tools-for-business.

Kindig, D. 2015 (April 6). What are we talking about when we talk about population health? Health Affairs blog. http://healthaffairs.org/blog/2015/04/06/what-are-we-talking-about-when-we-talk-about-population-health.

Kindig, D., and G. Stoddart. 2003. What is population health? *American Journal of Public Health*. 93(3):380–383. http://www.ncbi.nlm.nih.gov/pmc/articles/PMC1447747.

Leventhal, R. 2014 (October 13). Report: Health IT leaders say their infrastructure isn't prepared for the evolution of EHRs. *Healthcare Informatics*. http://www.healthcare-informatics.com/news-item/report-health-it-leaders-say-their-infrastructure-isn-t-prepared-evolution-ehrs.

Lewis, N. 2014 (March 19). Populations, population health, and the evolution of population management: Making sense of the terminology in US healthcare today. Institute for Healthcare Improvement. http://www.ihi.org/communities/blogs/_layouts/ihi/community/blog/itemview.aspx?List=81ca4a47-4ccd-4e9e-89d9-14d88ec59e8d&ID=50.

Miliard, M. 2015 (August 25). 18 health technologies poised for big growth. *Healthcare IT News*. http://www.healthcareitnews.com/news/18-health-technologies-poised-big-growth.

Miller, H.D. 2015 (April). The building blocks of successful payment reform: Designing payment systems that support higher-value health care. Network for Regional Healthcare Improvement (NRHI) Payment Reform Series no. 3. http://www.nrhi.org/uploads/nrhi_pymntrfrm_3_r9-2.pdf.

Mitchell, G. 2013. Long-term care and interoperable EHRs: A strategic match. *Leading Age*. 3(4). http://www.leadingage.org/Long-Term_Care_and_Interoperable_EHRs_A_Strategic_Match_V3N4.aspx.

Mitchell, R.L. 2014 (October 23). 8 big trends in big data analytics. *Computerworld*. http://www.computerworld.com/article/2690856/big-data/8-big-trends-in-big-data-analytics.html.

National Center for Health Statistics (NCHS). 2015 (November 6). Healthy People 2020. http://www.cdc.gov/nchs/healthy_people/hp2020.htm.

Normandeau, K. 2013 (September 12). Beyond volume, variety and velocity is the issue of big data veracity. *Inside Big Data*. http://insidebigdata.com/2013/09/12/beyond-volume-variety-velocity-issue-big-data-veracity.

Office for Civil Rights (OCR). 2012 (November 26). Guidance regarding methods for de-identification of protected health information in accordance with the HIPAA Privacy Rule. http://www.hhs.gov/hipaa/for-professionals/privacy/special-topics/de-identification/index.html.

Parker, C.D. 2015 (March/April). Update clinical communication strategy, not just the BYOD policy. *Patient Safety and Quality Healthcare*. http://psqh.com/online-first/update-clinical-communication-strategy-not-just-the-byod-policy.

Partners HealthCare. n.d. About population health management (PHM): So what exactly is population health management? http://www.partners.org/innovation-and-leadership/population-health-management/about-phm.

Pizzi, R. 2015 (May 29). Defining population health: What does population health truly mean? Who is responsible? What impact does it have on our current healthcare environment? *Healthcare IT News*. http://www.healthcareitnews.com/blog/defining-population-health.

Regard, D.L., and R. Hedges. 2015. Application of search analytics in the healthcare profession. *Journal of AHIMA*. 86(5):48–49.

Rossi, B. 2015 (August 21). How to measure the value of big data. *Information Age*. http://www.information-age.com/it-management/strategy-and-innovation/123460041/how-measure-value-big-data.

SAS Institute. n.d. Big data analytics: What it is and why it matters. http://www.sas.com/en_us/insights/analytics/big-data-analytics.html.

Scarfone, K., et al. 2007 (November). *Guide to Storage Encryption Technologies for End User Devices*. National Institute of Standards and Technology (NIST) special publication 800-111. http://nvlpubs.nist.gov/nistpubs/Legacy/SP/nistspecialpublication800-111.pdf.

Seife, C. 2013 (November 27). 23andMe is terrifying, but not for the reasons the FDA thinks. *Scientific American*. http://www.scientificamerican.com/article/23andme-is-terrifying-but-not-for-the-reasons-the-fda-thinks.

Shaw, J. 2014 (March–April). Why "big data" is a big deal. *Harvard Magazine*. http://harvardmagazine.com/2014/03/why-big-data-is-a-big-deal.

Spurlock, B., and M. Shannon. 2015 (October 13). The new era of narrow networks: Do they come at the cost of quality? Health Affairs blog. http://healthaffairs.org/blog/2015/10/13/the-new-era-of-narrow-networks-do-they-come-at-the-cost-of-quality.

Stedman, C. Analytical models in big data environments often best left small. TechTarget.com. http://searchbusinessanalytics.techtarget.com/feature/Analytical-models-in-big-data-environments-often-best-left-small.

Stratis Health. 2014. Population risk stratification and patient cohort identification. https://www.stratishealth.org/documents/HITToolkitcoordination/3-Population-Risk-Stratification-and-Patient-Cohort-Identification.pdf.

Varpio, L., et al. 2015. The EHR and building the patient's story: A qualitative investigation of how EHR use obstructs a vital clinical activity. *International Journal of Medical Informatics*. 84(12):1019–1028.

Webster, J. 2014 (December 8). Is it time for Hadoop alternatives? *Forbes*. http://www.forbes.com/sites/johnwebster/2014/12/08/is-it-time-for-hadoop-alternatives/#2715e4857a0b419fb0995975.

Wicklund, E. 2015 (September 10). IBM ramps up Watson with products and partnerships. *Healthcare IT News*. http://www.healthcareitnews.com/news/ibm-ramps-watson-products-partnerships.

Wiedemann, L.A. 2014. Nonsensical data input produces undesired output for data analysis. *Journal of AHIMA*. 85(6):50–51.

Wizemann, T., et al. 2015. *Spread, Scale, and Sustainability in Population Health: Workshop Summary*. Institute of Medicine Roundtable on Population Health Improvement. Washington, DC: National Academies Press. http://www.nap.edu/catalog/21708/spread-scale-and-sustainability-in-population-health-workshop-summary.

Wolfe, P. 2015 (October 19). Advanced analytics: Reimagining the power of data. *Executive Insight*. Advance Healthcare Network. http://healthcare-executive-insight.advanceweb.com/Features/Articles/Advanced-Analytics.aspx.

Woolf A., et al. 2013 (January). *U.S. Health in International Perspective: Shorter Lives, Poorer Health*. Institute of Medicine. Washington, DC: National Academies Press. http://www.nap.edu/catalog/13497/us-health-in-international-perspective-shorter-lives-poorer-health.

Zikopoulos, P.C., et al. 2012. *Understanding Big Data Analytics for Enterprise Class Hadoop and Streaming Data*. New York: McGraw-Hill.

Glossary and Index

Glossary

30-day readmission: Hospitals can be penalized 1 percent of their Medicare reimbursement when patients with myocardial infarction, congestive heart failure, or pneumonia were readmitted within 30 days of discharge

ABC Coding Solutions: A joint venture of the Foundation for Integrative Healthcare and Alternative Link. It provides more than 4,500 codes to describe complementary and alternative medicine and nursing services

Abstracting: The process of extracting information from a document or record, often to create a brief summary of a patient's illness, treatment, and outcome or enter them into an automated system for subsequent processing

Acceptance testing: Final review during EHR implementation to ensure that all tests have been performed and all issues have been resolved; usually triggers the final payment for the system and when a maintenance contract becomes effective

Accountability: A property that ensures that the actions of an entity can be traced solely to this entity

Accountable Care Organization (ACO): An organization of hospitals, physicians, and other healthcare providers that share responsibility for the quality, cost, and overall care of Medicare beneficiaries who are assigned to the program

Accredited Standards Committee X12 (ASC X12): A committee accredited by the American National Standards Institute (ANSI) responsible for the development and maintenance of electronic data interchange (EDI) standards for many industries. The ASC "X12N" is the subcommittee of ASC X12 responsible for the EDI health insurance administrative transactions such as 837 Institutional Health Care Claim and 835 Professional Health Care Claim forms

Acquisition strategy: The long-term process used to select and license software wherein a healthcare organization chooses, or defaults to using, either one primary vendor (considered a best-of-fit acquisition strategy) or many vendors (considered a bestof-breed acquisition strategy) for all healthcare information technology applications

Active (CDS) advice: A process of providing alerts and reminders to clinicians in which a specific action is required in response; in contrast, *see* **passive (CDS) advice**

Active Directory: The location within the Microsoft operating system where network access controls are set and authentication of users takes place

Actuarial models: Statistical techniques for predicting financial risk

Ad hoc information requirements analysis: Determination of the functions desired to be included in an EHR application performed in a nonstructured manner that may yield incomplete results

Adaptive case management (ACM): A process improvement technique most suitable for knowledge workers where processes performed are often not predictable and systems must be able to adapt to such situations

ADKAR model of communication: A model that encompasses the stages of awareness, desire, knowledge, abilities, and reinforcement and recognizes a continuum of messages for projects that introduce a great amount of change, and it illustrates the relationship between types of messages and project phases

Admissibility: The condition of being admitted into evidence in a court of law

Adoption: The phase after implementation in which intended users become acclimated to the EHR and regularly use more of its functionality

Adverse drug event: A patient injury resulting from a medication, either because of an anticipated pharmacological reaction to a normal dose or because of a preventable result occurring from an error

Adverse drug reaction (ADR): A harmful or unpleasant reaction produced by the use of a medication in the recommended manner. ADRs are a subset of adverse drug events and are nonpreventable

Aggregate data: Data from a population that are combined to form deidentified information that can be compared and analyzed

Agile modeling: A methodology for information modeling that is based on best practices, and it uses UML 2.x to envision a project, brainstorm through details, prioritize requirements, engage all stakeholders (including users), and produce an information model that is sufficient to develop software (Ambler 2014)

Agile Scrum: A technique where system-wide workflows are evaluated for the purpose of quickly and flexibly improving project management, software development, and managing value

Algorithm: A set of rules to be processed by a computer program that involves repetition of a finite number of steps

American National Standards Institute (ANSI): The US government's preferred accreditor of standards development organizations (SDOs). ANSI accreditation validates that organizations are representative of industry stakeholders and have produced standards that are not biased to any one group of the stakeholders they are attempting to represent

American Recovery and Reinvestment Act of 2009 (ARRA): A law, often called the economic stimulus package, enacted by the 111th United States Congress and signed by President Obama on February 17, 2009, intended to improve the economy and create jobs. It includes measures to improve use of health information technology to achieve greater healthcare value

Analytical database: *Also called* **data warehouse**, this is an organized collection of data that supports statistical analysis

Anecdotal benefits: Specific examples of events that occurred or were avoided when the EHR was used

ANSI Accredited Standards Committee X12: An SDO that develops messaging standards for electronic data interchange (EDI) of financial and administrative transactions

Application Programming Interfaces (APIs): Programs that allow internal functions to operate outside of their internal structure in a limited way (Raths 2014)

Applications inventory: Identifying all the applications that currently exist and how they may be related to one another (or not)

Architecture: The configuration, structure, and relationships of hardware (the machinery of the computer including input/output devices, storage devices, and so on) in an information system

ASC X12 999 Acknowledgement for Healthcare Insurance Transaction: Used to notify a provider that any functional group of *any* transaction set is accepted, accepted with errors, or rejected (that is, the ASC X12 999 is an acknowledgement for not only claims but also the end of any set of transactions). (Jackson 2010)

ASC X12 277CA Claim Acknowledgement: Used to acknowledge *each claim* received in a Functional Group only when the transaction set (of claims) is not rejected (Jackson 2010)

ASTM Continuity of Care Record (CCR): Standard specification, maintained by the ASTM International standards development organization, for a data set of the most relevant administrative, demographic, and clinical facts about a patient's healthcare that supports continuity of care when a patient is referred to another provider

ASTM International: Formerly known as the American Society for Testing and Materials, this organization is not ANSI-accredited, but its history predates ANSI and it follows the ANSI-prescribed SDO processes

Attributes: Properties or characteristics of data elements, such as their names (whether they are alphabetic, numeric, and so on), that are included in a relational database

Auditing: The performance of internal and/or external reviews (audits) to identify variations from established baselines (for example, review of users who accessed information as compared with the users' access privileges)

Authentication: 1. The process of identifying the source of health record entries by attaching a handwritten signature, the author's initials, or an electronic signature 2. Proof of authorship that ensures, as much as possible, that log-ins and messages from a person or system originate from an authorized source

Authorization: The giving of permission

Automated informed consent system: An application that provides patients a comprehensive and consistent set of information about the benefits and risks of a surgical or other procedure requiring a signed permission to perform

Availability: Data can continue to be able to be provided to authorized users at a required level of performance in situations ranging from normal through disastrous

Bad debt: A payment that is not collected from a party who was obligated to pay

Balance after insurance: May include the co-pay, any deductible amount that has not yet been fulfilled, and/or a co-insurance if the patient has a health insurance plan in which the patient owes a portion of the total bill, not just a co-pay and deductible (Matjucha and Giuliano 2011)

Balanced scorecard: A quality improvement technique that measures and manages defined metrics derived from institutional sources and aligns the metrics with the strategic goals of the organization

Bar code medication administration record (BC-MAR): System that uses barcoding technology for positive patient and drug identification during the process of giving a drug to a patient

Basic EHR: An EHR that includes computerized documentation but offers minimal or no clinical decision support that alerts clinicians of potential issues with their patients

Benefits portfolio: The set of quantitative and qualitative, financial and qualitative benefits that make the business case for making an investment

Benefits realization: The process of collecting and studying the same type of data about process performance—for the new process to determine that improvements have been achieved

Best of suite: A strategy used when purchasing HIT in which applications are acquired from only two primary vendors, usually the incumbent vendor providing the financial/administrative functions and another vendor providing the clinical functionality

Bidders' conference: A conference held by an organization to respond to questions about a submitted RFP which includes the specific date, time, and location

Big data: The massive amount of data available to study, which is often in unstructured formats

Big bang: An EHR implementation strategy where all components of the EHR are required to be used by all users starting at one time

Blue Button: A project sponsored by CMS and the Department of Veterans Affairs (VA) to make it easy for their beneficiaries to access claims data (and for veterans to create and maintain a web-based personal health record with the VA's MyHealth*e*Vet application)

Bundled payment: Also called episode-of-care payment; a method in which payments to providers are based on the expected costs for a clinically defined episode or bundle of related healthcare services, including cost associated with preventable complications

Business associate: A person who creates, receives, maintains, or transmits PHI on behalf of a covered entity or who provides services for a covered entity that involve the disclosure of PHI

Business case: An economic justification, usually for a capital expenditure

Business intelligence: *See* online analytical processing (OLAP)

Caching: A process wherein data and instructions that are used repeatedly are temporarily stored in a computer to speed up access

Capitation: A fixed payment amount given to providers for the care that patients may receive in a given time period, such as a month or year

Care coordination: Deliberate organization of patient care activities between two or more participants (including the patient) involved in a patient's care to facilitate the appropriate delivery of healthcare services. Care coordination may include facilitation among providers as well as social services (AHRQ 2007)

Care management: A function of a health plan or provider that attempts to improve medical practice and assist consumers to be more engaged in their healthcare in order to achieve quality of care and cost improvements

Care Map: A care-planning tool typically used by nurses in an acute care setting that outlines the steps and decision points in the management of a specific healthcare condition. A care map can be customized to represent care for a specific patient. Care maps, care pathways, and care plans, although similar, may be physically presented in different formats

Care pathway: A standardized, day-to-day course of care for patients with the same condition to achieve consistent outcomes. Pathways are often developed by a hospital, a long-term care facility, or a health plan; are modified for specific patients; and are more commonly used by nurses than by physicians

Care plan: The specific goals in the treatment of an individual patient, amended as the patient's condition requires. Used by physicians and nurses to communicate steps in a treatment regimen and assess outcomes of care; serves as a template for ongoing documentation of a patient's care, condition, and needs

Case management: The ongoing, concurrent review performed by clinical professionals to ensure the necessity and effectiveness of the clinical services being provided to a patient

Case mix: The distribution of patients into categories reflecting differences in severity of illness or resource consumption

Centers for Medicare and Medicaid Services (CMS): The division of the Department of Health and Human Services that is responsible for developing healthcare policy in the United States and for administering the Medicare program and the federal portion of the Medicaid program

Central processing unit: The circuitry of a computer that causes the electronic components to function

Certificate authority: Part of a public key authority, it issues and verifies a digital certificate that identifies the individual

Certified EHR technology (CEHRT): CEHRT moves beyond the basic EHR and is the subject of financial incentives encouraging hospitals and physicians to make meaningful use of it

Change agent: *See* change leader.

Change control: The process of performing an impact analysis and obtaining approval before modifications to a software application are made

Change leader: An individual who acts as catalyst for change. Change leaders have a clear vision that they can articulate to others, are patient and persistent, ask tough questions, are considered knowledgeable, and are able to lead by example

Change management: The formal process of introducing change, getting it adopted, and diffusing it throughout the organization

Charge capture: The entry of items charged into an accounting system as well as clinical documentation in the health record to substantiate the claim

Charge description master: Also called a chargemaster; the cataloging in a database of all the supplies and services provided to patients and the corresponding charges for those items

Chargemaster: *See* charge description master

Charity care: The provision of services at no cost to people who do not have the means to pay

Chart conversion: An EHR implementation activity in which data from the paper chart are converted into electronic form

Chief information officer: The chief information officer (CIO) is a member of executive leadership and is responsible for the overall management, implementation, and usability of information (Rouse 2015)

Chief medical informatics officer: Typically a practicing physician who volunteers to serve as the bridge between the medical staff and administration of a healthcare organization implementing health IT, as well as equivalent professionals in nursing, pharmacy, applied health, and public health.

Chief technology officer: The chief technology officer (CTO) reports to the CIO and is responsible for management, implementation, and maintenance of computer technologies (Rouse 2013).

Claim attachment: A set of transactions is intended to be used when a health plan finds it cannot adjudicate a claim without additional information

Classification: An organized structure for arranging objects, such as clinical terms or phrases, that aids in their definition, mapping, and use

Client/server architecture: A computer architecture in which multiple computers (clients) that store and process application software and data are connected to other computers (servers) that enter data and retrieve information

Clinical business intelligence: Terms relating to technologies for gaining a deeper understanding of a variety of business and clinical information, respectively, often through integration of financial and clinical information presented to applicable users

Clinical data analyst: Clinical data analysts configure information systems specific to organizational needs (Darling 2011)

Clinical data repository (CDR): *See* **data repository**

Clinical data warehouse (CDW): *See* **data warehouse**

Clinical decision support (CDS): A function of a computer application in which clinical data are compared with reference information (in a knowledge-base) or with previously entered clinical data of the same type to supply clinical reminders and alerts, contextsensitive templates and order sets, and other types of results

Clinical Documents for Payers: Created by HL7 and intended to be used for claims attachments or supporting documentation for prior authorization for referrals and other services needing approval from a payer for reimbursement

Clinical documentation systems: Systems in which clinicians enter documentation of clinical findings and services provided as they are taking care of patients

Clinical Laboratory Improvement Amendments (CLIA): Passed in 1988, the amendments established quality standards for all laboratory testing to ensure the accuracy, reliability, and timeliness of patient test results, regardless of where the test is performed. Under these regulations and similar state statutes, labs are restricted from providing patients with direct access to their test results; however, federal regulations to change this have been proposed

Clinical messaging: The function of electronically delivering data and automating the workflow around the management of clinical data

Clinical quality measures (CQMs): Measures that have been established to measure outcomes for many common disease conditions

Clinical research: A study carried out on a sample of patients, the quality of which varies with the degree to which there are controls designed to mitigate variation

Clinical support modeling: Focuses on things such as identification of patients who should be screened for fall risk, tracking systems to monitor compliance with treatment regimens, and modeling new processes needed for population health management, such as obtaining patient outcome information or integrating the EHRs of acute care, primary care, and LTPAC providers (Burton 2013; Mitchell 2013)

Clinical trial: A controlled research study involving human subjects that is designed to prospectively evaluate the safety and effectiveness of new drugs, tests, devices, or interventions

Clinically integrated network (CIN): A legal arrangement, often but not always including restructuring of an integrated delivery network with a single ownership, to improve and maintain the health of the people in their communities (Koppenheffer 2013)

Clinician: A healthcare professional, including physicians, nurses, and many others, who provides healthcare services

Closed system: A system that operates in a self-contained environment without input from other systems or the environment

Closed-loop medication management: A process that integrates all components of medication ordering, verifying, dispensing, and administering in order to provide safe and effective patient care

Cloud computing: A model for enabling convenient, on demand network access to a shared pool of configurable computing resources (e.g., networks, servers, storage, applications, and services) that can be rapidly provisioned and released with minimal management effort or service provider interaction

Code: In information systems, software instructions that direct computers to perform a specified action; in healthcare, an alphanumeric representation of the terms in a clinical classification or vocabulary

Code 39 bar code standard: An alphanumeric, self-checking, variable-length code that has been standardized by the Health Industry Bar Code Council (HIBCC); *also called* **linear bar code**

Code 128 bar code standard: A very high density code that encodes all alphanumeric and special characters, enabling bar codes to include upper- and lowercase and larger numbers

Code set: Under HIPAA, any set of codes used to encode data elements, such as tables of terms, medical concepts, medical diagnostic codes, or medical procedure codes; includes both the codes and their descriptions

Coding: In computer programming, the process of writing software using a specific computer language to encode instructions; in healthcare, the process of assigning numeric or alphanumeric representations to clinical documentation

Co-insurance: When a patient has a health insurance plan in which the patient owes a portion of the total bill, not just a co-pay and deductible (Matjucha and Giuliano 2011)

Comment fields: In a computer form or template, an area in which to record any nonstructured data; often used to further explain or embellish upon data that have been entered into structured data fields

Common framework: A set of principles that provides the foundation for managing personal health information within consumer-accessible data streams

Communication: Shared meaning

Communication plan: A tool that helps ensure that the communications about change are carried out

Community offering: A means for a physician's office or small hospital to acquire licenses to EHR software through, typically, a large hospital or integrated delivery system, rather than the vendor directly; this ensures consistency in use throughout the system

Companion guide: Provide the technical information and instructions for how providers must compile and transmit transactions to the specific health plan, such as the Internet Protocol (IP) address to use to submit a batch of claims, or who is the primary contact person at the claims processing site in the event of needing live technical support

Component producer: Producers who sell products that support the EHR and other types of health IT

Computer output to laser disks (COLD): The first optical disks used in healthcare that were used to store images of documents

Computerized provider order entry (CPOE): Electronic systems that support physicians and other applicable licensed healthcare professionals in developing and documenting instructions for the care of the patient, including the ordering of medications, diagnostic studies, food and nutrition, nursing services, and treatments. These systems contain some clinical decision support functionality that provides the user with standard order sets that reduce data entry time; alerts about the possibility of drug interactions, allergic reactions, or a potential overdose; warnings for potential duplicate diagnostic tests and therapies; reminders about the need to renew or discontinue an order; and other relevant information

Confidentiality: The treatment of information that an individual has disclosed in a relationship of trust and with the expectation that it will not be divulged to others in ways that are inconsistent with the understanding of the original disclosure unless the individual grants permission

Configuration management: The process of keeping a record of changes made in an information system as it is being customized to the organization's specifications; *also called* **change control**

Confounding variables: In statistics or other cause-and-effect studies, an extraneous variable whose presence affects the variables being studied, and thus the results do not reflect the actual relationship between the variables under investigation

Connectivity systems: Systems that support the ability of one computer system to exchange data with another computer system

Consent management: Policies, procedures, and technology that enable active management and enforcement of users' permission directives to control access to their electronic health information and allow care providers to meet patient privacy requirements

Consent2Share (C2S): An open-source tool for consent management and data segmentation designed to integrate with existing EHR and health information exchange (HIE) systems

Consolidated Clinical Document Architecture (C-CDA): A suite of templates for different types of health documents, including the CCD

Consolidated HIE Architecture: The manner in which an HIE enables the sharing of data across participants in which data are contributed to a central data repository, managed centrally, and shared in accordance with participant agreement and patient consent directives

Consumer access services: An emerging set of services designed to help individuals make secure electronic connections with health data sources (for example, providers, labs, pharmacies, health plans, disease management companies, health education)

Consumer-driven health: Consumers must manage their health savings accounts, high-deductible health plans, debit card payments, or direct account payments

Consumer empowerment: The investment of authority in those who purchase goods and services

Consumer-mediated exchange: The ability for consumers to aggregate and control the use of their health information among their different providers

Context sensitive: A feature of a software program that changes depending on the circumstances in which the program is used. For example, a context-sensitive help function provides information only about the specific function being performed; in healthcare, a template providing guidelines for documentation applicable to a given patient's diagnosis is offered for charting

Contingency plan: Documentation of the process for responding to a system emergency, such as a power failure, disaster, or other event that limits or eliminates access to an electronic system, including the performance of backups, the introduction of temporary paperbased processes and how they will be returned to electronic form after the emergency, the lineup of critical alternative facilities to support continuity of operations, and the process of recovering from a disaster

Continuity of care document (CCD): The result of ASTM's Continuity of Care Record standard content being represented and mapped into the HL7's Clinical Document Architecture specifications to enable transmission of referral information between providers; also frequently adopted for personal health records

Continuity of care record (CCR): *See ASTM Continuity of Care Record*

Controlled substances: Narcotics, depressants, stimulants, and hallucinogens as specified in the Comprehensive Drug Abuse Prevention and Control Act

Controlled vocabulary: A predefined set of terms and their meanings that may be used in structured data entry or natural language processing to represent expressions

Conversion strategy: An organization's plan for changing paper-based records to electronic form, or moving data from one electronic format to another

Coordination of benefits: A coordination that must be conducted between health plans, most often between a primary health plan (usually a commercial payer) and a secondary health plan, such as Medicaid

Copy and paste: A process wherein a clinician copies an entry from a previous note or a different patient and pastes it into a new entry. This is one of the most commonly used aids in data entry and one that poses considerable risk

Core clinical systems: Applications used by physicians, nurses, and other clinicians as they directly care for patients. These applications are considered to make up the electronic health record

Core measures: Standardized performance measures developed to improve the safety and quality of healthcare (used by the Joint Commission's ORYX initiative, CMS quality reporting program for hospitals, and others)

Corrective action: Implementation of solutions to mitigate risk and reporting on outcomes

Cost accounting: Identifies the costs of products and services so those costs can be accurately reported on financial statements and used to evaluate an organization's possible courses of action

Cost–benefit analysis: A process that uses quantitative techniques to evaluate and measure the benefit of providing products or services compared to the cost of providing them

Council for Affordable Quality Healthcare, Committee on Operating Rules for Information Exchange (CAQH CORE): The operating rules authoring entity for the HIPAA transaction standards, it includes providers and vendors, and is building consensus-based operating rules that enhance interoperability between providers and payers, streamline the use of the X12 transactions, and reduce the amount of time and resources providers spend on administrative functions

Covered entity: A health plan, healthcare clearinghouse, or healthcare provider who transmits any health information in electronic form in connection with a transaction covered by HIPAA (referring to transactions such as health insurance eligibility, claims submission, remittance advice, and other financial/administrative processes standardized under HIPAA)

Critical path: The sequence of tasks in a project in which there is no slack and therefore determines the project's finish date

Culture: Norms of behavior and shared values among a group of people

Customer relationship management (CRM): Helps healthcare providers manage physician credentialing and recruitment, referrals, clinical trials, and other information management tasks that require building and manipulating large contact databases (Microsoft Dynamics 2012)

Customer service: Activities performed before, during, and after the purchase of a product or delivery of a service that are designed to enhance customer satisfaction

Cybernetics: A theory of control systems based on communication (transfer of information) between components of systems with respect to their environment

Cyberspace: The virtual environment created by computer systems

Cyber threat: Malicious activity that can occur through cyberspace

DailyMed: A website provided by the National Library of Medicine offering information about marketed drugs, including the FDA product label information and excluding any advertisements

Dashboard: An application that displays key information. In healthcare, a dashboard may display key information from the EHR for a patient's care, may supply managers with reports of process measures, or may supply key indicators to help managers follow progress toward achievement of a strategic plan

Data: The dates, numbers, images, symbols, letters, and words that represent basic facts and observations about people, processes, measurements, and conditions

Data administrator: Apply domain expertise to the design of databases, establish policies for their creation and use, maintain data dictionaries, and manage the quality of data (Gillenson et al. 2008, 302)

Data architecture: The structure that must support the ability of IT to create the knowledge continuum

Data center: The location where computers and their components are housed

Data conversion: The task of moving data from one data structure to another, usually at the time of a new system installation

Data denormalization: A database in which there are redundant data in order to optimize analytical performance

Data dictionary: A descriptive list of the names, definitions, and attributes of data elements to be collected in an information system or database; the purpose of a data dictionary is to standardize definitions and ensure consistent use

Data discovery: The ability of end users to apply artificial intelligence tools to explore data for discovering trends.

Data Elements for Emergency Department Systems (DEEDS): A data set designed to support the uniform collection of information in hospital-based emergency departments

Data entry aid: A software features that helps users select the desired data to be input, such as a drop-down menu or copy-and-paste

Data governance: Addressing system inputs

Data infrastructure: The data needed to operate an enterprise, and how they are defined (vocabulary), structured and processed (architecture), and quality ensured

Data mapping: The process of identifying relationships between two distinct data models

Data mart: A wellorganized, usercentered, searchable database system that usually draws information from a data warehouse to meet the specific needs of users

Data mining: The process of extracting and analyzing large volumes of data from a database for the purpose of identifying hidden and sometimes subtle relationships or patterns and using those relationships to predict behaviors

Data modeling: The process of determining the users' information needs and identifying relationships among the data

Data normalization: In a relational database, it is the process of organizing data to minimize redundancy

Data provenance: Another type of administrative metadata that refers to where data originated and where data may have moved between databases

Data quality: The reliability and effectiveness of data for its intended uses in operations, decision making, and planning

Data quality management model: A graphic of the data quality management domains as they relate to the characteristics of data integrity and examples of each characteristic within each domain

Data repository: An open-structure database that is not dedicated to the software of any particular vendor or data supplier, in which data from diverse sources are stored so that an integrated, multidisciplinary view of the data can be achieved; *also called* **clinical data repository** when related specifically to healthcare data

Data reuse: A common data entry strategy in computer applications where data may be copied or supplied from a predefined set of content; strong caution must be applied to ensure that the entry is entirely applicable to the new situation

Data scientist: Combines mathematics, statistics, and software engineering

Data segmentation: The process of sequestering from capture, access, or view certain data elements that are perceived by a legal entity, institution, organization, or individual as being undesirable to share (Goldstein and Rein 2010)

Data sharing agreement: Data sharing agreements differ from data use agreements in that data sharing agreements have more expansive data governance requirements, often including certification and recertification of the de-identification of data being used and, where applicable, usage fees (Allen et al. 2014)

Data use agreement: Required under HIPAA for use of a limited data set, which includes PHI from which most—but not all—of the safe harbor de-identification requirements are applied

Data set: A list of recommended data elements with uniform definitions where the data are relevant for a particular use

Data stewardship: The responsibilities and accountabilities associated with managing, collecting, viewing, storing, sharing, disclosing, or otherwise making use of personal health information

Data Use and Reciprocal Sharing Agreement: An agreement that must be signed by all participants in a nationwide health information network in order to ensure that each abides by a common set of terms and conditions that supports the secure, interoperable exchange of health data between and among participants

Data visualization: A technique to actuate in information systems the human need for visual representations of information for easier understanding and improved retention (SAS n.d.)

Data warehouse: A database that is optimized for analytical query and report processing using data from multiple databases; *also called* **clinical data repository** when related specifically to healthcare data

Database administrator: Design and manage the technical implementation and maintenance of databases (Gillenson, et al. 2008)

Database management system (DBMS): Computer software that enables the user to create, modify, delete, and view the data in a database

Data-information-knowledge-wisdom (DIKW) continuum: The process of transforming raw facts and figures (data) into useful information and, by adding experiential information, into knowledge, and informed by context and experience into wisdom

DDI: Drug-drug interaction, which is a condition for an alert in many EHRs.

Decision Support Services (DSS): A standard that specifies a standardized interface for providing clinical decision support (CDS) as a software service

Default: 1. The status to which a computer application reverts in the absence of alternative instructions 2. Pertains to an attribute, value, or option that is assumed when none is explicitly specified

Denials: May include both denial of a current claim as well as a take-back of money from claims already paid where a review reveals issues

Dependency: The requirement that a step in a project must be performed before or simultaneously with another step or steps in order for subsequent steps to be undertaken

Designated record set: The medical and billing records used to make decisions about individuals

Diagnostic imaging reports: A dictated summary of findings with respect to the purpose of the study and the image

Digital certificate: An electronic document that establishes a person's online identity

Digital image: A representation of a two-dimensional image, such as a photograph, drawing, computed tomography, or other form, to enable it to be stored in a computer

Digital Imaging and Communication in Medicine (DICOM): A standard that promotes a digital image communications format and picture archive and communications systems for use with digital images

Digital signature: A type of electronic signature that binds a message to a particular individual and can be used by the receiver to authenticate the identity of the sender

Direct: A simple, secure, scalable, standards-based way for participants to send authenticated, encrypted health information directly to known, trusted recipients over the Internet

Direct Project: A simple, secure, scalable, standards-based way for participants to send authenticated, encrypted health information directly to known, trusted recipients over the Internet; a component of the Nationwide Health Information Network Exchange

Directed exchange: The ability to send and receive secure information electronically between care providers to support coordinated care

Discharge planning: Case management that focuses specifically on addressing consumers' health needs once discharged from a hospital or other inpatient setting (CMSA n.d.)

Disclosure: The release, transfer, provision of access to, or divulging in any other manner of information outside of the entity holding the information

Discrete data: *See* **structured data**

Discrete reportable transcription: Enables tagging elements in a document transcribed into an XML format so they can be placed into structured data collection templates

Disease management: A system of coordinated healthcare interventions and communications for populations with conditions in which patient self-care efforts are significant. Also called *integrated care* (URAC 2005)

Disk mirroring: A storage technique which mirrors data from a primary drive to a secondary in the event of a drive failure

Document imaging system (DIMS): Computer systems that capture, store, and reprint images of documents

Document repository: A database that stores indexed images of documents

Domain teams: Groups of people that work on special aspects of a project

Drug utilization review: Health plans, such as Medicaid, conduct prospective screening of prescription drug claims to identify therapeutic duplication, drug-disease contraindications, incorrect dosage or duration of treatment, drug allergy, and clinical misuse or abuse

Dual core (acquisition strategy): An acquisition strategy in which one vendor primarily supplies the financial and administrative applications and another vendor primarily supplies the clinical applications

Dual processor: Two separate physical computer processors, running in parallel

Due diligence: The actions associated with making a good decision, including investigation of legal, technical, human, and financial predictions and ramifications of proposed endeavors with another party; in EHR vendor selection, due diligence includes thorough analysis of responses to a request for proposal, product demonstrations, site visits, and reference checks

eHealth Exchange: Formerly known as the nationwide health information network. Spanning all 50 states, it was incubated by ONC and transitioned to function as an independent initiative with private sector responsibility for the stewardship of the network

Electronic content management (ECM) system: Software used to capture, manage, store, preserve, and deliver analog documents and digital records where specific content has been indexed for subsequent retrieval; ECM may also be referred to as a knowledge management system

Electronic data interchange (EDI): A standard transmission format using strings of data for business information communicated among the computer systems of independent organizations

Electronic document management (EDM) system: A storage solution based on digital scanning technology in which source documents are scanned to create digital images of the documents that can be stored electronically on optical disks

Electronic health record (EHR): An electronic record of health-related information on an individual that conforms to nationally recognized interoperability standards and that can be created, managed, and consulted by authorized clinicians and staff across more than one healthcare organization

Electronic Healthcare Network Accreditation Commission (EHNAC): It initially developed criteria for third-party review and accreditation primarily for healthcare clearinghouses, which helped the industry exchange HIPAA financial and administrative transactions providing accreditation services for other outsourced service organizations, such as printing companies, document imaging companies, media storage services, call centers, data centers, and network administrators

Electronic medical record (EMR): An electronic record of health-related information on an individual that can be created, gathered, managed, and consulted by authorized clinicians and staff within a single healthcare organization

Electronic medication administration record (EMAR): A system designed to reduce medication errors by supplying nursing staff with a legible printout or display of medications, their doses, route of administration, and time for administration; this is in contrast to barcode medication administration record (BCMAR)

Electronic prescribing (e-Rx): An application that supports the ability to electronically send an accurate, error-free, and understandable prescription directly to a pharmacy from the point of care

Electronic signature: A generic, technology-neutral term for the various ways that an electronic record can be signed, such as a digitized image of a signature, a name typed at the end of an email message by the sender, a biometric identifier, a secret code or PIN, or a digital signature

Electronic signature authentication (ESA): A system that utilizes a user ID and password to indicate review and approval of the content of a document

Electronic systems: Systems aided by computing devices

Eligibility inquiry and response: also referred to as the *eligibility verification process*; whenever a patient presents with insurance, the provider should use the ASC X12 270 Eligibility Inquiry in order to receive an ASC X12 271 Eligibility Response back to verify that the patient has insurance benefits as claimed

Emergent risk: Focuses on a tier of patients whose risk level is just below that of those patients who are at the highest level of risk for costly services

Encryption: The process of transforming text into an unintelligible string of characters that can be transmitted via communications media with a high degree of security and then decrypted when it reaches a secure destination

Enrollment and premium payment: An employer or other sponsor contracts with a health plan to provide health insurance benefits for its employees, or insurance beneficiaries. The employer may then use the ASC X12 834 Enrollment transaction to enroll its employees in real time and the employer/sponsor may make premium payments using the ASC X12 820 Premium Payment transaction

Enterprise content management system: Has workflow functionalities and other tools to manage documents in a logical manner; it goes beyond a scanning solution that only makes images of documents for retrieval or archival purposes

Enterprise content, collaboration, and communication management (EC3M) system: Systems that aid in the management of electronic content as well as the sharing and transmission of such content, especially among members of a team who may need to dynamically interact with documents as they are being created

Enterprise content and record management (ECRM) system: Convergence of enterprise-wide content management (ECM) and electronic record management (ERM) that provides functionality for managing all content across its lifecycle according to legal, regulatory, and operational requirements. Ability to imbed content classification and retention rules, and integrate with collaboration tools

Enterprise health information management professional: Provides perspectives on **information governance** and **data governance**, and ensures that the business processes, compliance, legal purposes, privacy protections, retention policies, and preservation of evidence are addressed in health IT strategic planning (Johns 2015; Washington 2015)

Enterprise resource planning: A suite of integrated tools that collect and interpret data from business activities for the purpose of planning improvements in operations, such as supply chain management, inventory management, patient relationship management, human resources, financing, and billing

Enterprise-wide MPI (EMPI): An index that provides access to multiple repositories of information from overlapping patient populations that are maintained in separate systems and databases

Environmental scan: A scan that focuses on factors that are external to, and often not under the control of, the organization conducting the strategic planning

e-prescribing (e-Rx): *See* **electronic prescribing**

Evaluation and management (E/M) codes: Current Procedural Terminology codes that describe patient encounters with healthcare professionals for assessment counseling and other routine healthcare services

Evidence-based medicine: Healthcare services based on clinical methods that have been thoroughly tested through controlled, peer-reviewed biomedical studies

E-visits: An evaluation and management service provided by a physician or other qualified health professional to an established patient using an electronic-based communication network for which the provider receives reimbursement

Executive decision support: A system that analyzes a large volume of aggregated data and provides trending information, used in healthcare to support strategic planning and management of the healthcare organization

Explanation of benefits: A document that health plans send their members when a claim has been filed by a provider

Extranet: A system of connections of private Internet networks outside an organization's firewall that uses Internet technology to enable collaborative applications among enterprises

Failover: In the event of a component failure, the ability of a redundant compontent to pick up the function of the system

Fast Healthcare Interoperability Resources (FHIR): Addresses the transition from HL7 V2.x and second platform technology to HL7 V3 and third platform technology; recognizes the need to not only share views of documents (as made possible by the CDA) but also have structured and standardized data from these documents that can to be exchanged so that the recipient of any such data can incorporate the data into their own EHRs, data repositories, or data warehouses

Favorites list: As used in EHRs, commonly used drugs, problems, or other values for data fields; these may be pre-populated by the user and/or compiled by the computer based on the frequency with which terms are selected for use

Federated HIE Architecture: The manner in which an HIE enables the sharing of data across participants in which data are retained and managed locally at each participant site, and shared in accordance with participant agreement and patient consent directives

Fee for service (FFS): A method of payment for healthcare in which doctors and other healthcare providers are paid for each service performed (CHPQR n.d.)

File formats: Include those used in word-processing software (e.g., .DOC or .DOCX), as PDF files (.PDF), as .JPG or other image structures, and other formats

Financial benchmarking: The process that establishes spending levels used to determine the VBP rates for providers (HCP-LAN 2016)

Financing and acquisition strategy: How HIT is acquired and paid for

Five rights of medication administration: A patient safety process that checks that (1) the right medication to be administered for (2) the right patient is given in (3) the right dose, (4) right route, and (5) right time

Free software: 1. Software that is distributed free of charge to the user, often in the form of web-based software paid for through advertising directed to the user 2. Free and open-source software is free of charge to the user, and the underlying program source code is able to be accessed by the acquirer of the software

Free text: The entry of narrative data via keyboarding, dictation, voice recognition, and/or handwriting recognition

Front-end speech (FES) recognition: Uses of speech recognition technology that rely on limited vocabularies and away from a point of care

Full redundancy: The state of a computer system in which all critical components, including hardware, software, power, and telecommunications capabilities, are duplicated as a contingency measure

Functional capabilities inventory: The result of a functional needs assessment that is used in a selection process to compare products

Functional needs assessment: An assessment that describes the key capabilities or application requirements for achieving the benefits of the EHR as the organization envisions them

Functional profile: Statements of functions and conformance criteria deemed important for EHR systems used in a given specialty

Gantt chart: A graphic tool used to plot tasks in project management that shows the duration of project tasks and overlapping tasks

General Equivalence Mappings (GEMs): A program created to facilitate the translation between ICD-9-CM and ICD-10-CM/PCS

Goal: A specific description of the goods or services to be provided as the result of a business process

Go-live: The first instance that a user logs onto the production system

Go-live rehearsal: Staff members take turns role-playing themselves and patients as they run through a typical workflow and process with the EHR in the test environment

Governance: The establishment of policies for the effective and efficient management of an organization's assets and the continual monitoring of how well those policies are working to achieve their stated ends (Johns 2015, xxii)

Granularity: The relative degree of detail, specificity, or size of components; in healthcare, granularity is often used to describe the specificity with which a diagnosis is made or how much detail is included in the workflow and process being mapped

Graphical user interface (GUI): The manner in which computer commands are displayed to a user to make using the computer easier; generally utilizing small images (icons) that represent tasks, functions, and programs performed by a software program

Group purchasing organizations (GPOs): Entities created to help providers achieve deep discounts by applying economies of scale to purchasing supplies

Groupware: An Internet technology that consolidates documents from different information systems within an organization to help people collaborate on specific tasks

Hadoop: Apache's open-source software that is currently most popular and serves as a basis for other software development

Health Breach Notification Rule: Regulation that requires commercial PHR vendors to notify individuals whose information was breached and file a report with the FTC

Healthcare clearinghouse: Manages the transmissions between providers and the standards, and implementation guides, but also with multiple different health plan companion guides, and transmit transactions in a point-to-point manner to many different locations

Healthcare Employer Data and Information Set (HEDIS): A set of performance measures developed by the National Commission for Quality Assurance (NCQA) that are designed to provide purchasers and consumers of healthcare with the information they need to compare the performance of managed care plans

Health data stewardship: The responsibilities and accountabilities associated with managing, collecting, viewing, storing, sharing, disclosing, or otherwise making use of personal health information

Health informatics professional: These professionals play a role in strategic planning and governance in health IT. These professionals are enlightened advocates of health IT and strong proponents of system usability (the efficiency, effectiveness, and satisfaction with which users achieve results from health IT) as well as **patient safety** (that is, preventing harm to patients, learning from errors, and building a culture of safety) (Pfister and Ingargiola 2014; Hughes 2008)

Health information exchange (HIE): The sharing of patient information among different provider organizations and others as authorized

Health information exchange organization (HIO): An organization that supports, oversees, or governs the exchange of health information among organizations according to nationally recognized standards

Health Information Technology: The application of information processing involving both computer hardware and software that deals with the storage, retrieval, sharing, and use of healthcare information, data, and knowledge for communication and decision making (HRSA n.d.)

Health Information Technology for Economic and Clinical Health Act (HITECH): Legislation enacted in 2009 to stimulate the adoption of EHR and supporting technology in the United States

Health insurance exchange (HIX): An online marketplace where individuals can shop for insurance coverage and thereby avoid the shared responsibility payment requirement under ACA that is paid via the federal income tax return (Healthcare.gov 2016)

Health intelligence: Data collected by dashboards and other aids that are used to monitor quality, cost, and experience of care measures (Burke 2013)

Health Level 7 (HL7): An ANSI-accredited standards development organization dedicated to creating standards for the exchange, management, and integration of electronic health information

Health plan: An individual or group plan that provides, or pays the cost of, medical care

Health record banking: A PHR model in which patients and healthcare providers make deposits of health information into an organization that acts like a bank, protecting the privacy and security of the health information while affording the ability to share information with those authorized

Health record integration: The integration of personal health record (PHR) data (potentially from multiple PHRs) into a health record compiled by a provider

Heuristic thought: Exploratory thinking that aids learning, discovery, understanding, or problem solving through experimentation, trial and error, applying intuitive judgment, or other techniques

HIE data sharing agreement: A documented arrangement between providers and others to comply with specific requirements for sharing often aggregated health data for purposes other than direct patient care or payment for care

HIO participation agreement: A documented arrangement between participants in an HIO to comply with specified requirements for utilizing the services of the HIO

HL7 Functional Profiles: A standardized description and common understanding of functions sought or available for special uses of HIT, such as for an intensive care unit, cardiology practice, or others

HL7 PHR System Functional Model: Identifies the features and functions in a system necessary to create and manage an effective PHR

Home monitoring: Devices that enable patients, caregivers, or healthcare providers to monitor the patient's vital signs and other physiological indicators from the patient's home; examples include diabetes kits, home pregnancy tests, or transtelephonic pacemaker monitoring

Human systems: Systems that are organized relationships among people

Human–computer interface: The combination of input device and user interface software used by humans to access and enter data into a computer system

Hybrid HIE Architecture: The manner in which an HIE enables the sharing of data across participants, which is a combination of the consolidated and federated models, so that some data are contributed to a central repository managed by the HIO and other data are retained and managed locally at each participant site; data shared in accordance with participant agreement and patient consent directives

Hybrid record: A system with functional components that (1) include both paper and electronic documents and (2) use both manual and electronic processes

Icon: A small image that represent tasks, functions, and programs performed by a software program

Identity management (IdM): A security control process of identifying individuals and systems that are authorized access to computer networks, addressing how individuals and systems are identified, how their identity is protected, and the technologies supporting that protection (such as network protocols, digital certificates, and passwords)

Identity matching: A process that analyzes information relating to individuals and/or entities and applies probability scoring to determine which identities are most likely the same

IEEE: *See* **Institute of Electrical and Electronics Engineers**

IEEE 802.11: A set of standards developed by IEEE for implementing wireless local area network (WLAN) computer communication

Implementation: The process of installing hardware and software, configuring them to meet specific user needs, testing that they work properly, training users, and supporting users' initial use of an information system application

Implementation guide: A part of each ASC X12 standard that explains intended usage and technicalities for the standard

Implementation plan: The sequence of tasks to be taken to accomplish an implementation; for EHR and other HIT systems, implementation plans may have hundreds or even thousands of tasks

In-basket: A function that provides users with information on the current status of workflow and tasks to be performed, such as a reminder to sign a document or place a followup call to a patient

Incidental uses or disclosures: Those made pursuant to an otherwise permitted or required use or disclosure

Infection surveillance system: Aggregates information from multiple sources and notify an infection control nurse of a possible infection in real time

Inference engine: Specialized computer software often used in clinical decision support systems that looks for matches between conditions in rules to data elements entered into a repository; when a match is found, the engine executes the rule, which results in an alert or other specified action

Influencer: Those who attempt to influence behavior (encourage) rather than change behavior (force)

Information: Data that have been deliberately selected, processed, and organized to be useful

Information governance: Addressing system outputs and uses.

Information models: Used to describe how types of data (often referred to as *objects* may be used together to provide value

Information security analyst: Plan and carry out information security measures to protect an organization's computer networks and systems (BLS 2014–2015)

Information silo: Information that does not readily communicate with other information systems due to lack of technical, semantic, or process interoperability; in healthcare, the connotation is that information silos exist in specific disciplines by intent for fear of losing control over the data

Information systems theory: The explanation that information is generated by data that are processed in predictable ways that contribute value

Informed consent: Permission to perform a treatment (often governed by state law [ACS 2014]) or engage an individual in a clinical trial or research study

Inputs: Data entered into an information system (for example, the patient's vital signs entered by a nurse or monitoring device, the admitting clerk's interview of the patient to obtain demographic information)

Installation: The process of loading software onto applicable servers

Institute for Safe Medication Practices (ISBT): A nonprofit organization devoted to medication error prevention and safe medication use through providing education and newsletters and its voluntary Medication Errors Reporting Program (MERP) to learn about errors occurring, understand their causes, and share "lessons learned" to help prevent future errors

Integrated delivery network (IDN): Also called integrated delivery system (IDS), a group of healthcare organizations under a single parent holding company intended to improve the continuity of care for patients; some IDNs are limited to provider components, while others have a health maintenance organization (HMO) component as well

Integrating the Healthcare Enterprise (IHE): An initiative that brings healthcare stakeholders together to develop profiles that provide precise definitions of how DICOM, HL7, W3C, and security standards can be implemented to improve the sharing of information across disparate systems in order to meet specific clinical needs

Integration: The complex task of linking information system components together so that they communicate and act as a uniform entity. Information systems built on the same design platform are built to be integrated; otherwise, systems integrators use various programming and process techniques to integrate disparate systems

Integration profiles: Provide a reliable way of specifying a level of compliance to existing standards that is sufficient to achieve truly efficient interoperability

Integrity: 1. The state of being whole or unimpaired 2. The ability of data to maintain its structure and attributes, including protection against modification or corruption during transmission, storage, or at rest. Maintenance of data integrity is a key aspect of data quality management and security

Intelligent character recognition (ICR): An advanced form of OCR in which the system learns to recognize a specific person's handwriting and, over time, increases its accuracy (Vasudeva et al. 2012; Templeton 2015)

Interface: The zone between different computer systems across which users want to pass information (for example, a computer program written to exchange information between systems or the graphic display of an application program designed to make the program easier to use)

Interface engine: A software tool that manages many interface connections among many disparate systems

Internal rate of return (IRR): A calculation that does not take into consideration interest rate or inflation and that is used in capital budgeting to measure and compare the profitability of investments

International Classification of Functioning, Disability, and Health (ICF): A health and health-related classification system maintained by the World Health Organization (WHO) that reports body functions and structures, activities and participation, and environmental factors

International Health Terminology Standards Development Organisation (IHTSDO): The organization that owns the intellectual property rights to SNOMED CT

Internet of Things: The burgeoning phenomenon of commonplace consumer products and services that connect to the Internet (Han 2015)

Interoperability: The ability of different information systems and software applications to communicate and exchange data

Interoperability Standards Advisory: First issued by the ONC in 2015, the interoperability standards are characterized as vocabulary/code sets/terminology, content/structure, and services in 2016.

Intranet: A private information network that is similar to the Internet but whose servers are located inside a firewall or security barrier so that the general public cannot gain access to information housed within the network

Issues management: The process of identifying causes, resolving unexpected occurrences, and maintaining a level of problem or error control

Just culture: A culture that ensures a balanced approach to error, recognizing that a "trust, report, and improve" cycle promotes proactive and reactive risk reduction because staff are willing to report errors, close calls, and unsafe situations and solve problems before patients are harmed

Key differentiator: A tool used to summarize the key elements most likely to separate vendors with the desired key elements from those without

Key performance indicator: Area identified for needed improvement through benchmarking and continuous quality improvement

Key selection criteria: A set of initial vendor screening criteria drawn from the planning activities and considering elements such as vision, functionality, technology, acquisition policies, implementation strategy, operations and maintenance support, and viability

Knowledge: The information, understanding, and experience that give individuals the power to make informed decisions

Knowledge base: A database that contains reference data that may be integrated with patient care data for clinical decision support

Knowledge management: A management strategy that promotes an integrated and collaborative approach to the process of information asset creation, capture, organization, access, and use

Knowledge sources: Various types of reference material and expert information that are compiled in a manner accessible for integration with patient care information to provide clinical decision support and improve the quality and cost-effectiveness of healthcare provision

Knowledge worker: An employee whose job includes tasks of developing or using experiential-based information in new and different ways; formerly considered in contrast to tasks, which are considered manual labor or performed without autonomous thought. All employees, however, are encouraged to contribute their experience and expertise

Kubler-Ross grief cycle: This theory is named after its original theorist, Elizabeth Kubler-Ross and is frequently cited as a way to understand the emotional stages people often experience when grieving a death. Many have also applied the model to any type of loss, including the loss experienced when change requires moving from doing things the old way to doing things a new way

Laboratory information system (LIS): An information system that manages the laboratory in its performance of diagnostic studies and generation of their respective results

Laboratory outreach services: Services for care coordination with patients who have not had recent necessary laboratory tests performed, physician checkups, and monitoring treatment regimens (Miliard 2015)

Learning health system: A system which "aligns science, informatics, incentives, and culture for continuous improvement and innovation" (IOM 2012)

Leasing: A contractual arrangement in which regular, periodic payments are made to use an asset, such as computer equipment

Legacy systems: An old technology, computer system, or application that continues to be used, even though newer technology is available, because it represents a large investment, still provides basic functionality, and is familiar

Lexicon: 1. The vocabulary used in a language or a subject area or by a particular speaker or group of speakers 2. A collection of words or terms and their meanings for a particular domain

Limited data set: Includes PHI from which most—but not all—of the safe harbor de-identification requirements are applied

Logical Observation Identifiers, Names and Codes (LOINC): A database protocol developed by the Regenstrief Institute for Health Care aimed at standardizing laboratory and other data observed about a patient, such as vital signs or symptoms, outcomes management, and research

Long-term and post-acute care (LTPAC): Healthcare services provided in a nonacute care setting, often following an acute episode of care for those who are chronically ill, aged, disabled, or mentally handicapped

Longitudinal data: Data collected from a sample population over different points in a long period of time (NLS n.d.)

M technology: A programming language, database management system, and related protocols developed in the 1970s and still widely used today in (parts of) healthcare information system applications; formerly Massachusetts General Hospital Utility Multiprogramming System (MUMPS)

Macro: A command that a user can create and retrieve later that produces a specific set of terms, phrases, or sentences. In EHRs, macros are sometimes called smart text or dot phrases

Mainframe: A computer architecture built with a single central processing component to which terminals and/or personal computers without extensive processing capability of their own are connected

Maintenance costs: The fees paid to vendors to respond to software issues that arise during use as well as to keep the software upto-date

Management services organizations (MSOs): Businesses that provide nonclinical services (such as practice management) for physician offices (Anderson and Grey 2013)

Managing: Carrying out a project plan

Manual systems: Systems that entail humans performing certain processes

MAP Keys: HFMA's key performance indicators which have become the industry standard for measuring revenue cycle performance, with MAP awards being given for high-performing hospitals and physician practices (HFMA 2016)

Massachusetts General Hospital Utility Multiprogramming System: *See* **M technology**

Maturity model: Descriptions of how EHR and health IT efforts might change over time.

Meaningful use (MU): A regulation that was issued by the Centers for Medicare and Medicaid Services (CMS) on July 28, 2010, outlining an incentive program for professionals (EPs), eligible hospitals, and critical access hospitals (CAHs) participating in Medicare and Medicaid programs that adopt and successfully demonstrate meaningful use of certified electronic health record (EHR) technology

Measure: Used to refer to both the metric [noun] and the process of measurement [verb]

Mechanical systems: Systems developed by humans but can operate without human intervention

Medical Dictionary for Regulatory Activities (MedDRA): A vocabulary that has been developed within the regulatory environment as a pragmatic, clinically validated medical terminology with an emphasis on ease-of-use data entry, retrieval, analysis, and display, with a suitable balance between sensitivity and specificity

Medical director of information systems: A physician who provides clinical support for EHR configuration and training

Medical identity theft: The inappropriate or unauthorized misrepresentation of individually identifiable health information for the purpose of obtaining access to property or services, which may result in long-lasting harm to an individual interacting with the healthcare continuum

Medical necessity: Healthcare services that a physician, exercising prudent clinical judgment, would provide to a patient for the purpose of evaluating, diagnosing or treating an illness, injury, disease or its symptoms, and that are: 1. In accordance with the generally accepted standards of medical practice (i.e., based on credible scientific evidence, physician specialty society recommendations, view of physicians practicing in the relevant clinical areas, and any other relevant factors); 2. Clinically appropriate, in terms of type, frequency, extent, site and duration, and considered effective for the patient's illness, injury or disease, and; 3. Not primarily for the convenience of the patient or physician, or other physician, and not more costly than an alternative service or sequence of services as likely to produce equivalent therapeutic or diagnostic results (Cigna 2016)

Medication five rights: *See* **five rights of medication administration**

Medication list: An ongoing record of the medications a patient has received in the past and is taking currently; includes names of medications, dosages, amounts dispensed, dispensing instructions, prescription dates, discontinued dates, and the problem for which the medication was prescribed

Medication management systems: Systems including CPOE and electronic medication administration record (EMAR) or BC-MAR systems

Medication reconciliation: Process that monitors and confirms that the patient receives consistent dosing across all facility transfers, such as on admission, from nursing unit to surgery, and from surgery to intensive care unit (ICU)

Meta-analysis: A statistical technique in which the results of two or more studies are mathematically combined in order to improve the reliability of the results

Metadata: Descriptive data that characterize other data to create a clearer understanding of their meaning and to achieve greater reliability and quality of information. For example, metadata about the term *temperature* used in healthcare would specify that it must be in numeric form and within a specified range of values. With respect to EDiscovery laws, metadata includes not only attributes of data but other data associated with its use, such as the identity of the person or device that recorded the temperature, the date and time the temperature was recorded, the last access date and time, and even information about whether the metadata itself had been changed, such as the date and who gave approval to change temperature from being a required data element to one that is optional

Metrics: The measurement used to describe performance, such as the number of times patient medications were administered more than 30 minutes late

Migration path: A strategic plan that identifies the major applications, technology, and operational elements to move from one situation level to another, such as from having no clinical systems, to having an EMR, to having an EHR

Milestone: In project management, the event that marks the completion of a set of tasks or a phase, such as the fact that all computers have been installed or a negotiated contract has been signed

Minimum necessary use standards: One of the requirements in the HIPAA Privacy Rule that requires covered entities to identify classes of persons who need access to protected health information (PHI), categories of PHI to which access is needed, and any conditions appropriate to such access

Mobile devices: Small, handheld computing devices with a display screen and touch input and/or keyboard, weighing less than 2 pounds; earlier devices focused on data storage and display, with newer devices adding communication and processing capabilities

Mobile telehealth: Services using mobile technology placed in a patient's home or offered through a specially equipped vehicle (Siwicki 2016)

Motivational interviewing: A counseling approach first made popular by clinical psychologists Rollnick and Miller in the treatment of individuals who abuse or misuse alcohol; it is now recommended as a supportive communication technique to engage patients in important lifestyle changes and as a technique that can be used for eliciting behavior change in other contexts (Rollnick and Miller 1995; Stratis Health 2014a)

MUMPS: *See* **Massachusetts General Hospital Utility Multiprogramming System**

MyHealth*e*Vet: A gateway to veteran health benefits and services, providing links to federal and VA benefits and resources, a personal health summary, health logs for recording blood pressure and other vital signs, medications, allergies and immunizations, medical events, food and activity journals, online VA prescription refill, wallet health information card, health calendar, trusted health education information, self-assessment tools, mental health resources (including online courses), and secure messaging (at selected VA sites)

MyPHR.com: Website that offers information about PHRs and PHR vendors, created and maintained by the American Health Information Management Association

NACHA: Previously National Automated Clearing House Association; a not-for-profit membership organization that comprises most of the nation's financial institutions and administrator of the ACH (Automated Clearing House) Network

National Drug Codes (NDC): Codes that serve as product identifiers for human drugs, currently limited to prescription drugs and a few selected over-the-counter products

National Quality Forum: A private, not-for-profit membership organization created to develop and implement a nationwide strategy to improve the measurement and reporting of healthcare quality

National Quality Forum (NQF) Health Outcomes Policy Priorities: An output of the NQF National Priorities Partnership (NPP) that offers consultative support to the Department of Health and Human Services on setting national priorities and goals for the HHS National Quality Strategy. This work guided the development of the meaningful use (M.U.) criteria

Natural language processing: A technology that converts human language (structured or unstructured) into data that can be translated then manipulated by computer systems; branch of artificial intelligence

Navigational devices: Keyboards, handwriting recognition pads and pens (or stylus), and voice recognition microphones associated with them for data entry and retrieval as well as various token slots, biometrics, and other devices for security

Negotiation: In the context of project management, a discussion that resolves an issue in a way that all parties find acceptable

Net present value (NPV): A formula used to assess the current value of a project when the monies used were invested in the organization's investment vehicles rather than expended for the project; this value is then compared to the allocation of the monies and the cash inflows of the project, both of which are adjusted to current time

Nomenclature: A recognized system of terms used in a science or art that follows preestablished naming conventions; a disease nomenclature is a listing of the proper name for each disease entity with its specific code number

Nonrepudiation: The claim that guarantees that the source of documentation cannot deny later that he or she was the author

Nurse staffing by patient acuity: The determination of how many nurses are needed to treat the hospital's patients, given the nature of their illnesses

Object: The basic component in an objectoriented database that includes both data and their relationships within a single structure

Objectives and measures for earning MU incentives: The Centers for Medicare and Medicaid Services (CMS), which funds the MU incentive program, develops objectives and measures for eligible hospitals, critical access hospitals, and eligible professionals (CMS 2016)

Office for Civil Rights (OCR): Department in HHS responsible for enforcing civil rights laws that prohibit discrimination on the basis of race, color, national origin, disability, age, sex, and religion by healthcare and human services entities over which OCR has jurisdiction, such as state and local social and health services agencies, and hospitals, clinics, nursing homes, or other entities receiving federal financial assistance from HHS. This office also has the authority to ensure and enforce the HIPAA Privacy and Security Rules; OCR is responsible for investigating all alleged violations of the Privacy and Security Rules and the Patient Safety and Quality Improvement Act of 2005 (PSQIA) Patient Safety Rule

Office of the National Coordinator for Health Information Technology (ONC): The principal federal entity charged with coordination of nationwide efforts to implement and use the most advanced health information technology and the electronic exchange of health information. The position of National Coordinator was created in 2004, through an Executive Order, and legislatively mandated in the Health Information Technology for Economic and Clinical Health Act (HITECH Act) of 2009

Omnibus Rule: A composite of several rules finalized in 2013, contributed further to addressing the privacy enhancements called for under HITECH

On-demand computing: Provision of computing resources to users as needed, either within the user's organization or, more commonly in healthcare, through a service provider often using cloud computing. For example, data analytics processing may only be needed occasionally for special projects, so the organization would only need to pay for such resources as used; *see also* **cloud computing**

Online analytical processing (OLAP): A methodology that supports complex analysis on a large set of data from multiple sources retained in either a multidimensional or relational database; in contrast, *see* **online transaction processing**

Online transaction processing (OLTP): A methodology that supports dayto-day entry of data and immediate retrieval of data from a relational database; *also called* a **transactional database**. In contrast, *see* **online analytical processing**

Ontology: A common vocabulary organized by meaning, allowing for an understanding of the structure of descriptive information that facilitates a specific topic or domain

Open system: A system that permits other parties to produce products that interoperate with it

Open systems interconnection (OSI): Rules developed by the International Standardization Organization (ISO) that describe the seven layers with which data pass through, such as in human readable form at the highest layer to the electrical pulses or wave forms at the lowest level, in order to be communicated from one system to another

Open-source software: Software in which the underlying program source code is able to be accessed by the acquirer of the software; open-source does not imply the software is free

Operating rules: The necessary business rules and guidelines for the electronic exchange of (HIPAA transaction) information that are not defined by a standard or its implementation specifications; mandated for adoption under the Affordable Care Act of 2010

Operating system: Software that provides instructions that cause application programs to work by performing basic tasks such as recognizing input from the keyboard, sending output to the display screen, keeping track of files and directories on a disk, and controlling peripheral devices such as disk drives and printers

Optical character recognition (OCR): A method of encoding text from analog paper into bit-mapped images and translating the images into a form that is computer readable

Optical mark recognition (OMR): The oldest form of optical recognition and requires pre-printed forms to contain locations for marking specific, limited information that is then read by a scanning system and content incorporated into an EDM, ECM, or any other system capable of receiving such information

Optimization: The fine-tuning of the EHR and other types of health IT in a systematic way, including assessment and improvement of the systems' hardware, software, people, policy, and process aspects, in order to improve its value (HCI Group 2014)

Opt-in: Originally used in email advertising and marketing, adopted in HIOs to enable patients to be excluded from HIE unless they provide express permission for inclusion; in contrast, *see* **opt-out**

Optionality: Where a data element or associated process may be used at the discretion of the vendor in developing software using the protocol

Opt-out: Originally used in email advertising and marketing, adopted in HIOs to enable patients to be included in HIE unless they expressly request not to be included; in contrast, *see* **opt-in**

Order communication: An information system used by nursing staff to transcribe orders written on paper in order to transmit them to their respective destinations, such as to the lab, pharmacy, dietary department, and other departments; there is no clinical decision support in an order communication system, in contrast to CPOE

ORYX: *See* **ORYX initiative**

ORYX initiative: The Joint Commission's initiative that supports the integration of outcomes data and other performance measurement data into the accreditation process; often referred to as ORYX

Outputs: The outcomes of inputs into a system (for example, an output of the entry of a medication order is the receipt of the order by the pharmacy information system)

Outsourcing: The deployment of an individual or a company that is not an employee of the organization to perform a function either on-site or off-site

Passive (CDS) advice: A process of providing clinical decision support to clinicians where a specific action is not required in response, such as a message that additional information is available but does not require a specific action or hinder action

Patient-centered medical home (PCMH): A physician practice and patient partnership that provides accessible, interactive, family-focused, coordinated, and comprehensive care and is reimbursed under FFS with reimbursement for care coordination and sometimes pay for performance bonuses. Also known as *healthcare home* (NCQA n.d.)

Patient clinical summary: An after-visit summary that provides a patient with relevant and actionable information and instructions, the generation of which is required to earn M.U. incentives

Patient empowerment: *See* patient engagement

Patient engagement: The combination of patient activation ("a patient's knowledge, skills, ability, and willingness to manage his or her own health and care") with interventions designed to promote positive patient behavior (Health Affairs 2013)

Patient safety: Preventing harm to patients, learning from errors, and building a culture of safety

Patient satisfaction survey: The process of collecting information from patients about their experience in a hospital or provider office

Patient-flow management system: The ability to determine where a patient is at all times in a facility and to link staff requirements to patient location

Patient-provided documentation: Information supplied by the patient to the provider that may be in paper or electronic format, initiated by the patient or the provider, and completely unstructured or structured via an industry standard or patient portal application; the decision whether to accept the patient-provided documentation or request that the patient use it as personal reference material is often a matter of provider preference

Payback period: A financial method used to evaluate the value of a capital expenditure by calculating the time frame that must pass before inflow of cash from a project equals or exceeds outflow of cash

Payer: A business that is engaged by a health plan to process payments on claims submitted by providers

Payment and remittance advice: A provider receives this advice, reconciles the amounts with the provider's accounts receivables, and post payments, which should then reconcile with the provider's statement of deposits from a bank or other financial institution.

Payment schedule: The dates or events that trigger a payment; for EHR, the recommended payment schedule is one that spreads payments over time, triggered by successful achievement of implementation milestones

Person identification: Process that can be anything from a basic comparison of data elements using an exact match of demographic information (for a very small, stable environment) to the use of sophisticated mathematical or statistical algorithms (as in most HIE environments)

Personal health record (PHR): An electronic or paper health record maintained and updated by an individual for himself or herself; a tool that individuals can use to collect, track, and share past and current information about their health or the health of someone in their care

Pharmacy information system (PIS): An information system that manages the pharmacy in its performance of filling orders or prescriptions for medications, including evaluating patient safety issues, dispensing medications, managing medication inventories, affording special security over controlled substances, and managing formulary information

Phasing strategy: A plan in which an information system is implemented and users go live in separate steps; these steps, or phases, may be structured by the components of the application to be implemented or the location, specialty, or other user-based factor

Physician extender (PE): A professional such as a physician assistant or nurse practitioner who can perform a variety of services under the direction of a physician and be reimbursed for those services to free up the physician to focus on more complex cases and to help reduce the overall cost of care

Picture archiving and communication system (PACS): An integrated computer system that obtains, stores, retrieves, and displays digital images (in healthcare, radiological and other diagnostic study images)

Pilot testing: When an information system will be tested with one group of users, and if they do not like it, use of the system will be discontinued. If the term is used to describe a roll-out strategy, it more commonly means that one group of users will go live first, and how they use the system will be evaluated for lessons learned prior to rolling out other groups of users

Planning: The preparation done as part of a project.

Platform: The combination of the hardware and operating system (OS), such as Windows, Mac OS, and mobile OS, on which an application program can run

Point-of-care (POC) charting: Also called point-of-care documentation, the process of entering data into the health record at the time and location of service; often refers to an application that supports specific types of documentation, such as nurse assessments or emergency care services

Point of care (POC) documentation: *See* Point-of-care (POC) charting

POISED: *preparing* to see patients by reviewing the record in advance; *orienting* the patient to the physician's use of the computer; gathering *information* while the patient is talking; *sharing* information with the patient by turning the computer screen to them; *educating* patients using graphical representations of information from the system; and *debriefing* with the patient to ensure understanding (Hirsch 2015a)

Population health: A cohesive, integrated, and comprehensive approach to health that considers the distribution of health outcomes in a population, the health determinants that influence the distribution of care, and polices and interventions that impact and are impacted by the determinants (Jacobson and Teutsch 2012)

Population health management: The collection of activities, not reimbursable in the fee-for-service model, but important in care, including primary care, specialty care, non-hospital care, patient engagement, and analytics and technology (Partners HealthCare n.d)

Population medicine: The design, delivery, coordination, and payment of high-quality healthcare services to manage the Triple Aim for a population using the best resources available (Lewis 2014)

Portal: An application that provides the ability to interact and communicate with another application via the Internet; often used to provide physicians access to patients' health records and to provide patients the ability to request or schedule an appointment, pay bills, and/or access their EHR or PHR

Positive patient identification: A method of matching a patient to their information, such as requiring the use of government-issued photo identification

Practice guidelines: Protocols of care that summarize and evaluate evidence for the most current best practices about disease prevention, diagnosis, and therapy that guide the clinical care process; may be embedded into templates and other forms of clinical decision support. Practice guidelines are similar to care maps, but *practice guidelines* is generally the term used for guidance directed to physicians

Precision/personalized medicine: A medical practice that aims to customize health care, with decisions and treatments tailored to each individual patient in every way possible, often including pharmacogenomics in which drugs are targeted to specific genomes (Mayo Clinic 2015)

Predictive modeling: A process used to identify patterns that can be used to predict the odds of a particular outcome based on the observed data

Pre-load: The entry of (some) existing data from paper health records into the EHR in advance of a clinician's first use; a process intended to prepopulate an EHR prior to golive so the user has at least key information from previous visits already in and ready to be processed by the EHR

Print file: Output from a computer system that generates a file containing an image of information that can be printed

Privacy: The right to control the uses and disclosures of protected health information (PHI), and for individuals to be assured of certain rights in their health information.

Pro forma: A statement about something, usually an estimate, that is "provided in advance" of having actual results

Process: A systematic series of actions taken to create a product or perform a service

Process interoperability: The degree to which the integrity of workflow can be maintained between systems and includes maintaining and conveying information such as user roles, data protection, and system service quality between systems

Processor: Also called a CPU. The area of the computer where data in machine-readable form are processed according to specific instructions (software) that also are in machine-readable form; made of semiconductor material etched on a small electronic device called a (silicon) *chip* or an integrated circuit

Program: A group of related projects managed in a coordinated way to obtain benefits not available from managing them individually (PMI 2013)

Project: A temporary endeavor undertaken to create a unique product, service, or result (PMI 2013)

Project champion: A physician, chief medical informatics officer (CMIO) or medical director of information systems (MDIS) who supports colleagues in their adoption of a new technology or program

Project charter: Provides further detail about the exact boundaries and agreements that surround any given EHR or other health IT project

Project management: A formal set of principles and procedures that help control the activities associated with implementing usually a large undertaking to achieve a specific goal, such as an information system project

Project management office: Consists of multiple project managers with direct responsibility to the director of the PMO and also responsibility to the project sponsor as each different project is worked on

Project manager: An individual who aids an organization in planning the tasks required to achieve the project goals and objectives, determining what resources are needed, associating budgets and timelines for completion, and then managing the project according to plan

Project plan: *See* implementation plan

Project risk: An uncertain event or condition that, if it occurs, has an effect on at least one project goal (PMI 2013)

Project scope: The embodiment of the work that needs to be accomplished so that the specified features and functions are in place

Project sponsor: The person who provides resources and support for the project and is accountable for enabling success (PMI 2013)

Protected health information: Individually identifiable health information transmitted by electronic media, maintained in electronic media, or transmitted or maintained in any other form or medium (including paper, voice, image, and other)

Protocol: In healthcare, a detailed plan of care for a specific medical condition based on investigative studies; in medical research, a rule or procedure to be followed in a clinical trial; in a computer network, a rule or procedure used to address and ensure delivery of data

Provider: Physician, clinic, hospital, nursing home, or other healthcare entity that delivers and is reimbursed for healthcare services

Public key infrastructure (PKI): A system of digital certificates and other registration authorities that verify and authenticate the validity of each party involved in a secure transaction

Pull technology: Query-based exchange

Push technology: A provider pushing information to another provider known to need the information

Quantifiable benefits: Tangible benefits described by a numeric representation, such as a percent of improvement, a number of full-time equivalent staff reduction, or cost savings from not having to purchase paper record folders

Query-based exchange: A query is released, usually to an HIO, that then uses its registry, patient ID matching, and record locator services to determine where information may be located

Quick response (QR) codes: A matrix form of bar code that can be read by a smart phone app, which will take the holder of the phone to a specific URL

Radio frequency identification (RFID): An automatic recognition technology that uses a device attached to an object to transmit data to a receiver and does not require direct contact

Radiology information system (RIS): An information system that manages a radiology department or clinical imaging center as it collects, stores, and provides information on radiological tests such as ultrasound, magnetic resonance imaging, positron emission tomography, and other procedures

Record locator service (RLS): A service provided by a health information exchange organization that indicates where among its participants a given patient may have health information

Redundant arrays of independent (or inexpensive) disks (RAID): A form of data storage that combines multiple disk drives into a logical unit to improve access performance and reliability

Reference Information Model (RIM): Provides the grammar for HL7 messages, specifying the basic building blocks of the language and their permitted relationships

Refreezing: Helping people establish a new stability

Registration: The act of enrolling, such as adding a patient to a healthcare organization's list of patients it treats

Registration Authority (RA): Verifies the validity of the request for a digital signature to a certificate authority

Registry: A collection of healthcare information related to a specific disease, condition, or procedure that makes the information readily available for analysis and comparison

Registry functionality: Refers to functions that can be performed on a panel of patients simultaneously, rather than functions typically performed in an EHR, which relate to only one patient at a time

Registry service: A process to qualify an identified participant

Report wizard: A special type of software application that enables a computer user to run routine reports or make small modifications to standard reports themselves

Report writers: An application that enables compilation of data into various reports

Reporting systems: Systems that generate visit summaries, referral letters, quality reporting, patient follow-up lists, and other patient care–related reports

Reports inventory: A component of a functional needs assessment in which every report produced electronically or manually is reviewed, first for whether the report is actually needed, and second for the information produced

Request for information (RFI): A written communication sent to a comprehensive list of vendors during the early stages of vendor selection to ask for general product information; largely replaced now by researching vendor information on the web

Request for proposal (RFP): A formal communication asking vendors for very specific product and contract information that is generally sent to a small number of vendors that have been preselected after a review of requests for information or other research during the vendor selection process

Request for quote (RFQ): A formal communication asking a vendor to deliver pricing information for a specific product or service or set of products and services

Resolution: 1. The sharpness and clarity of an image on a display screen 2. The solution or settlement of a problem or issue

Resolution amount: In a privacy complaint, a fee intended to cover the government costs of the investigation and subsequent monitoring

Resource leveling: A project management technique used to balance resources (usually people or equipment) over time in order to avoid having too many or two few resources at a given time in a project

Results management: An application that supports retrieval of diagnostic studies and other clinical results and permits viewing and manipulation of data, such as graphing, trending, and comparing with other data

Results review: An application that supports retrieval of diagnostic studies and other clinical results and permits only viewing and potentially printing, but no manipulation of the data

Retail clinics: Clinics that treat uncomplicated minor illnesses and injuries and provide some preventive healthcare services under physician oversight

Retrospective analysis of decision making: A component of a functional needs analysis in which data needs are determined by reviewing past efforts at making decisions

Return on investment (ROI): The financial analysis of the extent of value a major purchase will provide

Rip-and-replace: An information technology acquisition strategy in which virtually all older technology is replaced with new technology over a relatively short period of time

Risk analysis: The process of identifying possible threats that may exploit an organization's vulnerabilities and identifying which risks should be proactively addressed and which risks are lower in priority. The HIPAA Security Rule requires covered entities to perform a security risk analysis, and a similar process may be a prudent exercise with respect to EHR configuration and use

Risk management: *See* issues management

Risk stratification: Tools that periodically and systematically review a population of patients served by a provider to categorize them according to risk factors (Stratis Health 2014b)

Role-specific training: Instruction provided to persons that is specific to their unique job needs

Roll-out strategy: Describes whether an organization will phase in or follow a "big bang" approach to implementing an EHR or its components

Rules engine: A computer program that applies sophisticated mathematical models to data that generate alerts and reminders to support healthcare decision making

RxNorm: A clinical drug nomenclature developed by the Food and Drug Administration, the Department of Veterans Affairs, and HL7 to provide standard names for clinical drugs and administered dose forms that links to many of the drug vocabularies commonly used in pharmacy management and drug interaction software, including those of First Databank, Micromedex, MediSpan, Gold Standard, and Multum

Safe harbor: A provision that affords protection from liability under specified circumstances

SAFER: The Safety Assurance Factors for EHR Resistance Guides for EHR, which are issued by the ONC

Scheduling system: An application used to determine and record the time for an event, such as when a patient is to be seen at a physician's office or to be brought to surgery

SCODF typing model: A model that identifies traits that individuals may have relative to their project contributions and helps distinguish roles such as starters, creators, overseers, doers, and finishers

Screen real estate: The size of the screen, especially with respect to the amount of data that can be viewed from a single screen

Scribe: Employee who follows a physician and performs documentation for him or her

SCRIPT: The National Council for Prescription Drug Program standard for eprescribing that communicates prescription information (including new prescriptions, refill requests, fill-status notifications, and cancellation notifications) between prescribers and pharmacies and has been regulated for use under the Medicare Modernization Act (MMA) of 2003, Medicare Part D eprescribing

Scripting language: A high-level programming language that is used primarily to add functionality, such as dynamic advertisements, to a web page or other browser-based technology

Secondary storage: The permanent storage of data and programs that are directly accessible to the central processing unit of a computer

Security: Measures that complement privacy and also afford certain legal and usability assurance

Self-administered history assessment: The process of obtaining a health history about a patient in which the patient or caregiver completes a paper-based or online form to structure and collect a comprehensive—and consistent—set of data about the patient; some are integrated within the EHR or are part of a PHR

Semantic interoperability: The degree to which there is mutual understanding of the meaning of data exchanged between information systems

Semantic normalization: Translation among different terminology standards

Semantics: The meaning of a word or term; sometimes refers to comparable meaning, usually achieved through a standard vocabulary

Sequoia Project: formerly known as Healtheway; provides support for the eHealth Exchange, which in 2016 served 40 percent of all US hospitals

Service Level Agreement (SLA): A contract between a customer and a service provider that records the common understanding about service priorities, responsibilities, guarantees, and other terms, especially related to availability, serviceability, performance, operation, or other attributes of the service like billing and penalties in the case of violation of the SLA

Service-oriented architecture (SOA): A logical way of designing software in modular and flexible components, called services; services are often, though not always, provided over the Internet or an intranet

Settlement agreement: A resolution agreement signed by HHS and a covered entity or business associate in which the covered entity or business associate agrees to perform certain obligations and make reports to HHS, generally for a period of three years

Shared decision making: A collaborative process that allows patients and their providers to make health care decisions together, taking into account the best scientific evidence available, as well as the patient's values and preferences (Informed Medical Decision Making Foundation n.d.)

Shared risk: Adds the dimension of the provider being at risk for the same portion of spending over the target as the health plan.

Shared savings: An arrangement in which all providers are reimbursed based on FFS and are then eligible to receive shared savings payments (incentive) after they meet quality performance and risk-adjusted standards.

Situational data: Required only when the situation (such as purpose or nature of other data) calls for the data

Smart bed: Combines medical device technology that is embedded in patient beds to adjust bed angle, assist in turning patients, and so on, with an interface to the EHR to support real-time monitoring and compliance

SMART goals: Statements that help an organization establish expectations that are specific, measurable, achievable, realistic, and time-based

Smart peripherals: Medical devices that are able to be directly connected to an information system to enable capture of their information into the EHR

Smartphone: A mobile device that supports both telephone calls and features of a computer, such as access to the Internet, web browsing, and many applications modified for use on a smartphone

SNOMED CT (Systematized Nomenclature of Medicine—Clinical Terms): A computer-processable clinical vocabulary that in 2011 includes more than 311,00 clinical concepts and over 1.3 million relationships to represent virtually all healthcare processes; originally developed by the College of American Pathologists and now managed by the International Health Terminology Standards Development Organization (IHTSDO), based in Denmark, it is designed to index, store, retrieve, and aggregate clinical data in a standardized manner

SOAP: Simple Object Access Protocol; was replaced by the REST APIs

Software as a Service (SaaS): Software based on a web-services architecture that is provided through an outsourcing contract and is deployed over the Internet

Solicted attachment: If the provider does not submit additional information with the claim and the health plan determines additional information is necessary to adjudicate the claim, the plan will deny the claim and send the provider a request for additional information

Source code: The underlying software running the hardware or applications

Source system: 1. A system in which data were originally created 2. Independent information system application that contributes data to an EHR, including departmental clinical applications (for example, laboratory information system, clinical pharmacy information system) and specialty clinical applications (for example, intensive care, cardiology, labor and delivery)

Specialty EHR: A type of EHR that is specific to the needs of a particular healthcare discipline, such as behavioral health or dental care

Stages of change: Based on a model by Prochaska and DiClemente, this model (also called the *transtheoretical model*) focuses on the decision-making of the individual experiencing intentional change

Standalone: Independent of any sponsor; a standalone information system is self-contained and can operate on its own without reliance on other systems

Standard message protocols: Provide the tools to map proprietary formats to one another and more easily accomplish the exchange of data

Standard order set: A set of instructions for a specific diagnosis, developed by a team of physicians and following evidence-based guidance, intended to increase physician efficiency, enhance documentation, and improve the quality of care

Standards and certification criteria requirements for certified EHR technology (CEHRT): CEHRT are developed by ONC and, ultimately, after soliciting public comment, codified in regulations. Vendors are required to have their EHR products tested in order to be certified

Standards and Interoperability (S&I) Framework: An open, collaborative community made up of stakeholders from the public and private sectors with a mission to find technical solutions to facilitate standardized, interoperable health information exchange

Standards development organization (SDO): A private organization or government agency involved in the development of standards at a national or international level

State HIE Cooperative Agreement Program: Enacted under HITECH, a program that provides federal support for states to promote rapid building of capacity for exchanging health information across the health care system both within and across states

State-Level Health Information Exchange Consensus Project: A federally funded initiative, managed through the AHIMA Foundation, to guide field research and contribute to analysis and recommendations regarding HIE development across states

Steering committee: A committee composed of representative stakeholders that advises the project manager and others on matters relating to the project implementation overall

Stewardship: Personal responsibility for taking care of something one does not own

Storage area network (SAN): Storage devices organized into a network so that they can be accessible from any server in the network; a type of storage system

Storage management program: with experts who can identify the appropriate storage media for different types of data, information, knowledge, and content (documents and images), and manage various retention requirements, retrieval strategies, and storage

Storage system: *See* storage area networks (SANs)

Storage virtualization: A process that creates a virtual version of an operating system, server, storage device, or network resources by decoupling these applications from their host resources—reducing the number of devices required and using less energy and maintenance (Daly 2012)

Strategic plan: The document in which leadership of an organization identifies the organization's overall mission, vision, and goals to help set the long-term direction of the organization

Structured data: Computer-processable data

Supply chain management system: An application that can help manage an organization's selection, acquisition, inventorying, invoicing and payment, usage tracking, contract compliance, and rebate attainment for supplies

Support costs: Expenditures associated with helping users use the EHR

Supporting infrastructure: Technology that integrates data from applications internal to a given care delivery organization

SWOT analysis: An analysis that focuses on the organization and its strengths, weaknesses, opportunities, and threats

Syntactic interoperability: Data being structured in a manner that enables exchange between two software applications

Syntax: A term that refers to the comparable structure or format of data, usually as they are being transmitted from one system to another

System: A set of related and highly interdependent components that are operating for a particular purpose

System build: The customization of data dictionaries, tables, decision support rules, templates for data entry, screen layouts, and reports used in a system to meet specific organizational requirements; also called system configuration

System configuration: *See* **system build**

System documentation: Detailed information about how a computer system is configured, including its architecture, design, data flow, and programming logic as well as instructions for configuration, troubleshooting, and use

System integrator: Companies or persons that specialize in getting disparate vendor products to work together, primarily through acquiring a large body of interface knowledge and experience

Systems development life cycle: A model used to represent the ongoing process of developing (or purchasing) information systems

T-lines: Also known as trunk lines; are the backbone of long-distance network transmission that transmits data in digital form.

Tablet: Computers that are characterized by a writing slate

Taxonomy: The principles of a classification system, such as data classification, and the study of the general principles of scientific classification

Team building: A subset of all other interpersonal skills required of a project manager consisting of recognizing what help a project needs and then dividing up the work into various components that individual teams can address. The second part relates to helping each person in a team work together as a team

Technical interoperability: The degree to which networks, systems, devices, or components are able to exchange and use data in the manner for which they have the basic capability

Telehealth: The delivery of health-related services and information via telecommunications technologies. Telehealth may support local care to those who are homebound or in difficult-to-access places (such as prisons) as well as remote care around the world

Template: A preset format for documenting data in a computer application so that the user is reminded of what data to capture and in what format

Terminal: A term used to describe the hardware in a mainframe computer system by which data may be entered or retrieved

Terminology: A set of terms representing the system of concepts of a particular subject field; a clinical terminology provides the proper use of clinical words as names or symbols

Tethered: The sharing of a connection between devices or applications; for example, tethered PHRs may be connected to a provider, payer, or other sponsor

Thick client: A computer with full processing capability and persistent storage that accesses data and applications on a host server

Thin client: A computer with processing capability but no persistent storage (disk memory) that relies on data and applications on a host server it accesses to enter, retrieve, and have data being used processed

Threat agent: An individual with the motivation and resources to carry out a threat (for example, a computer-savvy disgruntled employee or a cybercriminal)

Threat event: The results of a threat

Threat intelligence: The active use of reliable sources to monitor trends and implement appropriate controls

Threat target: The objects of a threat

Throughput: The movement of inputs and outputs through a production process; often studied to achieve more rapid processing

Topology: In networking terms, the physical or logical arrangement of a network

Total cost of ownership (TCO): The set of all costs associated with EHR, not only those paid to the vendor to license or subscribe to the product

TPO (treatment, payment, and operations): The three core types of healthcare activities for which covered entities are permitted to use and disclose PHI (except when an authorization or prohibition is explicitly required by the Privacy Rule).

Transaction: Any operation performed on a database, such as entering of an order for a patient, retrieving vital signs of a patient, or sending a claim for healthcare services; under HIPAA, transactions refer specifically to financial and administrative transactions that occur between a provider and a payer, sometimes with the support of a healthcare clearinghouse, such as sending a claim and verifying eligibility for benefits

Transactional database: A database that enables data to be entered, retrieved, updated, modified, trended, and deleted by the user

Transitions of care: A continuous process in which a patient's care shifts from being provided in one setting of care to another (Health Affairs 2012)

Transparency: In healthcare, the degree to which individual patients are made aware of how their personal health information is or has been dispersed to secondary medical databases

Triggered review: A more comprehensive investigation that occurs when a monitoring system identifies an event that could be a potential risk

Triple Aim: Three priorities for healthcare, including 1. improve the experience of care—provide care that is effective, safe, and reliable—to every patient, every time; 2. Improve the health of a population, reach out to communities, manage chronic conditions, and so forth; and 3. Decrease per capita costs of healthcare

Trust: Feeling confident that one can rely on others to act as they should and achieve what is expected of them

Trust agent: Some examples of trust agents in the Direct model are HISPs, certificate authorities (CAs) and registration authorities (RAs)

Trust bundle: Provides a common set of policies and procedures for different types of health information exchanges (HIEs)

Turnover strategy: A plan for releasing a new application to users, wherein considerations are given to whether the paper system will cease on golive (with access to former documents) or whether it will be run parallel (documenting in both paper and electronic systems) for some period of time after go-live

Two-dimensional bar code: A barcode in which data are encoded in both the height and the width of the barcode symbol; the amount of data that can be contained in a two-dimensional barcode symbol is significantly greater than that stored in a one-dimensional symbol

Two-factor authentication: The use of two electronic signature components (such as PIN, password, biometric, or token) together

Unfreezing: Preparing people to be change-ready

Unified Code for Units of Measure (UCUM): A system of codes for unambiguously representing the magnitude of a physical quantity, defined and adopted by convention and/or by law, that is used as a standard for measurement of the same physical quantity

Unified Medical Language System (UMLS): A program initiated by the National Library of Medicine to build an intelligent, automated system that can understand biomedical concepts, words, and expressions and their interrelationships; includes concepts and terms from many different source vocabularies. UMLS integrates and distributes key terminology, classification and coding standards, and associated resources to promote creation of more effective and interoperable biomedical information systems and services, including electronic health records

Unified Modeling Language (UML): Provides a standard that can help modelers share their work with others and enables models to be used across different programming situations

Uniform Hospital Discharge Data Set (UHDDS): A core set of data elements adopted by the US Department of Health and Human Services that are collected by hospitals on all discharges and all discharge abstract systems

Unique Device Identification (UDI): A unique identifier for medical devices required by the Food and Drug Administration that contributes to patient safety by helping to identify counterfeit products, improving the ability of staff to distinguish between devices that are similar in appearance but serve different functions, facilitating the recall process, tracking infection exposure and allergic reactions to devices, and improving studies on medical device effectiveness

Units of measure: Three different standards deployed by various laboratories (and imaging centers), including ANSI X3.50, ISO 2955, and the Unified Code for Units of Measure (Schadow 2009)

Universal Medical Device Nomenclature System (UMDNS): A standard international nomenclature and computer coding system for medical devices, developed by ECRI

Universal serial bus (USB): An industry standard developed in the mid-1990s that defines communications protocols used to connect computer peripherals, such as keyboards and storage devices (for example, USB drives, also called thumb drives or flash drives), with computers

Unsolicited attachment: Some providers may be able to anticipate the need for additional information and send the information with the claim

Unstructured data: Narrative or imaged data that are human readable and able to be stored and displayed in a computer but not uniquely processable by a computer

Usability: The extent to which a product can be used by specified users to achieve specified goals with effectiveness, efficiency, and satisfaction in a specified context of use (ISO9241).

Use: The sharing, employment, application, utilization, examination, or analysis of PHI within an entity that maintains such information

User functional needs survey: A process to define system functionality requirements in which users are asked to identify needed functionality, and perhaps priority rank them

User ID: Used to identify the user for purposes of triggering access controls

User interface: The technology that enables humans to interact with a computer, primarily referring to the display of information and tools to facilitate data entry and retrieval

User satisfaction survey: A tool to solicit feedback from those engaging in, typically, a new process or using a new information system application

Uncompensated use: Use of data about patients or other consumers without asking their permission or offering them compensation may be viewed as a privacy violation, even if the data are used to benefit the individuals or society as a whole

Utilization management: The evaluation of the medical necessity, appropriateness, and efficiency of the use of healthcare services, procedures, facilities under the provision of the applicable health benefits plan. Also called *medical management* (URAC 2005)

Value: 1. An attribute associated with a characteristic—for example, "Mary," "Jose," and "Pat" are values of the variable "first name" 2. The quality of outcomes for the level of spending

Value-based payment: Models including include shared savings, shared risk, bundled payments, and capitation. In these models, providers assume some degree of financial risk as a stimulus to improving care

Value-driven healthcare: A focus of the federal government on ways to achieve better quality outcomes per dollar spent on healthcare, such as providing incentives for use of EHR, affording consumers transparency, and introducing risk sharing and greater accountability among providers for continuity of care, along with other health reform measures

Value stream maps for clinical service delivery and patient safety processes (lean enterprise tools used to document, analyze and improve the flow of information or services required to produce a product or service effectively and efficiently) (Barry 2013)

Variable: A characteristic or property that may take on different values; for example, the variable "diagnosis" is a storage location for each patient's diagnosis, such as hypertension, diabetes, or many other values, and "temperature" is the variable field in which 98.6 degrees Fahrenheit, 38 degrees Celsius, or other values would be recorded

Vendor-neutral archive: An integrated platform on which multiple different EDM and ECM systems can exchange content

Virtual Medical Record (vMR): A standard that is a data model for representing the data that are analyzed or produced by CDS rules engines

Virtual private network (VPN): An encrypted tunnel through the Internet that enables secure transmission of data

Volatility: How long data and the information derived from data will remain useful

Vocabulary server: Has the ability to use multiple vocabularies across different applications in an EHR system

Walk-through: A process where managers engage workers on-the-job in a meaningful discussion about the work being performed in order to identify opportunities for improvement; similar to rounding, where, in a teaching setting, physicians walk through patient care areas to discuss cases with students

Web services architecture (WSA): An architecture that utilizes web-based tools to permit communication among different software applications

Wireless (or workstation) on wheels (WOW): Notebook computers mounted on carts that can be moved through the facility by users

Work breakdown structure: A hierarchical structure that decomposes project activities into levels of detail

Workflow engine: A system that takes care of the management of workflow, including task assignment generation, resource allocation, activity performance, case preparation and modification, launching of applications, and the recording of logistical information (Andrew and Bruegel 2005)

Workflow management: The planning, organizing, directing, and controlling of the workflow

Workflow management system: A system that stores workflow definitions as a collection of tasks, resources, and conditional logic

Workflow modeling: Helps identify efficiencies and targets processes associated with diagnostics, substance therapeutics, ambulatory care, emergency care, and invasive diagnostics and therapeutics.

Workflow technology: Technology that automatically routes electronic documents into electronic in-baskets of its department staff for disposition decisions

Workgroup on Electronic Data Interchange (WEDI): A multi-stakeholder, nonprofit organization dedicated to improving administrative efficiency, quality, and cost-effectiveness of healthcare information; acts as an advisor to HHS on HIPAA transactions and code sets

Workstation: A computer designed to accept data from multiple sources in order to assist in managing information for daily activities and to provide a convenient means of entering data as desired by the user at the point of care

X.509: The standard under which digital certificates are standardized

XML (extensible markup language): A standardized computer language that allows the interchange of data as structured text

References

Agency for Healthcare Research and Quality (AHRQ). 2007. *Closing the Quality Gap: A Critical Analysis of Quality Improvement Strategies: Volume 7—Care Coordination.* Rockville, MD: AHRQ. http://www.ncbi.nlm.nih.gov/books/NBK44015.

Allen, C., et al. 2014. Data governance and data sharing agreements for community-wide health information exchange: Lessons from the Beacon Communities. *eGEMS (Generating Evidence and Methods to Improve Patient Outcomes).* 2(1):1057. https://www.ncbi.nlm.nih.gov/pmc/articles/PMC4371395.

Ambler, S.W. 2014b. Home page. Agile Modeling: Effective Practices for Modeling and Documentation. http://www.agilemodeling.com.

American Cancer Society (ACS). 2014 (July 28). What are the legal requirements of informed consent? http://www.cancer.org/treatment/findingandpayingfortreatment/understanding financialandlegalmatters/informedconsent/informed-consent-legal-requirements-of-consent.

Anderson, G.D., and E.B. Grey. 2013 (February 11). The MSO's prognosis after the ACA: A viable integration tool? Presentation at Physicians and Physician Organizations Law Institute, Phoenix, AZ. Bureau of Labor Statistics, US Department of Labor (BLS). 2014–2015. Informational security analysts. Occupational Outlook Handbook. http://www.bls.gov/ooh/computer-and-information-technology/information-security-analysts.htm.

Andrew, W.F., and R.B. Bruegel. 2005. EHR workflow management review and survey results. *ADVANCE for Health Information Executives.* 9(2):34–50.

Barry, C. 2013 (February 27). How to use value stream maps in healthcare. Minitab blog. http://blog.minitab.com/blog/real-world-quality-improvement/how-to-use-value-stream-maps-in-healthcare.

Burton, D.A. 2013. White paper: Population health management: Implementing a strategy for success. Health Catalyst. https://www.healthcatalyst.com/WhitePaper_PopulationHealthManagement.html.

Case Management Society of America (CMSA). n.d. What is a case manager? http://www.cmsa.org/HOme/CMSA/WhatisaCaseManager/tabid/224/Default.aspx.

Center for Healthcare Quality and Payment Reform (CHQPR). n.d. The payment reform glossary, first edition. http://www.chqpr.org/downloads/paymentreformglossary.pdf.

Centers for Medicare and Medicaid Services (CMS). 2016 (July 14). Electronic health records (EHR) incentive programs. https://www.cms.gov/Regulations-and-Guidance/Legislation/EHRIncentivePrograms/index.html?redirect=/ehrincentiveprograms.

Cigna. 2016. Cigna Healthcare definition of medical necessity for physicians. http://www.cigna.com/healthcare-professionals/resources-for-health-care-professionals/clinical-payment-and-reimbursement-policies/medical-necessity-definitions.

Daly, J. 2012 (October 8). What is virtualization? *Ed Tech Magazine.* http://www.edtechmagazine.com/higher/article/2012/10/what-virtualization.

Darling, G. 2011. What does a clinical informatics data analyst do, exactly? Healthcare IT Today blog. http://healthcareittoday.com/2011/11/08/clinical-informatics-data-analyst.

Gillenson, M., P. Ponniah, A. Kriegel, B. Grukhnov, A. Taylor, and G. Powell. 2008. *Introduction to Database Management.* Hoboken, NJ: John Wiley & Sons.

Goldstein, M.M., and A.L. Rein. 2010 (September 29). Data segmentation in electronic health information exchange: Policy considerations and analysis. Prepared for Office of the National Coordinator for Health Information Technology. https://www.healthit.gov/sites/default/files/privacy-security/gwu-data-segmentation-final-cover-letter.pdf.

Han, C. 2015 (April 28). Using consumer health data: Some considerations for companies. Federal Trade Commission business blog. https://www.ftc.gov/news-events/blogs/business-blog/2015/04/using-consumer-health-data-some-considerations-companies.

HCI Group. 2014 (April 7). EHR optimization: Planning for success. http://blog.thehcigroup.com/ehr-optimization-planning-for-success.

Health Affairs. 2012 (September 13). Improving care transitions. Health policy brief. http://www.healthaffairs.org/healthpolicybriefs/brief.php?brief_id=76.

Health Affairs. 2013 (February 14). Patient engagement. Health policy brief. http://www.healthaffairs.org/healthpolicybriefs/brief.php?brief_id=86.

Healthcare.gov. 2016. If you don't have health insurance: How much you'll pay. https://www.healthcare.gov/fees/fee-for-not-being-covered.

Healthcare Financial Management Association (HFMA). 2016. About MAP. https://www.hfma.org/MAP/AboutMap.

Health Care Payment Learning and Action Network (HCP-LAN). 2016. White paper: Accelerating and aligning population-based payment models: Financial benchmarking. Mitre Corporation. http://hcp-lan.org/workproducts/fb-whitepaper-final.pdf.

Health Resources and Services Administration, US Department of Health and Human Services (HRSA) n.d. What is health IT? http://www.hrsa.gov/healthit/toolbox/oralhealthittoolbox/introduction/whatishealthit.html.

Informed Medical Decisions Foundation. n.d. What is shared decision making? http://www.informedmedicaldecisions.org/what-is-shared-decision-making.

Institute of Medicine (IOM). 2012. *The Learning Health System Series.* http://www.nap.edu/catalog/13301/the-learning-health-system-series.

Jackson, J. 2010 (September 29). HIPAA version 5010: Tenth national provider call—acknowledgement transactions. Centers for Medicare and Medicaid Services. https://www.cms.gov/Regulations-and-Guidance/Administrative-Simplification/Versions5010andD0/Downloads/Acknowledgements_National_Presentation_9-29-10_final.pdf.

Jacobson, D.M., and S. Teutsch. 2012. An environmental scan of integrated approaches for defining and measuring total population health by the clinical care system, the government public health system, and stakeholder organizations. National Quality Forum. http://www.qualityforum.org/Publications/2012/06/An_Environmental_Scan_of_Integrated_Approaches_for_Defining_and_Measuring_Total_Population_Health.aspx.

Johns, M.L. 2015. *Enterprise Health Information Management and Data Governance.* Chicago: AHIMA.

Koppenheffer, M. 2013 (April 15). Clinical integration, demystified. Advisory Board Company Care Center Transformation Blog. https://www.advisory.com/research/care-transformation-center/care-transformation-center-blog/2013/04/clinical-integration-defined.

Lewis, N. 2014 (March 19). Populations, population health, and the evolution of population management: Making sense of the terminology in US healthcare today. Institute for Healthcare Improvement. http://www.ihi.org/communities/blogs/_layouts/ihi/community/blog/itemview.aspx?List=81ca4a47-4ccd-4e9e-89d9-14d88ec59e8d&ID=50.

Matjucha, K., and C. Giuliano. 2011 (December). Improving your bottom line through bad debt management. Deloitte Consulting, LLP. http://www.njhfmainstitute.org/pdf/Oct13/Improving%20Your%20Bottom%20Line%20Through%20Effective%20Bad%20Debt%20Management.pdf.

Mayo Clinic. 2015 (January 5). Personalized medicine and pharmacogenomics. http://www.mayoclinic.org/healthy-lifestyle/consumer-health/in-depth/personalized-medicine/art-20044300.

Microsoft Dynamics. 2012. Microsoft Dynamics CRM: healthcare providers. http://crm.dynamics.com/en-us/healthcare-providers.

Miliard, M. 2015 (August 25). 18 health technologies poised for big growth. *Healthcare IT News.* http://www.healthcareitnews.com/news/18-health-technologies-poised-big-growth.

Mitchell, G. 2013. Long-term care and interoperable EHRs: A strategic match. *Leading Age.* 3(4). http://www.leadingage.org/Long-Term_Care_and_Interoperable_EHRs_A_Strategic_Match_V3N4.aspx.

National Committee for Quality Assurance (NCQA). n.d. Patient-centered medical home. http://www.ncqa.org/home/patient-centered-medical-home.

National Longitudinal Surveys (NLS). n.d. What are longitudinal data? US Bureau of Labor Statistics. https://www.nlsinfo.org/content/getting-started/what-are-longitudinal-data.

Partners HealthCare. n.d. About population health management (PHM): So what exactly is population health management? http://www.partners.org/innovation-and-leadership/population-health-management/about-phm.

Pfister, H.R., and S.R. Ingargiola. 2014 (February 20). ONC: Staying focused on EHR usability. iHealthBeat. http://www.ihealthbeat.org/insight/2014/onc-staying-focused-on-ehr-usability.

Project Management Institute (PMI). 2013. *A Guide to the Project Management Body of Knowledge (PMBOK Guide)*. Newton Square, PA: PMI.

Raths, D. 2014 (February 19). Top ten tech trends: Catching FHIR. *Healthcare Informatics*. http://www.healthcare-informatics.com/article/top-ten-tech-trends-catching-fhir.

Rollnick S., and W.R. Miller. 1995. What is MI? Motivational Interviewing. http://www.motivationalinterview.net/clinical/whatismi.html.

Rouse, M. 2013. Chief technology officer (CTO) definition. TechTarget website. http://searchcio.techtarget.com/definition/Chief-Technology-Officer-CTO.

Rouse, M. 2015. Chief information officer (CIO) definition. TechTarget website. http://searchcio.techtarget.com/definition/CIO.

SAS. n.d. Data visualization: What it is and why it is important. http://www.sas.com/en_us/insights/big-data/data-visualization.html.

Schadow, G. 2009 (July 18). The unified code for units of measure. http://www.unitsofmeasure.org.

Shareableink.com. 2011. Shareable ink physician progress notes. http://www.shareableink.com/applications-physician-progress-notes.html.

Siwicki, B. 2016 (April 14). Cleveland Clinic inks deal with CVS, doctors to conduct telehealth visits through MinuteClinics. *Healthcare Finance News*. http://www.healthcarefinancenews.com/news/cleveland-clinic-inks-deal-cvs-doctors-conduct-telehealth-visits-through-minute-clinics.

Stratis Health. 2014a. Supportive communications. *Community-Based Care Coordination: A Comprehensive Development Toolkit.* https://www.stratishealth.org/documents/HITToolkitcoordination/4-Supportive-Communications.pdf.

Stratis Health. 2014b. Population risk stratification and patient cohort identification. https://www.stratishealth.org/documents/HITToolkitcoordination/3-Population-Risk-Stratification-and-Patient-Cohort-Identification.pdf.

Templeton, G. 2015 (October 12). Artificial neural networks are changing the world. What are they? ExtremeTech. http://www.extremetech.com/extreme/215170-artificial-neural-networks-are-changing-the-world-what-are-they.

URAC. 2005. Trends and practices in medical management: 2005 industry profile. http://www.urac.org/resources/careManagement.aspx.

Vasudeva, N., et al. 2012. Offline character recognition system using artificial neural network. *International Journal of Machine Learning and Computing.* 2(4):449–452.

Washington, L. 2015 (November 12). Information governance provides the framework for data governance. Journal of AHIMA blog. http://journal.ahima.org/2015/11/12/information-governance-provides-the-framework-for-data-governance.

Index